CLINICAL MRI

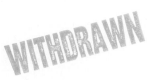

Val M. Runge, M.D.

Robert and Alma Moreton Centennial Chair in Radiology
Scott and White Clinic and Hospital
Texas A&M University Health Science Center
Temple, Texas

W.B. SAUNDERS COMPANY
Philadelphia London New York St. Louis Sydney Toronto

W.B. SAUNDERS COMPANY

The Curtis Center
Independence Square West
Philadelphia, Pennsylvania 19106

Library of Congress Cataloging-in-Publication Data

Runge, Val M.

Clinical MRI / Val M. Runge.—1st ed.

p.   cm.

ISBN 0–7216–8036–4

1. Magnetic resonance imaging.   I. Title.

RC78.7.N83 R86 2002

616.07'548—dc21   2001041120

Acquisitions Editor: Lisette Bralow

Developmental Editor: Gwen Wright

Project Manager: Mary Anne Folcher

Illustration Specialist: Peg Shaw

Book Designer: Lynn Foulk

CLINICAL MRI   ISBN 0–7216–8036–4

Printed in the United States of America

Last digit is the print number: 9   8   7   6   5   4   3   2   1

To my two daughters,
Sadie and Valerie,
with all my love

Contributors

Mark H. Awh, MD
President, Radiology Alliance, PC
Medical Director, OrMed (Orthopedic Medical Imaging Management)
Director of MRI, St. Thomas Hospital
Nashville, Tennessee, USA
Musculoskeletal System

Günther Schneider, MD, PhD
Department of Diagnostic Radiology
Saarland University Hospital
Homburg/Saar, Germany
Chest, Abdomen, and Pelvis

Michael E. Stadnick, MD
Chief of Musculoskeletal Imaging, St. Thomas Hospital
Associate Medical Director, OrMed (Orthopedic Medical Imaging Management)
Nashville, Tennessee, USA
Musculoskeletal System

Preface

Clinical MRI is intended to serve as a practical educational textbook for clinical magnetic resonance imaging (MRI). The bulk of the text is organized along anatomic lines and discusses disease entities commonly encountered in clinical practice. The final two chapters discuss in depth contrast media and contrast-enhanced MRI angiography, two topics deserving additional attention because of their clinical importance today. MRI physics per se is not discussed in a separate chapter, and the reader is referred to the many available texts for detailed reviews of this topic.

Emphasis is placed on disease entities that are routinely seen in the clinical practice of MRI. The focus is on common examinations, covering briefly in each area important points relative to imaging technique and discussing in depth clinical interpretation. Clinical cases serve as the backbone of this discussion.

The clinical applications of MRI continue to expand owing to both greater availability and advances in instrumentation. Progress in MRI has largely dominated the field of diagnostic radiology for the past 20 years. Today, MRI stands as a major diagnostic subspecialty. The sophisticated application of this technique and further advances dictate that MRI will continue to play a dominant role in clinical medicine for a long time to come.

VAL M. RUNGE, M.D.

Contents

Brain: Neoplastic Disease

The value of magnetic resonance imaging (MRI) for assessing intracranial disease was quickly recognized after its clinical introduction in the early 1980s. Advantages of MRI over computed tomography (CT) include superior soft tissue contrast, absence of bone artifact, and ability to acquire high-resolution images in any plane. These features, combined with the variety of available scan types, lead to a highly sensitive and versatile imaging technique. As a result, MRI has become the principal imaging modality for intracranial tumor detection and evaluation.

The sensitivity of unenhanced MRI to detect brain neoplasms is primarily due to its ability to visualize small differences in extracellular fluid. Both T_1 and T_2, the two time constants describing the relaxation process of protons, are prolonged in most tumors. This leads to a decrease in lesion signal intensity on T_1-weighted images and an increase on T_2-weighted images. In clinical practice, it is the change on T_2-weighted images that is most useful. Detection is possible even when lesions are small or isodense on CT. However, some brain tumors, such as neurofibromas, have only a small increase in water content. These lesions have less pronounced prolongation of T_1 and T_2.

Despite the sensitivity of unenhanced MRI, the visualization and characterization of many tumors were not possible before the introduction of intravenous MRI contrast media. Clinical examples of diagnostic difficulties encountered before the advent of contrast media include separation of tumor from surrounding edema, visualization of vascular extra-axial tumors, and detection of small metastatic lesions. The availability of MRI contrast media has largely overcome these drawbacks by providing information about blood-brain barrier (BBB) integrity and tissue vascularity.

CONTRAST MEDIA

The iodinated contrast agents that play an essential role in x-ray-based imaging are not effective at clinical doses in MRI. This would be anticipated because of the difference in physical principles between the two imaging modalities. Iodinated contrast agents attenuate the x-ray beam, whereas MRI contrast agents change (decrease) T_1 and T_2. It is the shortening of T_1 that is most important for contrast enhancement in clinical MRI.

Three MRI contrast agents dominate the worldwide market: Magnevist (gadolinium [Gd] DTPA), ProHance (Gd HP-DO3A), and Omniscan (Gd DTPA-BMA). No difference exists between these agents in contrast effect when given at the same dose. The gadolinium ion is the active ingredient. The ligand (DTPA, HP-DO3A, or DTPA-BMA) serves only to tightly bind (chelate) the gadolinium ion. This ensures complete renal excretion. It is possible that small differences exist in safety between the agents. The stability of the chelate is very important because of the toxicity of the free gadolinium ion (Gd). In this regard, ProHance has the greatest safety margin followed by Magnevist. Minor adverse reactions occur in a small percentage of patients with all three agents. Nausea and hives are the most common. Anaphylactoid reactions are rare but necessitate close monitoring and adequate safety measures.

The gadolinium chelates are distributed in the extracellular space after intravenous injection. Excretion is rapid and occurs by glomerular filtration. There is no hepatobiliary excretion. Patients with poor renal function (creatinine <2.5 mg/dL) should not receive contrast unless arrangements are made for repeated dialysis. To date, the preparations sold commercially are formulated at a concentration of 0.5 mol/L. The solutions are clear and colorless. The agents are given by weight; the standard dose is 0.1 mmol/kg. This equates to a 15-mL injection in a 75-kg individual. Injections are typically given as a fast infusion (over 10 to 20 seconds). Rates up to 10 mL/second have been used for specific applications, in particular first-pass studies of the brain. High dose (0.3 mmol/kg) is indicated in specific situations. High dose is particularly important for screening and follow-up of brain metastases.

The mechanisms of lesion enhancement with gadolinium chelates are similar to that with iodinated contrast agents in CT. Enhancement can occur on the basis of either disruption of the BBB or a difference in vascularity. MRI is much more sensitive to soft tissue changes than CT. Thus, it should come as no surprise that abnormal contrast enhancement is better seen on MRI than on CT. Lesion detectability, when based on contrast enhancement, is higher on MRI. Enhancement is

Portions of this text are reprinted in revised form, with permission, from VM Runge (ed): *Clinical Magnetic Resonance Imaging*, Philadelphia, JB Lippincott, 1990; VM Runge, MA Brack, RA Garneau, JE Kirsch (eds): *Magnetic Resonance Imaging of the Brain*, Philadelphia, JB Lippincott, 1994; VM Runge, MH Awh, DF Bittner, JE Kirsch (eds): *Magnetic Resonance Imaging of the Spine*, Philadelphia, JB Lippincott, 1995; VM Runge (ed): *Review of Neuroradiology*, Philadelphia, WB Saunders, 1996; VM Runge (ed), *Contrast Enhanced Clinical Magnetic Resonance Imaging*. Lexington, University Press of Kentucky, 1997.

also seen in some pathologies on MRI and not on CT, providing a further improvement in diagnostic efficacy.

Whether an intra-axial neoplasm displays contrast enhancement depends largely on the degree of BBB disruption. Histologic studies reveal a structural alteration in the capillary walls in most neoplastic disease that allows interstitial accumulation of contrast. Generally, the more aggressive the tumor, the greater is the degree of BBB breakdown and thus contrast enhancement. The degree of vascularity plays an important role in tumors that occur outside the normal BBB (extra-axial neoplasms), including meningiomas, schwannomas, pituitary-origin tumors, and some parasellar tumors such as chordomas. Highly vascular lesions show strong enhancement. Enhancement of intra-axial lesions with BBB disruption occurs more slowly than that for extra-axial lesions with high vascularity. Thus, scans obtained at 5 to 10 minutes postcontrast may best show enhancement in intra-axial lesions (e.g., metastatic disease) as opposed to scans 1 to 2 minutes postcontrast in extra-axial lesions (e.g., acoustic schwannomas).

IMAGING SEQUENCES

Scans in MRI can be T_1-, T_2-, or proton density weighted. The latest hardware is also capable of acquiring images with diffusion weighting. Note that all scans are "weighted" in character. This provides, on any one scan, a sense of the parameter in question. However, the appearance of tissues can still be substantially influenced by the other parameters. Construction of an image that is a calculated map of one parameter, for example T_1, is possible but rarely done in clinical practice. T_1 is defined as the spin-lattice relaxation time and reflects the time required for a proton (a "spin") to return (or relax), once excited, by the process of giving off energy to the surrounding structure (the "lattice"). T_2 is defined as the spin-spin relaxation time and reflects the time required for a proton to relax by giving its energy to a neighboring proton (thus "spin-spin"). Proton or spin density is the quantity of mobile protons (hydrogen atoms), principally water. Diffusion relates to the thermal (random) motion of protons at the molecular level.

Most scans currently in use fall within one of two general categories: spin echo or gradient echo. A third category, inversion recovery, also exists. However, scans of this type are used much less frequently. In a spin echo scan, a radiofrequency pulse is used to generate (refocus) the magnetic resonance (MR) signal from the patient. In a gradient echo scan, a small magnetic field gradient is used to generate the MR signal. TE (time to echo) and TR (time to repetition) are operator-selected parameters that specify in spin echo scans the parameter weighting (T_1, T_2, or proton density). A short TE (<25 milliseconds) and short TR (<800 milliseconds) produces T_1-weighting. A long TE (>60 milliseconds) and long TR (>2000 milliseconds) produces T_2-weighting. Combining a short TE with a long TR gives a proton density-weighted scan. For inversion recovery scans, an additional parameter TI (time to inversion), which highly influences tissue contrast, must be specified along with TE and TR. T_1-weighted scans can be recognized by the high signal intensity (white) of fat and low signal intensity (black) of cerebrospinal fluid (CSF). T_2-weighted scans can be recognized by the high signal intensity of CSF. Proton density-weighted scans appear in between, with low overall tissue contrast. Proton density-weighted scans are not commonly used today in brain imaging.

The terms fast spin echo and turbo-spin echo refer to a more recent imaging development, a variant of spin echo imaging. With this technique, scan times are generally shorter. Overall image quality is usually also better, as judged by signal-to-noise and spatial resolution. The use of fast spin echo scans does make the interpretation of tissue contrast more difficult. Fat is generally high signal intensity on fast spin echo scans. Thus, whereas on a conventional spin echo T_2-weighted scan fat will appear as intermediate to low signal intensity, on a fast spin echo scan it will be high signal intensity. A better marker of T_1- and T_2-weighting is the gray-white matter ratio. In adults, white matter is of higher signal intensity than gray matter on a T_1-weighted scan. The reverse is true on a T_2-weighted scan, with gray matter of higher signal intensity.

Correct identification of T_1- and T_2-weighting, by visual image inspection, has become even more difficult with the advent of a technique known as fluid-attenuated inversion recovery (FLAIR) scanning. In the clinical use of FLAIR in the brain, with the pulse parameters specified to obtain T_2-weighting, CSF signal is attenuated (black). This provides markedly improved sensitivity to T_2 abnormalities (such as edema), which are seen with high signal intensity. Gray and white matter are relatively isointense, both with lower signal intensity but not as dark as CSF. FLAIR is a type of inversion recovery scan.

With gradient echo scans, in addition to TE and TR, the "tip" or "flip" angle must be specified. Gradient echo scans typically have much shorter TEs and TRs than spin echo scans, with the relationship among TE, TR, and tip angle complex. Both T_1- and T_2-weighted scans can be produced with gradient echo technique. Only two common applications of gradient echo scans exist in the brain. The first is for improved sensitivity to iron, such as that in deoxyhemoglobin and hemosiderin. The second is for high-resolution three-dimensional (3D) imaging. In the latter application, images can be acquired with a spatial resolution of 1 mm $\times$ 1 mm $\times$ 1 mm. This allows postacquisition high-resolution image reformatting in any desired plane.

Contrast enhancement is best visualized on T_1-weighted scans. The presence of the gadolinium ion causes a reduction in the T_1 of nearby water protons. This leads to an increase in signal intensity or equivalently positive lesion enhancement. It should be noted that the presence of the gadolinium ion actually causes a reduction in both T_1 and T_2. This is of relevance in first-pass brain imaging, in which the T_2 effect of the agent is actually visualized. Although both T_1 and T_2 are shortened, the T_1 shortening is of larger magnitude.

One can only visualize the T_2 effect at high concentrations, which occur during the first pass of the bolus through the brain (immediately after intravenous injection).

To appropriately identify all signal intensity abnormalities, both T_1- and T_2-weighted scans should be obtained before contrast administration. Acquisition of a postcontrast T_1-weighted scan then completes the imaging set, with high efficacy for the evaluation of all brain disease. It is strongly recommended that all three scans be acquired in the same plane because this facilitates correlation between images of different weighting. Precontrast T_1-weighted scans are also important for the differentiation of lesion enhancement from hemorrhage (methemoglobin) or fat (e.g., a corpus callosum lipoma). Supplemental scans in the coronal and sagittal planes are often useful for further lesion evaluation.

INTRA-AXIAL TUMORS (SUPRATENTORIAL SPACE)
Astrocytoma

Astrocytomas are the most common brain tumor, accounting for 50% of all intracranial neoplasms. As the name implies, astrocytomas arise from the astrocyte or its primitive precursor. These tumors occur in white matter, where astrocytes are abundant. In adults, astrocytomas are more frequent above the tentorium in the cerebral hemispheres. In children, these arise more commonly in the cerebellar hemispheres and brainstem.

Astrocytomas are classified histologically according to several scales: World Health Organization (WHO) grades I to IV, Kernohan grades I to IV, and Rubenstein grades I to III. Higher grade equates with greater malignancy. The Rubenstein classification is simpler to remember and is easier to correlate with imaging findings.

According to this scale, a grade I astrocytoma is low grade, grade II is an anaplastic astrocytoma, and grade III is a glioblastoma multiforme (GBM). In the 1993 WHO classification, a distinction is made between lesions that are histologically well circumscribed (grade I) as opposed to diffuse (grades II-IV). Low-grade (grade I) astrocytomas are further divided into specific tumor subtypes, recognizing the favorable prognosis of these lesions, which include juvenile pilocytic astrocytoma and subependymal giant cell astrocytoma. Other WHO grade I nonastrocytic tumors include gangliocytoma, meningioma, and choroid plexus papilloma. In the WHO classification, the best possible grade for a diffuse astrocytoma (the "ordinary" type of astrocytoma seen in adults) is grade II. In this classification scheme, a low-grade astrocytoma is grade II, an anaplastic astrocytoma grade III, and a glioblastoma grade IV.

Although a lower grade (for an astrocytoma) implies a lesser degree of malignancy, the outcome of even these tumors is generally poor because of the infiltrative pattern of growth. Complete tumor resection is often impossible. Grade I astrocytomas carry a uniquely favorable prognosis; the juvenile pilocytic astrocytoma (referred to in the older literature as the cystic cerebellar astrocytoma of childhood) is the most common such lesion. Surgical removal of these tumors usually produces a clinical cure. MRI is the most sensitive imaging modality for detection of astrocytomas. Increased extracellular fluid occurs as a result of abnormal capillary walls. This is easily identified on T_2-weighted scans as an area of increased signal intensity. On precontrast scans, this change may be the only or most convincing indication of the presence of a tumor. The change on T_1-weighted scans (a decrease in signal intensity) may be subtle. CT, particularly in low-grade astrocytomas, may be nearly normal or show only subtle mass effect.

GBM has the most profound as well as characteristic imaging findings (Fig. 1–1). Thus, it is the most readily

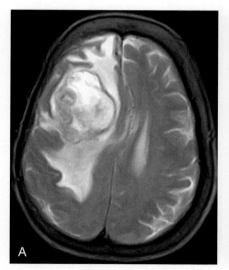
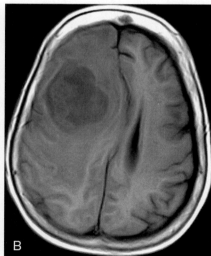
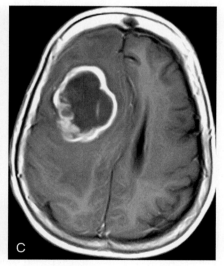

FIGURE 1–1. Glioblastoma multiforme (World Health Organization grade IV). A large right frontal lobe mass is noted on precontrast T_2- (*A*) and T_1-weighted (*B*) scans. There is extensive surrounding edema, which is high signal intensity on the T_2-weighted scan. Substantial mass effect is noted, with obliteration of sulci, compression of the right lateral ventricle, and displacement of the falx. Irregular rim enhancement is present on the postcontrast T_1-weighted scan (*C*), with no enhancement of the central necrotic portion of the tumor.

diagnosed tumor and the least frequently confused with other lesions. GBM usually has substantial mass effect, margin irregularity, and signal intensity heterogeneity on both T_1- and T_2-weighted scans. Low signal intensity on T_1-weighted scans corresponds to necrotic and cystic areas. Necrosis occurs as the tumor outgrows its blood supply. High signal intensity on T_2-weighted scans corresponds to associated, vasogenic edema, typically marked in amount. Hemorrhage may occur in higher grade tumors, frequently petechial in nature. GBMs spread via white matter tracts and frequently cross the corpus callosum to the opposite hemisphere (Fig. 1–2). Bifrontal corpus callosum tumors are referred to as "butterfly" gliomas.

Irregular enhancement of the tumor periphery ("rim") is seen after contrast administration in many higher grade astrocytomas and reflects the greater degree of BBB disruption. Other patterns of enhancement include homogeneous, garland-shaped, mixed or patchy, linear, and central. These enhancement patterns may occur in any tumor and thus are not grade specific. Occasionally, high-grade tumors will show little or no contrast enhancement. Thus, a completely accurate prediction of tumor grade by imaging appearance is not possible.

Contrast administration should, however, be routinely used in the assessment of all tumors. Because contrast use improves visualization, localization, and tumor margin delineation, a higher level of diagnostic confidence results. This is in part due to the separation of tumor nidus from surrounding edema, the former enhancing and the latter not. Unfortunately, histologic studies show that abnormal contrast enhancement in astrocytomas does not outline the entire extent of the tumor but simply the maximal site of BBB disruption (the area of greatest neovascularity). Astrocytomas are infiltrating lesions, with tumor often present beyond the border indicated by either precontrast T_2-weighted or postcontrast T_1-weighted scans. The area of maximal enhancement does identify the best site for diagnostic stereotactic biopsy. The irregular, finger-like growth pattern of these tumors produces many areas that are relatively uninvolved. If these areas are selected by chance for biopsy, the histologic diagnosis may be normal, although the imaging changes are consistent with tumor. This produces a management dilemma for the surgeon or radiation oncologist.

Contrast enhancement can also be used to separate viable tumor from frank necrosis. On postcontrast T_1-weighted scans, areas of necrosis remain low signal intensity without evidence of enhancement. Central tumor necrosis may be difficult to distinguish from cystic change. With necrosis, the interface between viable and nonviable tissue is often irregular or ragged. With cyst formation, a fairly well-circumscribed area is seen, with a smooth inner margin and enhancement at the periphery. T_1 and T_2 are typically prolonged in both cystic and necrotic areas, with low signal intensity on T_1-weighted scans and high signal intensity on T_2-weighted scans. Cysts may demonstrate a fluid-debris level or a contrast-fluid level, the latter resulting from diffusion of contrast from adjacent tumor with BBB disruption.

As with most brain disease, the primary plane for imaging should be axial. Coronal images can provide important additional information in temporal lobe abnormalities. Sagittal images assist in evaluation of brainstem and craniovertebral junction abnormalities. For preoperative evaluation, sagittal images are important, providing the neurosurgery team with improved visual localization of a lesion and thus assisting in craniotomy placement.

WHO grade III or anaplastic astrocytomas usually present with less severe imaging changes compared with GBM (Fig. 1–3). The margins are not as irregular, there is less mass effect, and the signal intensity changes on

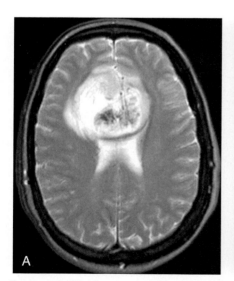 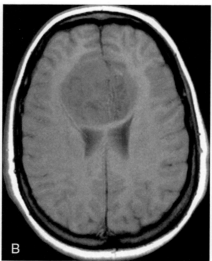 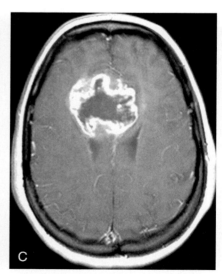

FIGURE 1–2. Glioblastoma multiforme with corpus callosum involvement. A large bifrontal lesion involving the genu of the corpus callosum is well seen on precontrast T_2- (*A*) and T_1-weighted (*B*) scans. *C*, There is irregular rim enhancement postcontrast. The enhanced scan also demonstrates a nonenhancing central component, which corresponds to necrotic debris and fluid. Glioblastomas are highly malignant, widely infiltrative lesions that grow along white matter tracts. A thick, irregular enhancing rim with central necrosis is characteristic.

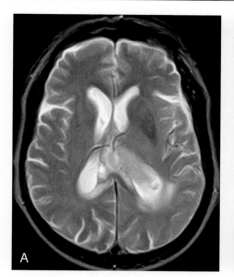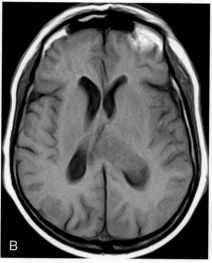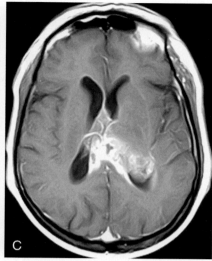

FIGURE 1–3. Anaplastic astrocytoma (World Health Organization grade III). *A,* On the precontrast T_2-weighted scan, a midline lesion with intermediate signal intensity is noted. There is subtle low signal intensity on the precontrast T_1-weighted scan (*B*). Neither scan depicts the lesion itself or its margins well. There is enhancement of the mass on the postcontrast scan (*C*), which also demonstrates involvement of the splenium of the corpus callosum. On magnetic resonance imaging, anaplastic astrocytomas (WHO grade III), as compared with low-grade astrocytomas (WHO grade II), tend to be less well defined and heterogeneous, with moderate mass effect, and may demonstrate contrast enhancement.

T_1- and T_2-weighted images are not as profound or heterogeneous. Hemorrhage is less frequently found. The degree of enhancement is variable. If the tumor lies near a convexity, enhancement may be difficult to assess without imaging in a second plane. Contrast enhancement often assists in differential diagnosis. Infarction, abscess, and resolving hematoma should be considered in the differential diagnosis of an anaplastic astrocytoma.

WHO grade II, or low-grade, astrocytomas have the least severe imaging changes (Fig. 1–4). The tumor margin, as identified on imaging, may be relatively smooth or slightly irregular. Mass effect is typically minimal. Cystic changes and necrosis are infrequent, and contrast enhancement usually does not occur. Calcifications are more frequent, as assessed by CT. However, these are not usually seen on MRI. Low-grade astrocytomas may go undiagnosed by CT, particularly if they are located in the temporal lobe. Thus, a patient with temporal lobe seizures and a normal CT should have an MRI for complete evaluation. On occasion, it may be difficult to distinguish these low-grade tumors from infarcts on a single study. Serial studies may be necessary to establish the diagnosis. Infarctions show a decline in mass effect over time and an increase in encephalomalacic changes. Tumors may show little change or a progression in mass effect with time. The major arterial territories should be kept in mind because both anterior and posterior cerebral artery infarctions, being less common, can be mistaken for an astrocytoma.

Oligodendroglioma

Oligodendrogliomas are relatively rare, accounting for about 5% of all intracranial neoplasms. These slow-growing tumors are often large at diagnosis. Oligodendrogliomas tend to involve the anterior cerebrum. They

are typically round or oval with fairly well-defined margins (Fig. 1–5).

Calcifications are more common in oligodendrogliomas than in other glia-origin tumors, occurring in more than 50% of cases. Because of the presence of calcification, CT has a diagnostic advantage. If the tumor is not calcified, it may be difficult to distinguish from other glia-origin tumors.

Ganglioneuromas (Gangliocytomas) and Gangliogliomas

Ganglioneuromas (gangliocytomas) and gangliogliomas share common characteristics in respect to incidence, macroscopic features, and biological behavior. These tumors are composed of mature ganglion cells with varying glial components. At one end of the spectrum is a tumor with mature neurons and scanty stromal glial cells. At the other end is a tumor that at first glance microscopically appears to be a glioma. Ganglioneuromas and gangliogliomas occur most frequently in children and young adults. The temporal lobe is the most common site. These tumors are usually small and well circumscribed. They are often cystic. Occasionally the cystic element dominates, with the tumor itself confined to a mural nodule (Fig. 1–6). These tumors grow slowly. Malignant change is rare. Their small size and good demarcation permit surgical resection in most cases. Prognosis is relatively good. By the WHO classification, gangliocytomas are grade I (with no malignant potential) and gangliogliomas grade I-II.

Primitive Neuroectodermal Tumor (PNET)

The term primitive neuroectodermal tumor (PNET) is controversial and refers to a group of tumors thought to originate from undifferentiated neuroepithelial cells.

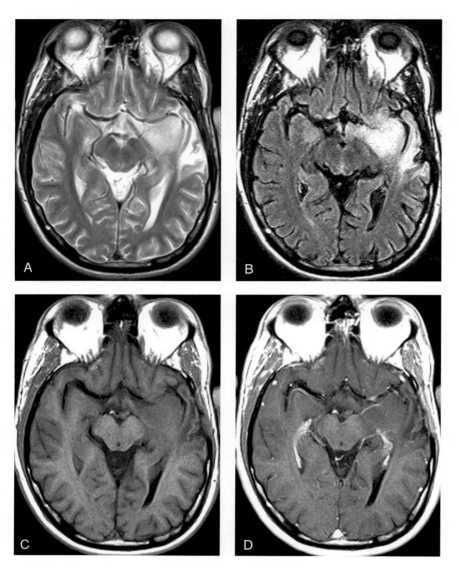

FIGURE 1–4. Low-grade astrocytoma (World Health Organization grade II). On precontrast T₂-weighted (*A*) fast spin echo and (*B*) fluid-attenuated inversion recovery scans, a high-signal-intensity abnormality is noted involving the left temporal lobe. The lesion is low signal intensity on the precontrast T₁-weighted scan (*C*) and does not demonstrate abnormal enhancement (*D*) postcontrast. On magnetic resonance imaging, low-grade astrocytomas appear well defined without substantial mass effect. Unlike higher grade tumors, these lesions usually do not enhance after contrast administration.

FIGURE 1–5. Oligodendroglioma. A large, hyperintense frontal lobe lesion is noted on the precontrast T₂-weighted scan (*A*). The mass demonstrates moderate low signal intensity on the postcontrast T₁-weighted scan (*B*). There is no abnormal contrast enhancement. Calvarial erosion resulting from location and slow growth is clearly depicted on both scans. Contrast enhancement is seen in about half of all oligodendrogliomas, which are typically being mild in degree and inhomogeneous.

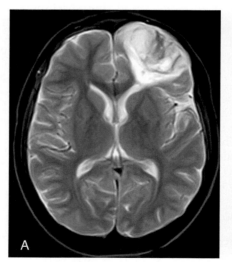

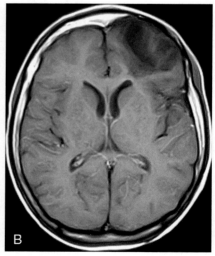

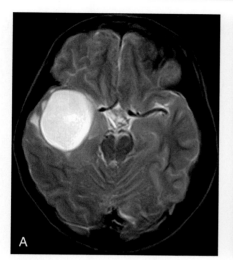 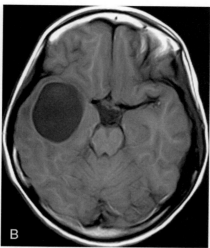 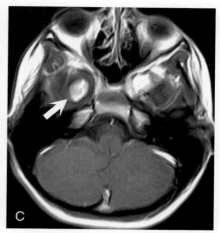

FIGURE 1–6. Ganglioglioma. A large cystic lesion is noted in the right temporal lobe on precontrast T$_2$- (*A*) and T$_1$-weighted (*B*) scans. There is mild mass effect on the brainstem. A small amount of edema is seen lateral to the lesion on the T$_2$-weighted scan. The signal intensity of the cyst is slightly different from that of cerebrospinal fluid on both images. *C*, The postcontrast T$_1$-weighted scan, obtained at a level several centimeters lower, reveals an enhancing nodule (*arrow*) along the inferior wall of the cyst.

There is considerable histopathologic heterogeneity. These tumors are highly malignant and carry a poor prognosis. Local spread, dissemination via the subarachnoid space, and distant metastases are frequent. When cerebellar in location (the most common type), the term medulloblastoma has also been used (this tumor is discussed in detail later). When supratentorial in location, the terms cerebral neuroblastoma and cerebral medulloblastoma have also been used.

Supratentorial PNETs are typically large, well-circumscribed frontal or parietal lesions. The lesion is often dominated by a cystic component, with enhancing tumor located around the periphery (Fig. 1–7). Hemor-

rhage into the cyst is not uncommon and often leads to clinical presentation.

Lymphoma

There has been a marked increase in the last decade in the incidence of primary central nervous system (CNS) lymphoma. This tumor, once rare, is now quite common. The increase in incidence has occurred in both immunosuppressed and immunocompetent patient populations. Also known as reticulum cell sarcomas or microgliomas, these tumors are derived from microglial cells that histologically resemble lymphocytes. The basal

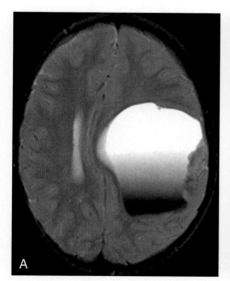 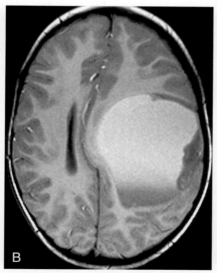 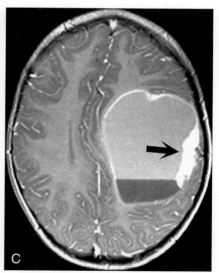

FIGURE 1–7. Supratentorial primitive neuroectodermal tumor (PNET). A large well-demarcated cystic frontoparietal mass is seen on precontrast T$_2$- (*A*) and T$_1$-weighted (*B*) scans. Within the lesion, there is a fluid-fluid level representing separation of different hemoglobin degradation products. The body of the left lateral ventricle is completely obliterated by mass effect. *C*, The postcontrast T$_1$-weighted scan reveals enhancement of a soft tissue component (*arrow*) along the lateral aspect of the mass as well as enhancement of the entire lesion rim.

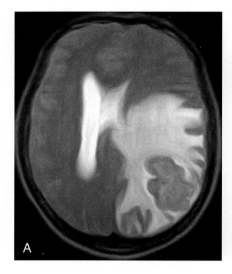

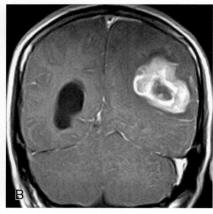

FIGURE 1–8. Primary central nervous system lymphoma. A mass with intermediate signal intensity and extensive surrounding high-signal-intensity edema is noted on the axial T$_2$-weighted scan (A). B, The postcontrast coronal T$_1$-weighted scan demonstrates prominent peripheral enhancement with central hypointensity. Before the advent of AIDS, the majority of cerebral lymphomas were primary in origin with prominent homogeneous contrast enhancement. In AIDS, primary and secondary lymphomas occur with equal frequency, and enhancement is typically ringlike in nature with central lesion necrosis.

ganglia, thalamus, and corpus callosum are the most frequently affected sites. There is an increased incidence of primary CNS lymphoma in the immunocompromised patient population. Thus, lymphoma should be considered in the differential diagnosis of brain lesions in patients who underwent organ transplantation and in those with AIDS.

Lesions not associated with AIDS are typically homogeneous in signal intensity and periventricular in location and enhance (uniformly) after contrast administration. In AIDS, lymphoma may have ring enhancement (Fig. 1–8). Lymphomas may be difficult to distinguish from abscesses, metastases, or glial tumors. Periventricular location and minimal mass effect (little edema) favor lymphoma. Some solid lymphomas have mild hypointensity on T$_2$-weighted scans.

Metastasis

Metastases comprise almost 40% of all intracranial tumors. The most common tumors that metastasize intracranially are lung, breast, melanoma, colon, and kidney. Multiplicity is the hallmark that distinguishes metastases

from gliomas or other primary tumors (Fig. 1–9). Other imaging findings that suggest metastasis are a gray-white matter junction location, a small tumor nidus with a large amount of associated vasogenic edema, and less margin irregularity. MRI is markedly superior to CT for detecting metastatic disease. Contrast administration is mandatory (Fig. 1–10). In one published study, enhanced MRI revealed three times the number of lesions seen by enhanced CT. High-dose contrast administration on MRI provides a further improvement in sensitivity (Fig. 1–11). The multi-institutional study that examined contrast dose found that high dose (0.3 mmol/kg) revealed 32% more metastases compared with standard dose (0.1 mmol/kg). If stereotactic radiation therapy is an option (depending on geographic location of the patient and hospital), high-dose thin-section (5 mm or less) imaging in both the axial and coronal planes should be performed. This approach maximizes lesion detection. Small single metastases can also be missed on a standard dose (0.1 mmol/kg) exam.

The mechanism of enhancement for intra-axial metastases is similar to gliomas in that BBB disruption is

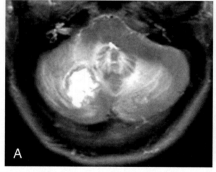

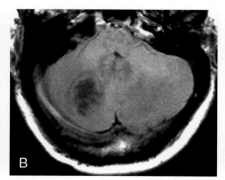

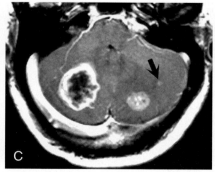

FIGURE 1–9. Brain metastases (varied appearance). A cystic or necrotic mass is noted in the right cerebellum on the precontrast T$_2$-weighted scan (A). Vasogenic edema, with abnormal high signal intensity, is seen bilaterally. Comparison of pre- (B) and postcontrast (C) T$_1$-weighted scans reveals three enhancing lesions: large necrotic right-sided metastasis, a 1-cm-diameter solid left-sided metastasis, and a smaller pinpoint metastasis (arrow) just anterior and lateral to this lesion. The case illustrates the value of contrast enhancement in identification of metastatic lesions. Although the left cerebellar hemisphere appears abnormal precontrast, focal lesions cannot be identified. Also illustrated are the multiple patterns of lesion enhancement that can be seen in metastatic disease, including rim, solid, and pinpoint.

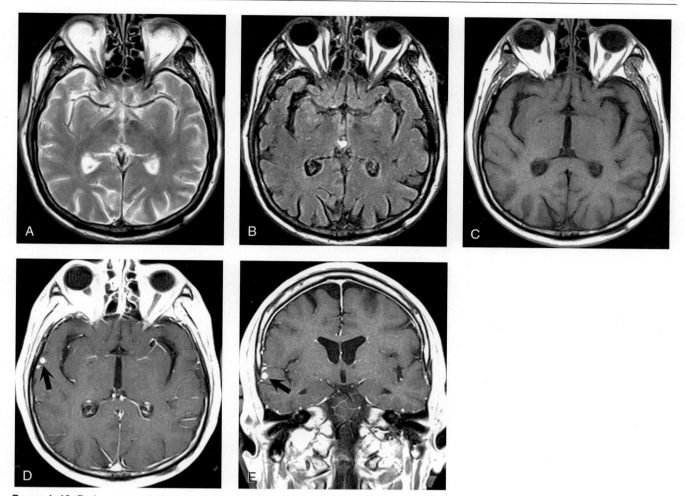

FIGURE 1–10. Brain metastasis (seen only postcontrast). Precontrast T_2-weighted fast spin echo (*A*) and fluid-attenuated inversion recovery (*B*) scans are normal, as is the precontrast T_1-weighted scan (*C*). *D*, Postcontrast, a single small enhancing lesion is noted (*arrow*), which is confirmed on the coronal scan (*E*). Small brain metastases may not elicit sufficient surrounding vasogenic edema to be recognized on precontrast magnetic resonance scans. Identification of blood-brain barrier disruption, provided by intravenous contrast administration, permits diagnosis of such lesions.

marked and separates the tumor nidus from surrounding edema. Various types of enhancement are seen, including focal dotlike, larger rounded, and variable sized areas of ring enhancement. Perhaps the greatest importance of contrast use in evaluating metastatic disease is the greater number of lesions depicted. The diagnostic and therapeutic impact is immense. The demonstration of multiple lesions may dictate radiation or chemotherapy, whereas a solitary lesion may be more effectively treated with surgical resection. Stereotactic radiation is often used in patients with only a few brain metastases. Contrast enhancement is particularly critical in elderly individuals with age-related white matter ischemic changes. These areas of increased signal intensity on T_2-weighted images may be impossible to distinguish from the signal intensity change of a metastatic lesion with surrounding edema.

Although T_2-weighted scans are quite sensitive in demonstrating vasogenic edema (as an area of increased signal intensity), not all metastatic lesions have sufficient edema to be detected on this basis alone. The lesions not visualized on unenhanced MRI are typically small (<5 mm). Common locations for metastases missed on T_2-weighted scans include the temporal lobes and the cortical-subcortical regions. Small lesions may also be missed when adjacent to the ventricles or a larger metastatic lesion. Thus, a complete evaluation for metastatic disease requires precontrast T_2-weighted, precontrast T_1-weighted, and postcontrast T_1-weighted scans. As with most brain disease, acquisition of two different T_2-weighted scans is suggested: one using FLAIR and one with fast spin echo technique. On precontrast T_1-weighted scans, large metastases are seen as low-signal-intensity lesions. Small metastases are often not visualized on these scans. The primary purpose of precontrast T_1-weighted imaging is to distinguish areas of enhancement from subacute hemorrhage (which also has high signal intensity on T_1-weighted scans).

MRI also surpasses CT in its demonstration of subacute hemorrhage. Metastases with a propensity toward hemorrhage include melanoma, choriocarcinoma, lung carcinoma (oat cell), and kidney, colon, and thyroid

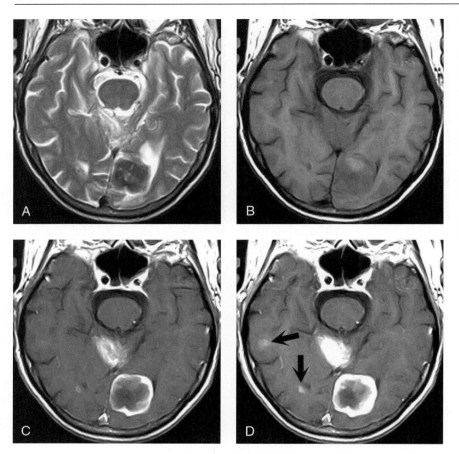

FIGURE 1–11. Brain metastases (improved lesion detection with high contrast dose). Precontrast T_2- (*A*) and T_1-weighted (*B*) scans are compared with postcontrast T_1-weighted scans using doses of 0.1 mmol/kg (standard dose) (*C*) and 0.2 mmol/kg (high dose) (*D*). The contrast agent used in this instance was gadolinium (Gd BOPTA) (MultiHance), which has improved relaxivity compared with Gd DTPA (Magnevist) because of weak protein binding. In this patient, higher contrast dose improves the enhancement of all lesions and makes two small lesions (*arrows, D*) more evident, one near the right occipital horn and the other in the right temporal lobe. (Reprinted with permission from Runge VM, Nelson KL: Contrast agents. In Stark DD, Bradley WG Jr (eds): Magnetic Resonance Imaging, 3rd ed. St. Louis, CV Mosby, 1999, pp 257–275).

carcinoma (Fig. 1–12). Petechial hemorrhage may be seen in metastases following radiation therapy. Patients receiving chemotherapy occasionally develop coagulopathies. Ensuing intracranial hemorrhage may produce a sudden decline in mental status similar to the effect of a significant hemorrhage into an intracranial metastasis. These hemorrhages may remain undiagnosed by CT, as do many subacute hemorrhages.

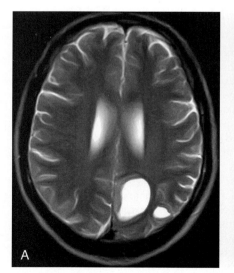
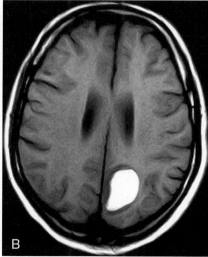
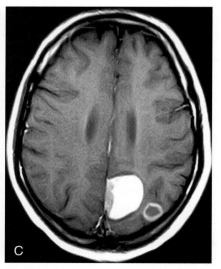

FIGURE 1–12. Hemorrhagic brain metastases. *A*, The precontrast T_2-weighted scan reveals (posteriorly) two hyperintense lesions. On the precontrast T_1-weighted scan (*B*), the larger of the abnormalities is also hyperintense, whereas the smaller is difficult to identify. This appearance is compatible with two intraparenchymal hematomas of slightly different composition. *C*, Postcontrast, there is enhancement of abnormal soft tissue along the medial border of the larger lesion, with a thick circumferential rim of enhancement surrounding the smaller lesion. Both abnormalities were confirmed to represent metastatic disease. In the presence of acute and subacute hemorrhage, careful inspection of postcontrast scans is mandated to rule out an underlying abnormality, such as metastatic disease in this instance.

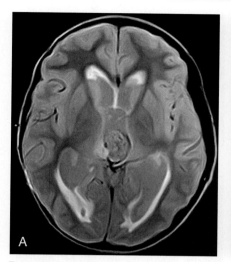
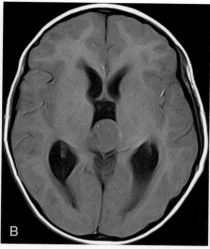
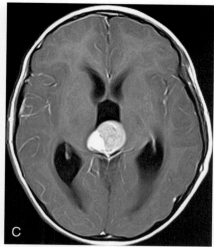

FIGURE 1–13. Mixed germ cell tumor. A soft-tissue mass is identified just posterior to the third ventricle on precontrast T₂- (*A*) and T₁-weighted (*B*) scans. There is mild internal signal inhomogeneity. A striking finding on the mildly T₂-weighted scan (*A*) is the abnormal high signal intensity surrounding the ventricles. This is consistent with transependymal flow secondary to acute obstructive hydrocephalus. *C*, Postcontrast, there is intense enhancement of the lesion. Although contrast enhancement improves lesion identification, imaging characteristics for pineal region tumors on magnetic resonance imaging are nonspecific in regard to lesion type.

Pineal Region Tumors

Pineal region tumors are classified by cell of origin (pineal or germ cell). Germ cell tumors include germinoma, teratoma, and teratocarcinoma. The occurrence of mixed germ cell tumors, with various cellular elements, is common (Fig. 1–13). All occur more frequently in males. Germinoma is the most common of these abnormalities and occurs almost exclusively in males. These tumors may be large and engulf the normal pineal gland. Less heterogeneity in signal intensity is seen in germ cell tumors compared with pineal cell tumors. Intense, homogeneous enhancement occurs. MRI defines the tumor margins better than CT.

Pineal cell tumors include pineocytoma and pineoblastoma (Fig. 1–14). These are less common than other pineal region tumors, particularly germinoma. There is no sex predilection. These tumors may calcify. Pineoblastoma is the more malignant of the two and

arises from a more primitive cell type. MRI is particularly helpful in assessing the extent of these rather large, bulky tumors and the degree of involvement of adjacent structures.

Metastases and gliomas may also occur in the pineal region. Obstructive hydrocephalus may accompany large tumors. All but teratomas are notorious for seeding by CSF pathways. Pineal cysts, which are benign, can cause difficulty in differential diagnosis. Typical pineal cysts have signal intensity only slightly different from CSF and demonstrate mild rim enhancement (Fig. 1–15).

INTRA-AXIAL TUMORS (INFRATENTORIAL SPACE)

Since its introduction, MRI has been well known for its efficacy in the diagnosis of posterior fossa lesions. CT is a poor imaging modality for evaluating the posterior

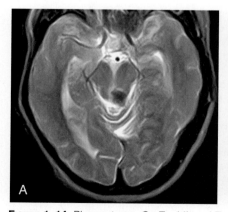
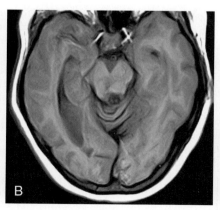
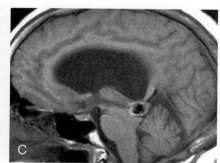

FIGURE 1–14. Pineocytoma. On T₂- (*A*) and T₁-weighted (*B*) axial scans, a well-demarcated very-low-signal-intensity mass is noted near the quadrigeminal plate. There is no associated edema. *C*, The precontrast sagittal T₁-weighted scan reveals the lesion to be pineal in location. The lateral ventricles are dilated. Noncontrast computed tomography (not shown) demonstrated a 1-cm-diameter extremely dense calcification in the region of the pineal gland.

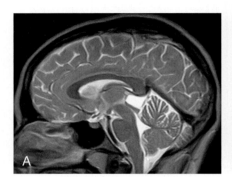
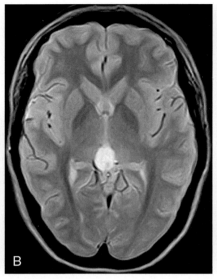
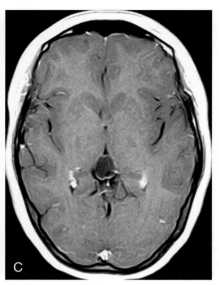

FIGURE 1–15. Pineal cyst. *A,* The sagittal fast spin echo T₂-weighted scan reveals a cystic midline pineal lesion with mild mass effect on the colliculi. On the intermediate T₂-weighted spin echo scan (*B*), the lesion is hyperintense. *C,* Postcontrast, a faint rim of enhancement can be identified. Pineal cysts are common normal variants. These cysts are round, smoothly marginated, and rarely larger than 15 mm in diameter and have a thin wall that may demonstrate contrast enhancement.

fossa. The absence of bone artifacts and the ability to acquire images in multiple planes are the two main reasons that MRI is so effective in the posterior fossa.

Astrocytoma

Cerebellar astrocytomas are predominantly tumors of early life (the first two decades). They are one of the most common posterior fossa tumors. Cerebellar astrocytomas are often well circumscribed and tend to be grossly cystic (Fig. 1–16). Anaplasia is uncommon in these lesions. This subtype is usually amenable to surgery. However, some cerebellar astrocytomas are solid tumors; infiltration of surrounding tissues is noted microscopically. Anaplastic change is more common in older patients.

Astrocytomas can involve any part of the cerebellum. If a tumor is located in the cerebellar hemispheres, the incidence of different tumor types favors diagnosis of an astrocytoma. Medulloblastomas and ependymomas are more likely to be midline.

In large cystic lesions, tumor tissue may be confined to a mural nodule, which enhances. In other instances, the cyst is lined circumferentially with tumor. Cerebellar astrocytomas consistently display contrast enhancement. This aids in differentiation between lesions with just a small tumor nidus (mural nodule), lesions with central cystic change or necrosis, and solid lesions. Caution is indicated when a cystic mass in the cerebellum is noted on MRI. The tumor nidus in a cerebellar astrocytoma may be quite small and go unrecognized without contrast enhancement. Imaging in two planes, in addition to careful examination of the postcontrast scans, is highly recommended.

Brainstem Glioma

Brainstem gliomas generally occur in older children and young adults. Most gliomas of the brainstem are dif-

fusely infiltrating astrocytomas. Symptoms include progressive cranial nerve palsies, extremity weakness, and respiratory difficulty. MRI is markedly superior to CT for visualizing these lesions. With CT, only large extensive lesions are usually recognized. In more aggressive tumors, necrotic or cystic changes can be seen, with low signal intensity on T₁-weighted scans and very high signal intensity on T₂-weighted scans. The tumor itself, specifically the soft tissue component, is best seen on T₂-weighted scans with high signal intensity but not that of CSF or fluid (Fig. 1–17). Contrast enhancement is variable.

Medulloblastoma (Cerebellar PNET)

Medulloblastomas are one of the most common posterior fossa tumors in childhood, with a predilection for males. These embryonal tumors arise in the roof of the fourth ventricle or less commonly in the cerebellar hemisphere of older patients. They are difficult to distinguish from ependymomas, unless the ependymoma extends into the cerebellopontine angle. As with most brain tumors, medulloblastomas have slightly low signal intensity on T₁-weighted scans and moderately high signal intensity on T₂-weighted scans (Fig. 1–18). Intense contrast enhancement is characteristic. Medulloblastomas are highly malignant and CSF spread is common.

Hemangioblastoma

Hemangioblastomas are histologically benign neoplasms of vascular structures. They may occur at any age but are more frequent in young and middle-aged adults. These tumors are usually solitary and located in the cerebellum. They can occur sporadically or as part of von Hippel-Lindau disease. In the latter, the tumors are typically multiple and patients present in childhood. About half of all hemangioblastomas are cystic, and half

FIGURE 1–16. Pilocytic astrocytoma (cystic cerebellar astrocytoma, World Health Organization grade I). A large cystic lesion is seen within the cerebellum on precontrast T$_2$- (*A*) and T$_1$-weighted (*B*) axial scans. A small soft tissue component along the right lateral wall is noted to enhance (*C, D*) postcontrast. Enhancement of the nodule (*arrow*) is better seen on the coronal scan (*D*). With this type of tumor, the enhancing mural nodule corresponds to neoplastic tissue. The cyst wall, which does not enhance, is nonneoplastic.

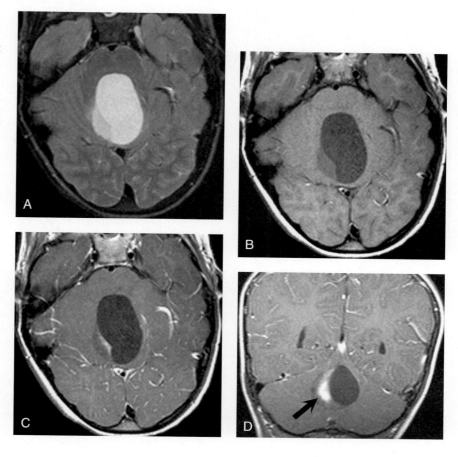

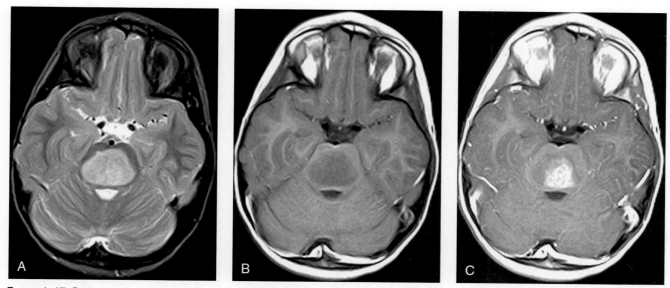

FIGURE 1–17. Brainstem (pontine) glioma. *A,* The T$_2$-weighted axial scan demonstrates a high-signal-intensity expansile mass. The lesion occupies almost the entire pons, leaving only a residual rim of normal tissue. The mass is low signal intensity on the precontrast T$_1$-weighted scan (*B*). *C,* Postcontrast, the more posterior portion of the lesion enhances. On histologic exam, brainstem (pontine) gliomas are often low-grade astrocytomas but have a tendency to undergo anaplastic change. Exophytic extension and cerebrospinal fluid seeding are common.

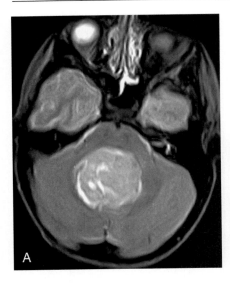

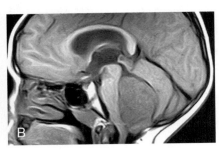

FIGURE 1–18. Medulloblastoma. A midline mass with heterogeneous, although predominantly high, signal intensity is noted on the T_2-weighted axial scan (A). B, The midline T_1-weighted sagittal scan demonstrates the mass to fill the fourth ventricle. The brainstem is displaced anteriorly and the inferior aspect of the cerebral aqueduct widened. Leptomeningeal metastases were noted on the thoracic and lumbar magnetic resonance examinations performed on the same date (images not shown).

are solid. A characteristic feature is an enhancing mural nodule (Fig. 1–19). Because these tumors involve the cerebellar hemisphere, the main differential diagnosis is a cystic astrocytoma. Cystic astrocytomas tend to be larger tumors and occur in a younger population.

INTRAVENTRICULAR TUMORS
Colloid Cyst

Colloid cysts are benign congenital lesions and occur in the anterior third ventricle. These cysts are well defined and vary in diameter from a few millimeters to several centimeters. Larger colloid cysts may produce hydrocephalus by obstruction of the foramen of Monro. Growth is slow, and the lesion may not become symptomatic until adult life.

Colloid cysts are easily diagnosed by MRI because of their location and appearance. Signal intensity characteristics cover the entire spectrum from low to high on both T_1- and T_2-weighted scans (Fig. 1–20). If the contents are predominantly lipid, the signal intensity will be high on T_1-weighted scans and fade to low on T_2-weighted scans. Colloid cysts do not enhance.

Choroid Plexus Papilloma

Choroid plexus papillomas originate from the ependyma (the lining of the ventricles). These are more common during the first decade of life and show a slight male predominance. Choroid plexus papillomas most frequently arise in the lateral ventricle in children, particularly the left lateral ventricle, and in the fourth ventricle in adults. In the lateral ventricles, hydrocephalus is asymmetric but bilateral and results from outlet obstruc-

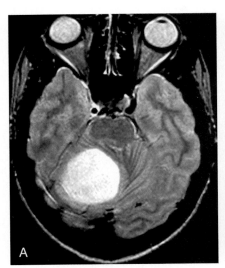

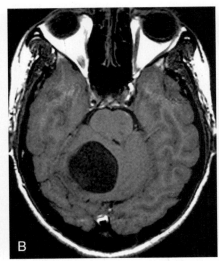

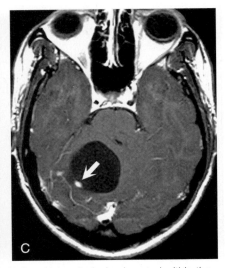

FIGURE 1–19. Hemangioblastoma. On the axial scan with intermediate T_2-weighting (A), a high-signal-intensity lesion is noted within the posterior fossa. There is mass effect with compression of the fourth ventricle. The lesion is slightly higher in signal intensity than cerebrospinal fluid on this scan and the precontrast T_1-weighted scan (B), suggesting a neoplastic origin. C, Postcontrast, there is enhancement of a small mural nodule (arrow), with a large prominent vein also identified adjacent to the mass. The most common appearance for a hemangioblastoma is that of a cystic mass with a peripheral mural nodule. Tumor vessels may also be apparent. Less commonly, these lesions present as solid masses.

FIGURE 1–20. Colloid cyst. A large round mass with signal intensity slightly lower than cerebrospinal fluid is noted on the axial T_2-weighted scan (*A*). The mass is very high signal intensity on the axial T_1-weighted scan (*B*). The lateral ventricles are enlarged, suggesting obstructive hydrocephalus. Comparison with sagittal and coronal scans (not shown) confirmed the location of the cyst at the anterior third ventricle. No abnormal contrast enhancement was noted (not shown).

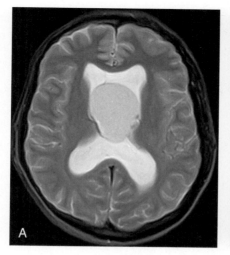
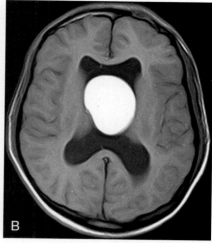

tion of the ventricle, overproduction of CSF, or a combination of these two factors. Intermittent hemorrhage into these tumors is not uncommon and may contribute to the obstructive hydrocephalus. In fourth ventricular lesions, hydrocephalus is symmetric.

Choroid plexus papillomas are frequently lobulated. Focal calcifications are common. Contrast enhancement is intense. There is little difference in appearance between choroid plexus papilloma and choroid plexus carcinoma, although the latter is much less common. Differential diagnosis includes ependymoma, meningioma, and metastases, all of which are more common in the adult population.

Ependymoma

Ependymomas are derived from ependymal cells that line the ventricles or from cell rests in the adjacent periventricular white matter. In adults, these tumors arise in the trigone of the lateral ventricle or near the foramen of Monro. Ependymomas can be periventricular or intraventricular in location. They can grow through the septum pellucidum and involve both lateral ventricles. In children, ependymomas occur more commonly in the posterior fossa, arising in the fourth ventricle. These frequently extend through the foramen of Luschka into the cerebellopontine angle. Recognition of this feature, if present, improves differentiation from other posterior fossa tumors, such as medulloblastoma and astrocytoma.

Because of their intraventricular origin, seeding via the CSF is common. The prognosis is poor with the occurrence of drop metastases. Hydrocephalus is very common, particularly with ependymomas in the posterior fossa. Whether supra- or infratentorial in location, ependymomas are usually calcified, and about half have areas of cystic change.

MRI is helpful in confirming the intraventricular location, particularly if these tumors occur in the lateral ventricles. Ependymomas usually present as large, bulky, soft tissue masses. Cystic changes or dense calcifications appear as focal areas of low signal intensity on T_1-weighted images. Ependymomas have high signal intensity on T_2-weighted images (in both cystic and noncystic regions). These lesions do show contrast enhancement, which is variable in pattern.

Meningioma

Intraventricular meningiomas are rare, occurring in the atrium of the lateral ventricle more commonly than in the third or fourth ventricles. They can occur at any age but show a predilection for older adults. As with all meningiomas, there is an increased incidence in neurofibromatosis. Intraventricular meningiomas are usually large, lobulated masses. There may be slight ventricular dilatation, either unilateral or bilateral. The signal intensity precontrast may be heterogeneous as a result of vascularity or dense calcifications. Enhancement is intense after contrast administration. MRI is more accurate in the assessment of intraventricular location than CT because of the availability of multiplanar imaging. The differential diagnosis should include other enhancing intraventricular tumors.

EXTRA-AXIAL TUMORS
Meningioma

Meningiomas are the most common extra-axial adult tumor, comprising about 15% of all intracranial neoplasms. These tumors are more frequent in women between the ages of 40 and 70 years. The most common location is high over the convexity adjoining the superior sagittal sinus in its middle or anterior third (Fig. 1–21). Other sites, in decreasing order of frequency, are the lateral convexity, sphenoid ridge, olfactory groove, suprasellar-parasellar region, and posterior fossa (petrous bone, clivus, and foramen magnum). When these tumors are multiple or occur in childhood, they are usually associated with neurofibromatosis. Meningiomas are typically benign, slow-growing tumors that compress rather than invade adjacent brain tissue. Occasionally, more aggressive changes are seen such as dural sinus or bone invasion. With such changes, complete resection

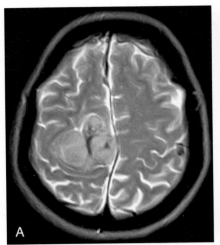
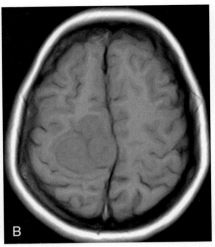
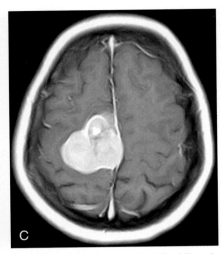

FIGURE 1–21. Falx meningioma. A soft tissue mass that is isointense to the brain is noted adjacent to the falx on precontrast T_2- (A) and T_1-weighted (B) scans. There is mild mass effect. C, Postcontrast, the mass is easily identified as a result of intense enhancement.

may not be possible, and recurrences are more likely to occur.

Regardless of location, meningiomas usually have a broad base that lies along a bony or dural margin. Features characteristic of extra-axial lesions are seen, including arcuate bowing of the white matter resulting from compression of the brain, a low-signal-intensity interface with brain on T_1-weighted scans (caused in part by displacement of pial vessels), and a CSF cleft between the lesion and brain, seen best on T_2-weighted images (Fig. 1–22). Displacement of the dura at the lateral margin of the lesion can be seen on occasion, more commonly with cavernous sinus lesions. Meningiomas are typically highly vascular; calcifications and cystic changes produce intrinsic tumor mottling. These findings are more obvious at higher field strengths perhaps because of differences in magnetic susceptibility. Meningiomas have a variable amount of associated edema. Occasionally, this edema will be the only evidence for the presence of a lesion on precontrast scans.

Unlike most intracranial tumors, meningiomas tend to be isointense with adjacent brain on both T_1- and

T_2-weighted scans. Thus, small lesions and en plaque meningiomas can be difficult to detect without contrast administration. Contrast enhancement is intense because of the lack of a BBB. On occasion, a more intensely enhancing thin rim is present, surrounding the bulk of the tumor, which shows less but still substantial enhancement). Contrast use aids in lesion visualization, accurate localization, and assessment of lesion vascularity.

Meningiomas often invade adjacent dural sinuses (Fig. 1–23). MRI venography and postcontrast T_1-weighted imaging are two effective ways to demonstrate sinus invasion. MRI venography is usually performed before contrast administration. Two-dimensional (2D) time-of-flight technique is used, depicting venous flow as high signal intensity. Sinus invasion is diagnosed on the basis of the irregular contour of the sinus, presence of a signal void within the sinus, or absence of flow (with occlusion). On postcontrast T_1-weighted scans, the venous sinus also has high signal intensity. Signs of sinus invasion are similar to that on MRI venography, except that the tumor is depicted as an enhancing soft tissue

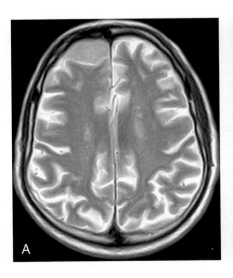
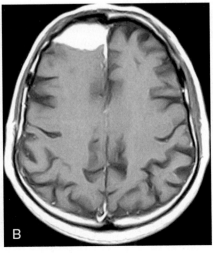

FIGURE 1–22. Convexity meningioma. A soft tissue frontal lesion of slightly higher signal intensity than adjacent brain is noted on the precontrast T_2-weighted scan (A). The mass is adjacent to both the falx and the calvarium. Erosion of the calvarium is evident on comparison of the diploic space from side to side. A cerebrospinal fluid cleft is seen posterior to the lesion, demarcating its extra-axial location. Intense uniform enhancement is seen on the postcontrast T_1-weighted scan (B).

FIGURE 1–23. Posterior fossa meningioma with dural sinus invasion. Sagittal (*A*) and axial (*B*) T_2-weighted scans reveal a subtle mass adjacent to the tentorium. The lesion is difficult to detect because it is isointense with adjacent brain. The lesion remains isointense on the T_1-weighted precontrast scan (*C*). *D*, Postcontrast, the lesion is easily seen as a result of homogeneous enhancement. The lesion is also noted to invade the adjacent transverse sinus. With extra-axial lesions in particular, precontrast scans alone may fail to diagnose an abnormality or grossly underestimate its extent.

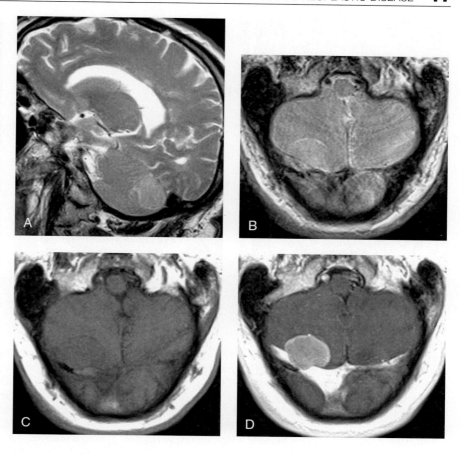

mass (although with lower signal intensity than that of venous blood). MRI is more sensitive in detecting sinus invasion than either CT or x-ray angiography.

When meningiomas arise in the cavernous sinus or secondarily extend into this structure, encasement and displacement of the carotid artery are common. MRI offers improved evaluation of this type of vascular involvement over CT and angiography. Angiographically, it may be difficult to determine whether the change in vessel caliber is atherosclerotic in nature or caused by vascular encasement. With MRI, the soft tissue mass encasing the vessel, with narrowing of its caliber, is directly visualized. Contrast enhancement more clearly shows the enlargement of the cavernous sinus when meningiomas arise within or extend into it. The displaced lateral hypointense dural line also becomes more evident. For small tumors and greater detail of involvement, thin section (<3 mm) imaging is necessary.

En plaque meningiomas represent a special and often clinically frustrating type of meningioma (Fig. 1–24). These may become extensive, with involvement of the tentorium, cavernous sinus, brainstem, and cranial nerves. Transdural and subperiosteal spread may also occur. Total resection is often not possible, leading to recurrence and relentless enlargement. These lesions are also often not well seen, or go undetected, by CT.

Meningiomas in the cerebellopontine angle can be difficult to differentiate from acoustic schwannomas. Widening of the orifice of the internal auditory canal (IAC) favors an acoustic schwannoma. A wide dural base favors a meningioma. Although meningiomas can involve the sheath of cranial nerve VIII (and thus extend into the IAC), they typically do not cause focal enlargement within the canal.

CT often depicts osseous changes (secondary to a meningioma) better than MRI. However, MRI may detect osseous change not noted by CT because of the acquisition of scans in multiple planes; CT is restricted to the axial plane. Calcifications within lesions are better shown by CT. However, MRI rarely has difficulty with differential diagnosis because of the enhancement and extra-axial location of the lesion.

Acoustic Schwannoma

Acoustic schwannomas (commonly and incorrectly referred to as "neuromas") are benign tumors that arise from the neurilemmal sheath of the vestibular division of cranial nerve VIII. Patients are usually 40 to 60 years of age and have unilateral sensorineural hearing loss and tinnitus. Larger tumors with brainstem involvement cause unsteadiness, ataxia, vertigo, and diminished corneal reflexes (Fig. 1–25). Acoustic schwannoma is the most common benign extra-axial tumor of the posterior fossa.

On its clinical introduction, MRI rapidly replaced other imaging techniques for the diagnosis and evaluation of these tumors. Polytomography, iophendylate cisternography, and air-contrast CT were former techniques that involved significant radiation to the patient.

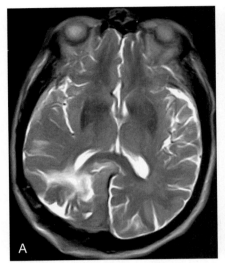
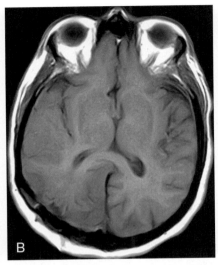
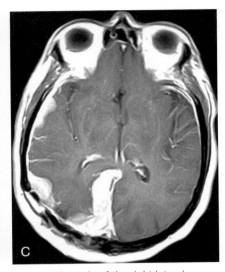

FIGURE 1–24. En plaque meningioma. *A,* The precontrast T₂-weighted scan reveals edema adjacent to the atria of the right lateral ventricle. Sulcal effacement is seen in the right hemisphere on the precontrast T₁-weighted scan (*B*). *C,* Postcontrast, an extensive homogeneous enhancing mass is identified extending along the posterior falx and right cerebral convexity. The mass follows the planes of the leptomeninges.

The latter two were also invasive, adding to patient morbidity. With MRI, the lack of signal from the adjacent dense bone allows direct visualization of cranial nerves VII and VIII. Thin-section (≤3 mm), high-resolution images are, however, necessary for appropriate diagnosis and evaluation of IAC tumors.

On precontrast scans, the tumor (if visualized) is isointense with brain on T₁-weighted scans and iso- to slightly hyperintense on T₂-weighted scans. The lesion may be extracanalicular in location, intracanalicular, or both. Necrosis and hemorrhage are not uncommon in large extracanalicular lesions, causing further variability in signal intensity. Of all sequences, postcontrast scans best demonstrate both the intracanalicular and extracanalicular extent. Accurate knowledge of tumor extent is important in operative planning.

Contrast enhancement is important not only for assessing tumor extent but also for detecting small intracanalicular acoustic schwannomas (Fig. 1–26). Precontrast scans alone may miss small lesions within the IAC. Postcontrast, these are seen as brightly enhancing small soft tissue masses. The normal cranial nerve VIII does not enhance. Thus, any contrast enhancement in this region is abnormal. The degree of enhancement seen with acoustic schwannomas is greater than that for any other intracranial tumor. Enhancement is due to intrinsic lesion vascularity.

For accurate assessment, thin-section T₁-weighted scans pre- and postcontrast in both the axial and coronal planes are highly recommended in addition to a precontrast thin-section T₂-weighted scan. MRI without contrast enhancement can produce both false-negative and

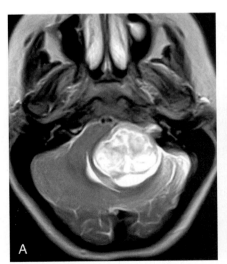
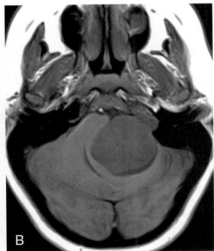
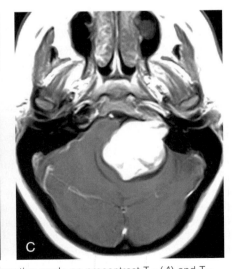

FIGURE 1–25. Acoustic schwannoma. A large soft tissue mass is noted in the left cerebellopontine angle on precontrast T₂- (*A*) and T₁-weighted (*B*) scans. *C,* Postcontrast, there is intense lesion enhancement consistent with a vascular extra-axial mass. Enlargement of the internal auditory canal (IAC) by the mass, with extension into the canal, favors diagnosis of an acoustic schwannoma. A meningioma, the other major consideration in differential diagnosis, is unlikely to enlarge the IAC.

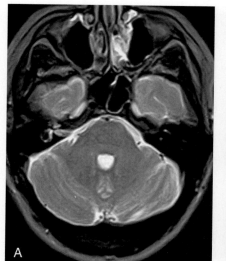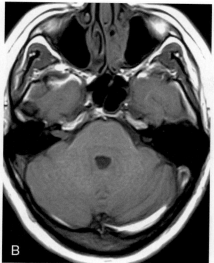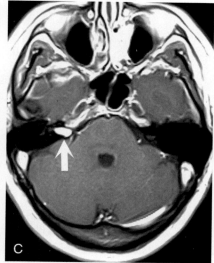

FIGURE 1–26. Intracanalicular acoustic schwannoma. On precontrast T_2- (*A*) and T_1-weighted (*B*) scans, the question of a right-sided intracanalicular lesion is raised. *C*, Postcontrast, there is intense lesion enhancement (*arrow*), permitting definitive diagnosis. The clinical presentation was that of right-sided sensorineural hearing loss. Other entities to be considered in differential diagnosis include facial (seventh) nerve tumor and inflammatory disease, although the latter should not result in a mass lesion.

false-positive results. In one series, the combination of these errors affected 10% of patients studied. Small intracanalicular tumors that went undetected without contrast could be seen with contrast. More alarming is the prospect of suggesting a tumor on precontrast scans when none can be found postcontrast. This can occur when the nerve appears (erroneously) to be enlarged on T_1-weighted scans. Also, ectasia of the IAC can produce signal intensity on T_2-weighted scans indistinguishable from that of intracanalicular tumor.

T_1-weighted 3D gradient echo scans are used in some institutions for evaluating the IAC (replacing 2D axial and coronal T_1-weighted spin echo scans). A high-resolution 3D scan can be acquired in less than 5 minutes. This approach offers high-resolution imaging in any desired plane, with postacquisition image reconstruction. Advantages over conventional spin echo technique include thinner slices (typically 1 mm) and the absence of a gap between slices (true contiguous sections).

T_2-weighted scans are not essential for the imaging evaluation of acoustic schwannomas. However, they are important for the differential diagnosis. Many abnormalities can mimic cranial nerve VIII disease clinically, and these are often better visualized with T_2-weighted scans. Examples include multiple sclerosis, mastoiditis, and vascular brainstem compression.

A special word of caution is offered for evaluating postsurgical recurrence. In the translabyrinthine approach, the resected portion of the mastoid bone is often packed with an autologous graft that contains fat. The graft may be superimposed over the course of the nerve on axial scans. Coronal scans are then necessary to separate recurrent enhancing tumor from high-signal-intensity graft. Dural enhancement may also occur after surgery. Careful evaluation in both the axial and coronal planes is important for differentiation. Dural enhance-

ment should be linear in character, with recurrent tumor presenting as a globular soft tissue mass.

Epidermoid

Epidermoids (cholesteatomas) result from incomplete cleavage of neural from cutaneous ectoderm, with inclusion of ectodermal elements at the time of neural groove closure. Both midline (suprasellar and intraventricular) and more eccentrically located (cerebellopontine angle) lesions occur; the latter result from an inclusion at a slightly later stage of embryogenesis (Fig. 1–27). Epidermoids grow by desquamation of epithelial cells, which break down into keratin and cholesterol within the tumor capsule. These fatty elements are soft and pliable, and in the slow accumulation process they conform to the shape of the subarachnoid space or ventricle. The lesions are fairly well demarcated. Compression of adjacent structures occurs late. These congenital tumors may not become symptomatic until patients are 25 to 30 years old. Rupture occasionally produces chemical meningitis. As with other lipid tumors, their appearance on MRI depends on the type of fat and its physical state. Many contain cholesterol and show a prolongation of both T_1 and T_2 relaxation times. Such lesions are low signal intensity on T_1-weighted images and high signal intensity on T_2-weighted images. A difference in the fat content or physical state yields brighter signal intensity on T_1-weighted images. These tumors do not enhance. Thus, contrast administration is of little diagnostic value, except to exclude other cerebellopontine angle lesions with similar precontrast signal intensity (e.g., some meningiomas).

Dermoid

Dermoids are congenital tumors, like epidermoids, that arise from inclusion of ectodermal elements at the time

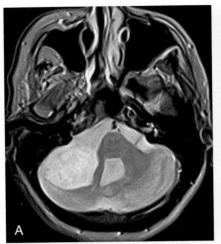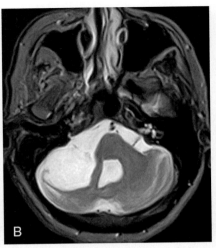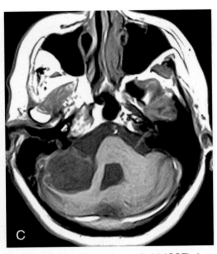

FIGURE 1–27. Epidermoid. An extra-axial mass with heterogeneous, but slightly higher signal intensity than cerebrospinal fluid (CSF), is noted in the right cerebellopontine angle cistern on an intermediate T₂-weighted scan (*A*). The difference in signal intensity between the lesion and CSF is not apparent on a heavily T₂-weighted scan (*B*). The mass is best demarcated on the precontrast T₁-weighted scan (*C*). On this scan, the mass can again be differentiated from adjacent CSF, the latter with slightly lower signal intensity. The mass compresses the right middle cerebellar peduncle and right cerebellar hemisphere. There was no enhancement postcontrast (not shown).

of neural groove closure. The presence of hairs and other skin appendages differentiates a dermoid from an epidermoid tumor. Dermoids arise near the midline and are less common than epidermoids. Most intracranial dermoids are located in the posterior fossa. Most spinal canal dermoids occur in the lumbosacral region. Dermoids may contain fat, hair follicles, and glandular elements (sebaceous and apocrine). Those containing a large amount of fatty elements have high signal intensity on T₁-weighted scans and lower signal intensity on conventional T₂-weighted scans (Fig. 1–28). Dermoids are not vascular tumors and do not cause BBB disruption. Thus, they do not enhance after contrast administration.

Arachnoid Cyst

Arachnoid cysts are benign lesions that contain CSF. Most are congenital in origin. Less common causes include inflammation, trauma, and subarachnoid hemorrhage. Their importance lies in differentiation from other masses, including epidermoids, dermoids, subdural hygromas or hematomas, and cystic tumors. Arachnoid cysts most frequently occur in the middle cranial fossa. Other common locations include the posterior fossa (retrocerebellar) (Fig. 1–29), the suprasellar region, the quadrigeminal plate, and the cerebral convexities. The cyst is lined by arachnoid membrane and filled with fluid

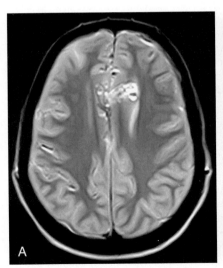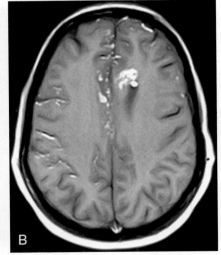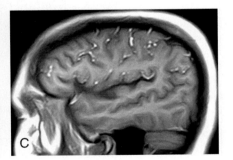

FIGURE 1–28. Ruptured dermoid. *A,* The intermediate T₂-weighted scan reveals scattered areas of abnormal hyperintensity, with many exhibiting a low-signal-intensity border along the frequency encoding direction (chemical shift artifact). Axial (*B*) and sagittal (*C*) precontrast T₁-weighted scans confirm the presence of scattered abnormalities, which remain hyperintense. The more peripheral globules are noted to lie within cortical sulci. By recognition of chemical shift, high signal intensity resulting from fat (as in this case) can be differentiated from methemoglobin. This case also illustrates the importance of obtaining precontrast T₁-weighted scans to identify fat or blood that might otherwise be mistaken for abnormal contrast enhancement.

FIGURE 1–29. Posterior fossa arachnoid cyst. Sagittal (*A*) and axial (*B*) T$_2$-weighted scans reveal a lesion, with cerebrospinal fluid signal intensity, posterior to the vermis and right cerebellar hemisphere. Mass effect is evident both by the anterior displacement of the vermis and the upward bowing of the posterior portion of the tentorium.

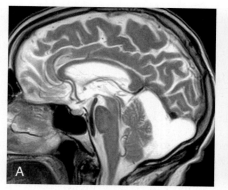
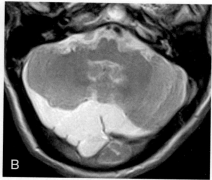

that is usually clear but on occasion slightly xanthochromic. The margins of an arachnoid cyst are sharply defined. The signal intensity is usually identical to that of CSF. No contrast enhancement occurs.

Leptomeningeal Metastases

Tumors that have access to the subarachnoid space may spread via the CSF or along the meninges. Tumors that, because of their origin in or near the ventricular system, spread via the CSF include ependymomas, medulloblastomas, pineal region tumors, and occasionally glioblastomas. Metastases from these primaries, often called "drop metastases," seed more commonly to the spine. Tumors that spread via cortical or meningeal involvement include metastatic breast carcinoma, melanoma, lymphoma, leukemia, and calvarial metastases with secondary meningeal involvement. Diffuse meningeal changes may be monitored by parenchymal deposits. These occur after the malignant meningeal lesions dip into the perivascular spaces of Virchow-Robin and spread to the parenchyma, forming nodular metastases.

Leptomeningeal metastases are not well seen by CT. Before approval of the gadolinium chelates, the same was true for MRI. Currently, contrast-enhanced MRI is the technique of choice for the diagnosis of leptomeningeal disease. In the brain, leptomeningeal metastases are visualized as abnormal contrast enhancement, linear or

nodular in character, lining the meningeal surface and extending into sulci and cisterns (Fig. 1–30).

PITUITARY AND PARASELLAR REGION TUMORS

After its clinical introduction, MRI rapidly replaced CT for evaluating the pituitary and parasellar region. The inherent advantages of MRI are of even greater importance in this small region. High-resolution imaging is possible in all planes without the need for image reformatting. Dental amalgam causes no artifacts. On CT, this often restricts the use of direct coronal scans. CT also poses the problem of radiation dose. Serial exams are often required in younger patients with hormonally active, but predominantly benign, lesions. Perhaps the greatest advantage of MRI is the superior depiction of soft tissue (without the presence of bone artifacts). This is particularly important in the imaging of such a small anatomic region situated in the dense skull base. Normal anatomic structures, including the cavernous sinus, internal carotid artery, and cranial nerves, are well visualized. Intrinsic abnormalities within the pituitary are easily recognized. Furthermore, the distinction between parasellar aneurysms and intrasellar tumor, a major pitfall with CT, is not a problem with MRI.

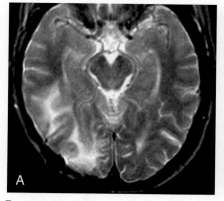
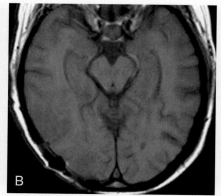
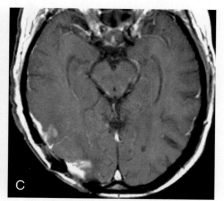

FIGURE 1–30. Meningeal carcinomatosis. Scans were taken 1 year after surgical resection and whole brain radiation for a right occipital metastasis from breast carcinoma. Abnormal high signal intensity, without a specific focal lesion, is noted in the right parietal and occipital lobes on the precontrast T$_1$-weighted scan (*A*). No additional information is provided by the precontrast T$_1$-weighted scan (*B*). *C*, After contrast administration, recurrent tumor is identified, marked by intense enhancement, along the surface of the brain in the area of prior resection.

The identification and characterization of lesions in the sella and parasellar region require thin-section imaging (≤3 mm). Spin echo technique typically can provide no thinner than 2-mm sections, whereas 3D gradient echo technique can provide 0.5- to 1-mm sections. The latter technique is also advantageous in that the slices are truly contiguous without an intervening gap. Images from a high-resolution 3D data set can be reformatted in multiple planes, further improving the diagnostic value of the exam. For gradient echo scans, TEs should be short (1 – 5 milliseconds) to avoid susceptibility ("blow-out") artifacts at the air-soft tissue interface between the sella and the sphenoid sinus.

Regarding the relative utility of T_1- and T_2-weighted scans, the first provide excellent delineation of anatomy. T_2-weighted scans are useful for recognizing necrosis and cystic changes and for characterizing areas of high signal intensity on T_1-weighted scans. Necrosis and cystic changes within the pituitary, as in the brain, are low signal intensity on T_1-weighted scans and high signal intensity on T_2-weighted scans. High signal intensity on precontrast T_1-weighted scans corresponds to subacute hemorrhage or high lipid content; the latter is seen in some craniopharyngiomas. Extracellular methemoglobin is high signal intensity on both T_2- and T_1-weighted scans. Lipid has high signal intensity on T_1-weighted scans yet low signal intensity on conventional T_2-weighted scans. With the exception of these changes, pituitary abnormalities are characterized using T_1-weighted scans before and after contrast administration. Most protocols call for precontrast T_2-weighted coronal or sagittal scans (one plane only) and T_1-weighted coronal and sagittal images (both planes) before and after contrast administration. Abnormalities are identified as a result of greater enhancement of normal adjacent structures, as in the case of many microadenomas, or of enhancement of the lesion itself (on the basis of intrinsic vascularity), as in the case of macroadenomas.

Normal Pituitary Gland

The size of the normal pituitary gland varies widely. A height of 10 mm is considered the upper limit of normal, with two exceptions. During puberty and the early childbearing years, the gland may be up to 12 mm in height. The upper surface of the gland may be flat, concave, or convex in the midline.

T_1-weighted images provide excellent anatomic definition. In the coronal plane, the pituitary is localized as a soft tissue structure lying between the rounded areas of signal void from the internal carotid arteries. The signal intensity of the gland is similar to the white matter of brain. In the sagittal plane, the anterior and posterior lobes of the pituitary can be distinguished by the high signal intensity of the posterior lobe. Immediately posterior to the pituitary itself is the high-signal-intensity marrow of the dorsum sellae. Frequently, there is a normal area of increased signal intensity on T_1-weighted images at the base of the pituitary. This may be mistaken for an abnormality but actually represents fatty marrow in the upper extreme of a sphenoid sinus septum.

The optic chiasm and pituitary stalk are outlined by low-signal-intensity CSF in the suprasellar cistern on T_1-weighted images. These structures are easy to identify in both the sagittal and coronal planes. The coronal plane is more useful for assessing gland symmetry. The cavernous sinus, with the internal carotid artery, cranial nerves III through VI, and the lateral dural margin, is also best evaluated in the coronal plane. The anteroposterior dimension of the sella turcica is obtained from sagittal images, which also provide an important second view for lesion visualization. Postcontrast, the pituitary gland, stalk, and cavernous sinus show intense enhancement, greatly facilitating the diagnosis of sellar and parasellar disease.

On T_2-weighted images, the gland is isointense with white matter (as on T_1-weighted images). CSF in the suprasellar cistern is high signal intensity. The low signal intensity of the lateral dural margin of the cavernous sinus is better defined than on T_1-weighted images.

Microadenoma

Microadenomas are defined as lesions smaller than 10 mm in diameter. Production of hormones brings these lesions to clinical attention early and thus when small. The most common microadenoma is the prolactinoma. These tumors secrete prolactin and present with infertility, amenorrhea, and galactorrhea in women and galactorrhea and impotence in men. Imaging findings include focal asymmetry of the gland surface, displacement of the pituitary stalk to the contralateral side, and a low-signal-intensity focal mass on T_1-weighted scans. Hemorrhage within the lesion may cause high signal intensity on precontrast T_1-weighted scans. On T_2-weighted scans, prolactinomas can be hypo-, iso-, or hyperintense. On early postcontrast scans, most prolactinomas are hypointense compared with the normal pituitary and infundibulum (which both enhance intensely). Contrast injection thus facilitates lesion detection (Fig. 1–31). A small number of tumors are isointense to the normal pituitary precontrast and hypointense postcontrast. With thin-section, high-resolution (small field of view) scans, evaluation of these tumors by MRI is superior to that by CT.

Cushing's syndrome is caused by adrenocorticotropic hormone (ACTH)-producing adenomas of the pituitary in 60% of cases. If not in the pituitary, these tumors arise in the adrenal gland or in ectopic sites. Clinical symptoms include truncal obesity, abdominal striae, moon facies, acne, hypertension, psychiatric disturbances, and amenorrhea and hirsutism in women. These occur because of excess cortisol production. Clinical symptoms usually bring these tumors to attention while still small. Detection on CT is difficult; less than half of all lesions are diagnosed. Presurgical localization still relies in some cases on petrosal vein sampling, an invasive and technically difficult angiographic procedure. Limited experience with MRI indicates a very high detection rate (80 – 100%).

Macroadenoma

Large pituitary adenomas are rarely a diagnostic dilemma for CT or MRI. These bulky tumors are usually

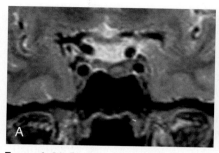
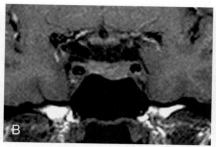
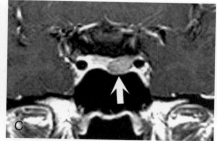

FIGURE 1–31. Pituitary microadenoma (prolactinoma). Asymmetry of the sellar floor is noted on the T₂-weighted coronal scan (*A*). A definite mass cannot be identified on either this scan or the T₁-weighted coronal scan (*B*). *C*, Postcontrast, the normal pituitary demonstrates intense enhancement, revealing a large, hypointense, left-sided pituitary microadenoma (*arrow*).

hormonally inactive, with a few tumors secreting prolactin. Because of the improved depiction of soft tissue, MRI can better assess suprasellar and lateral temporal extension (Fig. 1–32). The cavernous sinus can be displaced by tumor or on occasion can be invaded with encasement of the internal carotid artery. Macroadenomas are isointense with white matter on T₁-weighted images, unless there is associated hemorrhage. Subacute hemorrhage in most tumors, including macroadenomas (with high signal intensity on T₁-weighted images), is better demonstrated by MRI than CT. Hemorrhage within macroadenomas is more common than was once thought based on CT and clinical criteria. Pituitary apoplexy is defined as spontaneous hemorrhage into or ischemic necrosis of a normal pituitary or an adenoma. Before MRI, pituitary apoplexy was equated with severe neurologic symptoms, including sudden alteration in mental status and occasionally blindness. It is now known from MRI that small hemorrhages may be accompanied by no more than a severe headache.

On T₂-weighted images, macroadenomas have intermediate, homogeneous signal intensity. Necrosis causes foci of high signal intensity. If the necrotic portion is substantial in size, differentiation from a craniopharyngioma can be difficult. A distinguishing feature is the size of the sella, usually substantially enlarged with a macroadenoma.

Macroadenomas demonstrate substantial enhancement postcontrast. The presence of liquefaction or necrosis, which does not enhance, produces patchy enhancement postcontrast. Tumor margins are better seen after contrast administration. Tumor extent can be underestimated precontrast, with greater extent demonstrated postcontrast. Involvement of the cavernous sinus is easier to assess postcontrast, with the sinus enhancing to a greater degree than the macroadenoma.

Craniopharyngioma

Craniopharyngiomas are benign, slow-growing tumors that arise from nests of epithelium derived from Rathke's pouch. In regard to age of presentation, there are two peaks: one in childhood and the other in adults older than 50 years. These tumors most often are suprasellar in location; thus, the sella will not be enlarged. Occasionally, a portion of the tumor may extend into the sella, causing slight enlargement. However, the sella typically does not attain the size seen with macroadenomas. Although rare, a craniopharyngioma can arise within the sella. Intrasellar lesions are smaller at presentation than the more common suprasellar tumor and are difficult to differentiate from prolactinomas or Rathke's cleft cysts (a benign congenital cyst that can be intrasellar or suprasellar in location). Intrasellar craniopharyngiomas are usually accompanied by amenorrhea and galactorrhea resulting from low levels of prolactin.

Craniopharyngiomas are usually predominantly cystic with a small soft tissue component (Fig. 1–33). Most craniopharyngiomas are very low signal intensity on T₁-weighted scans because of a large cystic component containing relatively clear fluid. High signal intensity on precontrast T₁-weighted scans can also be seen resulting from high cholesterol content or byproducts (methemoglobin) from previous hemorrhage. The cystic portion

FIGURE 1–32. Pituitary macroadenoma. A large pituitary mass, with suprasellar extension, is identified on coronal pre- (*A*) and postcontrast (*B*) T₁-weighted scans. The lesion is isointense to gray matter precontrast and demonstrates homogeneous enhancement postcontrast. The optic chiasm is markedly thinned as a result of compression by the suprasellar portion of the mass.

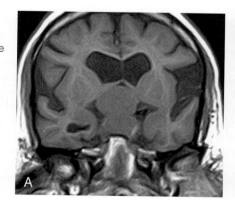
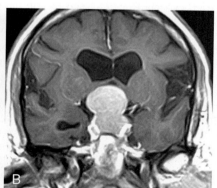

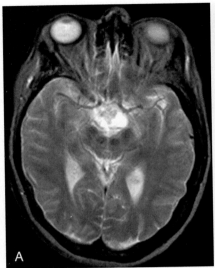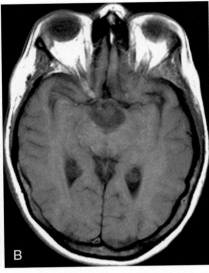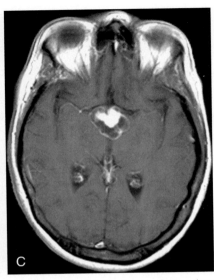

FIGURE 1–33. Craniopharyngioma. *A*, A high-signal-intensity suprasellar lesion is noted on the precontrast T_2-weighted scan. Comparison of pre- (*B*) and postcontrast (*C*) T_1-weighted scans reveals a solid enhancing nidus anteriorly and a cystic rim-enhancing component posteriorly. Craniopharyngiomas are complex heterogeneous masses with both cystic and solid components. Contrast administration aids in the differential diagnosis and definition of lesion extent.

of the tumor is usually very high signal intensity on T_2-weighted scans.

Suprasellar craniopharyngiomas vary from small lobulated to large multicystic septated lesions. Tumor margins are usually smooth and rounded. Craniopharyngiomas in children tend to be larger and contain more calcification. Postcontrast, the cyst walls of a craniopharyngioma enhance. There may also be areas of nodular enhancement. Contrast-enhanced scans aid in differential diagnosis. The normal pituitary, which enhances brightly, can be separated from suprasellar tumor or from tumor that partially extends into the sella. Contrast-enhanced scans also aid in visualization of craniopharyngiomas that are not large enough to obliterate the suprasellar cistern. In this case, the signal intensity of the tumor blends with the signal intensity of the suprasellar cistern on T_2-weighted studies. Although calcifications are not well visualized on MRI, the location of the lesion and dominant cystic component, along with the presence of septations and lobulations, enables correct diagnosis in most instances.

Other Parasellar Tumors

MRI, especially when used in conjunction with contrast media, is particularly effective in visualizing and clearly localizing other parasellar tumors. MRI also well defines the relationship of these lesions to important adjacent structures, such as the cavernous sinus, brainstem, and optic chiasm. These tumors include chordomas, hypothalamic gliomas, and meningiomas. With the exception of the hypothalamic glioma, which shows variable enhancement, these tumors show excellent enhancement.

Because of their propensity to invade adjacent sinuses and encase arterial structures, meningiomas produce special imaging problems, particularly in view of their variable delineation on T_2-weighted images. In the parasellar region, these tumors generally require thin-section

imaging for definition of venous and arterial involvement. Examination of other parasellar tumors is also benefited by thin-section imaging because of the compact regional anatomy and proximity of crucial structures.

TUMORS OF BONE
Chordoma

Chordomas are rare, slow-growing primary bone tumors that originate from remnants of the primitive notochord. The primitive notochord extends from Rathke's pouch to the clivus, continuing along the vertebral column. Remnants of the notochord can occur at any location along this line.

Thirty-five percent of chordomas are intracranial, and most of these arise from the clivus. Fifty percent are sacrococcygeal, and 15% arise from within a vertebral body. Within the calvarium, chordomas may involve the posterior or middle fossa by extension through the dura. The majority of these tumors cause extensive destruction of bony structures. Chordomas rarely metastasize to distant sites but are locally aggressive. Total surgical resection is rarely possible. Although locally invasive, chordomas are histologically benign. Macroscopically, chordomas are soft gelatinous tumors that frequently result in destruction of the clivus and skull base. They occur most commonly in men in the third and fourth decades. Patients present with headaches, facial pain, progressive cranial nerve palsies, and nasal stuffiness.

Calcification is identified in 50% to 60% of cases on CT. On MRI imaging, chordomas are usually well-defined, extra-axial tumors that show isointensity or mild hypointensity on T_1-weighted images and moderate to extreme high intensity on T_2-weighted images. Approximately 70% of chordomas have septations of low signal intensity separating lobulated areas of higher signal intensity on T$_2$-weighted images. Chordomas typically enhance after contrast administration.

Metastases

The normal diploic space does not enhance, except for diploic veins and the meninges near pacchionian granulations. Diploic veins appear as linear or small round (if cut in cross-section) foci of low to moderate signal intensity on precontrast MRI images, with enhancement postcontrast. The diploic space can appear inhomogeneous with areas of increased (resulting from fatty marrow) and decreased (caused by bony sclerosis or suture lines) signal intensity on precontrast scans. However, the diploic space should be symmetric from side to side. Gross asymmetry is highly suggestive of calvarial disease, even in the absence of appreciable destruction of the inner or outer table. Calvarial metastases enhance after intravenous contrast administration (Fig. 1–34).

Eosinophilic Granuloma

Langerhans cell (eosinophilic) granulomatosis is the term currently preferred for eosinophilic granuloma syndromes. This replaces older nomenclature, including histiocytosis X, which referred to a spectrum of diseases now known to include this benign entity and malignant lymphoma.

Unifocal Langerhans cell granulomatosis is a disease of children and young adults, predominantly males, who present with a solitary osteolytic lesion (most often in the femur, skull, vertebrae, ribs, or pelvis). Diagnosis requires biopsy; treatment is simple excision. The typical presentation in neuroradiology is that of a solitary skull lesion. MRI demonstrates a soft tissue mass, centered in the diploic space, with adjacent bone destruction (Fig. 1–35). The lesion may extend into the epidural or subga-

leal space. Eosinophilic granulomas enhance prominently postcontrast.

Multifocal Langerhans cell granulomatosis also presents in childhood, with multiple bony lesions in virtually any site. Diabetes insipidus occurs in one third as a result of hypothalamic involvement. The term Hand-Schüller-Christian syndrome was previously used to refer to the disease triad of destructive bone lesions, diabetes insipidus, and exophthalmos. However, only 25% of patients with multifocal Langerhans cell (eosinophilic) granulomatosis have this triad, which can also be caused by malignant lymphoma and carcinoma. Although benign, multifocal disease is treated with methotrexate, vinblastine, or prednisone.

POSTOPERATIVE TUMOR EVALUATION

The evaluation of tumors that recur after surgery is difficult without contrast administration. Subtle mass effect and postsurgical encephalomalacia are difficult to assess in regard to the question of tumor recurrence. Differentiation of encephalomalacia from edema associated with tumor recurrence is also difficult. Both have increased signal intensity on T$_2$-weighted scans. Extension of abnormal high signal intensity into the corpus callosum, without volume loss, is, however, specific for tumor. Edema does not track into corpus callosum because of the compact nature of the nerve fibers. Cystic, necrotic, and hemorrhagic changes are well seen on precontrast T$_1$-weighted scans. However, underlying tumor may be difficult to detect. Contrast-enhanced MRI is markedly superior to enhanced CT for demonstrating tumor recurrence (Fig. 1–36). One study demonstrated that 50% of postoperative tumor recurrences were primarily or more conclusively shown by contrast-

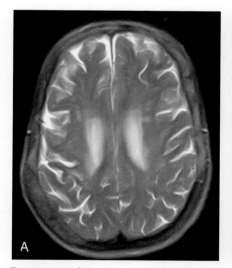
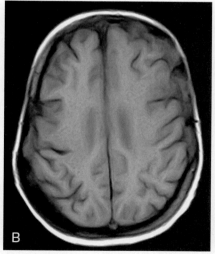
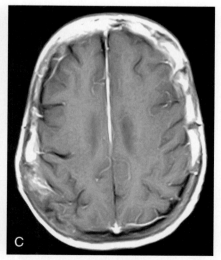

FIGURE 1–34. Calvarial metastases. There is widening of the diploic space in the right parietal and left frontal regions on *A*, the precontrast T$_2$-weighted scan. *B*, The marrow space in the left frontal region appears enlarged on the precontrast T$_1$-weighted scan. The soft tissue here is also of lower signal intensity than normal marrow fat. *C*, Postcontrast, there is intense enhancement of soft tissue within the diploic space in the right parietal and left frontal regions consistent with bony metastatic disease. Contrast administration, as in this case, can improve recognition of metastatic involvement of the diploic space as a result of the enhancement of neoplastic tissue. Comparison with precontrast scans is mandatory.

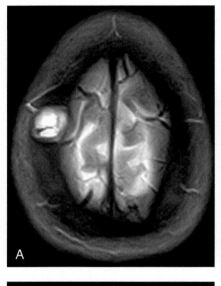

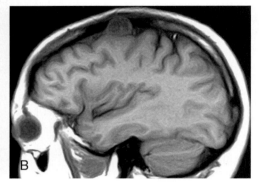

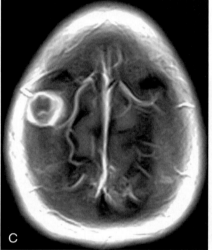

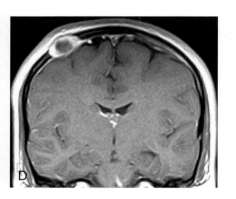

FIGURE 1–35. Eosinophilic granulomatosis. An expansile diploic space mass is identified on axial T_2- (*A*) and sagittal T_1-weighted (*B*) images. On axial (*C*) and coronal (*D*) postcontrast scans, there is a thick peripheral rim of abnormal contrast enhancement. The sagittal and coronal scans demonstrate focal expansion of the diploic space. Differential diagnosis plays an important role in scan interpretation in this instance, with imaging findings (a solitary lesion) and clinical information (a young man with headaches and a "bump" on his head) favoring a diagnosis of eosinophilic granuloma (proven by subsequent resection).

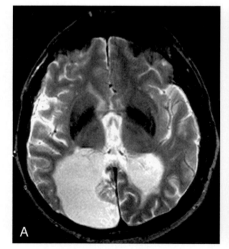

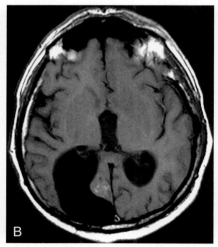

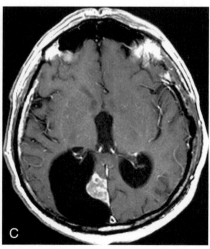

FIGURE 1–36. Recurrent astrocytoma. A large postsurgical defect, communicating with the atria of the right lateral ventricle, is noted on precontrast T_2- (*A*) and T_1-weighted (*B*) scans. The exam was performed to rule out tumor recurrence in this elderly patient with resection of an astrocytoma 4 years earlier. Medial to the postsurgical defect is soft tissue with signal intensity similar to that of normal brain. The question of tumor recurrence is raised by the slight hyperintensity of this soft tissue on the precontrast T_1-weighted scan. *C,* After contrast administration, there is intense enhancement, making possible definitive diagnosis of recurrent tumor.

enhanced MRI. Identification of recurrent tumor and delineation of the margin of tumor extent were both improved. Caution should be used, however, in the interpretation of tumor recurrence after radiation therapy. Both recurrent tumor and radiation necrosis can present as an enhancing lesion with surrounding edema and mass effect. These two entities cannot be differentiated on the basis of conventional MRI techniques. Regional cerebral blood volume (CBV) studies do offer the capability of distinguishing recurrent tumor (with high CBV) from radiation necrosis (with low CBV). This advanced type of study is performed by acquiring rapid images (on the order of one per second) after bolus contrast injection using a power injector during the first pass of the contrast agent through the brain.

2 | Brain: Hemorrhage and Vascular Anomalies

Cerebrovascular disease includes both structural vascular anomalies (aneurysms and vascular malformations) and ischemia. Vascular anomalies are discussed in this chapter; ischemia is discussed in Chapter 3. Cerebrovascular disease is often accompanied by intracranial hemorrhage. Knowledge of the appearance of hemorrhage on magnetic resonance imaging (MRI) is critical for scan interpretation, and this is discussed first. MRI is markedly more sensitive than computed tomography (CT) for the detection of cerebrovascular disease, including specifically hemorrhage, vascular anomalies, and ischemia. MRI often obviates the need for cerebral angiography, an invasive examination with accompanying increased risk.

HEMORRHAGE

MRI provides exquisite identification of intracranial hemorrhage. Understanding the appearance of hemorrhage requires knowledge of how the different forms of blood affect the local proton environment. Time to repetition (TR), time to echo (TE), type of imaging sequence, field strength, oxygen tension, hemodilution, rate of clot formation, and integrity of the blood-brain barrier (BBB) and the red blood cell membrane all affect the MRI appearance. Evolving hemorrhage follows an orderly progression of changes, although the exact timing of these changes is variable from patient to patient.

To understand the effects of different forms of hemoglobin, proton relaxation enhancement must be considered. In each water molecule, there are two hydrogen atoms. The nucleus of each hydrogen atom is a single proton. This unpaired proton possesses angular momentum or spin, producing a magnetic moment. The latter is a vector quantity with direction and magnitude and defines a magnetic dipole (or, more simplistically, a tiny bar magnet). Proton-proton dipole-dipole interaction describes the behavior or interaction that occurs between the magnetic dipoles of different protons.

The human body is largely composed of water protons that are in constant motion (on a microscopic level). This motion is characterized by rotational, translational, and vibrational components. In pure water, T_1 and T_2 relaxation occurs by proton-proton dipole-dipole interactions. T_1 is the characteristic time constant for spins to align with the external magnetic field. T_2 is the characteristic time constant for loss of transverse magnetization or, equivalently, loss of phase coherence among spins. Water is a small molecule with a high frequency of motion compared with the Larmor (resonance) frequency used for imaging. In pure water there is inefficient T_1 and T_2 relaxation, resulting in long T_1 and T_2 relaxation times. A long T_1 relaxation time yields low signal intensity on images with T_1-weighting (short TR and short TE). A long T_2 relaxation time yields high signal intensity on images with T_2-weighting (long TR and long TE).

Many of the breakdown products of hemoglobin are paramagnetic substances, which have unpaired electrons. An unpaired electron is the dominant factor in a magnetic moment created by a proton (positive charge) and an electron (negative charge). An electron has a mass equal to 1/1000 of the mass of a proton. It thus has a magnetic moment 1000 times that of a proton. The addition of a paramagnetic substance to the water environment can change the predominant proton relaxation mechanism from a proton-proton dipole-dipole interaction to a proton-electron dipole-dipole interaction. For a proton-electron dipole-dipole interaction to occur, the water proton must approach extremely close (within 0.3 nm) to the paramagnetic center. If this occurs, the frequency of motion of water decreases (the complex is bulkier), which yields a more efficient energy transfer (relaxation), shortening both T_1 and T_2. This process is called proton-electron dipole-dipole proton relaxation enhancement.

If a paramagnetic substance is confined within a red blood cell by the red blood cell membrane, the distribution in tissue will be heterogeneous. A high intracellular concentration of a paramagnetic substance causes local magnetic field inhomogeneity. The precession rate of water molecules (Larmor frequency) is proportional to the local field strength, and the local field strength varies with local magnetic inhomogeneity. Water protons diffusing through this local magnetic inhomogeneity precess at different rates and lose coherence. These dephased protons cannot be refocused by the 180-degree spin echo (SE) pulse, and transverse phase coherence is lost. This causes a shorter transverse relaxation time (T_2) without affecting T_1. This process is called preferential T_2 proton relaxation enhancement. T_2 proton relaxation enhancement is proportional to the square of the magnetic field and, therefore, is more pronounced at higher field strengths. T_2 proton relaxation enhancement is also proportional to the square of the concentration of the paramagnetic substance and is increased by lengthening the interecho interval (the time between the 180-degree refocusing pulses in a SE sequence). Lengthening the interecho interval allows the diffusing water molecules to encounter greater local magnetic inhomogeneity, which increases dephasing and further shortens T_2.

Using knowledge about T_2 proton relaxation enhancement, it is possible to predict the appearance of hemorrhage on SE and gradient echo sequences. The principal component of hemorrhage is hemoglobin, which occurs in several different forms, some of which are paramagnetic. As a hemorrhage ages, the hemoglobin molecule undergoes the following degradation pattern: oxyhemoglobin to deoxyhemoglobin to methemoglobin to hemosiderin.

Before describing each of these forms of hemoglobin, a brief discussion of MRI terminology is appropriate. Sequences with relative T_1 weighting (short TR and short TE) are called T_1-weighted images. Sequences with relative T_2 weighting (long TR and long TE) are called T_2-weighted images. Long TR, short TE sequences are called proton density images. Even though a sequence is called "T_1-weighted" or "T_2-weighted," the signal intensity derives from both T_1 and T_2 effects. Either effect may predominate and yield a particular signal intensity on a given image. Cranial lesions are described as hypointense (low signal intensity), isointense (signal intensity close to that of a reference tissue), or hyperintense (high signal intensity). Gray matter and white matter are typically used as reference tissues for signal intensity on T_1- and T_2-weighted images.

Oxyhemoglobin

A simple intraparenchymal hemorrhage initially is composed of intact red blood cells containing oxygenated hemoglobin. Oxyhemoglobin contains iron in the ferrous state (Fe^{2+}) and has no unpaired electrons. Oxyhemoglobin is thus not paramagnetic but rather diamagnetic. It has, for practical purposes, no magnetic moment and no proton relaxation enhancement. A hyperacute hematoma containing oxyhemoglobin exhibits long T_1 and T_2 relaxation times and is hypointense or isointense on T_1-weighted images and high signal intensity on T_2-weighted images. This is the expected MRI appearance of a protein-containing fluid. Oxyhemoglobin is often isointense with other intracranial mass lesions. Fortunately, oxyhemoglobin is quickly degraded in intra-axial hematomas, lasting only a few hours. It is thus uncommon to visualize oxyhemoglobin within an intraparenchymal bleed. However, the poor discrimination of oxyhemoglobin accounts for the limited ability of conventional SE sequences to detect acute subarachnoid hemorrhage.

Deoxyhemoglobin

In a few hours, the red blood cells become desaturated, and oxyhemoglobin is converted to deoxyhemoglobin. Iron remains in the ferrous state (Fe^{2+}) but with four unpaired electrons, making deoxyhemoglobin paramagnetic. Intracellular deoxyhemoglobin is confined by the red blood cell membrane and is heterogeneously distributed. Water protons cannot approach within 0.3 nm of the paramagnetic center, probably because of a slight change in configuration of the hemoglobin molecule. Preferential T_2 proton relaxation enhancement shortens T_2 but not T_1. As a result, intracellular deoxyhemoglobin is slightly hypointense or isointense on T_1-weighted images and has low signal intensity on T_2-weighted images (Fig. 2–1). The low signal intensity on T_2-weighted images becomes more pronounced with increasing field strength, increased interecho interval, and greater amounts of the paramagnetic substance (deoxyhemoglobin).

Methemoglobin

Intracellular deoxyhemoglobin within a hemorrhage is oxidized to methemoglobin. This process depends on

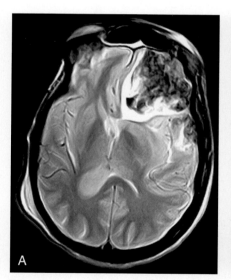
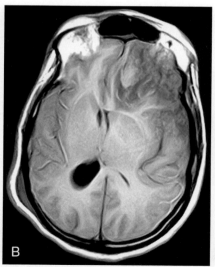
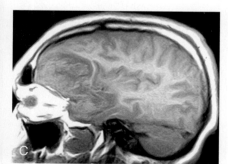

FIGURE 2–1. Acute hematoma (deoxyhemoglobin). A large left frontal lobe mass is noted on precontrast T_2- (*A*) and T_1-weighted (*B*) scans. The mass is predominantly low signal intensity on the T_2-weighted scan and intermediate to low signal intensity on the T_1-weighted scan (consistent with deoxyhemoglobin). Increased signal intensity, representing vasogenic edema, is seen surrounding the low-signal-intensity bleed on the T_2-weighted scan. There is substantial mass effect. The bleed extends into the left temporal lobe, a finding evident on close inspection of the sagittal T_1-weighted scan (*C*).

the partial pressure of oxygen. The rate of oxidation decreases substantially at very low or very high oxygen tensions. In certain circumstances, the formation of methemoglobin can thus be delayed. However, methemoglobin is usually seen by 2 days and persists for several weeks.

In the formation of methemoglobin, the heme iron is oxidized to the ferric state (Fe^{3+}). Methemoglobin has five unpaired electrons and is highly paramagnetic. The molecular configuration of methemoglobin allows the water protons to approach within 0.3 nm of the protein's paramagnetic center. A proton-electron dipole-dipole interaction shortens both T_1 and T_2. The heterogeneous distribution of methemoglobin in the intracellular state accentuates T_2 relaxation (T_2 proton relaxation enhancement), causing intracellular methemoglobin to appear as high signal intensity on T_1-weighted images and low signal intensity on T_2-weighted images (Fig. 2–2).

Soon after methemoglobin forms within the red blood cell, glucose reserves become depleted, which causes a loss of red blood cell integrity and subsequent lysis. Extracellular (free) methemoglobin then accumulates in the hematoma. The distribution of methemoglobin is no longer heterogeneous (no longer partitioned by a red blood cell membrane), causing a loss of T_2 proton relaxation enhancement. With red blood cell lysis, extracellular methemoglobin produces proton-electron dipole-dipole proton relaxation enhancement, which decreases T_1. Extracellular methemoglobin is thus high signal intensity on T_1-weighted images, like intracellular methemoglobin. The T_1 shortening and the effects of the high proton density of free methemoglobin overwhelm the T_2 shortening produced by the proton-electron dipole-dipole interaction. Thus, on proton density and T_2-weighted images, extracellular methemoglobin appears as high signal intensity. As methemoglobin is resorbed, a protein-containing fluid is formed, and actual prolongation of T_2 occurs, which also accounts for increased signal intensity on T_2-weighted images.

The signal intensity of extracellular methemoglobin on T_1-weighted images is also affected by concentration (dilution). The signal intensity of free methemoglobin can vary from hyperintense to hypointense, depending on dilution, on a given T_1-weighted image. As free methemoglobin is progressively diluted, its proton-electron dipole-dipole proton relaxation enhancement is lost. Its signal characteristics then approach those of cerebrospinal fluid (CSF).

Hemosiderin and Ferritin

Extracellular methemoglobin is oxidized to a series of compounds called hemichromes, which are degraded into hemosiderin. Hemosiderin is phagocytized and accumulates in the lysosomes of macrophages. Hemosiderin contains iron in the ferric state (Fe^{3+}) and is strongly paramagnetic. Hemosiderin is insoluble in water; therefore, no dipole-dipole interaction occurs. However, because hemosiderin has an inhomogeneous distribution, T_2 proton relaxation enhancement causes low signal intensity on T_2-weighted images. This strong T_2 effect may be appreciated as slightly low signal intensity on T_1-weighted images.

Hemosiderin can be distinguished from dense calcification on the basis of its T_2 proton relaxation enhancement effect. Hemosiderin is slightly low signal intensity on T_1-weighted images, moderately low signal intensity on proton density weighted images, and very low signal intensity on T_2-weighted images. Because T_2 proton relaxation enhancement is proportional to the square of field strength, these effects are most pronounced at higher field strengths. If fast T_2-weighted images (high-speed radiofrequency [RF] refocused echo imaging) are used, the T_2 effect will be less. Calcium has no mobile protons and does not change in signal intensity on T_1-weighted, proton density, or T_2-weighted images. However, calcium is sometimes mixed with hemosiderin, and the iron in the mixture produces a T_2 proton relaxation enhancement effect.

Hemosiderin can persist indefinitely in a lesion with an intact blood–brain barrier (BBB) and is a landmark for identifying chronic hemorrhage. However, in lesions without an intact BBB, the hemosiderin-laden macrophages have access to the blood stream, and the hemo-

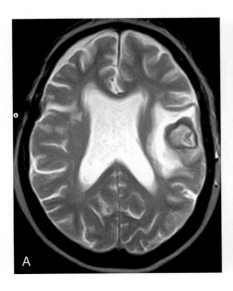

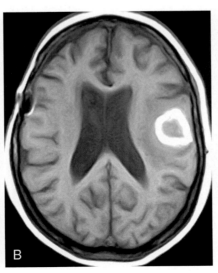

FIGURE 2–2. Subacute hematoma (intracellular methemoglobin rim). A left frontal lobe mass is noted on precontrast T_2- (*A*) and T_1-weighted (*B*) scans. The mass has a prominent low-signal-intensity rim on the T_2-weighted scan, with a thick high-signal-intensity rim on the T_1-weighted scan (findings consistent with intracellular methemoglobin). There is substantial surrounding vasogenic edema, best seen on the T_2-weighted scan as high signal intensity. The presence of edema supports the conclusion, based on the signal intensity of blood products, that the bleed is recent. The bleed was a complication of aneurysm clipping.

siderin is resorbed. The configuration of the hemosiderin rim can be an important feature in differentiating a simple intraparenchymal hematoma from intratumoral hemorrhage. In hemorrhage associated with neoplasm, hemosiderin deposition is discontinuous or inconspicuous because the BBB is not intact. In a simple intraparenchymal hematoma, the hemosiderin rim is well defined and continuous.

Intracerebral Hematoma

The evolution of an intraparenchymal hematoma is depicted by a characteristic sequence of MRI changes. These changes depend on many factors, including size, compartmentalization, oxygen tension, and BBB integrity. Therefore, the staging of intracerebral hematomas is not rigid. For example, several components of hemoglobin can be seen concurrently within a large hematoma. Although the timing and appearance of these changes are variable, a temporal sequence of changes can be described that provides a conceptual framework for identifying the stages of an intracerebral hematoma. Four stages in the evolving hematoma can be described: hyperacute (first few hours), acute (first few hours to 2 days), subacute (2 days to 4 weeks), and chronic (more than 4 weeks).

In the hyperacute stage, an intraparenchymal hematoma is composed of a mixture of oxyhemoglobin and deoxyhemoglobin. The formation of deoxyhemoglobin depends on the local oxygen tension. For example, hemorrhagic cortical infarcts are in a high local oxygen environment (resulting from arterial perfusion), and the formation of deoxyhemoglobin may be retarded. However, in hemorrhagic venous infarction or in a large intraparenchymal hematoma, the oxygen tension is lower and deoxyhemoglobin predominates. In a hyperacute intraparenchymal hematoma in which oxyhemoglobin predominates, the lesion is hypointense or isointense relative to brain on T_1-weighted images and hyperintense relative to brain on T_2-weighted images. A hyperacute intraparenchymal hematoma containing oxyhemoglobin is indistinguishable from other intracranial mass lesions, and its signal may be isointense with CSF. Fortunately, the hyperacute stage is not commonly imaged. CT does not have this limitation and is excellent for the diagnosis of hyperacute bleeds.

Within the first few hours of the formation of a hematoma, oxyhemoglobin is converted into deoxyhemoglobin. An acute intraparenchymal hematoma, which contains deoxyhemoglobin within intact red blood cells, is slightly hypointense to isointense on T_1-weighted images and hypointense T_2-weighted images. The degree of hypointensity on T_2-weighted images increases with the increasing field strength. Consequently, on low-field systems, an acute hematoma can be nearly isointense with brain on T_2-weighted scans. Acute hemorrhage is surrounded by extracellular water, which initially is serum extruded by the retracting clot and later is edema. This increased water content causes a low-intensity margin on T_1-weighted images and a high-intensity margin on T_2-weighted images.

During the subacute stage, intracellular deoxyhemoglobin is oxidized to intracellular methemoglobin, a process that depends on the local oxygen tension. The formation of intracellular methemoglobin begins at the periphery of the hematoma, where the conditions for its formation are optimal, and progresses inward toward the center of the hematoma. The presence of intracellular methemoglobin results in a hyperintense periphery of the hematoma on T_1-weighted images and a hypointense periphery on T_2-weighted images, which progress centrally as deoxyhemoglobin is oxidized (see Fig. 2–2). On T_1-weighted images, a subacute hematoma can have a low-intensity surrounding margin (edema), a hyperintense periphery (intracellular methemoglobin), and a hypointense or isointense center (intracellular deoxyhemoglobin). The corresponding appearance on T_2-weighted images is a high-intensity surrounding margin, a low-intensity periphery, and a hypointense center of the hematoma. With time, the entire hematoma fills in (with intracellular methemoglobin) and has uniform high signal intensity on T_1-weighted images (Fig. 2–3).

After 1 week to 1 month, red blood cell lysis occurs, and intracellular methemoglobin becomes extracellular. Free methemoglobin has high signal intensity on both T_1- and T_2-weighted images. Because of dilutional effects, the signal in the central of the hematoma (with dilute free methemoglobin) can be low or isointense on T_1-weighted images. At about the same time that methemoglobin becomes extracellular, the hematoma develops a peripheral rim of low intensity, which is more easily seen on T_2-weighted images and corresponds to hemosiderin in macrophages. The formation of the hemosiderin rim requires an intact BBB. As the hematoma resorbs, the hemosiderin rim increases in thickness. The edema surrounding the hematoma, just beyond the hemosiderin rim, begins to resolve. After the surrounding edema has resolved, the hematoma (now late subacute in stage) is characterized by a low-intensity rim of hemosiderin and central high-intensity area of extracellular methemoglobin. This appearance is similar on T_1-weighted and T_2-weighted images, except that the hemosiderin rim is more pronounced on T_2-weighted images.

In the chronic stage (more than 4 weeks), the methemoglobin within the center of the hematoma is broken down and resorbed. As this occurs, the T_1 shortening produced by the methemoglobin is lost. The remaining fluid contains some protein, without any iron, and is isointense with cerebrospinal fluid (CSF) (Fig. 2–4). This central fluid may be resorbed, leaving only a hemosiderin rim. Thus, a chronic hematoma can have several appearances. A chronic hematoma can have a center that is isointense or of high intensity (depending on whether methemoglobin is resorbed or present) with a low-intensity rim (hemosiderin). Alternatively, only a low-intensity hemosiderin cleft can be left, with complete resorption of any fluid.

Subdural Hematoma

Subdural hematomas result from a venous injury, with blood lying outside the brain parenchyma between the dura and arachnoid. Like intraparenchymal hematomas,

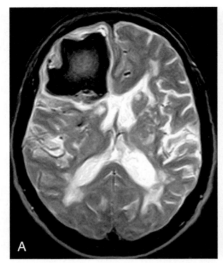
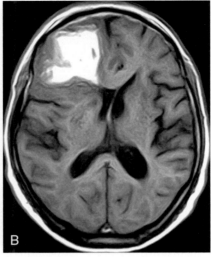

FIGURE 2–3. Subacute hematoma (intracellular methemoglobin). In this right frontal hemorrhage, the oxidation of deoxyhemoglobin to intracellular methemoglobin is nearly complete, resulting in almost uniform low signal intensity on the precontrast T_2-weighted scan (*A*) and high signal intensity on the precontrast T_1-weighted scan (*B*). There is a small rim of surrounding high signal intensity on the T_2-weighted scan consistent with vasogenic edema, confirming that the hemorrhage is still relatively recent. With time, red blood cell lysis will result in the intracellular methemoglobin becoming extracellular in location, with the hematoma then high signal intensity on both T_2- and T_1-weighted scans. The patient was predisposed to an intracranial bleed as a result of severe vascular disease. This is reflected on the T_2-weighted scan by the presence of chronic small vessel ischemic disease and several old lacunar infarcts.

four stages in the evolution of subdural hematomas can be described: hyperacute, acute, subacute, and chronic.

Hyperacute subdural hematomas are composed of a mixture of oxyhemoglobin and deoxyhemoglobin and are hypo- to isointense to brain on T_1-weighted images and hyperintense on T_2-weighted images. An acute subdural hematoma is composed of deoxyhemoglobin in intact red blood cells, causing preferential T_2 proton relaxation enhancement. An acute subdural hematoma is hypo- to isointense to brain on T_1-weighted images and hypointense on T_2-weighted images.

In a subacute subdural hematoma (Fig. 2–5), intracellular deoxyhemoglobin is oxidized to methemoglobin, which is hyperintense on T_1-weighted images and hypointense on T_2-weighted images. By 2 weeks, red blood cell lysis results in free methemoglobin, causing hyperintensity on both T_1- and T_2-weighted images. As methemoglobin is slowly broken down in the chronic phase, a subdural hematoma becomes intermediate in signal intensity between methemoglobin and CSF on T_1-weighted images and high signal intensity but lower than CSF on T_2-weighted images. These are the expected characteristics of a protein-containing extra-axial fluid collection. These characteristics distinguish a chronic subdural hematoma from the prominent CSF spaces seen with atrophy (Fig. 2–6).

In the subacute and chronic phases, the membrane delimiting a subdural hematoma may enhance with intravenous injection of a gadolinium chelate (see Fig. 2–6). Subdural hematomas may have a combination of

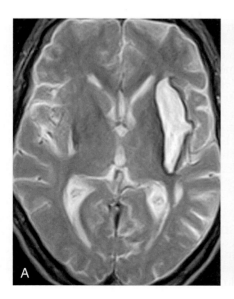
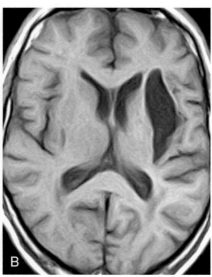

FIGURE 2–4. Chronic hematoma (hemosiderin rim) demonstrating the end result of a large basal ganglia hemorrhage. The hematoma has long since been resorbed, leaving a large cavity now filled with cerebrospinal fluid. This fluid collection has high signal intensity on the T_2-weighted scan (*A*) and low signal intensity on the T_1-weighted scan (*B*). The only direct evidence of previous hemorrhage is the low signal intensity (hemosiderin) rim, bordering the cavity, seen on the T_2-weighted scan.

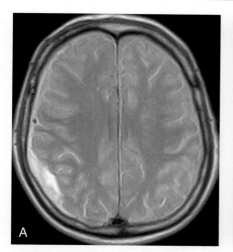 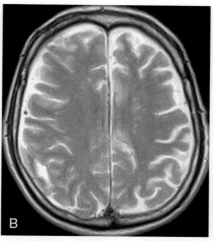 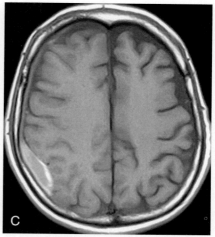

FIGURE 2–5. Subacute subdural hematoma. An extra-axial fluid collection is noted on the patient's right side, which is principally hyperintense on the proton density weighted scan (*A*), hypointense on the T$_2$-weighted scan (*B*), and hyperintense on the precontrast T$_1$-weighted scan (*C*). The signal characteristics are consistent with intracellular methemoglobin.

acute and subacute chronic components, which appear as fluid-fluid layers of the different forms of hemoglobin comprising the hematoma. Hemosiderin accumulation is typically absent in extra-axial fluid collections because of the lack of a BBB in the dura and access of hemosiderin-laden macrophages to the blood stream. On rare occasions, hemosiderin can be identified in patients with recurrent bleeds into chronic subdural hematomas.

MRI is very sensitive and superior to CT for detection of subacute and chronic subdural hematomas. Chronic extra-axial bleeds are low density on CT and may be indistinguishable from large CSF spaces seen with atrophy. Moreover, CT bone artifact can obscure small extra-axial fluid collections, even in the acute phase. In comparing the CTs and MRIs of a patient with a stable extra-axial fluid collection, the lesion will appear larger

on MRI because of bone artifact and soft tissue windowing on CT. These factors tend to reduce the apparent size of the fluid collection on CT. The hyperintensity of methemoglobin in the subacute and chronic phases makes extra-axial hematomas readily identifiable on MRI.

Epidural Hematoma

Epidural hematomas most often occur as a result of an arterial injury. Blood dissects between the calvarium and dura, producing a biconvex lentiform fluid collection (Fig. 2–7). Epidural hematomas follow the same pattern of evolution as subdural hematomas. An epidural hematoma can be distinguished from a subdural hematoma by its configuration and by the low-intensity fibrous

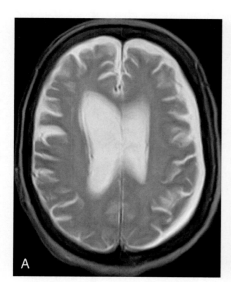 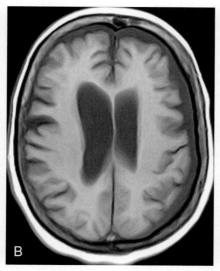 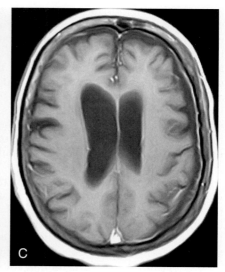

FIGURE 2–6. Chronic subdural hematoma. *A*, The T$_2$-weighted scan demonstrates an extra-axial fluid collection surrounding the left cerebral hemisphere. The fluid has high signal intensity on the T$_2$-weighted scan and low signal intensity on the T$_1$-weighted scan (*B*). The subdural fluid is, however, slightly higher in signal intensity on the T$_1$-weighted scan than the cerebrospinal fluid of the lateral ventricles. This difference was more evident on the proton density weighted scan (not shown). The adjacent dura is thickened and enhances postcontrast (*C*).

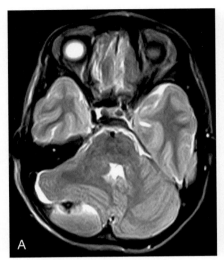
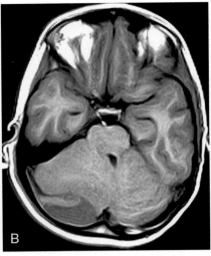
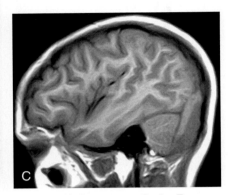

FIGURE 2–7. Acute epidural hematoma. There is compression of the right cerebellum by an extra-axial soft tissue mass. On the T_2-weighted scan (*A*), the mass has predominantly intermediate signal intensity, although a portion anteriorly has very low signal intensity. On the T_1-weighted scan (*B*), most of the lesion is slightly low signal intensity, with a more anterior component of intermediate signal intensity. This suggests a fluid composition, with layering of different components. Computed tomography (not shown) demonstrated a right occipital fracture. The imaging appearance of an epidural hematoma is that of a biconvex, elliptical fluid collection. Because of its epidural location, the fluid collection can cross the midline (falx) or the tentorium, unlike subdural fluid. On the sagittal T_1-weighted scan (*C*), the lesion is noted to cross the attachment of the tentorium posteriorly and thus can be localized to the extradural (epidural) space. An epidural hematoma accumulates between the dura and the inner table of skull. This lesion is typically caused by a skull fracture with laceration of blood vessels. The most common vessel involved is the middle meningeal artery resulting from a temporal or parietal bone fracture. Less common is laceration of the transverse sinus (as in the case presented) caused by an occipital bone fracture.

dura that demarcates the margin of the hematoma from the brain parenchyma. However, in the acute phase, the low-intensity dura may not be visualized as a separate structure from the low-intensity hematoma (deoxyhemoglobin). The differentiation of an epidural hematoma from a subdural hematoma can be difficult if the configuration of the fluid collection is atypical.

Subarachnoid and Intraventricular Hemorrhage

Subarachnoid hemorrhage, commonly secondary to rupture of an intracranial aneurysm or an arteriovenous malformation, is a potentially life-threatening event that requires prompt diagnosis and therapy. Hyperacute and acute subarachnoid hemorrhages are not well seen on conventional SE techniques. The conditions in the subarachnoid space are different from other intracranial locations, and the expected pattern of evolution of hemorrhage does not occur. The detection of subarachnoid hemorrhage on MRI requires the use of fluid attenuated inversion recovery (FLAIR) scan, a pulse sequence discussed later.

Acute subarachnoid hemorrhage occurs in, and is diluted by, CSF. This compartment has an average oxygen tension (PO_2) of 43 mm Hg, with 72% of the hemoglobin in the saturated oxyhemoglobin state. Oxyhemoglobin has signal characteristics that are isointense to CSF and, therefore, not well seen on conventional MRI scans. The contribution of deoxyhemoglobin, which causes preferential T_2 proton relaxation enhancement, to T_2 shortening during this phase is negligible. Because T_2 shortening is proportional to the square of the concentration of the paramagnetic compound, deoxyhemo-

globin in a concentration of 28% (100% − 72%) contributes only 8% (0.28^2) to T_2 shortening. The T_2 shortening of deoxyhemoglobin is also masked by dilution with CSF and CSF pulsation artifacts. Therefore, it is not surprising that oxyhemoglobin and deoxyhemoglobin in acute subarachnoid hemorrhage are not well demonstrated by conventional SE techniques.

FLAIR images have been shown to be virtually 100% sensitive to acute subarachnoid hemorrhage. With this pulse sequence, CSF is attenuated and thus black. In acute subarachnoid hemorrhage, there is a small decrease in T_1 caused by the higher protein content of the bloody CSF. This mild T_1 shortening leads to hypertense CSF on FLAIR. One problem with FLAIR is the high-intensity CSF inflow artifacts in the basal cisterns, which may simulate subarachnoid hemorrhage. This artifact is markedly lessened by the use of a FLAIR sequence in which the thickness of the 180-degree inverting RF pulse has been slightly increased.

In subacute subarachnoid hemorrhage, characteristic signal intensity changes can often be identified on T_1- and T_2-weighted images corresponding to methemoglobin within thrombus (Fig. 2–8). In rare instances, deoxyhemoglobin within thrombus in the acute phase is visualized. In chronic or recurrent subarachnoid hemorrhage, hemosiderin deposition can occur in a subpial location, which is called "superficial hemosiderosis" or "superficial siderosis." A thin rim of marked hypointensity on T_2-weighted images lines the parenchymal surface in superficial siderosis. This condition can be caused by hemorrhage from vascular abnormalities, intracranial tumors, ependymoma of the conus medullaris, or neonatal hemorrhage. Occasionally, patients develop hearing

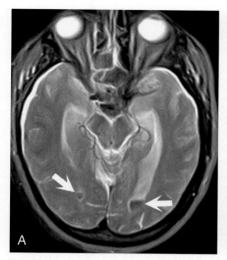
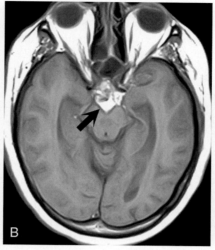
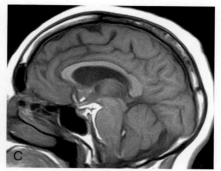

FIGURE 2–8. Subacute subarachnoid hemorrhage (intracellular methemoglobin). Clotted blood, containing methemoglobin, is well visualized in the interpeduncular cistern because of its low signal intensity on the T_2-weighted scan (A) and high signal intensity (*black arrow*) on the T_1-weighted scan (B). The bleed is 4 days old. C, The sagittal precontrast T_1-weighted scan reveals clotted blood, with high signal intensity, in the pontine, interpeduncular, and chiasmatic cisterns. A small amount of intraventricular blood is also present, layering posteriorly in the occipital horns. Subtle intraventricular hemorrhage can be missed without close inspection of the ventricles. In this instance, the blood is best detected in the ventricles on the T_2-weighted scan, with low signal intensity (*white arrows*).

loss with involvement of cranial nerve VIII, other cranial nerve abnormalities, and cerebellar ataxia.

Intraventricular hemorrhage is much like subarachnoid hemorrhage in signal characteristics and temporal evolution. Like subarachnoid hemorrhage and unlike intraparenchymal, subdural, or epidural hemorrhage, intraventricular hemorrhage mixes with CSF in an environment with high oxygen tension. Oxidative denaturation of hemoglobin to methemoglobin is delayed. Substantial amounts of methemoglobin, with high signal intensity on T_1-weighted scans (Fig. 2–9), are not formed for several days.

Gradient Echo Imaging in Hemorrhage

In gradient echo imaging, a reduced flip angle RF pulse and a subsequent applied gradient that refocus the echo are used rather than the 90-degree RF pulse and 180-degree refocusing pulse used in routine SE imaging. Gradient echo imaging is particularly sensitive to the magnetic susceptibility effects of paramagnetic substances.

Magnetic susceptibility is defined as the ratio of the induced magnetic field to the main magnetic field. Magnetic susceptibility occurs when substances are induced to form their own weak magnetic field under the influence of an externally applied field. Three classes of substances exhibit this type of magnetic behavior: paramagnetic, superparamagnetic, and ferromagnetic substances. Superparamagnetic and ferromagnetic substances can acquire large magnetic moments, even if exposed to very weak external magnetic fields. Ferromagnetic substances, unlike paramagnetic and super-

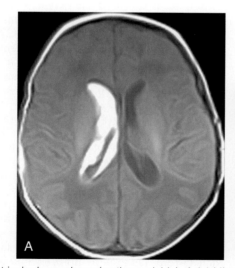
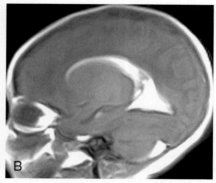

FIGURE 2–9. Intraventricular hemorrhage (methemoglobin). Axial (A) and sagittal (B) T_1-weighted scans demonstrate a high-signal-intensity (methemoglobin) blood clot filling the right lateral ventricle. The clot was also high signal intensity and thus not well distinguished from cerebrospinal fluid on the T_2-weighted scan (not shown). The signal characteristics are compatible with extracellular methemoglobin. The clot was approximately 2 weeks old.

paramagnetic substances, retain their magnetism after the external magnetic field is removed.

Paramagnetic substances have a high degree of magnetic susceptibility. Because many of the degradation products of hemoglobin (deoxyhemoglobin, methemoglobin, and hemosiderin) are paramagnetic, they are visualized with increased sensitivity on gradient echo imaging compared with SE imaging. Small amounts of these paramagnetic hemoglobin compounds can be detected with gradient echo imaging that may not be visualized with standard SE imaging or CT. For example, small cortical petechial hemorrhages or small amounts of residual hemosiderin from old hemorrhagic angiomas can be identified as areas of focal signal loss on gradient echo imaging. However, these susceptibility effects can also overwhelm other signal characteristics of a lesion and obscure important diagnostic features. For example, the central high-intensity area in a cavernous angioma (a distinguishing characteristic feature) can be obscured by the susceptibility effects of the hemosiderin rim. Furthermore, the boundary between deoxyhemoglobin or intracellular methemoglobin and surrounding brain appears as a hypointense rim on gradient echo imaging, which can obscure identification of a hemosiderin rim. Identification of the rim is important in evaluating hemorrhagic intracranial tumors, which typically have an incomplete surrounding hemosiderin rim because of the lack of an intact BBB.

VASCULAR ANOMALIES

Cerebrovascular anomalies can be divided into two major categories: intracranial aneurysms and vascular malformations. Clinical presentation of patients with cerebrovascular anomalies is variable. However, these patients not uncommonly present with acute intracranial hemorrhage, either secondary to subarachnoid hemorrhage or an intraparenchymal hematoma. In acute cases, detection of subarachnoid hemorrhage is critical, and the MRI exam must include a FLAIR sequence. MRI is very accurate for characterizing intracranial vascular disease. MRI has also replaced CT as the screening modality for detecting vascular malformations and intracranial aneurysms and associated mural thrombi.

Vascular malformations are congenital developmental abnormalities of the vascular system. Cerebrovascular malformations are divided into four major pathologic categories: arteriovenous malformation (AVM), venous angioma, capillary telangiectasia, and cavernous angioma. AVMs and venous angiomas can be routinely visualized with angiography, CT, and MRI. Capillary telangiectasias and cavernous angiomas are not directly visualized with current imaging modalities but are detected because of hemorrhage associated with the lesion. Thrombosed AVMs and venous angiomas may also be detected only by the presence of hemorrhage if their abnormal vessels become obliterated. These vascular malformations detected by the presence of recurrent or chronic hemorrhage, in which the vascular anomaly is not visualized angiographically, are called occult cerebrovascular malformations (OCVMs). Based on current imaging studies, the majority of vascular malformations are divided into three major radiologic groups: AVM, venous angioma, and OCVM.

Aneurysm

An aneurysm is a focal dilatation of a vessel. Aneurysms can be characterized by their configuration as fusiform (a spindle-shaped dilatation of a vessel) or saccular (a sharply circumscribed, spherical sac). Fusiform aneurysms are commonly secondary to arteriosclerosis and often involve the basilar artery and intracranial carotid arteries. The vast majority of aneurysms are saccular (berry aneurysms) and are thought to be congenital. They commonly arise at arterial branch points and are secondary to an inherent defect in the tunica media (Fig. 2–10). Mycotic infection, trauma, and neoplasm cause fewer than 5% of all aneurysms. These aneurysms typically occur at peripheral locations rather than branch points.

In the general population, the incidence of intracranial aneurysms is approximately 3%. The common congenital saccular aneurysm involves the anterior carotid circulation in 85% to 90% of cases and the posterior basilar circulation in 10% to 15% of cases. In the anterior circulation, the most common locations of saccular aneurysms are the anterior communicating artery (30%), the posterior communicating artery (25%), and the middle cerebral artery bifurcation/trifurcation (20%) (Fig. 2–11). In the posterior circulation, the basilar artery trunk and bifurcation (10%) (Fig. 2–12) and the vertebral-posterior inferior cerebellar artery (3%) are the most common sites. In 20% of patients, multiple aneurysms are identified at angiography.

A ruptured intracranial aneurysm is the most common cause (75%) of subarachnoid hemorrhage. Vascular malformations account for 5% of cases. Patients with a ruptured aneurysm commonly present with acute onset of a severe headache that may progress to coma. In the patient with a suspected acute subarachnoid hemorrhage caused by a ruptured aneurysm, CT still remains the screening modality of choice. CT readily visualizes acute hemorrhage as high density, and CT is more easily performed in the uncooperative patient.

MRI is often initially performed in patients without intracranial hemorrhage and in those with intracranial hemorrhage and atypical symptoms. In these patients, conventional MRI (without the use of magnetic resonance [MR] angiography) often demonstrates the aneurysm (Fig. 2–13). In approximately 20% of aneurysms that bleed, there is an associated intraparenchymal hematoma. Beyond the hyperacute stage, MRI exquisitely demonstrates intraparenchymal hematomas, and their location can suggest the diagnosis of a ruptured aneurysm. For example, an intraparenchymal hematoma adjacent to the anterior interhemispheric fissure suggests a ruptured anterior communicating artery aneurysm, and an intraparenchymal hematoma adjacent to the sylvian cistern suggests a ruptured middle cerebral artery aneurysm. In patients with known aneurysms, MRI can identify the bleeding site by demonstrating subacute hemorrhage adjacent to the aneurysm. Subacute or

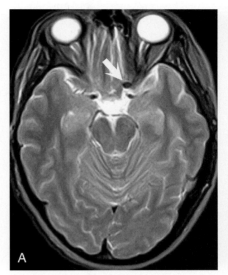
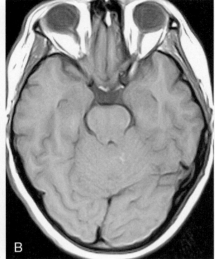
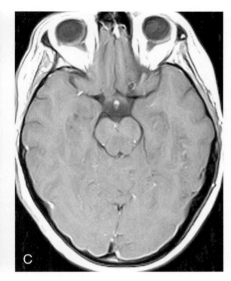

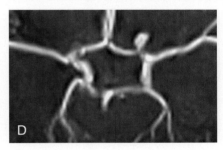

FIGURE 2–10. Ophthalmic artery aneurysm. On precontrast T_2- (A) and T_1-weighted (B) scans a small round signal void (*arrow*) is identified anterior to the supraclinoid segment of the left internal carotid artery. There is enhancement of the lesion rim on the axial T_1-weighted image postcontrast (C). D, A maximum intensity projection image from the three-dimensional time-of-flight magnetic resonance angiography examination reveals a small aneurysm just medial and anterior to the extracavernous intracranial segment of the left internal carotid artery.

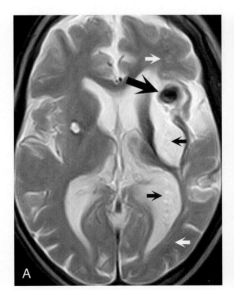
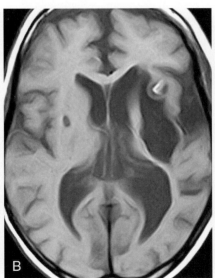
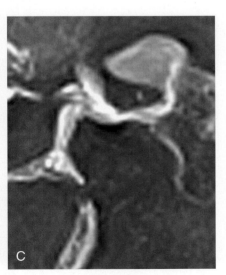

FIGURE 2–11. Middle cerebral artery bifurcation aneurysm. An abnormal low-signal-intensity flow void (*large black arrow*) is noted on the precontrast T_2-weighted scan (A). The pulsation artifact emanating from this structure anteriorly and posteriorly (*small black and white arrows*) in the phase encoding direction confirms that the structure is vascular in nature. The lesion has paradoxical high signal intensity, again because of the flow phenomenon, on the precontrast T_1-weighted scan (B). Also noted are chronic cavitated infarcts bilaterally: a small lacuna on the right and a larger hemosiderin-lined lesion on the left. Three-dimensional time-of-flight magnetic resonance angiography (C) confirms the presence of an aneurysm, at the middle cerebral artery bifurcation and approximately 1 cm in diameter. Also noted are multiple focal vessel stenoses.

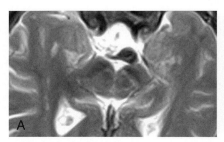
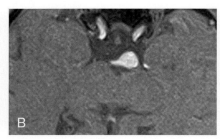
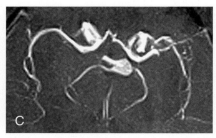

FIGURE 2–12. Basilar artery aneurysm. An oval flow void is identified on the precontrast T$_2$-weighted scan (*A*) in the prepontine cistern at the expected location of the basilar tip. *B*, A single slice from the three-dimensional time-of-flight magnetic resonance angiogram depicts the structure as high signal intensity and thus confirms it as a vascular structure. *C*, The maximum intensity projection image reconstructed from the three-dimensional examination, the image depicted in *B* being one of many slices in this data set, depicts a moderate-sized aneurysm arising from the tip of the basilar artery.

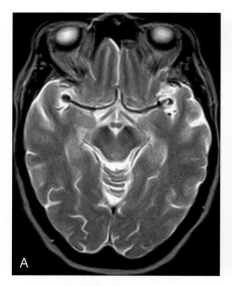
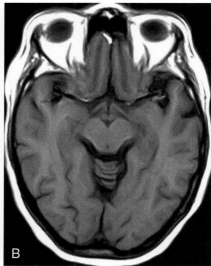
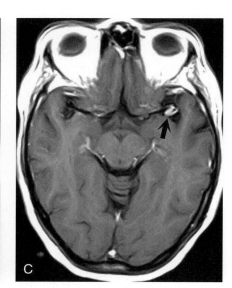

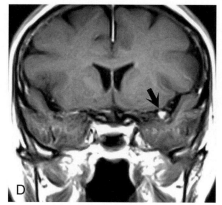

FIGURE 2–13. Left middle cerebral artery (MCA) aneurysm detected by conventional planar magnetic resonance imaging. *A*, The T$_2$-weighted scan is unremarkable. On the precontrast T$_1$-weighted scan (*B*), a question of abnormal hyperintensity, just posterior to the left MCA trifurcation, is raised. On the postcontrast axial (*C*) and coronal (*D*) T$_1$-weighted scans, enhancement of a small aneurysm (*arrow*) is seen, permitting detection. Slow flow within this berry aneurysm leads to marked contrast enhancement after intravenous gadolinium chelate administration. The lumen of the aneurysm is thus well depicted.

chronic subarachnoid hemorrhage resulting from a ruptured aneurysm is also clearly identified by MRI.

A unique feature of MRI is its ability to detect vascular flow, particularly in the arterial system. The appearance of flow on conventional (planar) MRI is presented first followed by a discussion of MRA. High-velocity flow in arteries or veins appears commonly as a flow void on MRI. This high-velocity signal loss occurs when protons in flowing blood do not remain within the selected slice long enough to acquire both the 90- and 180-degree pulses used to produce an SE. Saccular aneurysms appear as regions of flow void with a typical configuration and location. Pulsation artifact, propagating in the phase-encoding direction, is another supporting finding seen with pulsatile flow in patent aneurysms. Pulsation artifacts are more pronounced after contrast administration because of the increased signal within the vascular space.

Depending on the imaging parameters selected and the effects of turbulence and rephasing, slow-flowing blood within a vessel or an aneurysm can have high or mixed signal intensity rather than a flow void. Flow-related enhancement and even echo rephasing are two processes that cause increased signal intensity within vascular structures. Such phenomena should be recognized as possible pitfalls in the diagnosis of intracranial aneurysms. Another less common pitfall in the diagnosis of basilar artery aneurysms is CSF pulsation artifact in the prepontine cistern, which can simulate a basilar artery aneurysm. This artifact is more pronounced with increased slice thickness.

Small aneurysms are well depicted using 3D time-of-flight (TOF) MRA. This is particularly true for aneurysms at arterial branch points (Fig. 2–14). Diagnostic interpretation of MRA studies should be based on review of both the original thin-section axial images and the maximum intensity projection (MIP) images derived from this source data. The spatial resolution of current 3D TOF MRA is slightly better than $1 \times 1 \times 1$ mm, permitting detection of aneurysms as small as 2 to 3 mm. Aneurysms smaller than 3 mm are thought not to bleed and thus are of little clinical concern. On occasion, particularly with internal carotid artery lesions, the aneurysm neck may not be visualized. The use of targeted reconstruction, shorter TEs, and smaller voxels can substantially improve the quality of 3D TOF MRA exams. MRA should be considered complementary to conventional planar MRI scans, with the recommendation that both be acquired.

Conventional MRI routinely visualizes large intracranial aneurysms ($1.0 - 2.5$ cm in diameter) and giant aneurysms, which are defined as aneurysms larger than 2.5 cm in diameter (Fig. 2–15). These aneurysms commonly present with symptoms related to mass effect rather than subarachnoid hemorrhage. Large and giant aneurysms are often partially thrombosed and can be confused with an intraparenchymal hematoma. MRI provides an elegant, noninvasive method for diagnosing partially thrombosed giant intracranial aneurysms (Fig. 2–16). MRI is superior to CT and angiography in characterizing this type of aneurysm.

The MRI findings in partially thrombosed large or giant intracranial aneurysms include a flow void in the residual patent lumen of the aneurysm, with an adjacent high-signal-intensity rim. The rim is high intensity on both T_1- and T_2-weighted images and corresponds to extracellular methemoglobin. This finding contrasts with the formation of methemoglobin in an intraparenchymal hematoma, in which methemoglobin first forms at the periphery rather than centrally. Mixed, laminated signal intensity surrounds the high-signal-intensity methemoglobin rim, which represents different stages of organized clot in the thrombosed portion of the aneurysm. Perianeurysmal hemorrhage and adjacent edema within the brain may occur and can be distinguished from the aneurysm itself. Hemorrhage is typically high signal intensity on T_1-weighted images and either hypo- or hyperintensity on T_2-weighted images because of the presence of intracellular or extracellular methemoglobin. Edema within the adjacent brain is hypointense on T_1-weighted images and hyperintense on T_2-weighted images.

MRI can readily demonstrate complete thrombosis of large aneurysms. An old, organized thrombus will have a signal that is isointense with soft tissue or protein-containing fluid. Other soft tissue masses, including neoplasms, can have similar appearances and should be considered in the differential diagnosis. Patency or thrombosis of adjacent major intracranial vessels can be determined using MRA or, on conventional scans, by the presence or absence of arterial flow voids. MRI is also useful in evaluating aneurysm thrombosis after embolization.

MRI is contraindicated in the evaluation of the postsurgical patient with a ferromagnetic aneurysm clip. However, currently, most aneurysm clips are nonferromagnetic, and patients with these clips can be successfully imaged. Extreme care should be exercised in this area because at least one patient with a ferromagnetic

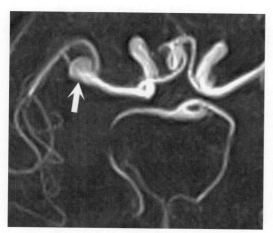

FIGURE 2–14. Right middle cerebral artery bifurcation aneurysm (*arrow*) detected on three-dimensional time-of-flight magnetic resonance angiography (MRA). The image presented is a maximum intensity projection derived from the thin-section axial three-dimensional MRA examination. Although aneurysms can be detected on conventional magnetic resonance imaging, as shown in FIGURE 13, MRA is far more sensitive for detecting small lesions and should be performed in all patients being evaluated for a possible intracranial aneurysm.

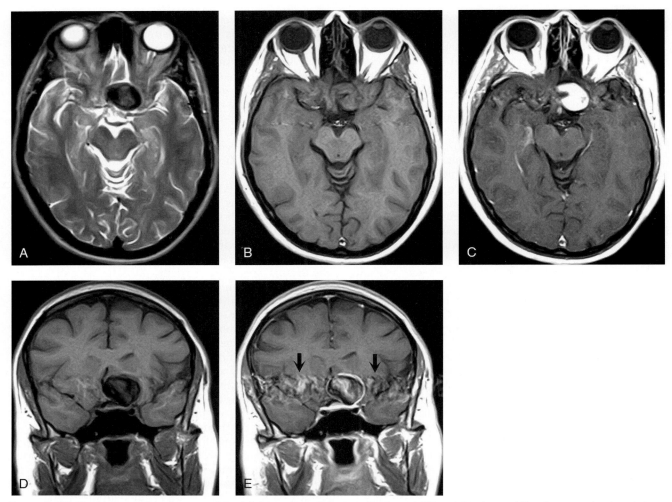

FIGURE 2–15. Giant intracranial aneurysm of the left internal carotid artery. On the axial T_2-weighted scan (*A*), a large predominantly low signal intensity mass is seen in the suprasellar region. The lesion is isointense with brain on the axial T_1-weighted scan (*B*). *C*, Post-contrast, enhancement is marked and homogeneous on the axial scan. On the coronal precontrast T_1-weighted scan (*D*), the lesion is predominantly low signal intensity. The variation of signal intensity with plane of acquisition (compare with *B*) is consistent with flow phenomena. On the coronal postcontrast scan (*E*), the intensity of the lesion is mixed, with much of the signal lost because of pulsation. A faint pulsation artifact can be identified in *D*, extending right to left across the scan. This artifact (*arrows*) is greatest on the postcontrast coronal scan (*E*), extending right to left and encompassing the entire height of the lesion. The imaging appearance of giant aneurysms on magnetic resonance imaging can be complex because of the presence of both flowing blood and thrombus (which may be layered). In the current case, there is no evidence of thrombus. The presence of pulsation artifacts, often accentuated on postcontrast scans, offers a clue to the nature of the lesion.

clip is known to have died after MRI. This occurred despite a program at the site involved designed to differentiate ferromagnetic and nonferromagnetic clips.

Vertebrobasilar Dolichoectasia

A dolichoectatic vessel is one that is both too long (elongated) and too large (distended). Basilar artery elongation is present, by strict criteria, when the artery lies lateral to either the clivus or dorsum sellae or terminates above the suprasellar cistern. A basilar artery larger than 4.5 mm in diameter is defined as ectatic (too large). The term "fusiform aneurysm" has, unfortunately, been used interchangeably in the scientific literature with dolichoectatic change and ectasia, all referring to diffuse tortuous enlargement and elongation of an artery. Dolichoectasia occurs with greatest frequency in the verte-

brobasilar system (Fig. 2–17) but may also involve the intracranial internal carotid and middle cerebral arteries.

A contour deformity of the pons resulting from basilar artery ectasia is a not uncommon incidental finding on MRI in the elderly population. Traction or displacement of cranial nerves can, however, lead to symptoms. Depending on the segment of the basilar artery involved, cranial nerve II, III, VI, VII, or VIII can be affected. The lower cranial nerves can be affected with vertebral artery involvement.

Symptomatic vertebrobasilar dolichoectasia exists in two different patient populations: those with isolated cranial nerve involvement and those with multiple neurologic deficits. The latter population includes patients with combinations of cranial nerve deficits (resulting from compression) and central nervous system deficits (resulting from compression or ischemia). A tortuous,

FIGURE 2–16. Partially thrombosed giant intracranial aneurysm. A large low-signal-intensity lesion is noted on the spin echo scan with intermediate T₂-weighting (A) in the region of the left cavernous sinus. A pulsation artifact (black arrows) is seen extending in the phase encoding direction posteriorly from the lesion but originating from only the more medial portion. Comparison of pre- (B) and postcontrast (C) T₁-weighted scans reveals enhancement in only the more anterior and medial portions of the lesion (white arrow). Three-dimensional time-of-flight magnetic resonance angiography depicts a patent lumen within the mass corresponding in position to that suggested by the pulsation artifact and contrast enhancement. The majority of this giant aneurysm of the cavernous and distal petrous carotid artery is thrombosed. Only a crescent of residual lumen remains. The precontrast scans are misleading because the clotted portion of the aneurysm has very low signal intensity on the T₂-weighted scan and intermediate to low signal intensity on the T₁-weighted scan.

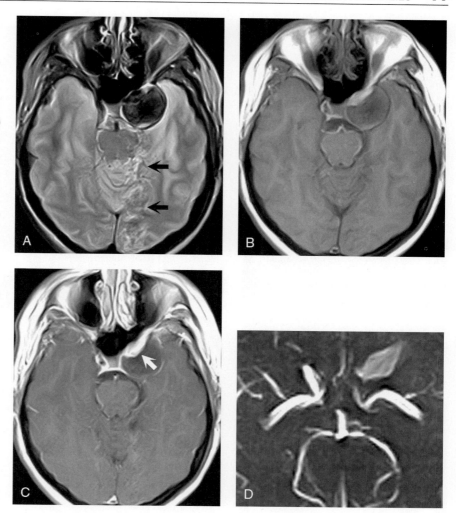

but normal-caliber, basilar artery is more likely to produce isolated cranial nerve involvement, whereas ectasia is more likely to cause multiple deficits of either compressive or ischemic cause.

Arteriovenous Malformation

AVMs are the most common type of vascular malformation, occurring in approximately 0.1% of the general population. The clinical presentation is variable and includes headaches, seizures, neurologic deficits, and symptoms related to hemorrhage. Occasionally, AVMs are discovered as incidental findings during the evaluation of an unrelated problem. All age groups are affected; most patients present with symptoms between the third and fourth decades.

AVMs occur throughout the central nervous system and are characterized pathologically by a direct communication between the arterial and venous circulations, without an intervening capillary bed. Intracranial AVMs are most commonly supratentorial (80%) and involve the peripheral branches of the middle cerebral artery. Angiographically, AVMs consist of a tangled nidus of dilated vessels supplied by enlarged tortuous feeding arteries and draining veins. Most commonly, the arterial

supply of AVMs is pial, arising from the cerebral or cerebellar arteries. In some AVMs, there is a mixed pial-dural or dural blood supply. Half of the infratentorial lesions and approximately 20% of the supratentorial lesions have a dural component to their blood supply. Aneurysms are associated with the feeding arteries of AVMs in approximately 10% of patients.

SE MRI accurately defines the vascular channels forming AVMs (Fig. 2–18). Typically, the arteriovenous shunting is so rapid that most of the vessels appear as flow voids rather than with increased signal (Figs. 2–18 and 2–19). The latter is seen in slow flow and many normal veins. As with intracranial aneurysms, pulsation artifacts may be seen with AVMs. Pulsation artifacts become more pronounced on contrast-enhanced images. Feeding arteries are often easy to identify (because of location and dilatation). Draining veins can be identified by their caliber (larger than the arteries) and drainage into deep or cortical veins. After the administration of intravenous contrast, many of the larger vessels involved will show prominent enhancement (Fig. 2–20). However, this effect is variable from patient to patient depending on flow rates and the pulse sequence used. Three-dimensional TOF MRA can be diagnostically useful in demonstrating feeding arteries, the nidus, and

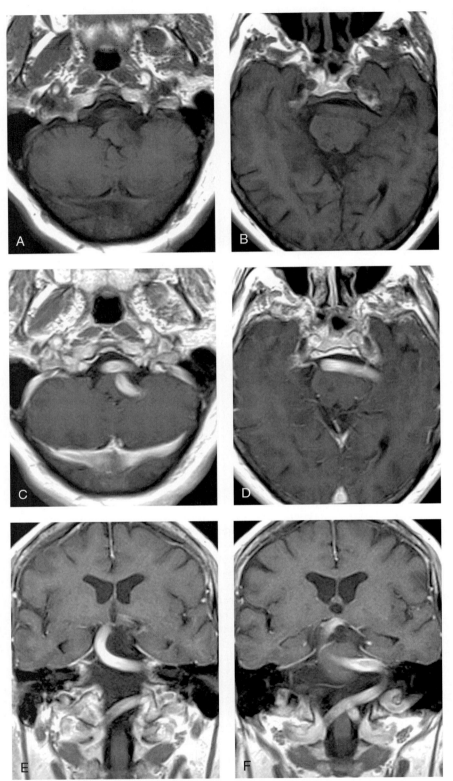

FIGURE 2–17. Vertebrobasilar dolichoectasia. *A* and *B*, Precontrast T₁-weighted axial scans reveal the vertebral and basilar arteries to be large in diameter, with the former causing a deformity of the medulla and the latter a deformity of the pons. *C* and *D*, Postcontrast, the vertebral and basilar arteries demonstrate uniform enhancement and are thus more readily identified. *E* and *F*, On coronal postcontrast T₁-weighted scans, the elongation of the vertebrobasilar system is clearly evident, with the basilar artery coursing lateral to the clivus and terminating above the suprasellar cistern.

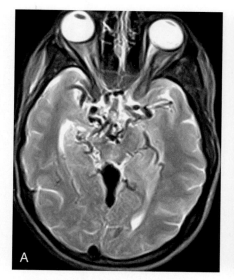
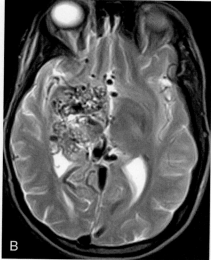
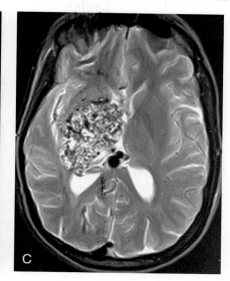

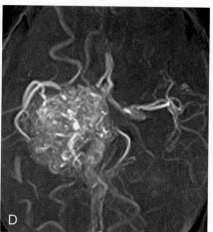

FIGURE 2–18. Arteriovenous malformation, depiction on T$_2$-weighted scans (*A–C*) and three-dimensional time-of-flight (TOF) magnetic resonance angiography (MRA). At the lower two anatomic levels (*A* and *B*), the T$_2$-weighted scans reveal multiple enlarged draining veins (including the vein of Galen) as well as enlargement of the anterior and middle cerebral arteries. At the highest anatomic level shown (*C*), the scan reveals a large heterogeneous mass in the expected location of the right basal ganglia and thalamus. The mass consists of innumerable serpiginous structures, most with low signal intensity because of fast blood flow. *D,* The maximum intensity projection from the three-dimensional TOF MRA exam shows the branches of the right middle cerebral artery to be enlarged and draping around the vascular malformation. Several enlarged draining veins are also visualized.

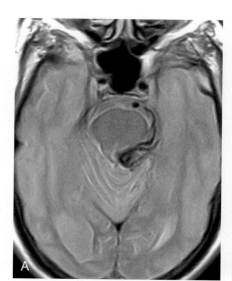
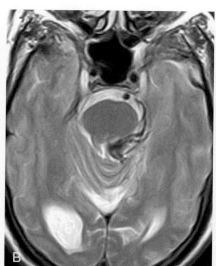
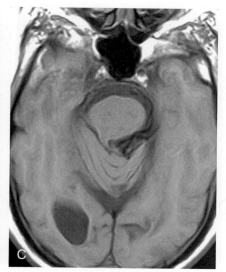

FIGURE 2–19. Perimesencephalic cistern arteriovenous malformation depicted on conventional spin echo scans. On proton density (*A*), T$_2$-weighted (*B*), and T$_1$-weighted (*C*) precontrast scans, a cluster of abnormal vessels is seen posterior and to the left of the pons, compressing the cerebral aqueduct. The vessels are low signal intensity on all sequences because of fast flow. The occipital horn of the lateral ventricle is dilated as a result of chronic compensated obstructive hydrocephalus.

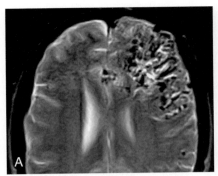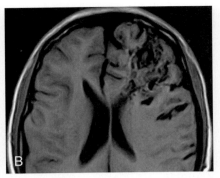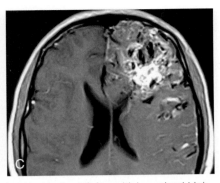

FIGURE 2–20. Arteriovenous malformation (AVM). On the T$_2$-weighted scan (*A*), a large lesion is noted in the left frontal lobe; mixed high and low signal intensity is suggestive of flow. Tubular-like signal voids are present on the precontrast T$_1$-weighted scan (*B*). *C*, Postcontrast, a large enhancing nidus is identified. Also seen is enhancement of multiple large draining veins. AVMs are well depicted on conventional planar spin echo magnetic resonance images because of flow phenomena. On precontrast scans, multiple serpiginous structures can be identified, most with low signal intensity because of rapid flow. After intravenous contrast administration, enhancement can be noted in areas of slower flow, particularly within draining veins.

draining veins (Fig. 2–21). MRA has several problems, including signal void in tortuous feeding vessels (as a result of complex flow), nonvisualization of some draining veins (resulting from spin saturation), and difficulty in differentiation of flow from blood clot (methemoglobin). Conventional MRI accurately depicts and stages (in regard to age) intraparenchymal hematomas associated with AVMs (Fig. 2–22). MRI, unlike CT, is also very sensitive for the detection of superficial siderosis related to chronic subarachnoid hemorrhage. Superficial siderosis is frequently associated with vascular malformations.

In contrast to congenital AVMs, pure dural-based AVMs are often secondary to trauma or inflammatory disease. These lesions drain into the venous sinuses or cortical veins and commonly have associated intracranial or subarachnoid hemorrhage. Planar MRI, without the

use of MRA, can have difficulty in detecting lesions adjacent to the inner table of the skull because vascular flow and cortical bone both appear as signal voids. CT also has difficulty in detecting such lesions. Hemorrhage complicating these lesions is clearly seen.

AVMs can have calcified components; CT is more sensitive in detecting these than MRI. Dense calcification has no mobile protons and appears as a signal void on MRI scan, which can be confused with flowing blood. In difficult cases in which accurate characterization of calcification, blood flow, and hemorrhagic components is desired, gradient echo techniques may be used as a helpful adjunct to SE imaging. On these sequences, flowing blood generally has increased signal intensity and can be distinguished from calcification or hemosiderin. Occasionally, however, flowing blood can have low signal intensity on gradient echo imaging as a result of

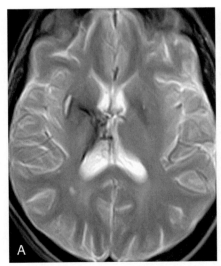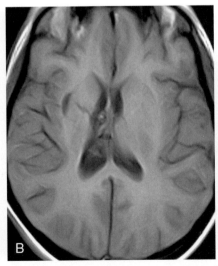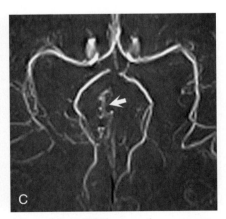

FIGURE 2–21. Thalamic arteriovenous malformation (AVM), best visualized on three-dimensional time-of-flight (TOF) magnetic resonance angiography (MRA). *A*, The precontrast T$_2$-weighted scan reveals abnormal iron deposition (with low signal intensity) in the right thalamus, along the border of the right lateral ventricle, and surrounding an old lacunar infarct in the right putamen. *B*, The precontrast T$_1$-weighted scan reveals slight ex vacuo dilatation of the right lateral ventricle. *C*, The maximum intensity projection image from the three-dimensional TOF MRA reveals an abnormal tangle of vessels (AVM, *arrow*) just to the right of the midline and medial to the right posterior cerebral artery. Viewing the T$_2$-weighted scan in retrospect, several abnormal vessels can be identified because of their flow voids medial to the hemosiderin staining along the margin of the lateral ventricle.

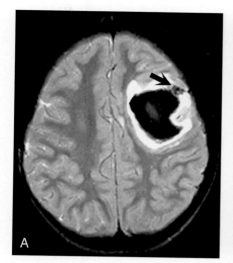
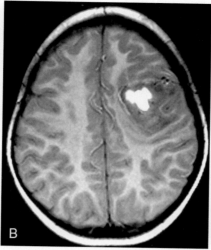
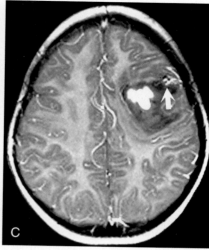

FIGURE 2–22. Small frontal lobe arteriovenous malformation (AVM) presenting clinically with intraparenchymal hemorrhage in a pediatric patient. T_2- (*A*) and T_1-weighted (*B*) precontrast scans reveal a large left frontal mass with marked hypointensity on the T_2-weighted image and hyperintensity centrally on the T_1-weighted image (the signal characteristics of intracellular methemoglobin). Surrounding cerebral edema, with high signal intensity, is well depicted on the T_2-weighted scan. Just lateral and anterior to the primary lesion, a second smaller serpiginous lesion is noted (*black arrow, A*). This has low signal intensity on both T_2- and T_1-weighted precontrast scans. The same area (*white arrow*) enhances on the postcontrast T_1-weighted scan (*C*). As with larger lesions, this small AVM is characterized by flow voids precontrast and enhancement postcontrast. Prospective identification on precontrast scans is difficult because of the lesion's small size and the large adjacent hematoma. The AVM was confirmed by x-ray angiography.

turbulent, in plane, or very slow flow, and this potential pitfall should be recognized.

Gliosis, edema, or ischemia can involve the brain adjacent to an AVM. These parenchymal changes are best detected as abnormal high signal intensity on T_2-weighted images. Although this high signal intensity is nonspecific, the absence of a soft tissue mass favors a benign process. AVMs also typically do not have substantial associated mass effect (unless accompanied by parenchymal hemorrhage).

Included in the spectrum of AVMs is a rare congenital anomaly, the vein of Galen aneurysm. Dilatation of the vein of Galen occurs if there is a downstream venous obstruction and increased flow through the vein of Galen secondary to an arteriovenous shunt. Hydrocephalus often develops. Infants usually present with cardiac failure, and older children present with hydrocephalus and increased intracranial pressure. MRI is useful in defining the anatomic extent of the abnormality and in evaluating blood flow patterns or thrombus within the aneurysm. Preoperative angiography remains essential because precise identification of the feeding arteries is necessary.

Multiple intracranial AVMs may be seen in patients with Wyburn-Mason's syndrome and Osler-Weber-Rendu disease. Wyburn-Mason's syndrome is rare and consists of a midbrain AVM, a facial cutaneous nevus in the distribution of the trigeminal nerve, and a retinal angioma ipsilateral to the facial nevus. MRI can noninvasively evaluate the retinal and midbrain components of this syndrome.

Venous Angioma

Venous angiomas are vascular malformations involving only the venous side of the circulation. They occur throughout the central nervous system but are most common in the frontal lobes and posterior fossa (Fig. 2–23). Patients with venous angiomas are most often asymptomatic. Although it was previously believed that venous angiomas had a high propensity to bleed, this is now generally regarded as an incidental finding. Venous angiomas consist of a group of dilated medullary venous tributaries, often arranged in a radial "spoke-wheel" pattern, draining into a large vein. This large transparenchymal vein drains into a venous sinus, a cortical vein, or a subependymal ventricular vein.

On SE MRI, venous angiomas appear as tubular flow voids with a radial configuration in the white matter. The enlarged draining vein and its site of drainage are often also visualized. Both T_1- and T_2-weighted images are used to detect venous angiomas; T_2-weighted sequences are often more sensitive compared with precontrast T_1-weighted scans. Because of slow venous flow, which can cause increased intravascular signal, these lesions may be inapparent (isointense to adjacent brain) on some imaging sequences. In particular, periventricular lesions can be difficult to identify on precontrast scans alone. Venous angiomas are best visualized on contrast-enhanced scans (Fig. 2–24).

Included in the spectrum of venous malformations is the Sturge-Weber syndrome (encephalotrigeminal angiomatosis). This syndrome consists of a cutaneous facial nevus (port-wine stain), usually in the ophthalmic distribution of the trigeminal nerve, ipsilateral leptomeningeal angiomatosis, and ipsilateral cortical atrophy with linear cortical gyral calcifications in a tram-track configuration. Dilated deep venous collaterals provide abnormal drainage. The leptomeningeal angiomatosis displays marked contrast enhancement. Gradient echo imaging can be useful for depiction of the cortical gyral calcifications.

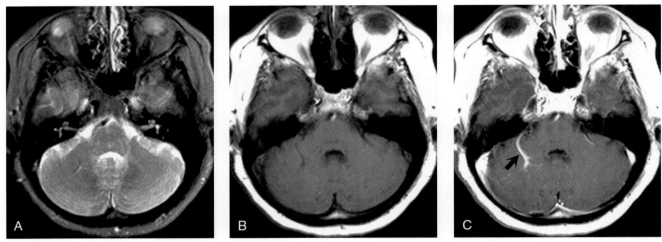

Figure 2–23. Infratentorial venous angioma. Precontrast T_2- (*A*) and T_1-weighted (*B*) scans reveal a linear, tubular flow void within the right cerebellar hemisphere. This is better seen on the T_1-weighted scan, in which there is also a suggestion of feeding branches. There is no surrounding edema or associated parenchymal abnormality. *C*, The postcontrast T_1-weighted scan reveals intense enhancement of the lesion (*black arrow*), with improved visualization of both the caput of dilated medullary veins and the large central draining vein.

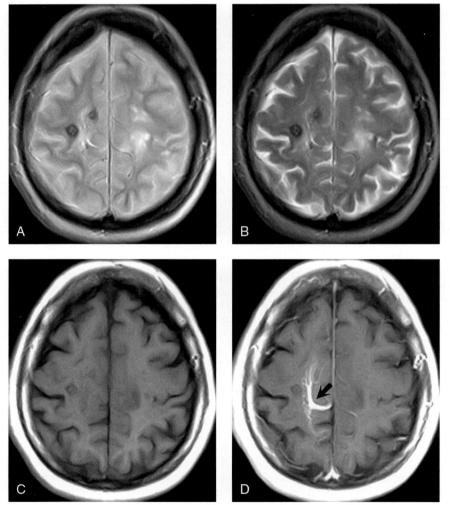

Figure 2–24. Supratentorial venous angioma. Two small round lesions with decreased signal intensity are noted in the right frontal lobe on the first (*A*) and second (*B*) echoes of the T_2-weighted scan. These two lesions have intermediate signal intensity on the precontrast T_1-weighted scan (*C*). The signal characteristics are compatible with hemosiderin. Abnormal contrast enhancement of numerous tiny veins and a solitary large draining vein (*arrow*) is identified in the right frontal lobe on the axial T_1-weighted postcontrast scan (*D*). The solitary draining vein extends to the midline and was noted on other images (not shown) to drain into the superior sagittal sinus.

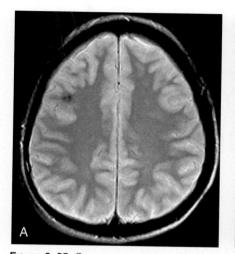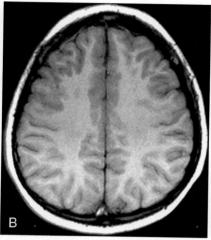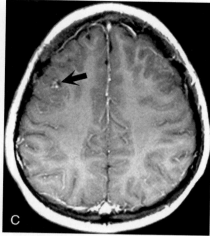

FIGURE 2–25. Cavernous angioma. A predominantly low signal intensity lesion is noted on the precontrast T_2-weighted scan (*A*). Comparison of pre- (*B*) and postcontrast (*C*) T_1-weighted scans reveals punctate enhancement of the lesion (*arrow*). On computed tomography (not shown) the lesion was calcified.

Cavernous Angioma and Capillary Telangiectasia

A cavernous angioma (cavernous malformation or cavernous hemangioma) is a collection of endothelial-lined vascular spaces with no intervening brain parenchyma between these vessels. These lesions occur throughout the central nervous system but are more common in a supratentorial, subcortical location. Cavernous angiomas are multiple in as many as 33% of cases. These lesions are usually asymptomatic, but some patients present with seizures. There are two forms of cavernous angioma: sporadic and familial. The familial form has a high incidence of multiple lesions, is autosomal dominant in transmission, and appears to have an increased frequency in Mexican American families. Cavernous angiomas display a well-defined low-signal-intensity border, caused by hemosiderin deposition, on T_2-weighted images (Fig. 2–25). Gradient echo imaging, using sequences with high sensitivity to T_2^* (susceptibility), often reveal more lesions than conventional imaging (in patients with multiple lesions). The internal architecture of cavernous angiomas is complex because of repeated hemorrhage. Multiple hyperintense, and often hypointense, round areas are seen separated by low signal intensity septations on both T_1- and T_2-weighted images. Because of the presence of large vascular spaces within the lesion, cavernous angiomas enhance after administration of intravenous contrast.

Capillary telangiectasias (capillary angiomas) are small, solitary lesions frequently found in the pons. In contrast to cavernous angiomas, capillary telangiectasia consists of dilated capillaries with intervening brain parenchyma between the vessels. Most of these lesions are asymptomatic clinically but can occasionally be associated with hemorrhage.

Occult Cerebrovascular Malformations

Any of the four previously described pathologic entities comprising cerebrovascular malformations can be categorized as an OCVM if the lesion is angiographically occult. MRI has become the primary screening modality for detection because of its exquisite ability to visualize the components of hemorrhage.

After an acute hemorrhage, OCVMs may be difficult to distinguish from an intraparenchymal hematoma, particularly those caused by neoplasm. Beyond this acute stage, OCVMs can be distinguished from hematomas of other causes by their continuous hemosiderin rim, absence of parenchymal mass effect or edema, location of the lesion, and expected temporal evolution of hemorrhage in a simple hematoma.

The detection of very small OCVMs by MRI depends on identifying the characteristic circumferential low-intensity hemosiderin rim. High-field MRI and gradient echo techniques are more sensitive in detecting hemosiderin and, therefore, OCVMs. Routine SE MRI may miss small OCVMs that can be detected by CT because of the presence of small focal calcifications.

3

Brain: Ischemic (and Atrophic) Disease

Cerebrovascular disease, with cerebral ischemia or infarction, is the most common disease affecting the brain. It is also the most common neurologic disease seen by the radiologist in daily practice. Cerebrovascular disease is an important health care problem, particularly in the older patient population. In the United States, it is the third leading cause of death after cancer and myocardial infarction. Half of the affected patients will have permanent neurologic deficits. There are more than 2 million survivors of cerebral infarction. Magnetic resonance imaging (MRI) is the modality that most completely characterizes cerebrovascular disease. MRI provides information regarding pathophysiology, anatomic location, and vascular patency.

CLINICAL CONSIDERATIONS

Stroke is a general term describing an acute neurologic insult, with a resulting permanent deficit, caused by a disease of the blood vessels. The term cerebrovascular accident (CVA) is synonymous with stroke. The clinical presentation of patients with stroke is variable and non-specific. Patients with a ruptured aneurysm, subdural hematoma, or hemorrhage into a tumor can present with strokelike symptoms similar to those of cerebral ischemia or infarction. The role of the radiologist is to determine the cause of the symptoms in the individual patient.

In patients with ischemia or infarction, there is often a disparity between pathophysiology (the derangement of function seen in the disease) and clinical manifestations. Therefore, the accurate use of terminology describing ischemic disease is important. Cerebral ischemia and infarction describe pathophysiologic processes. Cerebral ischemia describes global or regional reduction of blood flow to the brain. Cerebral infarction occurs when the reduction of blood flow causes irreversible cellular damage (i.e., cell death). The clinical terminology describing ischemic neurologic events is based on clinical presentation and evolution. A transient ischemic attack (TIA) is a transient loss of neurologic function that resolves in 24 hours. Reversible ischemic neurologic deficit (RIND) indicates loss of neurologic function that resolves within 21 days. A progressing stroke or stroke in evolution describes a changing neurologic state. A completed stroke indicates a permanent and fixed neurologic deficit. A patient with cerebral infarction may present with any of these clinical states, even though permanent tissue damage has occurred. MRI in particular often detects subclinical cerebral ischemia and infarction.

PATHOPHYSIOLOGY

In the normal state, the brain receives 15% to 20% of the cardiac output, and the brain extracts 50% of the available oxygen and 10% of the available glucose for cerebral metabolism. After an ischemic event, the tissue oxygen concentration decreases more than the glucose concentration. Prolonged lack of oxygen reduces energy production, decreasing adenosine triphosphate (ATP) levels and building lactic acid levels. The sodium-potassium pump fueled by ATP fails, and as sodium moves into cells potassium leaks out. Tissue osmolality increases because of the continued presence of glucose. Water accumulates in cells because of the osmotic gradient and increased intracellular sodium. This process, in which fluid accumulates in the intracellular spaces, is called cytotoxic edema. Within 30 minutes after the insult, mitochondria are destroyed. Disruption of cytoplasmic and endothelial membranes follows. These pathophysiologic changes suggest that reversible ischemia occurs within the first hour, before disruption of the blood-brain barrier.

Disruption of the blood-brain barrier, which occurs by 6 hours, causes leakage of water and protein into the extracellular compartment. Reperfusion of the infarcted region can occur within the first 30 minutes by reestablishing the native circulation or by development of collaterals. The degree of reperfusion of the infarcted region determines the amount of fluid that enters the extracellular compartment. This increase in extracellular fluid is called vasogenic edema. The amount of vasogenic edema can progress with continued reperfusion. The resulting mass effect causes compression of the adjacent microcirculation. There may be extension of the infarct by this process, with irreversible cellular damage (infarction) at the margins of the original ischemic region.

The mass effect caused by vasogenic edema progresses during the first 3 to 7 days, stabilizes during the second week, and begins to resolve by the third week. Blood-brain barrier disruption is commonly seen on imaging up to 8 weeks after the ischemic insult. The development of secondary hemorrhagic foci (i.e., petechial hemorrhage) occurs in up to 40% of cases, typically during the second week. These hemorrhages are usually clinically occult. Intraparenchymal hemorrhage can occasionally present clinically in the first few days, and in this situation the hemorrhage is commonly secondary to embolic infarction.

In the completed infarct, there is gliosis, loss of tissue, and associated focal atrophy. There may be residual cystic areas (i.e., macrocystic encephalomalacia) in the infarcted territory. If there has been associated hemorrhage, hemosiderin may be seen. Dystrophic calcification of the infarcted brain occurs rarely. In large supratentorial infarcts (and particularly those involving the motor cortex), anterograde degeneration of descending nerve pathways may be visualized and is called wallerian degeneration. MRI findings in wallerian degeneration include signal changes (gliosis) and loss of tissue volume. Changes can be noted in the posterior limb of the internal capsule, cerebral peduncles, anterior pons, and anterior medulla (where the fibers decussate).

MRI PRINCIPLES (ISCHEMIC DISEASE)

The prior description of pathophysiology provides a conceptual framework for understanding the appearance of cerebral ischemia and infarction on MRI. Before going into depth concerning the MRI appearance of ischemia and infarction, it is important to establish the terminology that is used regarding lesion dating. Unfortunately, there is no universal agreement regarding this terminology. The terminology presented here is one approach well accepted by both radiologists and neurologists. Hyperacute infarction is defined as that within the first 3 to 6 hours after onset of clinical symptoms. This is also the window of potential therapeutic reversibility with current treatment regimens. Acute infarction is defined as that within 6 to 24 hours after onset of symptoms. A TIA is defined as a sudden loss of neurologic function with complete recovery within 24 hours. If ischemia persists beyond 24 hours after onset of symptoms, the area of brain involved will be irreversibly injured and is unlikely to be rescued by reperfusion

attempts. Subacute infarction is defined as that from 24 hours to 6 weeks. This time period is subdivided into early subacute (from 24 hours to 1 week) and late subacute (from 1 to 6 weeks). Chronic infarction is defined as that more than 6 weeks after clinical presentation.

Cerebral ischemia and infarction produce fluid changes in the intracellular and extracellular spaces, as previously described (i.e., cytotoxic and vasogenic edema). The sensitivity of MRI for detection of cerebral ischemia is high because of its ability to detect small changes in tissue water. Cytotoxic edema, which occurs very rapidly after the onset of symptoms, can be visualized directly on diffusion weighted scans (Fig. 3–1). Diffusion imaging assesses the microscopic motion of water protons. The gradient magnetic fields used in imaging are used to achieve sensitivity to diffusion, with both a longer duration and higher amplitude of the gradients increasing such sensitivity. Higher (faster) diffusion produces greater signal attenuation. Diffusion is restricted (slower) in acute ischemia, a result of the intracellular shift of water (cytotoxic edema). Acute infarcts are markedly hyperintense on diffusion-weighted scans, with corresponding low intensity on apparent diffusion coefficient (ADC) maps. Diffusion-weighted scans are also typically T_2-weighted. Thus, without reference to a T_2-weighted scan, it cannot be said with certainty whether high signal intensity on a diffusion scan represents restricted diffusion or a long T_2. Clinical interpretation is aided by comparison with T_2-weighted scans and reference to ADC maps. Cytotoxic edema (alone, without accompanying vasogenic edema) is high signal intensity on a diffusion-weighted scan, isointense on a T_2-weighted scan (not detectable), and low intensity on an ADC map. Diffusion-weighted scans should be acquired when there is clinical suspicion of an acute or early subacute infarct. Some acute lesions will be visualized only by diffusion imaging. Such scans also permit the differentiation of acute and early subacute ischemia from chronic ischemic changes. Diffusion imaging permits detection of cerebral ischemia within minutes of onset. ADC values are initially low but progress with

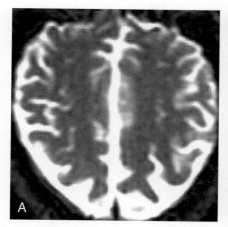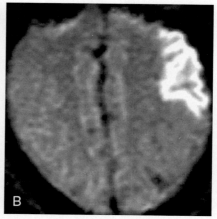

FIGURE 3–1. Hyperacute left middle cerebral artery infarction demonstrating the utility of diffusion imaging. *A,* The T_2-weighted axial scan is normal. *B,* The diffusion-weighted scan demonstrates abnormal high signal intensity because of the presence of cytotoxic edema. In very early infarcts, vasogenic edema is not present, and T_2-weighted scans will appear normal. Diffusion or perfusion scans are necessary to diagnose these early infarcts. (Courtesy of Dr. Larry Tanenbaum, New Jersey Neuroscience Institute.)

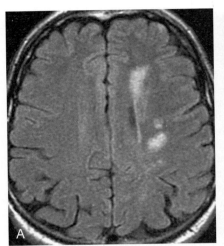
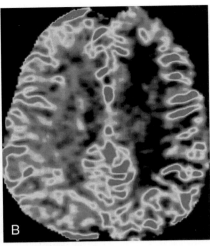
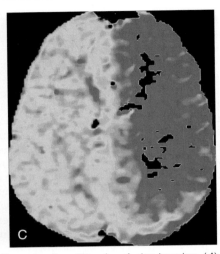

FIGURE 3–2. Infarction of the left hemisphere secondary to internal carotid artery occlusion, illustrating the utility of perfusion imaging. (*A*) On fluid-attenuated inversion recovery scan abnormal high signal intensity caused by vasogenic edema is confined to the periventricular white matter. A first-pass perfusion study was performed immediately after bolus injection of a gadolinium chelate. On the cerebral blood volume (CBV) (*B*) and mean transit time (MTT) (*C*) calculated images, the entire left hemisphere is noted to be involved (with reduced CBV and delayed MTT). (Courtesy of Dr. Larry Tanenbaum, New Jersey Neuroscience Institute.)

time to supranormal in irreversible ischemia. The transition from reduced to elevated ADC values is a current area of study; this change was reported by some investigators as early as 24 hours but by others not until 10 days after stroke onset.

Perfusion imaging is another major tool for the evaluation of brain ischemia; scan acquisition is recommended (in tandem with diffusion imaging) when acute or early subacute ischemia is suspected (Fig. 3–2). The T_2^*, or susceptibility, effect of a gadolinium chelate is visualized on perfusion imaging during first pass of the contrast agent through the brain. Perfusion imaging thus requires rapid image acquisition during bolus contrast injection, the latter typically performed with a power injector. From the dynamic change in signal intensity during first pass of the contrast agent, cerebral blood volume (CBV) and mean transit time (MTT) calculated images (or "maps") are produced. CBV relates to the area under the time-concentration curve and MTT to the timing of arrival of contrast. In early ischemia, CBV is reduced and MTT prolonged.

Vasogenic edema forms later, after cytotoxic edema, in cerebral ischemia. Although vasogenic edema can be seen as early as 30 minutes after the onset of ischemia, typically changes are not noted until 4 to 6 hours. Findings on conventional MRI within the first 24 hours may be subtle; correct diagnosis relies on the use of diffusion and perfusion imaging (for detection of cytotoxic edema and perfusion deficits) or close inspection of conventional images supplemented with MRI angiography (Fig.

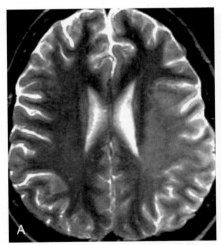
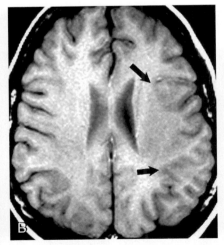
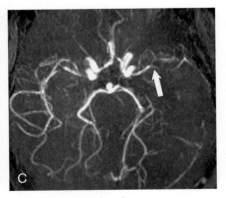

FIGURE 3–3. Acute (<24 h) left middle cerebral artery (MCA) infarction demonstrating the appearance of cytotoxic edema on conventional spin echo scans and the complementary role of magnetic resonance angiography (MRA). Subtle high signal intensity in the left MCA distribution on the T_2-weighted scan (*A*) is indicative of early vasogenic edema. *B*, The thickening and increased prominence (visibility) of cortical gray matter (*black arrows*) on the T_1-weighted scan is due to cytotoxic edema. These findings are subtle in distinction to those on diffusion imaging in early infarcts. *C*, The three-dimensional time-of-flight MRA exam reveals occlusion (*white arrow*) of the left MCA.

3–3). Once fully established, vasogenic edema is clearly seen with conventional MRI techniques. The increased water content causes prolongation of both T_1 and T_2. Vasogenic edema thus has low signal intensity on T_1-weighted scans and high signal intensity on T_2-weighted scans. T_2-weighted scans, however, are relied on in clinical practice for the visualization of vasogenic edema. Commonly used "T_1-weighted" spin echo sequences (i.e., short time to repetition [TR] and short time to echo [TE]) do not have optimal T_1 contrast. Such scans are only mildly T_1-weighted. The abnormal low signal intensity on these scans (as a result of vasogenic edema) is less obvious than the abnormal high signal intensity on T_2-weighted scans. Inversion recovery sequences or three-dimensional gradient echo T_1-weighted sequences (such as turbo-FLASH) are more heavily T_1-weighted. With the latter types of scans, the abnormal low signal intensity resulting from vasogenic edema is much better visualized than with conventional T_1-weighted spin echo scans.

Clinical studies demonstrated the marked superiority of MRI compared with CT for the detection of cerebral ischemia and infarction, particularly within the first few days. Using diffusion and perfusion imaging, cerebral ischemia can be detected by MRI within minutes of onset. CT is positive for infarction in only 20% of patients within the first 6 hours and in 80% within the first 24 hours. MRI is also markedly superior to CT in detecting posterior fossa and brainstem infarcts. These regions are not obscured on MRI, unlike CT, by beam-hardening artifacts.

The intravenous administration of gadolinium chelates with extracellular distribution provides important ancillary information in brain infarction. Paramagnetic contrast agents decrease T_1 relaxation times, increasing the signal intensity on T_1-weighted images. Contrast enhancement of vessels supplying the infarct ("vascular," "intravascular," or "arterial" enhancement) is seen in

more than half of all infarcts from 1 to 3 days after clinical presentation (Fig. 3–4). Vascular enhancement is more common in cortical lesions and is rarely seen in noncortical gray or deep white matter infarcts. Vascular enhancement occurs when perfusion is absent (complete ischemia). Vascular enhancement dissipates and parenchymal enhancement develops as collateral flow is established. Meningeal enhancement, which is less common than vascular enhancement, can be seen adjacent to large territorial infarcts from day 2 to day 6 (Fig. 3–5). In most cases, it is the adjacent dura that enhances. In some cases, the adjacent pia-arachnoid appears involved. Both vascular enhancement and meningeal enhancement are not seen after 1 week.

Parenchymal enhancement is consistently seen in late subacute infarcts and may persist for 8 weeks or more after clinical presentation (Fig. 3–6). Parenchymal enhancement occurs as a result of blood-brain barrier disruption. Scans should be not be taken immediately after contrast injection because parenchymal enhancement increases given a slight time delay. Lesion enhancement resulting from blood-brain barrier disruption will be substantially better on scans obtained 5 to 10 minutes postinjection as opposed to those obtained immediately after injection. MRI is slightly better than CT for the detection of abnormal contrast enhancement, partly because of the lack of beam-hardening artifact and the greater inherent sensitivity to the contrast agent.

Two types of parenchymal enhancement have been described: progressive enhancement and early or intense enhancement. In progressive enhancement, thin, faint enhancement is first seen at about 1 week near the margins of the lesion or the pial surface. The enhancement progresses over days and weeks to become thicker and more prominent, either in a gyriform pattern if cortical or uniform (solid) if noncortical. Progressive parenchymal enhancement, in both cortical and noncortical infarcts, typically lags behind (temporally) the

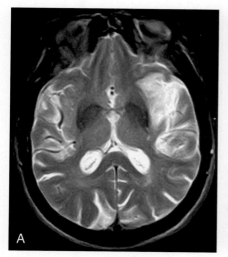
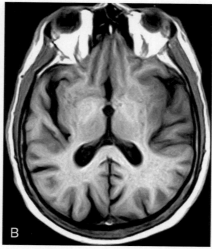
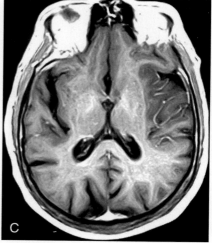

FIGURE 3–4. Intravascular contrast enhancement in an early subacute middle cerebral artery (MCA) infarction. *A,* Vasogenic edema is noted in the left MCA distribution on the T_2-weighted scan. Comparison of pre- (*B*) and postcontrast (*C*) T_1-weighted scans reveals enhancement of numerous vessels (intravascular enhancement) in the same region. This finding is particularly striking when comparison is made to the normal right side, where no vessels are apparent postcontrast.

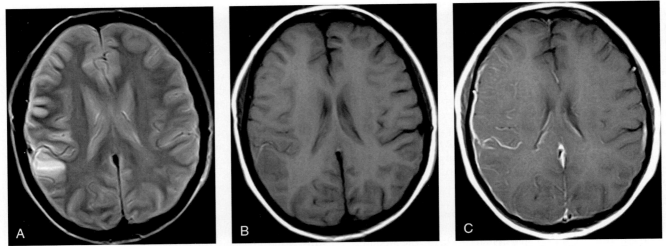

FIGURE 3–5. Meningeal contrast enhancement in an early subacute middle cerebral artery (MCA) infarction. *A*, A small amount of vasogenic edema is noted on the T_2-weighted scan in the right MCA distribution. There is extensive sulcal effacement on the precontrast T_1-weighted scan (*B*), indicative of a much larger lesion. Meningeal enhancement is present on the postcontrast T_1-weighted scan (*C*) along the surface of this entire area. Meningeal enhancement, although not common, is important to recognize as such in early subacute infarction. This sign provides supportive evidence for the diagnosis of an infarct and should not be misinterpreted as suggesting a different cause.

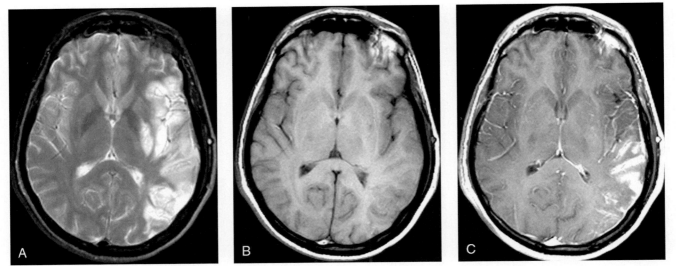

FIGURE 3–6. Subacute middle cerebral artery (MCA) infarction demonstrating gyriform contrast enhancement. There is abnormal high signal intensity consistent with vasogenic edema on the T_2-weighted scan (*A*) in the left MCA distribution (and putamen). Comparison of pre- (*B*) and postcontrast (*C*) T_1-weighted scans reveals gyriform (parenchymal) enhancement in part of the infarct resulting from blood-brain barrier disruption.

changes on T_2-weighted scans in both intensity and area of involvement. Early or intense enhancement is less common than progressive parenchymal enhancement. With early or intense enhancement, abnormal contrast enhancement is seen within 2 to 3 days of clinical presentation. The area involved equals or exceeds the size of the abnormality on T_2-weighted scans in most cases. Clinical outcome in patients with early or intense enhancement includes reversible and persistent neurologic deficits. Early parenchymal enhancement is thought to occur in cases of incomplete ischemia, allowing for delivery of substantial contrast material to the ischemic tissue.

In early subacute infarction, the MRI appearance is dominated by the presence of vasogenic edema. The latter is best seen on T_2-weighted scans, with abnormal high signal intensity. At this time, the blood-brain barrier is usually still intact and parenchymal enhancement is lacking. In the late subacute phase, cerebral infarction continues to be characterized by increased signal intensity on T_2-weighted images and moderately decreased signal intensity on precontrast T_1-weighted images. MRI accurately defines the mass effect associated with infarction, which is often most pronounced in the early subacute phase. These findings include compression and effacement of the sulci or ventricular system and displacement of midline structures.

In the chronic phase (after 6 weeks), edema subsides and there is glial proliferation with brain shrinkage. Gliosis is accompanied by increased brain water content and appears as high signal intensity on T_2-weighted images and low signal intensity on T_1-weighted images. Focal atrophy is identified as enlargement of adjacent sulci or portions of the ventricular system. Cystic changes (e.g., macrocystic encephalomalacia), if present, are character-

ized by a fluid intensity that follows that of cerebrospinal fluid (Fig. 3–7). Typically, disruption of the blood-brain barrier, detected after intravenous gadolinium chelate injection, is not visualized beyond 8 weeks.

MRI is particularly sensitive to petechial hemorrhage, which commonly complicates infarction, especially in the subacute phase. Petechial hemorrhage or cortical hemorrhagic infarction (Fig. 3–8) is most commonly identified as high signal intensity on T_1-weighted images because of methemoglobin (subacute stage). Acute and chronic petechial hemorrhage is also clearly depicted on MRI but has a distinct appearance compared with subacute blood. In the acute phase, cortical low signal intensity, resulting from the presence of deoxyhemoglobin, is seen on T_2-weighted images (Fig. 3–9). This is outlined by subcortical vasogenic edema with high signal intensity. The cortical signal changes produced by deoxyhemoglobin are isointense with brain on T_1-weighted images. In chronic hemorrhagic infarction, cortical low signal intensity is again seen on T_2-weighted images. This is due, however, in the chronic phase to the presence of hemosiderin and ferritin. Because the susceptibility effects of deoxyhemoglobin, hemosiderin, and ferritin (which lead to low signal intensity on T_2-weighted scans) are proportional to field strength, these findings are most pronounced at high field (1.5 T) and may not be detected at low field (0.5 T and below).

The cause of cerebral ischemia is often multifactorial. The efficiency of the heart, the integrity of vessels supplying the brain, and the state of the blood itself in supplying oxygen at the cellular level (e.g., oxygen-carrying capacity, viscosity, coagulability) are all contributory factors. Lesions of the vascular tree are commonly the dominant factor in the development of cerebrovascular insufficiency that leads to infarction.

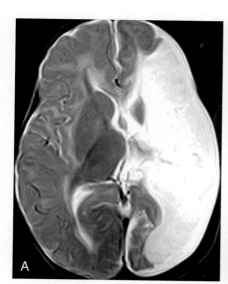
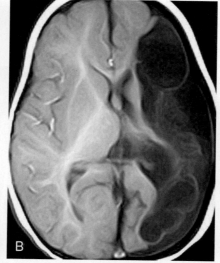
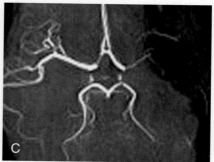

FIGURE 3–7. Chronic middle cerebral artery (MCA) infarction. Normal brain has been replaced by cystic encephalomalacia, with high signal intensity on the T_2-weighted scan (*A*) and low signal intensity on the T_1-weighted scan (*B*) in the entire left MCA distribution. Ex vacuo dilatation of the left lateral ventricle is also present. *C*, Three-dimensional time-of-flight magnetic resonance angiography demonstrates the left MCA to be small and without peripheral branches. The patient was a 10-month-old infant with a history of a neonatal cerebrovascular accident.

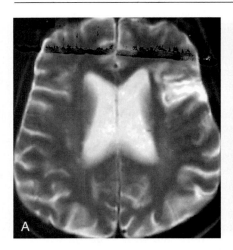

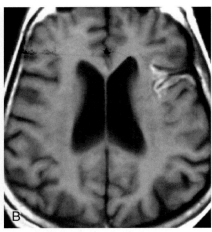

FIGURE 3–8. Hemorrhagic (methemoglobin) left middle cerebral artery (MCA) infarction. An infarct in the left MCA distribution (anterior division) is easily recognized because of abnormal high signal intensity on the T$_2$-weighted scan (A). The thin gyriform line of high signal intensity in the same region on the precontrast T$_1$-weighted scan (B) corresponds to petechial hemorrhage, in the form of methemoglobin, within cortical gray matter. There was marked gyriform enhancement postcontrast (image not shown), indicative of blood-brain barrier disruption in this late subacute infarct.

ARTERIAL VASCULAR TERRITORIES

The arterial vascular territories of the brain are shown in Figure 3–10. The middle cerebral artery (MCA) supplies the majority of the lateral surface of the cerebrum, the insular cortex, and the anterior and lateral aspects of the temporal lobe. It is the most common vascular territory involved by infarction. The lenticulostriate arteries originate from the M1 segment of the MCA and supply the basal ganglia and the anterior limb of the internal capsule. The sylvian triangle is composed of the MCA branches that loop over the insula deep in the sylvian fissure. Although MCA infarcts often involve a wedge-like section of brain, infarcts restricted to a small cortical distribution are not uncommon (Fig. 3–11).

The posterior cerebral artery (PCA) supplies the occipital lobe, the medial parietal lobe, and the medial temporal lobe (Figs. 3–12 to 3–14). PCA infarction follows MCA infarction in incidence. The thalamoperforating arteries arise from the P1 segment of the PCA and from the posterior communicating artery. These perforators supply the medial ventral thalamus and the posterior limb of the internal capsule.

The anterior cerebral artery (ACA) supplies the anterior two thirds of the medial cerebral surface, the corpus callosum, and 1 cm of superomedial brain over the convexity (Figs. 3–15 to 3–17). Of all cerebral hemispheric infarcts, ACA infarction is the least common and accounts for less than 3% of cases. The recurrent artery of Heubner originates from the A1 or A2 segment of the ACA and supplies the caudate head, the anterior limb of the internal capsule, and part of the putamen. Infarction of both the ACA and MCA territories occurs with thrombosis of the distal internal carotid artery in individuals with ineffective cervical collaterals or an incomplete circle of Willis (Fig. 3–18).

The anterior choroidal artery arises from the supraclinoid internal carotid artery. This vessel supplies the posterior limb of the internal capsule, portions of the thalamus, the caudate, the globus pallidus, and the cerebral peduncle.

In the posterior fossa, the posteroinferior cerebellar

Text continued on page 60

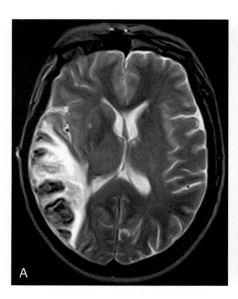

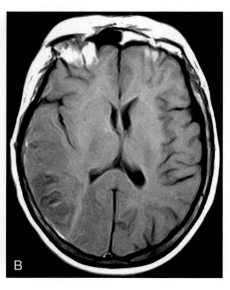

FIGURE 3–9. Hemorrhagic (deoxyhemoglobin) right middle cerebral artery (MCA) infarction. Abnormal high signal intensity is seen on the T$_2$-weighted scan (A) in the distribution of right MCA (posterior division), compatible with an early subacute infarct. The patient presented with clinical symptoms 6 days before the magnetic resonance scan. Gyriform low signal intensity within the region of high signal intensity is due to the presence of petechial hemorrhage. B, The precontrast T$_1$-weighted scan demonstrates substantial mass effect but adds little additional information in this instance.

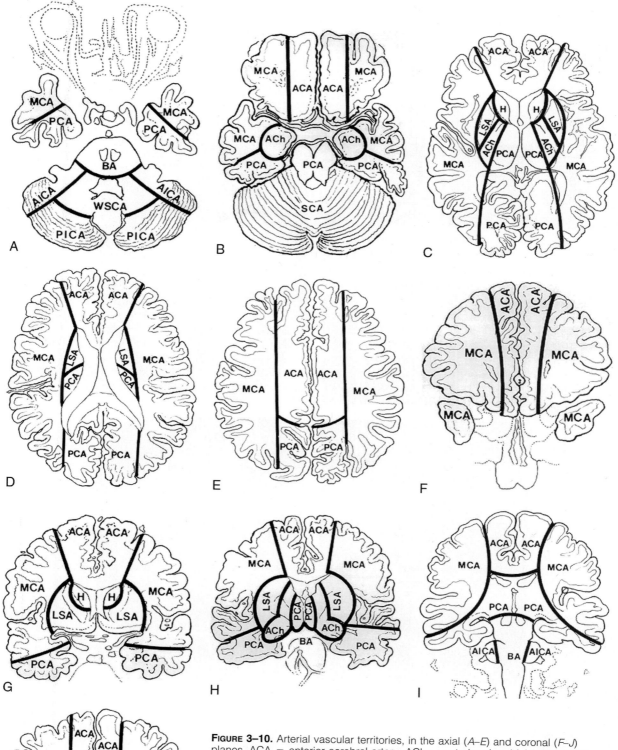

FIGURE 3–10. Arterial vascular territories, in the axial (*A–E*) and coronal (*F–J*) planes. ACA = anterior cerebral artery; ACh = anterior choroidal artery; AICA = anteroinferior cerebellar artery; BA = perforating branches of the basilar artery; H = recurrent artery of Heubner; LSA = lenticulostriate artery; MCA = middle cerebral artery; PCA = posterior cerebral artery; PICA = posteroinferior cerebellar artery; SCA = superior cerebellar artery; WSCA = watershed region supplied predominantly by the SCA.

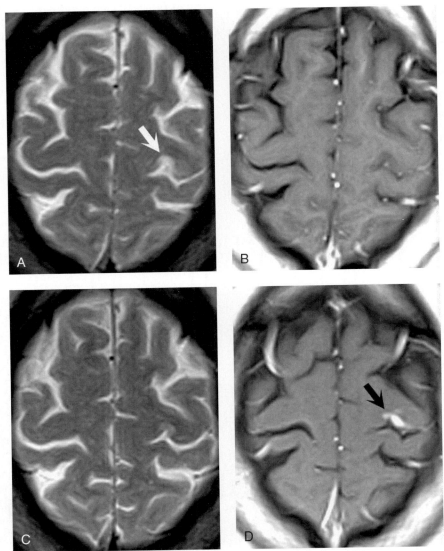

Figure 3–11. Cortical infarction, with progression from the early to the late subacute stage. On magnetic resonance imaging (MRI) performed within 1 week after clinical presentation, vasogenic edema is noted in a small section of cortical gray matter (*white arrow*), with abnormal hyperintensity on the T_2-weighted scan (*A*) and hypointensity on the postcontrast T_1-weighted scan (*B*). The MRI examination was repeated 9 days later, with the edema slightly less, as evaluated by the T_2-weighted scan (*C*). Abnormal contrast enhancement (*black arrow*) is now noted on the postcontrast T_1-weighted scan (*D*).

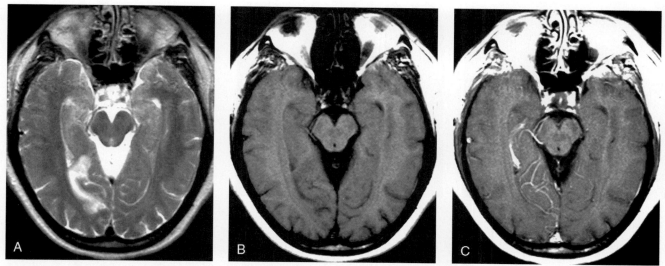

FIGURE 3–12. Early subacute posterior cerebral artery (PCA) infarction. The patient presented with a 2-day history of visual problems. Abnormal high signal intensity is noted in the right PCA distribution on the T_2-weighted scan (*A*). The same area demonstrates subtle low signal intensity on the T_1-weighted scan (*B*). *C*, Postcontrast, there is prominent intravascular enhancement in this region. This finding supports the leading diagnosis—cerebral infarction—and permits dating of the abnormality. Vascular enhancement is the earliest type of abnormal contrast enhancement identified on magnetic resonance imaging in cerebral infarction and is frequently seen in 1- to 3-day-old lesions.

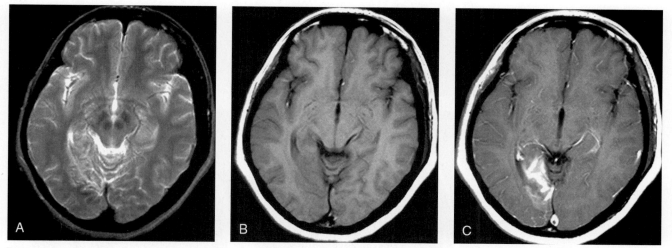

FIGURE 3–13. Late subacute posterior cerebral artery (PCA) infarction. The magnetic resonance (MR) scan was obtained 19 days after clinical presentation. Precontrast T_2- (*A*) and T_1-weighted (*B*) scans are unremarkable, at least at first glance. *C*, Postcontrast, gyriform enhancement is noted in the right PCA distribution. Parenchymal enhancement occurs because of blood-brain barrier disruption, identifying brain damaged by cerebral ischemia. In the subacute time frame, as with computed tomography, there may be sufficient resolution of vasogenic edema on MR imaging to render the lesion undetectable without intravenous contrast administration.

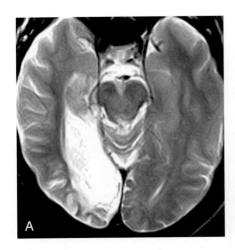

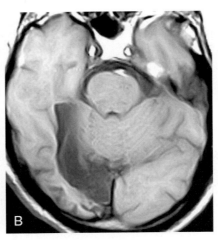

FIGURE 3–14. Chronic posterior cerebral artery (PCA) infarction. The patient, who has atrial fibrillation, presented clinically 2 years before the current magnetic resonance scan with confusion, unsteady gait, and difficulty reading. Cerebrospinal fluid signal intensity, consistent with cystic encephalomalacia, is noted in the distribution of the right PCA on both the T_2- (A) and T_1-weighted (B) scans.

FIGURE 3–15. Early subacute anterior cerebral artery infarction. There is abnormal high signal intensity in the genu and anterior body of the corpus callosum on the T_2-weighted sagittal scan (A) (obtained just to the right of midline). Involvement of gray matter (with similar abnormal hyperintensity) in the anteromedial frontal lobe is also noted on both the sagittal (A) and axial (B) T_2-weighted scans. The same medial strip of frontal lobe demonstrates sulcal effacement and abnormal hypointensity of cortical gray matter on the precontrast T_1-weighted axial scan (C). D, Postcontrast, intravascular and meningeal enhancement is seen along the 1-cm strip of right frontal lobe adjacent to the midline. This is most prominent posteriorly.

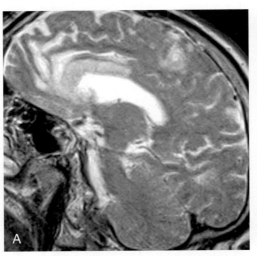

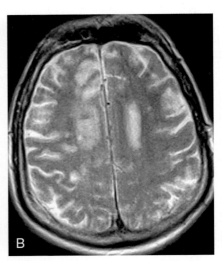

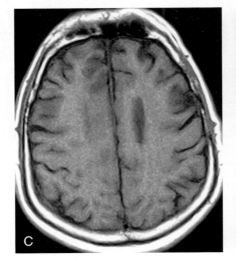

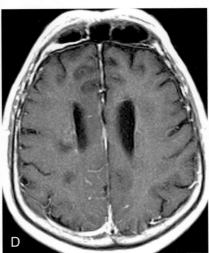

FIGURE 3–16. Late subacute anterior cerebral artery (ACA) infarction. On the T$_2$-weighted scan (A), abnormal high signal intensity is noted anterior to the left lateral ventricle and posterior to the right lateral ventricle. The latter finding relates to chronic ischemic changes previously documented in this patient. Comparing the pre- (B) and postcontrast (C) axial T$_1$-weighted scans, abnormal contrast enhancement is noted anteriorly, matching in position the lesion on the T$_2$-weighted scan. On the coronal postcontrast T$_1$-weighted scan (D), it is somewhat easier to recognize that the abnormal contrast enhancement lies within the ACA distribution. Enhancement is present because of blood-brain barrier disruption in this subacute lesion. Compared with middle and posterior cerebral artery infarcts, ACA infarcts are much less common. Familiarity with the arterial distribution of the vessel and greater awareness of this entity make misdiagnosis less likely.

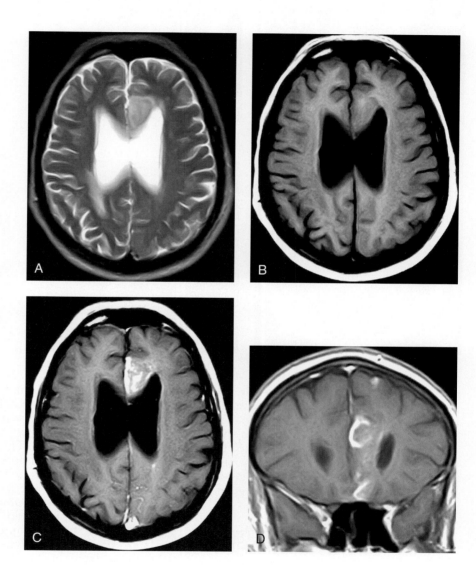

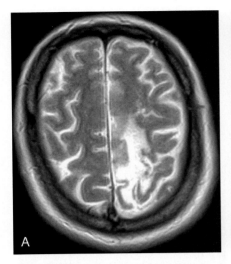

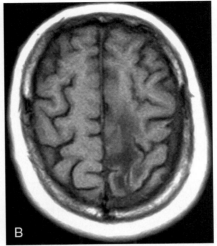

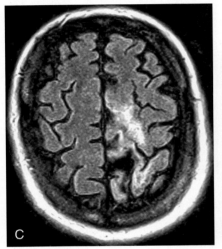

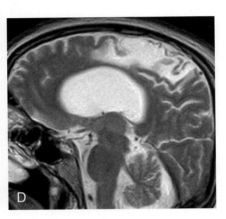

FIGURE 3–17. Chronic anterior cerebral artery (ACA) infarction. The posterior portion of the ACA territory on the left has abnormal hyperintensity on the T₂-weighted scan (*A*) and hypointensity on the T₁-weighted scan (*B*). *C*, The fluid-attenuated inversion recovery scan reveals the abnormality to be part gliosis (with high signal intensity) and part cystic encephalomalacia (with low signal intensity). *D*, The sagittal T₂-weighted scan just to the left of midline also clearly depicts the involvement of the posterior medial frontal lobe.

artery (PICA) supplies the retro-olivary medulla, the cerebellar tonsil, the inferior vermis, and the posterior lateral inferior cerebellum (Fig. 3–19). The anteroinferior cerebellar artery (AICA) supplies the anterolateral inferior cerebellum. Infarction restricted to the distribution of AICA is extremely rare. The superior cerebellar artery (SCA) supplies the superior cerebellum (Figs. 3–20 and 3–21). Cerebellar infarcts present with vertigo, nausea, poor balance, and dysarthria.

THROMBOTIC INFARCTION

Arterial thrombotic infarction occurs when the arterial lumen is narrowed significantly and blood clots form that occlude the artery. Degenerative atherosclerotic disease, inflammatory disease, or arterial dissection can cause arterial narrowing, although atherosclerotic disease is by far the most common cause. In atherosclerosis, there is degeneration of the intima and media of the arterial wall, with associated proliferation of these elements and lipid deposition. Atherosclerotic lesions or plaques occur at arterial branch points, which are the sites of greatest mechanical stress and turbulence. An atherosclerotic plaque slowly enlarges with time. A criti-

cal size is reached, and the surface of the plaque fissures and ulcerates. Platelets adhere to the irregular plaque surface and release prostaglandins, which promote deposition of additional platelet-fibrin plugs and clot on the plaque surface. Thrombosis then occurs, which results in arterial occlusion.

Atherosclerotic thrombotic infarction typically involves large arteries and causes major arterial branch distribution ischemic infarction. Atherosclerotic thrombosis most commonly involves the middle cerebral artery (50%), the internal carotid artery (25%), and the vertebrobasilar system (25%). The extent of infarction is determined by the location of obstruction (the more proximal the lesion, the less likely is the development of infarction), availability of collateral circulation, extent of occlusion, and state of the systemic circulation.

Atherosclerotic disease occurs more commonly in patients with hypertension, hypercholesterolemia, or hyperlipidemia and in those who smoke. Sex and race impact the distribution of lesions. In white men, atherosclerotic lesions predominate at the carotid bifurcation, at the carotid siphon, and in the vertebrobasilar system. White men also have a high incidence of vascular occlusive disease, hypertension, and hyperlipidemia. In women, blacks, and persons of Chinese or Japanese

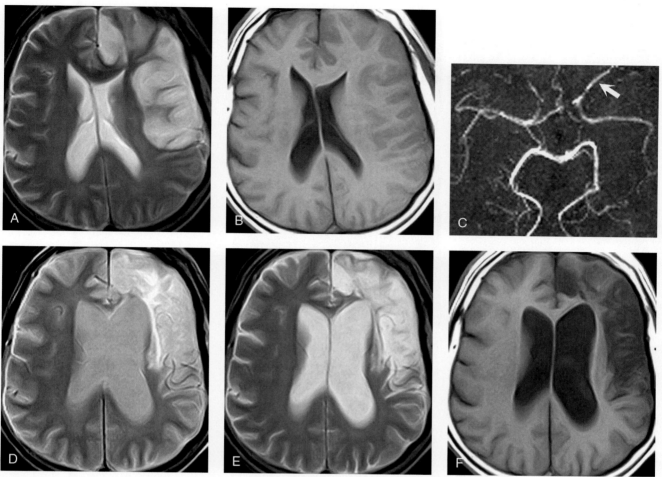

FIGURE 3–18. Combined anterior cerebral artery (ACA) and middle cerebral artery (MCA) infarction, progressing from early subacute to chronic. Vasogenic edema causes abnormal hyperintensity in both the left ACA and MCA territories on the T_2-weighted scan (A) at clinical presentation. B, The T_1-weighted scan demonstrates sulcal effacement in the corresponding region, with moderate mass effect on the frontal horn of the lateral ventricle. The magnetic resonance (MR) scan was repeated 18 months later (C–F). At this time, three-dimensional time-of-flight MR angiography reveals collateral flow from the external carotid artery to the supraclinoid internal carotid artery via the ophthalmic artery (*white arrow*). D, The axial scan with intermediate T_2-weighting reveals a mix of gliosis and encephalomalacia in the left ACA and MCA territories. The combined distribution of the two vessels is clearly depicted on the heavily T_2-weighted scan (E) with abnormal hyperintensity and the T_1-weighted scan (F) with abnormal hypointensity. Ex vacuo dilatation of the left lateral ventricle is also noted.

ancestry, atherosclerotic lesions predominate in the intracranial arteries. The common locations are the supraclinoid internal carotid arteries, the anterior, middle, and posterior cerebral arteries, and the vertebrobasilar branches supplying the cerebellum. These patients also have a high incidence of diabetes and hypertension.

The MRI findings in thrombotic cerebral infarction are an area of increased water content, with high signal intensity on T_2-weighted images and mild low signal intensity on T_1-weighted images, that is strictly confined to a major arterial vascular distribution. The distribution is that of the occluded artery. Characteristically, thrombotic infarcts are sharply demarcated, wedge-shaped lesions that extend to the cortical surface. However, depending on the extent and location of the occlusion and the status of the collateral circulation, thrombotic infarcts can have a variety of configurations. Regardless, the signal changes remain confined to a vascular distribution. For this reason, knowledge of the arterial territories of the brain is important.

The signal intensity characteristics of other brain abnormalities, in particular hyperacute hemorrhage, neoplastic disease, and inflammatory disease, can be similar to those of thrombotic infarction. Fortunately, additional findings on MRI assist in distinction of these entities. A hyperacute intraparenchymal hematoma is typically a round focal mass that is not localized to an arterial territory. Hematomas also have a characteristic temporal progression in signal intensity characteristics. Most thrombotic infarctions involve both gray and white matter. In contrast, neoplastic and inflammatory lesions (abscesses) are usually centered in the white matter. Neoplasms can on occasion extend to the cortex. The edema associated with a neoplasm extends diffusely into the adjacent white matter in finger-like projections, has ill-defined margins, and is unlikely to be restricted to an arterial distribution. Contrast enhancement adds further specificity to the MRI scan. A central enhancing mass is often seen with neoplastic and inflammatory disease. Contrast enhancement in cerebral infarction, although

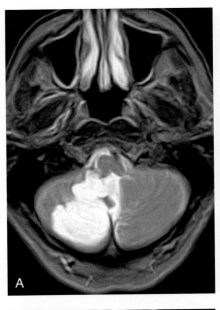

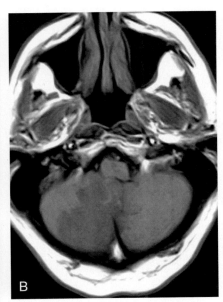

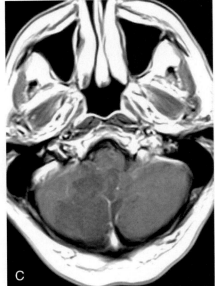

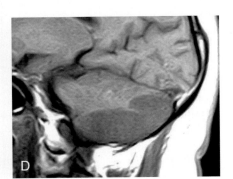

FIGURE 3–19. Early subacute posteroinferior cerebellar artery (PICA) infarction. There is abnormal hyperintensity on the T$_2$-weighted scan (A) and hypointensity on the T$_1$-weighted scan (B) in the posteroinferior cerebellum. Cerebellar tissue anteriorly and laterally, the distribution of anteroinferior cerebellar artery, is spared. C, The lesion is essentially unchanged postcontrast. The PICA distribution of this infarct is also well depicted in the sagittal plane (D) (precontrast, T$_1$-weighted).

FIGURE 3–20. Early subacute superior cerebellar artery (SCA) infarction. A, The T$_2$-weighted scan shows a wedge of vasogenic edema, with abnormal hyperintensity, in a portion of the left SCA territory. The scan plane is through the superior portion of the cerebellum and the occipital lobes. The outer edge of the lesion borders the tentorium. B, The postcontrast T$_1$-weighted scan demonstrates subtle abnormal hypointensity in the same region but no abnormal enhancement. There is mild mass effect, causing slight compression of the fourth ventricle.

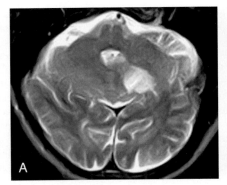

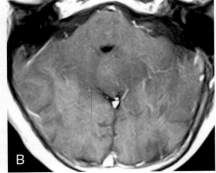

FIGURE 3–21. Late subacute superior cerebellar artery (SCA) infarction. The entire left SCA distribution is involved, with vasogenic edema noted on the T$_2$-weighted scan (*A*) and parenchymal enhancement on the postcontrast T$_1$-weighted scan (*B*). Although edema is present and the lesion is large, there is little mass effect, which would have resolved by this time in evolution of the lesion.

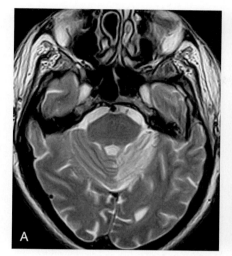
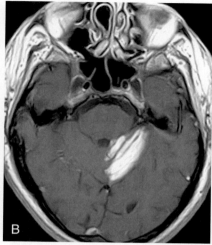

variable in type (depending on the age of the lesion), should conform to the wedge-shaped distribution of the arterial vessel. Despite these features, some lesions, particularly demyelinating disease, may be difficult to distinguish from bland thrombotic infarction.

MRI also provides substantial information about vascular patency. The major cerebral arteries are consistently visualized as signal voids because of rapid blood flow on spin echo scans. The absence of a normal flow void in a major cerebral vessel is presumptive evidence of occlusion. Three-dimensional time-of-flight MRA also elegantly displays the arterial vasculature. MRA clearly depicts vessel occlusions, segmental narrowing, and routes of collateral flow.

EMBOLIC INFARCTION

In embolic cerebral infarction, the occlusive material originates from an area proximal to the occluded artery. Emboli most frequently arise from the heart or from atherosclerotic plaques involving the carotid bifurcation or vertebral arteries. The common causes of cardiac emboli include thrombi associated with myocardial infarction or cardiac arrhythmias, valvular disease (including prosthetic valves), bacterial or nonbacterial endocarditis, and atrial myxomas. The ulceration of atherosclerotic plaques produces cholesterol or calcific emboli. Rare embolic causes of infarction are nitrogen emboli from rapid decompensation, fat emboli from long bone fractures, and iatrogenic air emboli.

The location and temporal evolution of embolic infarction differ from thrombotic infarction. Embolic particles shower the intracranial cerebral circulation, often causing multiple peripheral infarcts in different major arterial distributions. Embolic occlusions frequently fragment and lyse between the first and fifth days, which re-establishes normal circulation. These findings differ from the relatively permanent occlusion of a single major vascular distribution with atherosclerotic thrombotic infarction. Fragmentation and lysis of embolic occlusion produces a higher perfusion pressure than that seen with

simple occlusion (in which collateral vessels supply the circulation). There is also a loss of normal autoregulation of the cerebral vasculature, which can persist for several weeks. These factors produce hyperemia or luxury perfusion, with blood flow to the infarcted region greater than its metabolic requirements. This higher perfusion pressure can also cause hemorrhage into the infarct and conversion of a bland anemic infarct into a hemorrhagic one. This hemorrhage usually occurs between 6 hours and 2 weeks after the embolic event. Anticoagulant treatment of bland anemic infarcts can also result in hemorrhage.

Before lysis of the embolus, the MRI appearance of embolic infarction is similar to that of thrombotic infarction. However, in contrast to thrombotic infarctions, embolic infarctions are often multiple, may be located in more than one vascular distribution, and are approximately of the same age. After fragmentation of the embolus and the subsequent increase in perfusion pressure, a hemorrhagic infarction often develops. Most commonly, the hemorrhage in a hemorrhagic embolic infarction is petechial in nature and cortical in location. Occasionally, an intraparenchymal hematoma develops in the infarcted region. Development of secondary hemorrhage is characteristic of embolic infarction but can be seen with thrombotic or hemodynamic infarction.

HEMODYNAMIC INFARCTION

Hemodynamic infarction occurs because of the failure of the heart to pump sufficient blood to oxygenate the brain. Common causes of hypoperfusion include cardiac failure, cardiac arrhythmias, and hypovolemia after blood loss. Patients may have concomitant systemic hypertension, a subcritical arterial stenosis, or even arterial occlusion that had been adequately perfused by collaterals. With development of systemic hypoperfusion and decreased perfusion pressure to the brain, areas of the brain that were adequately perfused are now underperfused, leading to cerebral ischemia or infarction. In many patients, this ischemic event occurs at night while

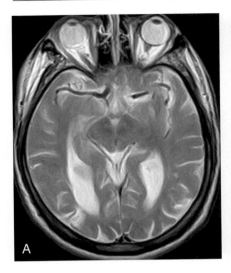
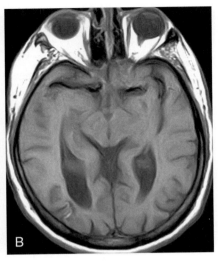

FIGURE 3–22. Chronic hemodynamic infarction. *A,* Gliosis and encephalomalacia are seen on the T₂-weighted scan at the junction of the right middle cerebral artery and posterior cerebral artery territories. *B,* The precontrast T₁-weighted scan reveals petechial hemorrhage (methemoglobin) in the same watershed distribution.

they are asleep, probably because of a nocturnal reduction in blood pressure.

The areas of the brain most commonly involved in hemodynamic infarction are the watershed regions located at the margins of the major arterial distributions (Fig. 3–22). These regions are the terminal areas supplied by each major artery. They have the lowest perfusion pressure in that vascular distribution. Watershed areas are more prone to ischemic insults caused by systemic hypoperfusion. Knowledge of the arterial vascular territories is necessary to recognize these hemodynamic watershed infarcts. In the cerebral cortex, these watershed areas are located at the junctions of the regions supplied by the anterior, middle, and posterior cerebral arteries. The parieto-occipital watershed region is particularly susceptible to hemodynamic ischemic injury because this region is at the peripheral junction of the anterior, middle, and posterior cerebral arterial distributions. In the cerebellum, a watershed region exists at the junction of the territories of the superior cerebellar and inferior cerebellar arteries.

The MRI findings in hemodynamic infarction are increased tissue water content in the distribution of the watershed or border zones of the major arterial vascular distributions. Often the deep periventricular white matter is preferentially involved. White matter receives less blood flow than gray matter and is probably more susceptible to ischemia with a decrease in perfusion. Common locations of white matter hemodynamic infarctions are superior and lateral to the body and trigone of the lateral ventricles. The deep basal ganglia supplied by the lenticulostriate arteries can be similarly affected.

Trauma, with brain contusion and secondary ischemia, can lead to an imaging appearance similar to hemodynamic or thrombotic infarction. Awareness of this entity and access to clinical information is important for appropriate diagnosis (Fig. 3–23).

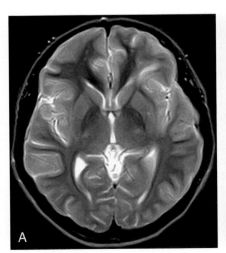
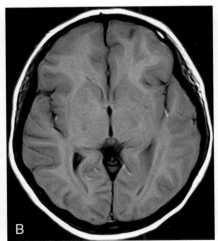
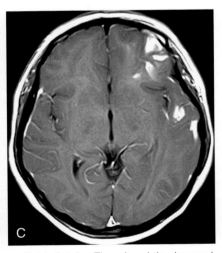

FIGURE 3–23. Cortical contusion. A young adult presents several days after a severe fall down a flight of stairs. There is subtle abnormal high signal intensity within the left frontal white matter on the T₂-weighted scan (*A*). The precontrast T₁-weighted scan (*B*) is unremarkable. *C,* Postcontrast, gyriform enhancement is noted in several locations, all within cortical gray matter of the frontal lobe. Contusion of the brain cortex has led to blood-brain barrier disruption, which better demonstrates (more so than vasogenic edema) the extent of injury in this case. It is important to note that gyriform contrast enhancement is not specific for infarction because of cerebrovascular disease and can occur in other situations such as trauma (in this instance).

LACUNAR INFARCTION

Lacunar infarcts or lacunes are small, deep cerebral infarcts involving the penetrating arteries that supply the basal ganglia, internal capsule, thalamus, and brainstem. These small arteries arise from the major cerebral arteries and include the lenticulostriate branches of the anterior and middle cerebral arteries, the thalamoperforating branches of the posterior cerebral arteries, and the paramedian branches of the basilar artery. These penetrating arteries are small end arteries (100-500 μm in diameter) that are difficult to evaluate angiographically. Most of these arteries are unbranching single vessels with essentially no collateral circulation. For these anatomic reasons, deep lacunar infarcts typically are spherical in shape and range from 0.3 to 2.5 cm in diameter (Fig. 3–24). The larger lacunes typically result from more proximal obstructions.

Lacunar infarcts are commonly seen in patients older than 60 years with hypertension. Because this population is also prone to chronic small vessel disease, identifica-tion of small recent lacunar infarcts superimposed on chronic disease can be difficult. Diffusion imaging is extremely helpful in acute and early subacute infarcts in this regard. Contrast enhancement is likewise extremely helpful in identifying late subacute infarcts (Fig. 3–25).

The pathogenesis of lacunar infarction is as follows. Chronic hypertension causes degeneration of the tunica media (i.e., arteriosclerosis), with hyalin deposition in the artery wall that narrows the lumen. Plaque or thrombosis, called microatheroma, may subsequently occlude these vessels, particularly the larger vessels. The weakened tunica media also predisposes to the formation of microaneurysms, which can rupture, causing an intraparenchymal hematoma. A hypertensive hemorrhage or hypertensive hemorrhagic infarction has a characteristic location in the deep cerebral structures supplied by these deep penetrating arteries. Other uncommon causes of lacunar infarction include secondary arteritis caused by meningitis, microemboli, and arterial dissection.

Lacunar infarction is often recognized by a distinctive clinical presentation. A pure motor stroke is the most

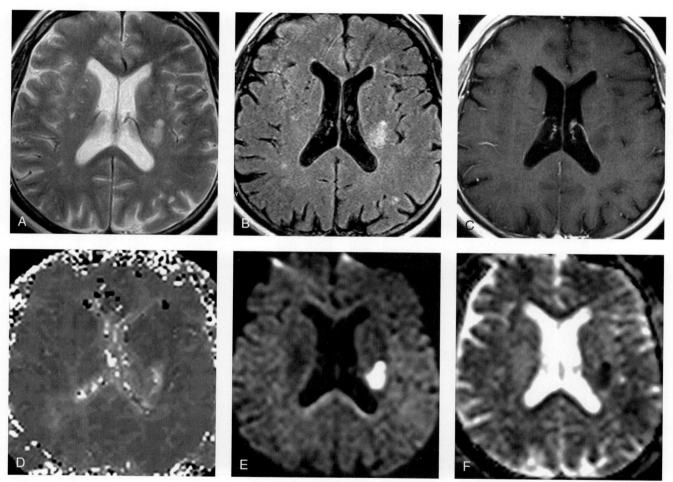

FIGURE 3–24. Early subacute lacunar infarction involving the posterior limb of the left internal capsule. Vasogenic edema is noted (with abnormal high signal intensity) on the T_2-weighted fast spin echo (A) and fluid-attenuated inversion recovery (B) scans. There is corresponding abnormal low signal intensity on the postcontrast T_1-weighted scan (C). However, there is no abnormal contrast enhancement (with disruption of the blood-brain barrier yet to occur). The mean transit time (MTT) for the lesion is prolonged, as seen on a calculated MTT image (D) from a first-pass perfusion study. E, Diffusion weighted imaging and the apparent diffusion coefficient map (F) reveal the presence of cytotoxic edema, as would be anticipated in an infarct less than 1 week old.

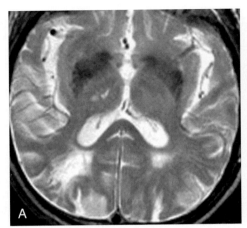 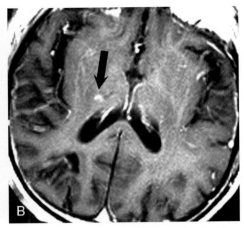

FIGURE 3–25. Late subacute lacunar infarction involving the posterior limb of the right internal capsule. The patient is an elderly diabetic who presented with acute hemiparesis. The magnetic resonance exam was obtained 10 days after presentation, at which time the hemiparesis had resolved. Multiple high signal intensity abnormalities are noted bilaterally on the T$_2$-weighted scan (A). The postcontrast T$_1$-weighted scan (B) reveals punctate enhancement (arrow) in the posterior limb of the right internal capsule. This corresponds to a high signal intensity lesion on the T$_2$-weighted scan. By identification of abnormal contrast enhancement, this subacute infarct can be differentiated from other chronic ischemic lesions, which are incidental to the patient's current medical problems.

common clinical syndrome, accounting for 30% to 60% of lacunar infarcts. A pure sensory stroke, combined sensorimotor stroke, ataxic hemiparesis, dysarthria (or "clumsy hand syndrome"), and brainstem syndromes are other characteristic clinical presentations of lacunar infarction. Patients with lacunar infarction often have a gradual progression of symptoms. An antecedent TIA occurs in approximately 25% of patients with lacunar infarction.

On MRI, lacunar infarcts appear as focal slitlike or ovoid areas of increased water content. They are high signal intensity on T$_2$-weighted images and isointense to low signal intensity on T$_1$-weighted images (Fig. 3–26). T$_2$-weighted scans are more sensitive than T$_1$-weighted scans for detection. In acute lacunar infarction, vasogenic edema may not be present; thus, diffusion-weighted scans are important for detection. Fluid-attenuated inversion recovery (FLAIR) scans are helpful in identifying small lacunes and differentiating them from spaces containing cerebrospinal fluid (CSF). If FLAIR is not an option, then spin echo scans with intermediate T$_2$-weighting provide similar information. On either type of scan, lacunar infarcts appear as small high-signal-intensity focal lesions and can be easily distinguished

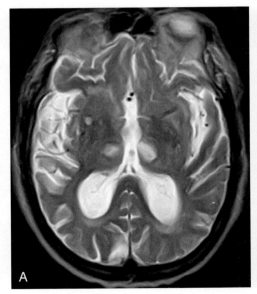 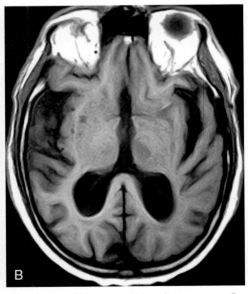

FIGURE 3–26. Early subacute thalamic infarction. A, Two round lesions, with abnormal high signal intensity corresponding to vasogenic edema, are noted medially on the T$_2$-weighted scan. The smaller lies in the right thalamus, the larger in the left thalamus. There is subtle low signal intensity in the corresponding areas on the T$_1$-weighted precontrast scan (B). There was no abnormal contrast enhancement (not shown). Thalamic lesions are easily missed by inexperienced film readers, leading to the recommendation that the thalamus be visually checked for abnormalities on each scan.

from the intermediate to low signal intensity of normal surrounding brain and CSF. MRI is much more sensitive than CT in detecting lacunar infarcts. Contrast enhancement of subacute lacunar infarcts, after intravenous gadolinium chelate administration, is consistently seen on MRI (Fig. 3–27). Enhancement occurs as a result of blood-brain-barrier disruption. Chronic lacunar infarcts are characterized by focal cavitation and a more pronounced decreased signal intensity on T_1-weighted images than in the earlier stages of lacunar infarction. These chronic (cavitated) lacunar infarcts are isointense with CSF on all imaging sequences.

Penetrating vessels from the basilar artery and adjacent segments of the posterior cerebral arteries supply the brainstem. Infarcts involving the pons are most frequently small, unilateral, and sharply margined at the midline. This location reflects the distribution of paramedian penetrating arteries, which consist of paired branches. Bilateral pontine infarcts do occur but are less common than unilateral infarcts. Lateral pontine infarction is extremely uncommon. The predominant finding on MRI in early subacute pontine infarction is

vasogenic edema (Fig. 3–28). Contrast enhancement is consistently seen in late subacute pontine infarction (Fig. 3–29).

In the elderly population with arteriosclerotic disease, lateral medullary infarction (Wallenberg's syndrome) is not uncommonly encountered (Fig. 3–30). This lesion is not clearly seen on CT. It is important for the radiologist to be familiar with the MRI appearance of this lesion and for the medulla to be included in the routine search pattern. Otherwise, a lateral medullary infarct may go unrecognized. Clinical presentation includes long-tract signs (contralateral loss of pain and temperature sensation, ipsilateral ataxia, and Horner's syndrome) and involvement of cranial nerves V, VIII, IX, and X. Acute respiratory and cardiovascular complications can occur. In addition to the more common presentation resulting from thrombotic occlusion, lateral medullary infarction has also been reported after chiropractic neck manipulation. The latter occurs as a result of dissection of the vertebral artery near the atlantoaxial joint. The arteries supplying the lateral medulla typically arise from the distal vertebral artery but can originate from the

FIGURE 3–27. Late subacute lacunar (basal ganglia) infarction. On adjacent T_2-weighted fast spin echo sections (*A* and *B*), abnormal high signal intensity is noted in the globus pallidus and body of the caudate nucleus on the right. Enhancement of both lesions is seen on the corresponding postcontrast T_1-weighted sections (*C* and *D*). The use of intravenous contrast assists in lesion recognition (conspicuity) and in dating lesions. Involvement of both the globus pallidus and caudate nucleus is not uncommon and points to involvement of the lenticulostriate arteries. These small perforating vessels arise from the superior aspect of the proximal middle cerebral artery (M1 segment) and supply the globus pallidus, putamen, and caudate nuclei.

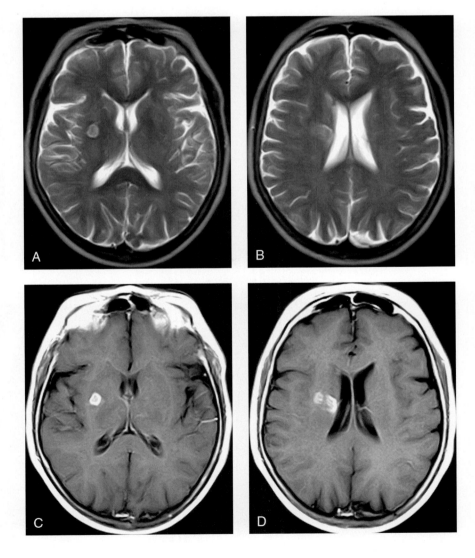

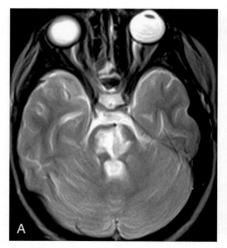
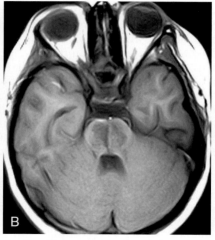
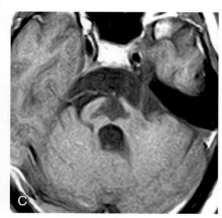

FIGURE 3–28. Early subacute bilateral pontine infarction. The central portion of the pons has abnormal high signal intensity on the T$_2$-weighted scan (*A*) and abnormal low signal intensity on the T$_1$-weighted scan (*B*). Despite the lesion being bilateral, there is some indication of a straight border along the midline. A follow-up T$_1$-weighted scan (*C*) performed 6 months later demonstrates cavitation of the lesion.

FIGURE 3–29. Late subacute pontine infarction. On the precontrast T$_2$-weighted scan (*A*), an area of abnormal hyperintensity is noted in the left pons, with a sharp line of demarcation along the median raphe. The lesion enhances on the postcontrast T$_1$-weighted scan (*B*). As with other lacunar infarcts, pontine infarcts will consistently demonstrate contrast enhancement after gadolinium chelate administration in the late subacute time period.

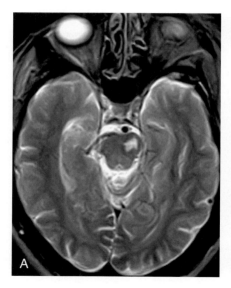
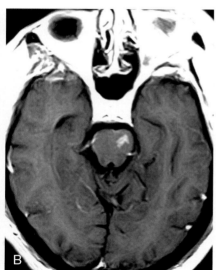

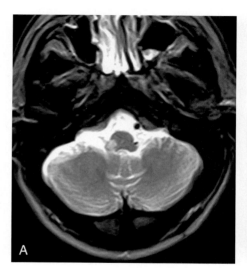
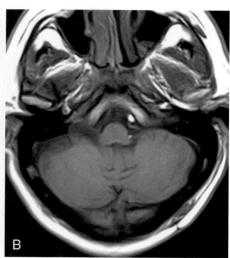

FIGURE 3–30. Lateral medullary infarction (early subacute). Abnormal hyperintensity is noted on the T$_2$-weighted scan in the right lateral medulla (*A*). The T$_1$-weighted scan (*B*) is grossly normal.

PICA. Thus, lateral medullary infarction can accompany PICA infarction. Medial medullary infarction is less common than lateral medullary infarction. The clinical presentation of medial medullary infarction is that of contralateral hemiparesis, sparing the face.

DILATED PERIVASCULAR SPACES

Dilated perivascular spaces (DPVSs) are invaginations of the subarachnoid (Virchow-Robin) space that surrounds vessels coursing through the brain. DPVSs are commonly found in the basal ganglia (Fig. 3–31) and in the periatrial and supraventricular white matter (Fig. 3–32). A third common location is the midbrain (Fig. 3–33), at the junction of the substantia nigra and cerebral peduncle. DPVSs are small, round, or linear fluid collections that lie along the distribution of penetrating vessels and have signal intensity that strictly follows CSF. Because of their location and appearance, they can mimic lacunar infarction. Therefore, correlation of the anatomic MRI abnormality with clinical history is important.

DPVSs that involve the lenticulostriate arteries supplying the basal ganglia are commonly located adjacent to the lateral aspect of the anterior commissure. Pathologically, focal fluid intensities in the region of the inferior one third of the putamen invariably prove to be DPVSs, but lesions in the upper two thirds are commonly lacunar infarctions. DPVSs that surround middle cerebral artery branches located in the white matter of the centrum semiovale are seen with equal frequency in

patients younger and older than 40 years. DPVSs in this location should be considered in the differential diagnosis of lacunar infarction, ischemic-gliotic white matter disease, and multiple sclerosis.

DPVSs often have MRI characteristics that allow their differentiation from lacunar infarction and other small focal lesions. DPVSs are commonly tubular in shape, and lacunar infarcts are slitlike or ovoid. On sagittal or coronal images, the tubular configuration of DPVSs along the course of the penetrating arteries can often be appreciated. DPVSs strictly follow CSF characteristics on T_1-weighted and T_2-weighted images, although volume averaging of small lesions with adjacent brain can alter signal characteristics. Acute and subacute lacunar infarcts will be higher signal intensity than CSF on T_1-weighted images, FLAIR, and spin echo scans with intermediate T_2-weighting.

CHRONIC SMALL VESSEL DISEASE

Punctate or confluent areas of increased signal intensity are commonly seen in the white matter of older patients on T_2-weighted scans (Fig. 3–34). The terms "small vessel disease" and "ischemic-gliotic disease" are used interchangeably. These hyperintense white matter foci can be seen in as many as 30% of asymptomatic patients older than 65 years. The majority of geriatric patients with cardiovascular risk factors and a history of com-

FIGURE 3–31. Dilated perivascular space (basal ganglia). A very large dilated perivascular space is noted, with cerebrospinal fluid (CSF) signal intensity on axial T_2- (*A*) and T_1-weighted (*B*) scans. This case illustrates the most common location for dilated perivascular spaces: within the inferior third of the basal ganglia and adjacent to the anterior commissure. On the sagittal T_1-weighted scan (*C*), lenticulostriate vessels can be identified coursing superior from this CSF space.

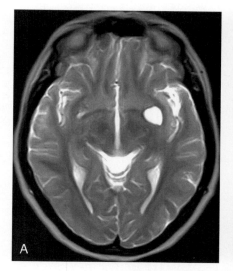
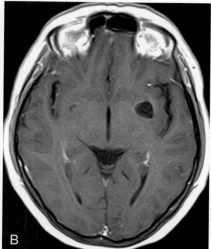
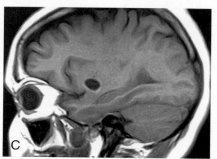

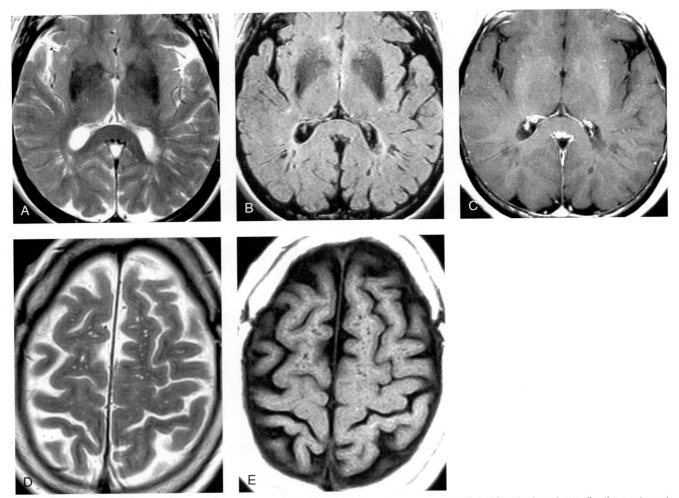

FIGURE 3–32. Periventricular (*A–C*) and high convexity (*D–E*) dilated perivascular spaces (DPVSs). After the basal ganglia, the next most common location for DPVSs is the white matter posterior and superior to the lateral ventricles. When adjacent to the trigones of the lateral ventricles (*A*, T$_2$-weighted fast spin echo; *B*, T$_2$-weighted fluid-attenuated inversion recovery; *C*, postcontrast T$_1$-weighted), DPVSs are linear in shape on axial sections. In the high convexity white matter, they appear as small pinpoints on axial sections (*D*, T$_2$-weighted fast spin echo; *E*, precontrast T$_1$-weighted).

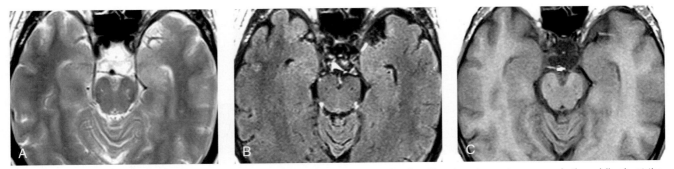

FIGURE 3–33. Midbrain dilated perivascular spaces. Another characteristic location for dilated perivascular spaces is the midbrain at the junction of the substantia nigra and cerebral peduncle. These may be unilateral or bilateral in location: the latter is illustrated here. Dilated perivascular spaces follow cerebrospinal fluid signal intensity on all pulse sequences, with high signal intensity on T$_2$-weighted fast spin echo scans (*A*) and low signal intensity on T$_2$-weighted fluid-attenuated inversion recovery (*B*) and T$_1$-weighted spin echo (*C*) scans. Dilated perivascular spaces are, however, best visualized on fast spin echo T$_2$-weighted scans.

FIGURE 3–34. Chronic small vessel ischemic disease. Multiple small foci with abnormal high signal intensity are noted in peripheral white matter on T$_2$-weighted fast spin echo (*A*) and fluid-attenuated inversion recovery (*B*) scans. The same disease process also accounts for the hyperintensity immediately adjacent to ("capping") the frontal horns and surrounding the atria of the lateral ventricles.

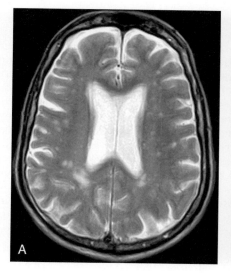
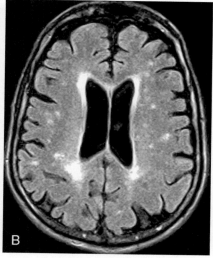

pleted stroke or ischemia (RIND or TIA) have hyperintense white matter foci. These lesions often create problems in diagnostic interpretation because of their prevalence, particularly in the asymptomatic patient, and their similarity to other lesions.

Pathologic evidence, correlated with MRI, suggests that ischemia and infarction produce the majority of these lesions. One study found white matter atrophy and gliosis surrounding thickened vessels in the region of the hyperintense MRI white matter foci. The authors postulated that increased extracellular water is responsible for the increased signal intensity on T$_2$-weighted scans. They also suggested the cause to be chronic, mild vascular insufficiency rather than thrombotic or embolic occlusive infarction. True white matter infarction was commonly the cause of hyperintense MRI white matter foci. Central necrosis, axonal loss, and demyelination were found to be compatible with true infarction.

Because ischemia and infarction appear to be the predominant causes of hyperintense white matter foci in older patients, and because infarction often has a significant component of gliosis, we refer to these lesions as ischemic-gliotic disease and describe the degree of involvement as mild, moderate, or severe. In mild cases, there are a few scattered, small, hyperintense, white matter lesions. In severe cases, there can be confluent increased signal intensity in the white matter on T$_2$-weighted scans. In moderate cases, the changes are intermediate in nature. In patients with diffuse white matter disease, diffusion imaging and postcontrast scans can be useful in distinguishing areas of acute and subacute infarction from chronic disease.

There are other, less common causes of hyperintense white matter lesions that should be recognized. Plaques of multiple sclerosis can occur with minimal clinical symptoms. In these subclinical cases, the lesions tend to be small and involve only the supratentorial white matter, sparing the brainstem and cerebellum. Brain cysts and congenital ventricular diverticula have increased signal intensity on T$_2$-weighted images but are uncommon. These lesions characteristically border the ventricular system or subarachnoid space, have a smooth rounded

configuration, and have CSF signal intensity on all pulse sequences. Occasionally, a cavitated infarct becomes cystic and displays similar signal intensity characteristics. Dilated perivascular spaces can also mimic other focal white matter lesions and lacunar infarcts. Binswanger's disease (subcortical arteriosclerotic encephalopathy) represents a distinct clinical entity with characteristic clinical findings in patients with hypertension, hydrocephalus, and dementia. These patients have rapid deterioration of their cognitive ability, gradual development of neurologic symptoms, and a lengthy clinical course with long plateau periods. MRI demonstrates focal or confluent white matter lesions on T$_2$-weighted images. Hypertensive encephalopathy is an acute neurologic syndrome with the clinical presentation, including headache, somnolence, convulsions, and vomiting. T$_2$-weighted images demonstrate hyperintense lesions in the white matter and cerebral cortex, particularly involving the occipital lobes. Reversibility of these lesions after treatment has been reported.

ARTERITIS

Cerebral arteritis can be classified as primary or secondary. In the primary form, the inflammatory process originates in the arteries. In the secondary form, the inflammatory process starts in the brain parenchyma or meninges, and the arteries are involved secondarily. Primary cerebral arteritis often presents with recurrent neurologic symptoms that may simulate multiple sclerosis. This disease tends to affect a younger age group than arteriosclerotic vascular disease. Primary cerebral arteritis is usually caused by systemic disorders. Causes include systemic lupus erythematosus (SLE), other collagen-vascular diseases, polyarteritis nodosa, giant cell arteritis, Behçet's disease, and sarcoidosis.

Both white and gray matter involvement can be seen in SLE. There are two patterns of white matter involvement. One pattern consists of large, confluent areas of high signal intensity on T$_2$-weighted images consistent with infarction (Fig. 3–35). The other pattern consists of small focal punctate white matter lesions, presumably corresponding to small microinfarcts. Lesions can also involve the gray matter. In some patients with gray matter involvement, clinical resolution may be accompanied by the resolution of these lesions on MRI.

Findings similar to SLE are seen in other vasculitides, including polyarteritis nodosa. Focal brainstem infarction has been described in Behçet's disease. Some MRI findings help to differentiate arteritis from multiple sclerosis. Periventricular white matter involvement is less extensive and may be absent in primary cerebral arteritis. Multiple sclerosis is typically characterized by extensive, punctate periventricular white matter involvement (which is not symmetric from side to side). A lesion in a major cerebral artery vascular territory, or cortical involvement, favors a vascular disease process.

The cause of secondary cerebral arteritis is commonly meningitis. Bacterial or fungal organisms, including *Mycobacterium tuberculosis*, are common causes. A contrast-enhanced MRI should be performed to identify the location and extent of meningeal disease. T_2-weighted scans demonstrate high-signal-intensity lesions compatible with ischemia or infarction in the vascular distribution involved by the meningeal process.

VASOSPASM AND MIGRAINE

Spasm of the intracranial arteries can be associated with subarachnoid hemorrhage or migraine headaches. Subarachnoid hemorrhage is commonly caused by a ruptured intracranial aneurysm (75% of cases). The arteries in the affected subarachnoid space can experience varying degrees of spasm, which may progress to complete occlusion. MRI demonstrates findings compatible with ischemia or infarction involving major arterial distributions or their watershed regions, corresponding to the distribution of the artery in spasm.

Migraine headaches are initiated by vasoconstriction of extracranial and intracranial arteries. This leads to ischemia, which produces neurologic deficits or an aura. Vasoconstriction is followed by vasodilatation, which produces the headache. CT and MRI findings consistent with ischemia or infarction have been described in these patients. MRI demonstrates focal lesions with increased signal intensity on T_2-weighted images, predominantly involving the periventricular white matter but also involving the cortex. Corresponding hypointensity is seen in some lesions on T_1-weighted images. Resolution of small focal lesions can be seen on MRI with time after resolution of symptoms.

Patients with the classic or common form of migraine, visual aura that responds to ergotamine followed by a unilateral throbbing headache, have focal periventricular lesions. Patients with neurologic deficits or complicated migraine have larger periventricular lesions and often have cortical lesions. Cortical lesions in general are associated with neurologic deficits.

ANOXIA AND CARBON MONOXIDE POISONING

Cerebral anoxia has many causes, including primary and secondary respiratory failure, drowning, and carbon monoxide poisoning. The cerebral ischemia or infarction that develops initially involves the regions of the brain in which the blood supply is most tenuous. The watershed regions of the cortex, periventricular white matter, and the basal ganglia are particularly prone to ischemic injury. In severe cases, the cortex, white matter, and basal ganglia can be diffusely involved (Fig. 3–36). Patients with irreversible injury demonstrate focal areas of necrosis or demyelination.

In children, the distribution of hypoxic-ischemic brain injury is related to the degree of development. In premature infants, the periventricular corona radiata is most predisposed to ischemic injury. These patients may later experience delayed myelination, periventricular leukomalacia (Fig. 3–37), cerebral atrophy, and hydrocephalus. In full-term infants and young children, the cortical and subcortical regions are most prone to infarction. The full-term infant and older child no longer have the collaterals between the meninges and cerebral arteries that protect the cortex as in the premature infant.

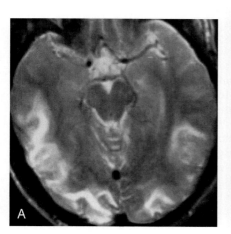
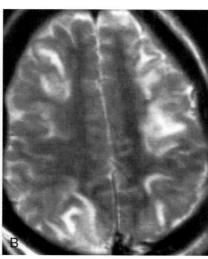

FIGURE 3–35. Systemic lupus erythematosus. *A* and *B*, T_2-weighted scans reveal multiple bilateral parenchymal abnormalities. These lesions, which correspond to territorial infarcts, involve both gray and white matter in both the anterior and middle cerebral artery distributions.

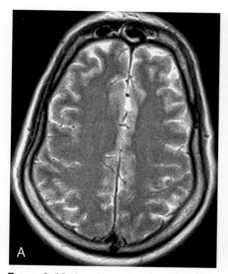
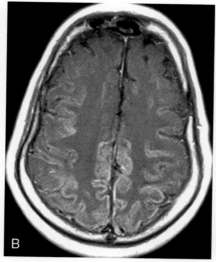
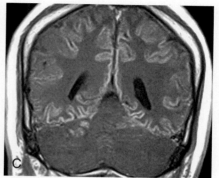

FIGURE 3–36. Anoxic brain injury. *A*, At first glance, the T$_2$-weighted scan appears normal. In retrospect, there is loss of the gray-white matter differentiation. Axial (*B*) and coronal (*C*) T$_1$-weighted scans show reversal of the normal signal intensity relationship of gray and white matter. White matter has abnormal low signal intensity as a result of global vasogenic edema.

MRI demonstrates increased signal intensity on T$_2$-weighted images and isointense or low signal intensity on T$_1$-weighted images in the ischemic or infarcted regions. In the infant, attention to imaging technique and scan interpretation are important to differentiate edema from the normal high water content of white matter at this age (Fig. 3–38). In the premature infant, ultrasonography may be a more useful modality for evaluating infarction. Increased iron deposition in infarcted regions in children who survive a severe ischemic-anoxic insult has been described. This iron deposition may be produced by disruption of normal axonal transport of brain iron by injury. It is more evident at higher field strengths and with gradient echo imaging.

Focal areas of ischemic necrosis are seen in carbon monoxide poisoning. Four types of lesions are described in pathologic studies: necrotic lesions of the globus pallidus, focal necrotic white matter lesions or confluent demyelination, spongy lesions in the cerebral cortex, and necrotic lesions of the hippocampus. Frequently, MRI demonstrates only abnormal high signal intensity in the globus pallidus bilaterally (on T$_2$-weighted images). All four types of lesions can, however, be seen on MRI.

ARTERIAL DISSECTION

Arterial dissection is often overlooked as a cause of cerebral ischemia or infarction. Arterial dissection may be caused by trauma, diseases intrinsic to the arterial wall, or local inflammatory disease, or it may have a spontaneous onset. Arteriography has been the best modality for diagnosing arterial dissection, but findings may be nonspecific. MRI is a sensitive and noninvasive method for identifying the hemorrhagic component of a dissection. MRI can provide a definitive diagnosis in patients with nonspecific arteriographic findings and is useful in monitoring the resolution of these lesions.

The temporal sequence of MRI changes in an arterial dissection with intramural hemorrhage is similar to that

FIGURE 3–37. Periventricular leukomalacia. Abnormal increased signal intensity, resulting from gliosis, is noted on the T$_2$-weighted scan in the periventricular white matter (*A*). The amount of periventricular white matter is also decreased, particularly in the periatrial region, as best seen on the T$_1$-weighted scan (*B*). The patient is a 17-month-old infant with mild paralysis affecting the lower extremities (paraparesis).

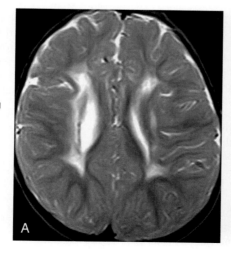
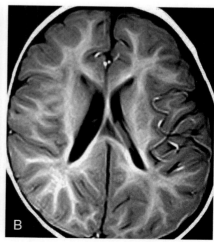

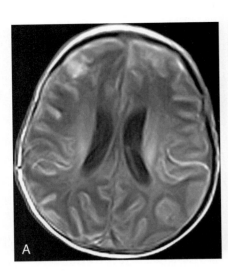
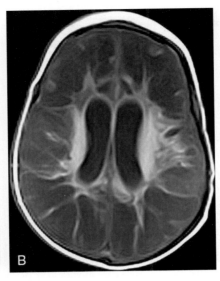

FIGURE 3–38. Neonatal infarction. *A*, On this T₁-weighted scan of a 1-month-old infant, gray and white matter appear normal at first glance. In the neonate, before myelinization, white matter will be of lower signal intensity than gray matter on T₁-weighted scans. However, in this case, a focus of abnormal hyperintensity is seen in the right frontal lobe corresponding to hemorrhage (methemoglobin). Alerted by this finding, and looking more closely, it is noted that the gray matter mantle is too thin and that the gray-white matter contrast is accentuated (with white matter of too low signal intensity). Global infarction is confirmed on the follow-up scan (*B*) 1 month later, which demonstrates cystic encephalomalacia sparing only the immediate periventricular white matter.

of an intraparenchymal hematoma. Hemosiderin is not deposited because the blood-brain barrier is not present. Subacute hemorrhagic dissection (containing extracellular methemoglobin) appears as a hyperintense lesion on T₁- and T₂-weighted images that expands the wall of the vessel and narrows its lumen. Axial images best demonstrate the intramural hemorrhage because the artery is visualized in cross-section. Sagittal images are difficult to interpret because of vascular tortuosity, volume averaging of the vessel, and the similarity of the linear, hyperintense intramural hematoma to an interstitial fat plane.

An acute intramural hemorrhage may be difficult to diagnose because deoxyhemoglobin has low signal intensity on T₂-weighted images, thus simulating a flow void. On T₁-weighted images, an absence of the normal flow void indicates thrombosis. Phase images, gradient echo scans emphasizing flow, and time-of-flight MRA are useful in detecting the presence or absence of flow in these cases.

MOYAMOYA

Moyamoya is an ischemic vascular disease of unknown cause. There is progressive stenosis or occlusion of the supraclinoid segments of the internal carotid arteries. This is accompanied by the development of lenticulostriate and thalamoperforate collaterals. The proximal portions of the anterior, middle, and posterior cerebral arteries may also be involved. There is endothelial hyperplasia and fibrosis but no evidence of inflammatory disease. The disease usually develops during childhood, and children typically present with ischemic symptoms. Adults with the disease commonly present with subarachnoid or intracranial hemorrhage. There is an increased incidence of moyamoya in the Japanese population.

Angiography has been the procedure of choice in confirming the diagnosis. Arterial stenoses and occlusions and the vascular blush of the collaterals are charac-

teristic of the disease. This vascular blush is called moyamoya, or "puff of smoke," in Japanese.

Characteristic MRI findings have been described for moyamoya. These include multiple bilateral infarctions involving the watershed regions of the carotid circulations, absence of the signal flow void in the supraclinoid internal carotid artery or middle cerebral artery, and visualization of the dilated collateral moyamoya vessels as multiple signal flow voids (Fig. 3–39).

AMYLOID ANGIOPATHY

Amyloid angiopathy is an uncommon cause of nonhypertensive hemorrhage in older patients. Amyloid deposits are identified in small and medium-sized arteries and arterioles in the cerebral cortex. The temporal, parietal, and occipital lobes are most frequently involved. In particular, the calcarine region of the occipital lobe is commonly involved. These pathologic findings probably reflect changes of aging. The amyloid deposition in the vessel wall presumably increases vessel fragility, which predisposes to rupture of the vessel and hemorrhage. The autopsy incidence of this disease is 40% in patients older than 70 years and 60% or greater in patients older than 80 years. Noncortical arteries of the brain are not involved. Cortical hemorrhages, which may extend into subcortical locations, suggest this disease in older patients. Subarachnoid hemorrhage is commonly an associated finding because of the peripheral location of the cortical hemorrhages.

VENOUS THROMBOSIS

Cerebral venous thrombosis may involve any of the cerebral veins, including the major venous sinuses, cortical veins, and deep veins. The clinical diagnosis of this disease is difficult because of nonspecific signs and symptoms. Because of the high incidence of morbidity and mortality, prompt recognition is important to improve patient outcome.

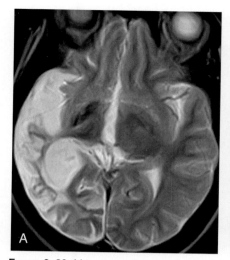
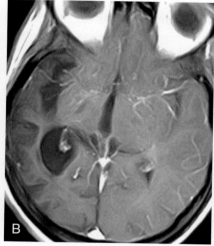
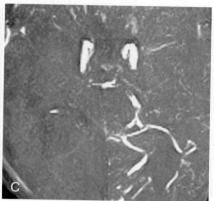

FIGURE 3–39. Moyamoya disease. An old right middle cerebral artery (MCA) infarct is noted on T$_2$- (*A*) and T$_1$-weighted (*B*) scans. The patient is only 27 years old. The perforating arteries feeding the basal ganglia appear prominent, particularly on the left, on the T$_1$-weighted scan (which is postcontrast). *C*, Three-dimensional time-of-flight magnetic resonance angiography demonstrates occlusion of both internal carotid arteries just before their division into the anterior cerebral artery and MCA.

Cerebral venous thrombosis can be divided into two major etiologic categories: inflammatory and noninflammatory. Before the advent of antibiotics, inflammatory causes, particularly mastoid sinus disease, were common causes of cerebral veno-occlusive disease. Inflammatory causes are relatively uncommon today, but there are many noninflammatory causes. Venous thrombosis associated with pregnancy and the puerperium, trauma, dehydration, neoplasm, the use of oral contraceptives, or L-asparaginase therapy are today the most common causes.

MRI provides a sensitive, noninvasive means for evaluating cerebral venous thrombosis. There is an orderly temporal evolution of MRI findings. Initially, the absence of a normal flow void is seen on T$_1$-weighted images. In this stage, the thrombus appears as intermediate signal intensity on T$_1$-weighted images. On T$_2$-weighted images, there is low signal intensity in the corresponding region. These findings are due to the presence of deoxyhemoglobin. The low signal intensity on T$_2$-weighted images is more pronounced with increased field strength. A supportive finding is the identification of venous collaterals bypassing the obstruction. Later, the thrombus becomes high signal intensity, initially on T$_1$-weighted images and subsequently on T$_2$-weighted images. These findings are due to the formation of methemoglobin (Fig. 3–40). Long-term, the vessel can recanalize, and flow voids are again visualized.

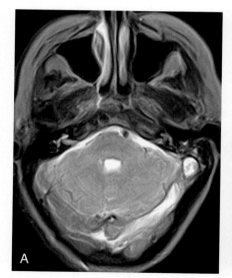
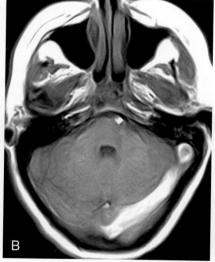
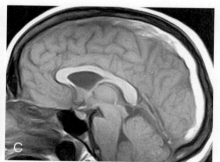

FIGURE 3–40. Superior sagittal and transverse sinus thrombosis. On precontrast T$_2$- (*A*) and T$_1$-weighted (*B*) scans, the left transverse sinus has abnormal hyperintensity. This suggests occlusion (with the signal intensity caused by extracellular methemoglobin), which is supported by the lack of venous pulsation artifacts. Thrombosis is confirmed by visualization of the same signal intensity within the sinus on an orthogonal plane; the sagittal T$_1$-weighted scan (*C*) is chosen to illustrate this and to show occlusion of the superior sagittal sinus as well.

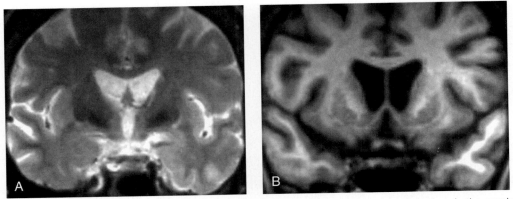

Figure 3–41. Huntington's disease. Coronal T_2- (*A*) and T_1-weighted (*B*) scans reveal substantial volume loss in the caudate nucleus bilaterally.

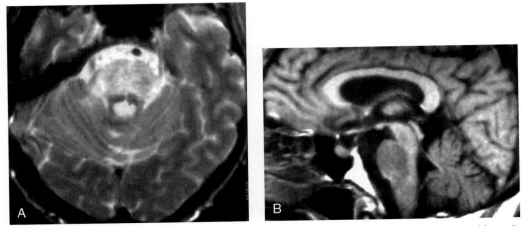

Figure 3–42. Central pontine myelinolysis. The pons and middle cerebellar peduncles have abnormal high signal intensity on the axial T_2-weighted scan (*A*). The pons also demonstrates abnormal low signal intensity on the sagittal T_1-weighted scan (*B*). In this instance, the pons is involved in its entirety. In mild cases, the abnormality may be confined to a smaller central triangular region.

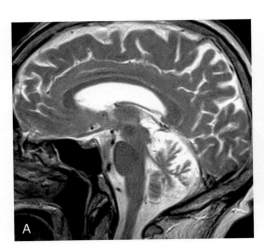

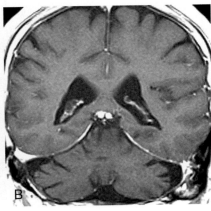

Figure 3–43. Cerebellar degenerative disease (alcoholic). *A*, The midline sagittal T_2-weighted scan demonstrates marked atrophy of the cerebellar vermis. The folia are small and the sulci enlarged. *B*, The coronal postcontrast T_1-weighted scan demonstrates atrophy of the cerebellar hemispheres as well. The cerebellar atrophy is disproportionate relative to the cerebral atrophy, which is mild at most.

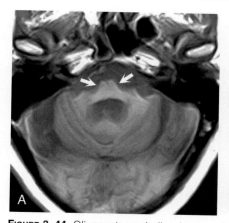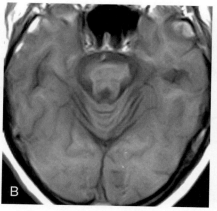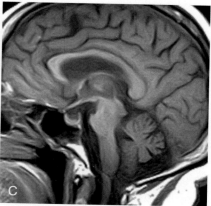

FIGURE 3–44. Olivopontocerebellar degeneration. *A*, The axial T$_1$-weighted scan at the level of the fourth ventricle demonstrates loss of the normal olivary bulge bilaterally (*arrows*) and atrophy of the middle cerebellar peduncles. Pontine and cerebellar atrophy is noted on additional axial (*B*) and sagittal (*C*) T$_1$-weighted scans.

Slow flow in a normally patent vein can produce high or intermediate signal intensity and can have the appearance of a thrombus on a single sequence. Flow-related enhancement and even-echo rephasing must be recognized as such and identified as representing normal venous flow. However, a thrombus will maintain the same signal characteristics in any plane and on sequences done at different times. These features generally distinguish a thrombus from slow flow with high signal intensity. MR venography, using time-of-flight techniques, can also be helpful in diagnosis. Care should be exercised, however, to prevent the interpretation of a methemoglobin clot as representative of flow (on MR venography).

Venous thrombosis is often associated with infarction. Venous infarction can involve the cortex and underlying white matter. A common pattern seen with superior sagittal sinus thrombosis is multiple bilateral, parasagittal, high-convexity infarcts. Gyral enhancement is seen in subacute venous infarcts as a result of blood-brain-barrier disruption. Hemorrhage commonly accompanies venous infarction. Hemorrhagic venous infarction most often involves the cortex, often in a gyriform manner. Hemorrhage can also occur in the white matter with or without associated cortical hemorrhage.

HUNTINGTON'S DISEASE

In Huntington's disease, there is premature death of certain neurons. Inheritance is autosomal dominant. Patients present clinically in the fourth to sixth decades with choreoathetosis and progressive dementia. MRI is substantially better than CT for demonstration of morphologic changes. Thin-section, coronal, heavily T$_1$- or T$_2$-weighted techniques are recommended. Findings include volume loss in the corpus striatum: the caudate nucleus, putamen, and globus pallidus (Fig. 3–41). Cortical atrophy is seen in long-standing disease.

CENTRAL PONTINE MYELINOLYSIS

Central pontine myelinolysis is an osmotic injury that occurs as a result of rapid correction of severe chronic hyponatremia (in alcoholism and severe malnutrition). There is symmetric destruction of myelin sheaths, starting at the median raphe of pons. Central pontine myelinolysis presents clinically with flaccid quadriplegia and facial, pharyngeal, and glottic paralysis. CT is usually negative. On MRI, abnormal high signal intensity is seen on T$_2$-weighted scans within the pons, extending to include the middle cerebellar peduncles in severe cases (Fig. 3–42). Differential diagnostic considerations include infarction, small vessel ischemic disease, metastasis, glioma, and radiation changes.

CEREBELLAR DEGENERATIVE DISEASE

Cerebellar atrophy can be either primary or secondary in type. The most common cause is alcoholism. The pathogenesis is twofold, with alcohol having a direct toxic effect and thiamine deficiency also contributing. The clinical presentation includes ataxia, impaired heel-to-toe walking, truncal instability, and a broad-based staggering gait. Atrophy of cerebellar vermis and hemispheres is seen in up to 40% of chronic alcoholics (Fig. 3–43). The atrophy is irreversible. Although much less common, phenytoin (diphenylhydantoin or Dilantin) can also cause global cerebellar atrophy.

Primary forms of cerebellar degenerative disease are much less common. Olivopontocerebellar degeneration is one primary form. This disease is differentiated by olivary atrophy, which is not present in alcoholism. The clinical presentation is that of ataxia, first in the lower and then the upper extremities. MRI findings include atrophy of the pons, middle cerebellar peduncles, olives, and cerebellar hemispheres (Fig. 3–44). There may also be accompanying gliosis.

4

Brain: White Matter Disease and Infection

Since the early 1980s, magnetic resonance imaging (MRI) has been the technique of choice for visualizing white matter lesions in the brain. This is especially true for the plaques found in multiple sclerosis (MS). Careful review of scans and the use of pattern recognition are critical for differential diagnosis. Although sensitive to disease, MRI cannot always provide a specific diagnosis. Clinical presentation is then critical for disease differentiation.

Other disease entities can easily be confused on MRI with MS. In MS, periventricular changes are typically punctate and asymmetric in distribution (from side to side). Postmortem studies have confirmed that the white matter abnormalities demonstrated by MRI correspond to MS plaques. Edema associated with acute lesions and gliosis with chronic lesions permit visualization. Demyelination by itself does not contribute significantly to alterations in proton density or relaxation, and thus is not directly visualized with conventional imaging techniques. In chronic small vessel ischemic disease, which can mimic MS, periventricular changes are often milder and smoother in contour. However, the white matter changes found in some patients closely resemble those of advanced MS.

In very ill, uncooperative patients with intracranial infection, computed tomography (CT) can be superior to MRI because of its shorter imaging times. However, MRI offers the advantage of direct, high-resolution, multiplanar imaging with superior sensitivity to inflammatory change. In a mature abscess, the capsule can often be differentiated from inner debris and surrounding edema on unenhanced MRI. CT offers advantages in detecting calcifications, such as those associated with chronic infections (e.g., cysticercosis) and end-stage congenital infection. However, MRI is more sensitive to parenchymal hemorrhage regardless of stage. MRI can detect hemorrhage long after CT scans become normal, allowing more complete characterization of certain infectious diseases. With meningeal disease, enhanced MRI is more sensitive than enhanced CT. In the encephalitides (e.g., herpes simplex type 1), MRI can also reveal widespread abnormalities simply not seen on CT.

MRI is favored in almost all instances over CT for the evaluation of patients with suspected white matter disease or intracranial infection. CT should be considered only if the detection of calcifications is important for diagnosis. MRI's strength lies in its superior demonstration of soft tissue abnormality because of its ability to gauge tissue water. In common with CT, differential diagnosis is largely based on the pattern of disease involvement.

WHITE MATTER DISEASE
Multiple Sclerosis

MS is characterized clinically by multiple neurologic episodes separated in time. Two thirds of patients are female. The disease progresses in a relentless stepwise fashion, marked by exacerbations and remissions. MS is highly variable in its course. A study from the Mayo Clinic documented that 75% of patients were alive 25 years after onset, 55% without significant disability. McAlpine's scale, based on clinical criteria, defines definite MS as that with characteristic transient neurologic symptoms and one or more documented relapses. Probable MS is defined as that with one or more attacks of disease and clinical evidence in the first attack of multiple lesions. Possible MS is defined as that with a similar history to probable disease but with a paucity of findings or unusual features. Dictation of films should avoid use of this terminology (definite, probable, or possible MS), a standard in the practice of neurology and based on clinical criteria alone. MRI is extremely sensitive for the detection of MS plaques in the brain and spinal cord. However, clinical assessment continues to be crucial for appropriate diagnosis.

The diagnosis of MS by MRI hinges on pattern recognition. Most lesions are small, 1 to 5 mm in diameter. The most common location of MS plaques is in the periventricular region, particularly adjacent to the superolateral angles of the lateral ventricles (Fig. 4–1). There is often a marked asymmetry in lesion distribution (comparing lesions in the right and left hemispheres), a factor distinguishing it from ischemic disease, which is often encountered in the elderly patient. Other common locations for lesions include the centrum semiovale, atrial trigone, occipital horns, forceps major and minor, colliculi, and temporal horns (Fig. 4–2). Approximately 30% of patients demonstrate brainstem and cerebellar lesions; the middle cerebellar peduncles are a preferred location. Corpus callosum involvement by MS is common (Fig. 4–3). Thirty percent of patients demonstrate focal lesions in this location, a percentage established both by imaging studies and pathologic exam. Callosal lesions with a flat border along the ependymal surface of the ventricles and otherwise a round or oval shape are relatively specific for MS. These are best visualized on sagittal images. Focal or diffuse atrophy of

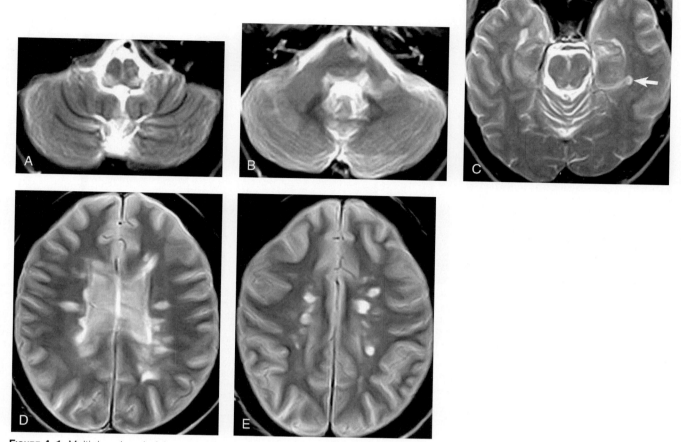

FIGURE 4–1. Multiple sclerosis (characteristic lesion locations). T_2-weighted scans from two patients, one man and one woman, both 38 years old, are presented. Each patient had intermittent weakness and numbness of the upper and lower extremities as well as problems with balance. Multiple punctate high-signal-intensity lesions are noted, located predominantly in the white matter. Lesions can be identified in the medulla (*A*), in the pons and middle cerebellar peduncle (*B*), adjacent to the temporal horn (*C, arrow*), and in the white matter immediately adjacent to the lateral ventricles (*D* and *E*). Only the periventricular and supraventricular lesions were clearly seen on the T_1-weighted images (not shown). In both patients, there was no abnormal enhancement noted on the postcontrast exam (not shown).

the corpus callosum is seen in 40% of patients. Thinning of the corpus callosum results from general cerebral atrophy and accompanying wallerian degeneration. Changes in the corpus callosum are most prominent in patients with long-standing and extensive disease. Although MS is commonly thought of as a white matter disease, 5% to 10% of plaques occur in gray matter. These can be seen in the cortex and in the basal ganglia. There are many pitfalls in the MRI diagnosis of MS. Differentiation from other clinical entities that mimic MS on MRI depends on pattern recognition and correlation with clinical history.

Fast spin echo scans with moderate T_2-weighting and fluid-attenuated inversion recovery (FLAIR) scans with heavy T_2-weighting are preferred for visualization of MS plaques in the brain. Both techniques depict lesions as high-signal-intensity foci, contrasting well against a background of intermediate to low-signal-intensity brain and cerebrospinal fluid (CSF). Conventional heavily T_2-weighted scans should not be used. These fail to detect some MS lesions because of their proximity to high-signal-intensity CSF. The primary plane for imaging is axial. This choice is often supplemented by T_2-weighted scans in the sagittal and coronal planes. The use of thin sections, 5 mm or less, is critical for lesion detection, minimizing partial volume effects.

MS plaques are characterized by prolonged T_1 and T_2 relaxation times and increased proton density. MS plaques are low signal intensity on T_1-weighted scans and high signal intensity on T_2-weighted scans. T_1-weighted scans are poor for lesion visualization, unless heavily T_1-weighted FLAIR scans are used. Even with these, only lesions entirely circumscribed by normal white matter are well seen. T_1-weighted scans, regardless of technique, are insensitive to lesions adjacent to the ventricles or gray matter, because of the lack of contrast with these structures. T_2-weighted scans, which depict plaques as high signal intensity foci compared with adjacent normal brain, are preferred for lesion detection. For visualization of brainstem and cerebellar lesions, compensation by software techniques (such as gradient moment nulling) for CSF motion is important. MRI is markedly more sensitive than CT for detection of lesions, regardless of location. CT detects only larger

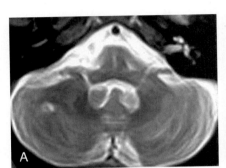
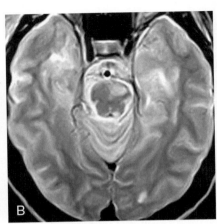
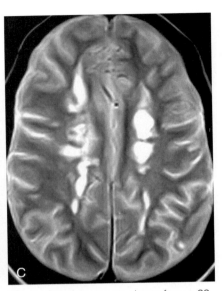

FIGURE 4–2. Multiple sclerosis (other characteristic lesion locations and imaging appearances). T$_2$-weighted scans are shown from a 32-year-old white woman with a 10-year history of disability. The patient initially presented with fatigue and unsteadiness. Clinical exacerbation of disease led to two previous hospital admissions. Ataxia of all extremities was noted 3 years before the current admission; the patient became wheelchair bound 1 year later. The patient now presents with increasing numbness of the extremities and urinary incontinence. However, neurologic exam does not reveal evidence of a new focal brain lesion. Lesions (which are predominantly punctate in configuration) are noted in the right cerebellar hemisphere (*A*), in the left pons and superior colliculus (*B*), and immediately adjacent to the lateral ventricles (*C*), with asymmetry of disease involvement when comparing the right and left hemispheres. Because of the large number of plaques immediately adjacent to the lateral ventricles, the disease appears somewhat confluent in this region. Other scans (not shown) revealed mild diffuse cortical atrophy and thinning of the corpus callosum. No abnormal enhancement was noted on postcontrast T$_1$-weighted scans (not shown).

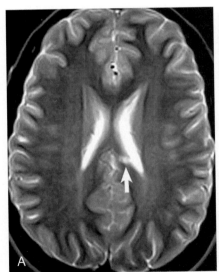
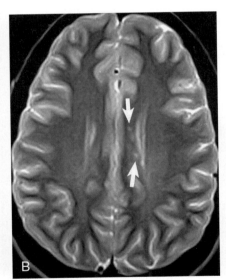
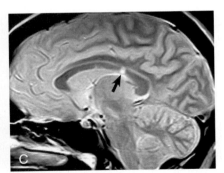

FIGURE 4–3. Multiple sclerosis (involvement of the corpus callosum). T$_2$-weighted scans are shown from an 18-year-old woman with new onset of left lower extremity paresthesia, which progressed to include the left upper extremity. A few days later, abnormal sensation developed in the right lower extremity. *A* and *B*, At the level of the lateral ventricles, at least four periventricular lesions (*white arrows*) are seen. The lesions lie medial to the lateral ventricle and thus lie within the corpus callosum. On a sagittal scan with intermediate T$_2$-weighting (*C*), the larger of the callosal lesions is well seen (*black arrow*). On the postcontrast exam (not shown), several other larger lesions were noted to enhance along with a cord lesion at C2.

lesions. Less severe disease is undetected by CT, with the scan appearing normal.

Acute MS lesions tend to be large, greater than 1 cm, with indistinct margins. Well-demarcated, small punctate lesions are much more common, and for the most part correspond to chronic (quiescent) disease. Lesions larger than 1 cm can represent confluent plaques of different ages or clinically active disease. Both acute and chronic lesions have high signal intensity on T_2-weighted scans. In acute disease, this corresponds to edema. In chronic disease, this corresponds to gliosis. Demyelination per se does not contribute significantly to the change in relaxation time.

MS plaques are also not necessarily homogeneous in appearance. The border of a lesion can, on occasion, be differentiated from the center on precontrast scans, an appearance more common with acute plaques. A thin line of moderately high signal intensity (T_1 shortening) can be seen at the edge of some MS lesions on T_1-weighted images. Postcontrast, this line corresponds to the edge of the enhancing region. On tissue pathology, an accumulation of myelin breakdown products is found in this region at the edge of active lesions.

The vast majority of MS plaques remain unchanged on follow-up MR scans. However, new lesions are often observed with the apparent resolution of older lesions. Confluent abnormalities in the periventricular region correlate with long-standing disease. Periventricular disease, when severe, has a characteristic irregular, "lumpy-bumpy" outer margin. This feature can be useful to distinguish MS from small vessel ischemic disease. The latter typically has a smooth outer margin in the immediate periventricular region. Involvement of the periventricular white matter in MS is also often markedly asymmetric, when the left hemisphere is compared with the right.

MRI is commonly used to assess disease activity and the effectiveness of medical therapy. Patients with more severe disease have a larger number of plaques and more confluent white matter disease. Thinning of the corpus callosum and generalized parenchymal atrophy are also seen in long-standing disease. Many of the lesions depicted by MRI are clinically silent. Consequently, MRI is more sensitive for detecting disease and demonstrating disease activity than physical examination. Studies with experimental allergic encephalomyelitis (EAE), an animal model of demyelinating disease, have advanced substantially our knowledge of imaging-pathologic correlation.

With regard to contrast administration, it is the minority of patients with MS who demonstrate enhancing lesions. The majority of lesions visualized on MRI are chronic in nature and thus do not enhance. Results from clinical trials reveal that contrast enhancement is more sensitive than clinical exam in detecting active disease. Enhancement after contrast administration is a consistent finding in new lesions. MS is a dynamic disease; lesions demonstrate dramatic changes during longitudinal study. Lesion enhancement is best seen on scans obtained within 5 to 10 minutes after contrast injection. Lesion enhancement is transient, persisting for fewer than 4 weeks in most cases. Some lesions demonstrate punctate enhancement (Fig. 4–4) and others ring enhancement (Fig. 4–5). Evolution in appearance, over days to weeks, from punctate to ring-like enhancement, has also been observed. Serial scans reveal some lesions reverting to normal signal intensity on T_2-weighted images, suggesting resolution of transient inflammatory changes.

MS plaques can also be visualized in the cervical and thoracic spinal cord. These lesions often do not respect gray-white matter boundaries, nor do they follow specific fiber tracks. Lesions are often elongated, paralleling the axis of the cord, and are more common dorsally and

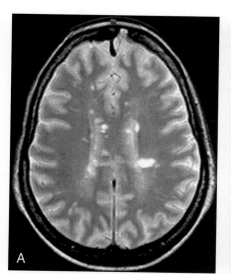
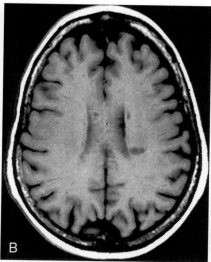
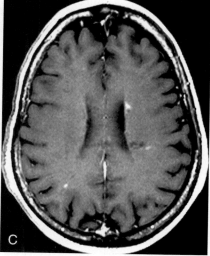

FIGURE 4–4. Multiple sclerosis (active disease). Bilateral punctate high-signal-intensity white matter lesions are noted in the periventricular white matter and in the body of the corpus callosum on the T_2-weighted scan (*A*). These findings are consistent with the diagnosis of multiple sclerosis. *B*, The precontrast T_1-weighted exam identifies only a few of these abnormalities. *C*, Postcontrast, several lesions demonstrate abnormal enhancement, signifying active disease. Contrast enhancement plays a specific role in multiple sclerosis for the demonstration of active lesions and for monitoring response to therapy.

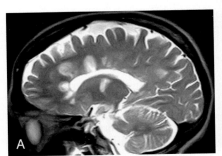
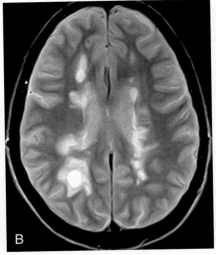
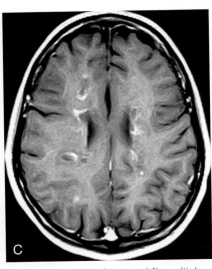

FIGURE 4–5. Multiple sclerosis (MS) mimicking metastatic disease. On the sagittal heavily T$_2$-weighted fast spin echo scan (*A*), multiple periventricular high-signal-intensity abnormalities are noted. Some involve the corpus callosum and have a broad base along the border of the lateral ventricle. The distribution of the lesions in the periventricular white matter is confirmed on the axial scan with intermediate T$_2$-weighting (*B*). On the corresponding postcontrast T$_1$-weighted scan (*C*), many of the lesions demonstrate ring enhancement. Focusing on the postcontrast exam alone, the multiplicity of lesions and ring enhancement could lead to an incorrect diagnosis of metastatic disease. The knowledge that MS plaques can demonstrate ring enhancement, together with recognition of the characteristic location of these lesions, leads to the proper diagnosis. The availability of pertinent clinical history is also paramount to film interpretation.

laterally within the cord. Before the advent of MRI, spinal cord lesions were rarely demonstrated radiologically. Cervical lesions are detected more commonly by MRI than thoracic lesions, a finding that may be related to technique. Imaging of the thoracic cord is still inferior to that of the cervical cord because of differences in coil design and problems caused by respiratory and cardiac motion. T$_2$-weighted imaging in both the sagittal and axial planes is recommended to confirm the presence of lesions. Although lesions can be demonstrated in the cervical and thoracic cord, brain MRI is advocated (in addition to spine imaging) for the evaluation of patients with primarily spinal cord symptoms. As an imaging modality, MRI is more sensitive for the detection of brain lesions in MS than spinal cord lesions. Furthermore, the demonstration of characteristic periventricular plaques can confirm the diagnosis of MS, whereas spinal imaging may reveal only one or two nonspecific lesions.

Optic Neuritis

For the study of patients with optic neuritis, both a screening examination of the brain and an examination focusing on the optic nerves are recommended. The actual demonstration of optic nerve lesions can be difficult, demanding attention to imaging technique. With good technique, optic nerve lesions are seen in more than 90% of symptomatic patients. However, visual evoked potentials remain more sensitive for isolated optic nerve lesions. Disseminated areas of demyelination in the brain can also be observed in patients with optic neuritis in a pattern similar to MS. The frequency with which patients with isolated optic neuritis subsequently acquire MS remains controversial.

The use of fat suppression is particularly important for the study of the optic nerves. Surrounding orbital

fat impedes recognition of optic nerve lesions because of chemical-shift artifact and loss of lesion contrast. T$_2$-weighted scans with fat suppression reveal nerve enlargement and edema. Postcontrast T$_1$-weighted scans with fat suppression show abnormal contrast enhancement of the nerve.

Small Vessel Ischemic Disease

Patchy white matter lesions, or small vessel ischemic disease (see Chapter 3), common in elderly patients and those with cerebrovascular disease, must be differentiated on MRI from MS. The lesions can be periventricular in location or situated more peripherally (Fig. 4–6). Involvement in the two hemispheres is usually relatively symmetric (Fig. 4–7). This is different from MS, in which involvement is often markedly asymmetric. When periventricular in location, the exterior margin of the involved region is often relatively smooth, providing another key for differentiation from MS.

Twenty percent to 30% of elderly patients in good general medical health demonstrate patchy white matter lesions on brain MRI. These correspond on postmortem study to areas of gliosis and demyelination, presumably caused by chronic vascular insufficiency. Larger lesions may demonstrate necrosis, axonal loss, and demyelination, thereby representing true infarcts. These lesions and those of frank infarction account for the majority of focal white matter lesions seen on MRI in the elderly population. CT commonly fails to reveal these abnormalities. The patchy white matter lesions seen in the elderly population should be distinguished from focal gliosis and encephalomalacia surrounding ventricular shunts.

In most patients, some degree of periventricular hyperintensity can be recognized on MRI. A fine line of

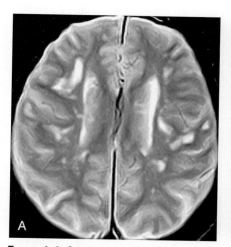
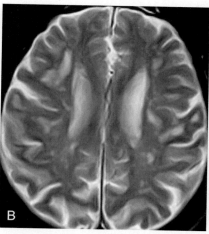
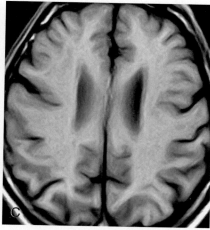

FIGURE 4–6. Small vessel ischemic disease with predominantly punctate lesions. The patient is a 72-year-old man with multiple medical problems. Numerous foci of increased signal intensity are present in the white matter (primarily the subcortical white matter, a distinguishing factor from multiple sclerosis) on the first (*A*) and second (*B*) echoes of the axial T$_2$-weighted scan. The lesions are not clearly seen on the axial T$_1$-weighted scan (*C*). Note the poor gray-white matter contrast on both the T$_1$- and T$_2$-weighted images. There was no abnormal contrast enhancement (not shown).

FIGURE 4–7. Small vessel ischemic disease, a mixture of punctate, and less well-defined white matter lesions. Multiple foci of abnormal high signal intensity are noted on the T$_2$-weighted scan (*A*) in the subcortical and periventricular white matter. The abnormal areas correspond pathologically to necrosis, infarction, demyelination, and astroglial proliferation. The lesions adjacent to cerebrospinal fluid are better seen on the fluid-attenuated inversion recovery scan (*B*). Note that the involvement is very symmetric, from side to side, one distinction from the typical imaging presentation with multiple sclerosis. The lesions are poorly visualized on the T$_1$-weighted scan (*C*) and do not demonstrate enhancement on the postcontrast scan (*D*).

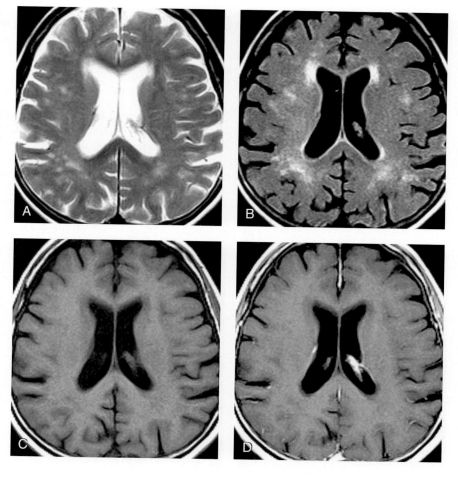

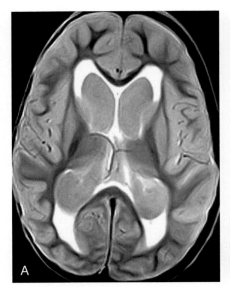
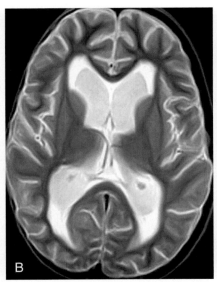
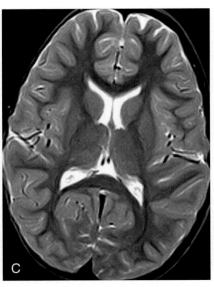

FIGURE 4–8. Transependymal cerebrospinal fluid (CSF) flow. There is dilatation of the lateral ventricles on the intermediate (*A*) and heavily (*B*) T₂-weighted scans. The patient is a 5-year-old girl who received radiation therapy for a brainstem glioma (not shown). A thick, smooth rim of periventricular white matter hyperintensity is identified surrounding the lateral ventricles, best seen on the scan with intermediate T₂-weighting (*A*). This involves only the periventricular white matter and does not extend into the basal ganglia. Ventricular size and periventricular signal intensity were normal on the axial T₂-weighted scan (*C*) performed 45 days earlier. At that time, there was no obstruction to CSF flow. The brainstem lesion subsequently hemorrhaged, enlarging and obstructing CSF outflow.

high signal intensity adjacent to the ventricular system, often more prominent surrounding the frontal horns, should be considered a normal finding and not indicative of demyelinating disease or hydrocephalus. This pattern must be distinguished from that seen with transependymal flow in obstructive hydrocephalus (Fig. 4–8).

Systemic Lupus Erythematosus

As with most other injuries to the brain, MRI demonstrates high sensitivity to the lesions of systemic lupus erythematosus (SLE) (see also Chapter 3). Patients with SLE demonstrate a broad range of disease involvement, from perivascular microinfarctions to discrete cerebral infarction. Partial or complete resolution of gray matter lesions can be seen on follow-up exams. The wedge shape of lesions in many patients and involvement of both gray and white matter assist in differentiation from MS. MRI is an important modality for detecting the extent of cerebral injury in SLE; CT is much less sensitive.

Hypoxemic Injury

Hypoxemic (subnormal oxygenation of arterial blood) injury (see also Chapter 3) to the brain can be the result of decreased concentration of functional hemoglobin (anemic hypoxia), hypoperfusion (ischemic hypoxia), or defective oxygenation (hypoxic hypoxia). Causes include carbon monoxide poisoning, cardiorespiratory arrest (Fig. 4–9), and near-drowning. All can produce irreversible brain damage. The white matter diseases discussed

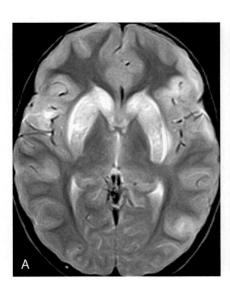
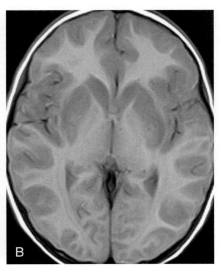

FIGURE 4–9. Hypoxemic injury (infarction). *A*, Abnormal high signal intensity is noted bilaterally on the T₂-weighted scan in the putamen, globus pallidus, and caudate nuclei. There is also patchy increased signal intensity in cortical gray matter. This is most prominent on the patient's left side, in the watershed regions between the anterior and middle cerebral artery territories, and between the middle and posterior cerebral artery territories. Findings are similar, but less evident, with abnormal low signal intensity on the T₁-weighted scan (*B*). The patient presented for imaging several days after respiratory arrest.

previously should not be confused with ischemic damage resulting from hypoxemia. Cortical gray matter, basal ganglia, and deep white matter are commonly involved. Care should be exercised in interpreting scans in the infant, when the question of hypoxic injury is raised, because of the normal prolonged T_1 and T_2 values of immature (nonmyelinated) white matter (Fig. 4–10).

The brain is not affected uniformly in hypoxemic injury. Gray matter (neurons) is more vulnerable than white matter; watershed zones between arterial circulations are particularly vulnerable. Highly susceptible regions include the hippocampus, cerebral cortex, cerebellum, caudate, and putamen. The globus pallidus, thalamus, hemispheric white matter, and brainstem are less susceptible but may also be involved.

Periventricular Leukomalacia

Periventricular leukomalacia (PVL) is the result of white matter hypoperfusion in watershed areas in the premature infant, which progresses to infarction. Clinical sequelae include spastic diplegia, quadriplegia, cerebral palsy, and mental retardation (in severe cases). MRI is often performed in the young child, visualizing chronic end-stage changes. These include decreased quantity of periventricular white matter and abnormal increased signal intensity (on T_2-weighted images) in the adjacent white matter (see Chapter 3, Fig. 3–37). The latter corresponds to gliosis. The areas most commonly affected include the white matter adjacent to the atrial trigone and frontal horn. Focal or generalized ventricular enlargement can be seen as a result of ex vacuo dilatation. There may also be thinning of the corpus callosum. Although neurosonography is used for evaluation of the neonate, the sensitivity of this modality is low in mild or moderate disease. Follow-up MRI in symptomatic infants can confirm the diagnosis of PVL despite a negative neonatal ultrasound examination. The pattern of white matter involvement in PVL in the young child can resemble that of small vessel ischemic disease in the elderly. Age and clinical history clearly differentiate these two populations.

Toxic Demyelination

Of the demyelinating diseases resulting from problems with nutrition or metabolites (with the exception of inborn errors of metabolism), central pontine myelinolysis (CPM) and Wernicke's encephalopathy are two that demonstrate characteristic findings on MRI. In CPM, there is symmetric destruction of myelin sheaths, which appears to start from the median raphe of the pons. The lesion can involve part of or the entire base of the pons. Contiguous spread into the dorsal pons (tegmentum) and superiorly into the mesencephalon (midbrain) has been reported. The cause is believed to be an osmotic injury secondary to rapid correction of severe chronic hyponatremia (see Chapter 3 for a further description). In Wernicke's encephalopathy, there is involvement of the periventricular structures at the level of the third and fourth ventricles. Patients with classic Wernicke's encephalopathy exhibit confusion, nystagmus (less commonly ophthalmoplegia), and truncal ataxia. These clinical findings reflect the localization of the lesions pathologically. MRI reveals lesions in these characteristic locations (Fig. 4–11). Untreated, Wernicke's encephalopathy is a progressive disease. The administration of thiamine reverses the disease over the course of days to weeks, although mortality even with treatment is 10% to 20%.

Radiation Injury

Symmetric periventricular white matter hyperintensity on T_2-weighted scans is a typical finding in radiation injury to the brain (Fig. 4–12). MRI evidence of injury is more likely to be seen in older patients, in cases involving higher radiation dose (and larger volume of radiated tissue), and when radiation is combined with chemotherapy. The injury to white matter by radiation consists of demyelination, edema, and fibrillary gliosis. The pattern may be focal, if radiation is restricted to a port, or diffuse. In diffuse disease, involvement of the white matter may extend to the interface with cortical gray matter. The scalloped appearance of radiation in-

FIGURE 4–10. Global hypoxia in the neonate. Hypoxemic injury (infarction) can be easily missed in the infant, particularly when it is symmetric in distribution, if one is not familiar with normal myelination and its appearance on magnetic resonance imaging. In the neonate, white matter on a T_2-weighted scan has higher signal intensity than gray matter, a reversal of the normal adult pattern. However, this is not as high as the abnormal signal intensity seen in this neonate on the T_2-weighted scan (*A*). Another striking finding is how thin the gray matter mantle is on both the T_2- and T_1-weighted scans. In the neonate, peripheral white matter is normally low signal intensity on a T_1-weighted scan but not as low as seen in *B*. Also, the posterior limb of the internal capsule should be high signal intensity, as a result of myelination, but is not in this infant (because of edema).

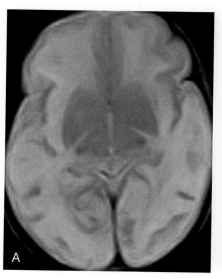
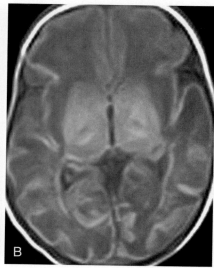

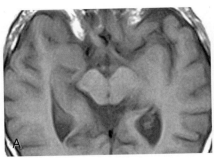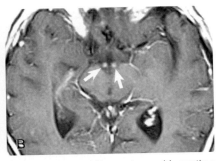

FIGURE 4–11. Wernicke's encephalopathy. T_1-weighted scans pre- (*A*) and postcontrast (*B*) are shown. Magnetic resonance findings include symmetric periventricular lesions that are hyperintense on T_2-weighted scans and enhanced after contrast administration (in the acute phase) on T_1-weighted scans. Bilateral involvement of the mammillary bodies, as seen in this case with enhancement postcontrast (*arrows*), is characteristic. This uncommon disorder is caused by thiamine deficiency. Clinical diagnosis is difficult; the disease is characterized by ophthalmoplegia, ataxia, and disturbances of consciousness. These clinical signs may or may not be present. Wernicke's encephalopathy is due to malnutrition or malabsorption (often after prolonged alcohol intake).

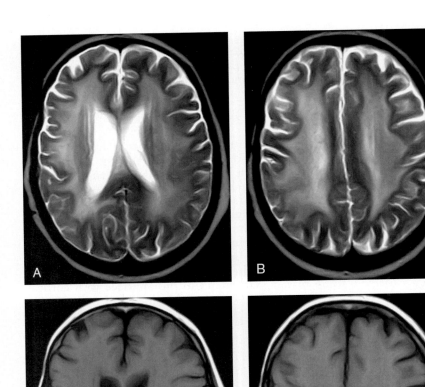

FIGURE 4–12. White matter changes as a result of therapeutic radiation. *A* and *B*, There is diffuse symmetric white matter hyperintensity on the T_2-weighted scans. The involvement extends to the cortical gray matter and is scalloped laterally. The corpus callosum is spared. The white matter changes are typically accompanied by cortical atrophy, also present in this case. *C* and *D*, The atrophy is clearly seen on T_1-weighted scans; the diffuse abnormality of white matter is less evident. Another typical finding is loss of gray-white matter differentiation, which is also present in this case.

jury at the gray-white matter junction represents extensive white matter damage involving the more peripheral arcuate fibers. This pattern can be differentiated from transependymal absorption, which does not extend to the gray-white matter junction and demonstrates a sharp, rounded margin. The corpus callosum is usually spared in radiation injury. Diffuse white matter disease can also be caused by inhalation of organic solvents. However, uniform involvement of both central and peripheral white matter is more characteristic of radiation injury. Radiation-induced changes can mask recurrent tumors and other pathologic findings. MRI demonstrates high sensitivity to radiation-induced changes but low specificity. CT is relatively insensitive for detecting radiation damage; visualization of abnormalities is confined primarily to patients with severe disease. Both MRI and CT demonstrate the late sequelae of radiation therapy, which include sulci enlargement and ventriculomegaly. Abnormal contrast enhancement is seen in areas of radiation-induced necrosis (Fig. 4–13). MRI, like CT, lacks specificity in discriminating recurrent tumor from radiation necrosis (using conventional imaging sequences). Both are seen as focal enhancing lesions with surrounding edema. First-pass studies, acquired during bolus intravenous contrast injection, do, however, permit differentiation of these two entities. Classically, radiation necrosis demonstrates very low cerebral blood volume (CBV), whereas recurrent tumor manifests high CBV.

Dilated Perivascular Spaces

Dilated perivascular spaces (see also Chapter 3) are a normal finding on MRI. They occur in three common locations. The perivascular space is an invagination of the subarachnoid space. Also known as the Virchow-Robin space, it surrounds perforating arteries entering the brain and contains CSF. The most common location for a dilated perivascular space is within the inferior one third of the basal ganglia adjacent to the anterior commissure and following the course of the lenticulostriate arteries. In this location, they are usually smaller than 5 mm in diameter but can be larger. Another common location is within the high convexity white matter of the centrum semiovale following the course of nutrient arteries (Fig. 4–14). Lesions in this location are usually less than 2 mm in diameter. A third common location is the midbrain, at the junction of substantia nigra and cerebral peduncle following the branches of collicular arteries (Fig. 4–15). In this location, they are usually less than 1.5 mm in diameter. Dilated perivascular spaces are commonly noted on MRI but rarely visualized on CT.

It is important to distinguish this common variant from other pathologic entities, such as lacunar infarction, that carry more serious clinical implications. Dilated perivascular spaces are isointense compared with CSF on all pulse sequences. Except for cavitated old lesions, lacunar infarcts do not have CSF signal intensity on all scans and are hyperintense to CSF on intermediate T_2-weighting. In general, dilated perivascular spaces are smaller than lacunar infarcts. The latter are often more slitlike and in the basal ganglia occur in the superior two thirds (as opposed to the inferior one third).

INFECTION

Infection may reach the intracranial contents by hematogenous spread, direct extension (e.g., from sinusitis), and spread along peripheral nerves (e.g., herpes enceph-

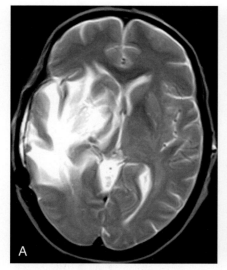
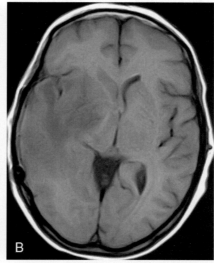
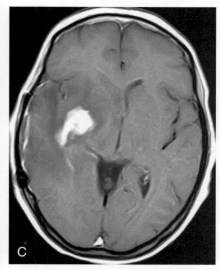

FIGURE 4–13. Radiation necrosis. This 65-year-old patient underwent resection of a right temporal lobe glioblastoma followed by stereotactic radiation therapy (7 months before the current scans). *A,* On T_2-weighted scan, there is abnormal high signal intensity in the right temporal lobe, confined mainly to white matter, consistent with edema. *B,* The T_1-weighted scan demonstrates mass effect, with sulcal effacement and compression of the frontal horn and atria of the right lateral ventricle. *C,* Postcontrast, a large enhancing mass is noted within the area of edema defined on the T_2-weighted scan. In the absence of a cerebral blood volume study (which can be acquired on magnetic resonance imaging during bolus contrast administration), an enhancing mass such as this could represent either recurrent tumor or radiation necrosis. On conventional scans such as that shown, there are no differentiating factors. The actual histologic diagnosis in this case, established by biopsy, was a mixture of recurrent tumor and radiation necrosis.

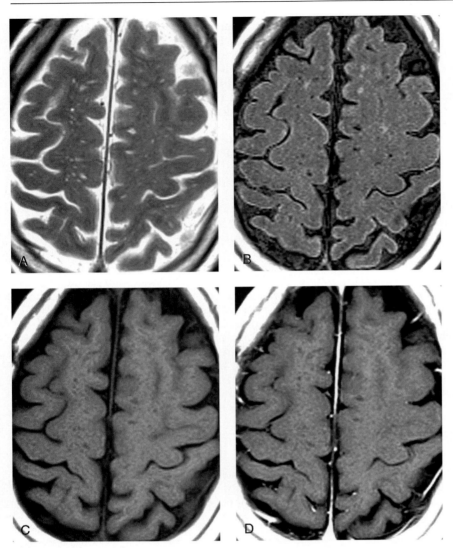

FIGURE 4–14. Supraventricular dilated perivascular spaces. T$_2$-weighted fast spin echo (A) and (B) fluid-attenuated inversion recovery scans, together with T$_1$-weighted pre- (C) and postcontrast (D) scans reveal multiple small punctate cerebrospinal fluid signal intensity lesions in the supraventricular white matter.

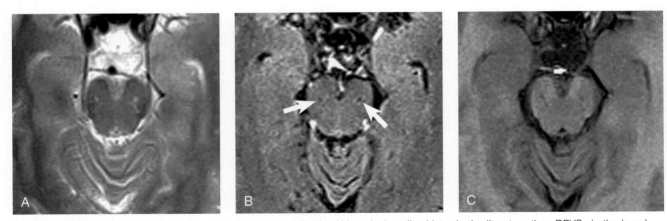

FIGURE 4–15. Dilated perivascular spaces (DPVSs) in the midbrain. Although described later in the literature than DPVSs in the basal ganglia and high convexity white matter, this normal variant is also not uncommon in the midbrain. Here, the location is very specific: at the junction of the substantia nigra and the cerebral peduncle. DPVS may be unilateral or bilateral, as in this case (arrows). The signal intensity is that of cerebrospinal fluid, as shown on fast spin echo T$_2$-weighted (A), fluid-attenuated inversion recovery (B), and precontrast (C) T$_1$-weighted scans.

FIGURE 4–16. Brain abscess. A mixed low- and high-signal-intensity abnormality, with a thin hypointense rim and surrounding high-signal-intensity edema, is noted on the T$_2$-weighted scan (A). On the postcontrast T$_1$-weighted scan (B), a thin uniform rim of abnormal enhancement is noted. Characteristic features of a brain abscess include location at the corticomedullary junction and the presence of a smooth, well-defined, enhancing capsule. Necrotic contents are typically heterogeneous in signal intensity. Cultures for the lesion shown were positive for gram-positive cocci.

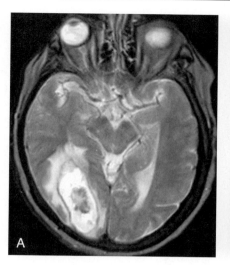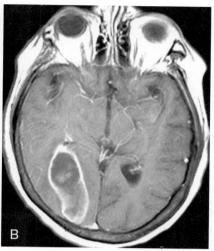

alitis). MRI is extremely valuable for early detection of parenchymal disease. Dystrophic calcification, which represents the primary finding on CT in chronic and congenital infection, is poorly visualized.

Parenchymal Disease

Staphylococcus, Streptococcus, and more recently *Toxoplasmosis* (in AIDS) are the common organisms responsible for focal parenchymal brain infections. The temporal evolution of brain infection has been carefully studied on both CT and MRI. An abscess evolves from an early focus of cerebritis to a more mature stage with a discrete capsule. Abnormal contrast enhancement occurs as a result of blood-brain barrier disruption (Fig. 4–16). Contrast enhancement on MRI permits early lesion identification (with sensitivity superior to that of unenhanced MRI and enhanced CT) and differentiation of

cerebritis and capsule stages. Cerebritis demonstrates focal enhancement, often ill defined, while the capsule stage demonstrates ring enhancement (Figs. 4–17 and 4–18). Enhanced MRI also provides more precise delineation of disease extension. The evolution of intracranial infection, whether treated by antibiotic therapy or neurosurgical drainage, is well evaluated by MRI.

Incidental sinus disease is commonly seen on MRI. The spectrum of disease includes retention cysts and mucosal inflammation. Much less common is active infection. Intracranial complications from sinus infection include meningitis, abscess, and sinus thrombosis. The presence of a true air-fluid level within the sinus, opacification of the sinus by soft tissue with intermediate signal intensity on T$_2$-weighted scans, and prominent abnormal contrast enhancement (Fig. 4–19), given the appropriate clinical presentation, point toward acute sinus infection.

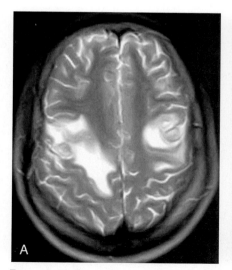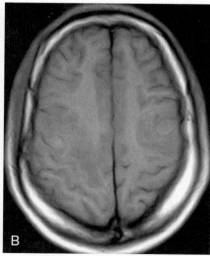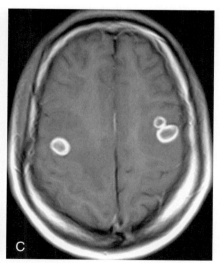

FIGURE 4–17. Cryptococcosis. Two areas of abnormal high signal intensity are noted on the T$_2$-weighted scan (A) consistent with cerebral edema. Comparison of pre- (B) and postcontrast (C) T$_1$-weighted scans reveals three ring-enhancing lesions, two of which (on the patient's left) are adjacent to one another. Cryptococcus is a ubiquitous fungus that grows in tissue as yeast cells and spreads hematogenously. This organism usually causes leptomeningitis, which may be either acute or chronic. Parenchymal lesions, as featured in this case, are less common.

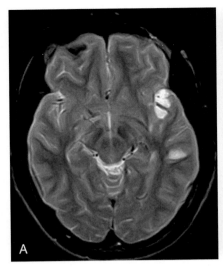

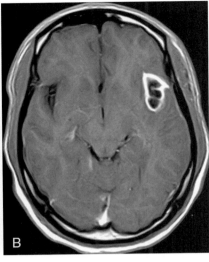

FIGURE 4–18. Neurocysticercosis. On the precontrast T₂-weighted scan (*A*), an ovoid area of abnormal high signal intensity is noted in the region of the sylvian fissure. On the T₁-weighted scan after contrast administration (*B*), there is ring enhancement of the lesion, with a suggestion of septations. In neurocysticercosis (infection by the larval stage of the pork tapeworm), the patient may present with either seizures, because of parenchymal cysts, or obstructive hydrocephalus, because of intraventricular cysts. On magnetic resonance imaging, the cysts have fluid signal intensity, with ring enhancement postcontrast of the cyst wall.

FIGURE 4–19. Mastoiditis, with transverse and sigmoid sinus thrombosis. The patient is a 7-year-old boy with right earache, nausea, vomiting, and low-grade fever. Physical exam revealed a right sixth nerve palsy and a very erythematous right tympanic membrane. On the precontrast T₂-weighted scan (*A*), there is abnormal mixed signal intensity in the right mastoid air cells and petrous bone. Note that this abnormal soft tissue does not have high signal intensity, which is a common finding as a result of inflammation (but without active infection). The presence of abnormal soft tissue is confirmed on the precontrast T₁-weighted scan (*B*); the postcontrast scan (*C*) reveals prominent enhancement (*white arrow*). The sigmoid sinus remains at low signal intensity on all scans, suggesting occlusion. On a follow-up precontrast T₁-weighted scan obtained 10 days later (*D*), there is abnormal hyperintensity (*black arrow*) in the right transverse sinus consistent with evolution of thrombus (in the transverse sinus) from deoxyhemoglobin to methemoglobin. Repeat exam 1 month later demonstrated recanalization of the sinus (scans not shown).

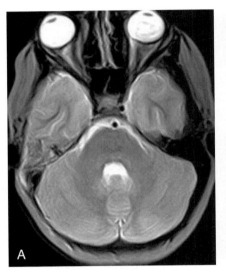

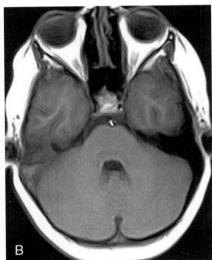

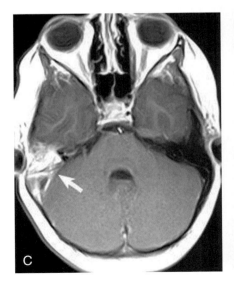

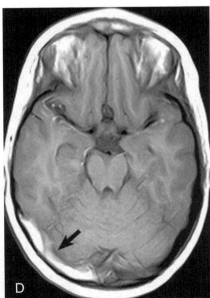

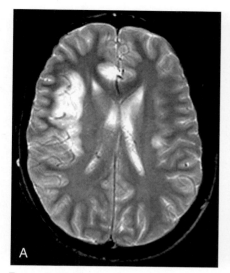 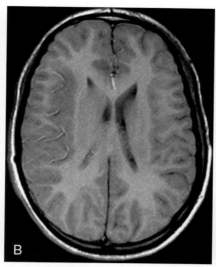 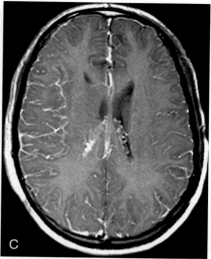

FIGURE 4–20. Herpes simplex type 1 encephalitis. *A,* The T$_2$-weighted scan reveals abnormal high signal intensity in the insula bilaterally and in the right frontal lobe. Comparison of pre- (*B*) and postcontrast (*C*) T$_1$-weighted scans reveals abnormal meningeal enhancement within the sylvian fissure on the right. Herpes encephalitis in the adult most often affects the temporal and inferior frontal lobes. Meningeal enhancement is seen in the acute phase of the disease.

The most common cause of diffuse parenchymal infection is viral. The brain responds to insult with an inflammatory infiltration of lymphocytes and mononuclear cells. Petechial hemorrhage can result from vascular necrosis. Herpes simplex type 1 encephalitis typically involves the temporal lobe, although involvement may extend to the frontal or parietal lobes (Fig. 4–20). The basal ganglia are usually spared. MRI allows early diagnosis and can document effective response to therapy. Coronal imaging is useful for improved visualization of temporal lobe disease in this and other diseases. Herpes simplex type 2 encephalitis can occur in the infant exposed at birth during vaginal delivery. Infection in the infant causes a widespread necrotizing meningoencephalitis. Early in the disease course, brain edema may be patchy or widespread. Areas of involvement increase rapidly in size. Late findings include cortical atrophy and multicystic encephalomalacia. On CT, punctate or gyral calcification can also be seen at this stage.

Acute disseminated encephalomyelitis is an inflammatory and demyelinating disorder of white matter, which can occur after a childhood viral infection. CT is usually nondiagnostic. MRI demonstrates multiple foci of demyelination in the brainstem, cerebellum, and cerebrum (Fig. 4–21). Lesions are relatively few and nonhemorrhagic, with asymmetric involvement of the left and right hemispheres. Follow-up MRI exams can demonstrate resolution of lesions in conjunction with clinical improvement. MRI is an important modality for diagnosing acute disseminated encephalomyelitis because of its ability to identify the sites and extent of involvement and response to therapy.

Two main patterns of brain involvement occur with sarcoidosis. Parenchymal disease presents with symptoms of an intracranial mass lesion. Periventricular and more peripheral white matter lesions can be seen. This pattern in certain instances is indistinguishable from that of MS. The parenchymal lesion, granulomatous in

FIGURE 4–21. Acute disseminated encephalomyelitis (ADEM). There are multiple high-signal-intensity white matter lesions, both infra- (*A*) and supratentorial (*B*) in location, on the T$_2$-weighted scans. In the supratentorial white matter, the lesions appear to be more peripheral than periventricular (unlike characteristic plaques in multiple sclerosis). The lesions also appear to have an indistinct margin (they appear "fluffy"). Computed tomography was within normal limits. ADEM is thought of as a monophasic illness and is known to occur after vaccination and minor viral infections.

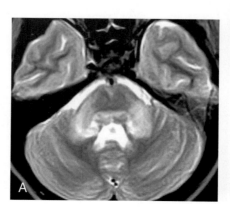 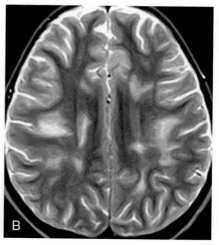

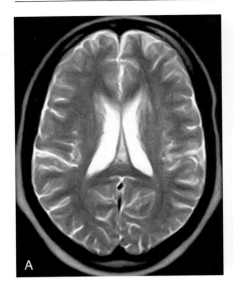
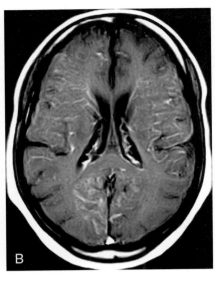

FIGURE 4–22. Neurosarcoidosis. *A,* The T$_2$-weighted scan appears to be normal. On the postcontrast T$_1$-weighted scan (*B*), there is diffuse enhancement of the leptomeninges. On imaging, two major patterns of brain involvement are seen with neurosarcoidosis: (1) granulomatous leptomeningitis and (2) parenchymal involvement because of spread along the Virchow-Robin spaces.

nature, is the result of disease spread via the Virchow-Robin spaces. Parenchymal involvement is typically accompanied by leptomeningitis. Meningeal disease can present with cranial nerve palsies, meningeal signs, and hypothalamic dysfunction. The granulomatous leptomeningitis seen in sarcoidosis involves the skull base and can be either focal or diffuse (Fig. 4–22). As with other brain infections, MRI is more sensitive than CT and better demonstrates the extent of disease.

Meningeal Disease

Contrast-enhanced MRI is markedly superior to CT for the detection of meningeal disease. Unfortunately, neoplastic, inflammatory, and traumatic changes often cannot be differentiated. Contrast-enhanced MRI is also more effective than CT in the identification of compli-

cations of meningitis, including ventriculitis and cerebritis. Abnormal areas of contrast enhancement correlate pathologically with inflammatory cell infiltration (Fig. 4–23). Pathology studies also reveal that inflammation can extend beyond the region identified by abnormal contrast enhancement.

Dural enhancement is common after intracranial surgery (Fig. 4–24). Head trauma is also recognized as a cause of dural enhancement. Once present, dural enhancement can persist indefinitely. Abnormal enhancement is likely the result of a chemical arachnoiditis caused by blood. Involvement of the pia-arachnoid (with or without dural involvement) (Fig. 4–25), indicative of acute meningitis, should be distinguished from involvement of the dura alone, the latter commonly chronic in nature.

MRI is also superior to CT for detecting extracerebral

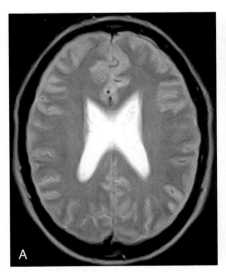
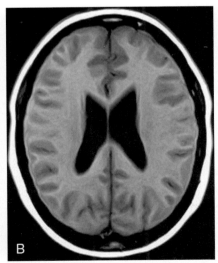
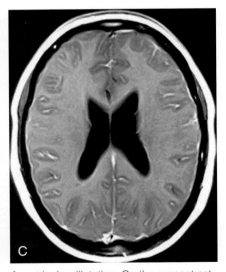

FIGURE 4–23. Viral meningitis. *A,* The T$_2$-weighted scan is grossly normal, with the exception of ventricular dilatation. On the precontrast T$_1$-weighted scan (*B*), the gray matter immediately adjacent to cortical sulci appears to have too low signal intensity. That the cortical gray matter is diffusely edematous is indirectly confirmed by the postcontrast T$_1$-weighted scan (*C*), which demonstrates diffuse abnormal leptomeningeal enhancement. The imaging appearance of viral meningitis, with diffuse enhancement of the pia arachnoid, is indistinguishable from that of bacterial meningitis.

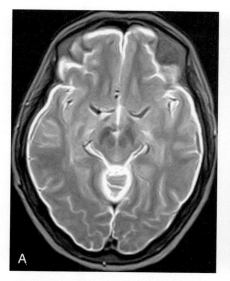

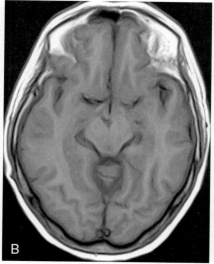

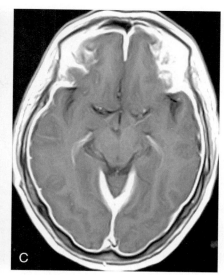

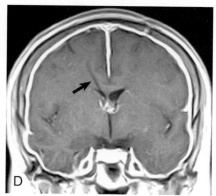

FIGURE 4–24. Postsurgical dural enhancement. Comparison of precontrast T$_2$- (*A*) and T$_1$-weighted (*B*) scans with postcontrast axial (*C*) and coronal (*D*) T$_1$-weighted scans reveals diffuse intense dural enhancement. Identification of a ventricular shunt (*arrow*) on the coronal scan (*D*) suggests the cause: recent surgery. Dural enhancement, once present, is likely to remain for life. Although typically representative of chronic disease, it can be seen in acute settings and with active infection.

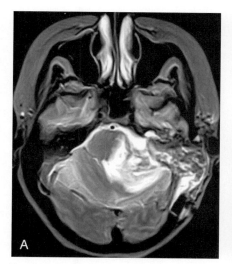

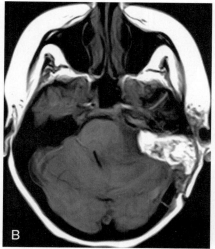

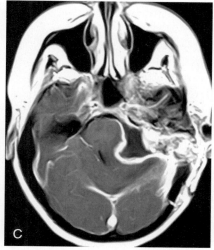

FIGURE 4–25. Bacterial meningitis (postoperative). *A*, On the T$_2$-weighted scan, edema in the pons, middle cerebellar peduncle, and cerebellar hemisphere is noted. Postoperative changes are present, including fat packing. The latter is best seen on the precontrast T$_1$-weighted scan (*B*). The patient is in the early postoperative period after resection of a large acoustic neuroma. There is mass effect on the brainstem and fourth ventricle. *C*, On the postcontrast T$_1$-weighted scan, there is intense enhancement of the dura, in particular at the site of recent surgery. Mild cases of meningitis may show no abnormality on magnetic resonance scans. Severe disease will display marked enhancement of the coverings of the brain.

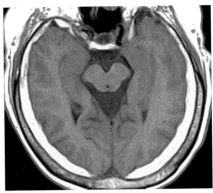

FIGURE 4–26. Bilateral subdural hematomas. On the T_1-weighted scan, high-signal-intensity extra-axial fluid collections are noted bilaterally. On the T_2-weighted scan (not shown), the collection on the right was also high signal intensity, but the collection on the left was low signal intensity. This indicated that the subdurals were of different ages: the one on the right was made up of extracellular methemoglobin and that on the left, intracellular methemoglobin.

fluid collections (Fig. 4–26). Epidural and subdural hematomas appear smaller on CT as a result of Hounsfield artifact. Contrast-enhanced MRI plays an important role in the diagnosis and follow-up of subdural and epidural empyemas (Fig. 4–27). Early diagnosis is critical with subdural empyemas because of the possible sequelae of cortical venous thrombosis and infarction. If all pulse sequences are compared, purulent fluid can be distinguished from CSF because of the shortening of T_1 and T_2. Contrast enhancement is marked, consistent with infection. Epidural empyemas can be caused by the extension of sinus or ear disease or can occur as a complication after neurosurgical intervention.

AIDS

Greater sensitivity to disease involvement makes MRI superior to CT for the examination of patients with AIDS and its central nervous system complications. White matter lesions are clearly visualized on T_2-weighted scans. Contrast enhancement is important for biopsy localization, judging lesion activity, and detecting small cortical lesions with minimal surrounding edema.

Diffuse periventricular hyperintensity on T_2-weighted scans is common in HIV encephalitis (Fig. 4–28). These changes are a result of a direct neurotrophic effect of the virus. Cortical atrophy and ventricular enlargement are found in virtually all patients with HIV encephalitis (Fig. 4–29), reflecting chronic infection and prolonged debilitation.

Toxoplasmosis is a ubiquitous obligate intracellular protozoan. Approximately 50% of the U.S. population have been exposed and have antibodies. Transmission is through insufficiently cooked meat and handling of cat feces. Toxoplasmosis is an important pathogen in the fetus and the immunocompromised patient. Transmission to the fetus occurs during acute infection of the mother.

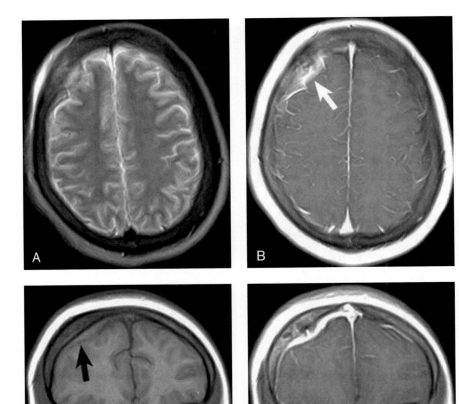

FIGURE 4–27. Epidural abscess (empyema), with accompanying osteomyelitis. A 24-year-old patient presented with progressive right-sided headache, fever, and vomiting for 3 weeks. Blood cultures were positive for *Salmonella*. Abnormal high signal intensity, representing subcutaneous soft tissue edema, is seen on the T_2-weighted scan (*A*) in the right frontal region. There is also a subtle abnormal increase in signal intensity of the adjacent diploic space (between the inner and outer tables of the skull). The presence of an extra-axial mass, together with involvement of the adjacent marrow, is confirmed by enhancement (*white arrow*) on the postcontrast T_1-weighted scan (*B*). The disease involvement is better demonstrated by comparison of the pre- (*C*) and postcontrast (*D*) coronal scans. *C*, Note the hypointense rim, corresponding to the dura (*black arrow*), separating the lesion from normal brain.

FIGURE 4–28. HIV encephalitis. A man in his 40s presented with dementia and was found to be HIV positive. On the T_2-weighted scans, there is diffuse increased abnormal high signal intensity in the white matter bilaterally. Diffuse periventricular white matter hyperintensity, on T_2-weighted scans, is a hallmark of HIV encephalitis.

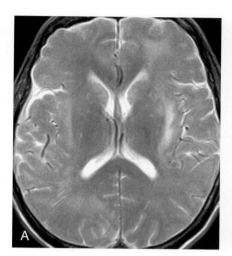
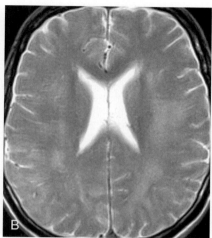

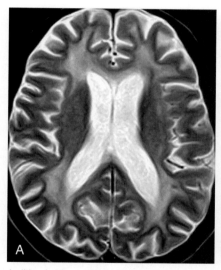
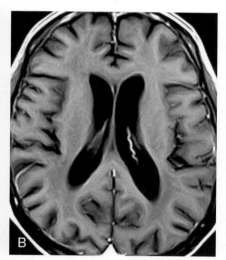

FIGURE 4–29. HIV encephalitis. A 33-year-old HIV-positive man with a CD4 count of 36 presented with progressive mental confusion over the past several years. *A,* The T_2-weighted scan demonstrates diffuse abnormal high signal intensity in the periventricular white matter. *B,* The T_1-weighted scan demonstrates central and peripheral (cortical) atrophy. There is also loss of the normal differentiation between gray and white matter (on the basis of signal intensity). There was no abnormal contrast enhancement (not shown). Atrophy is the most common magnetic resonance finding in the AIDS dementia complex. More severe grades of deep white matter abnormality are associated with the AIDS dementia complex. Distinguishing progressive multifocal leukoencephalopathy (PML), when extensive, from HIV infection can be problematic.

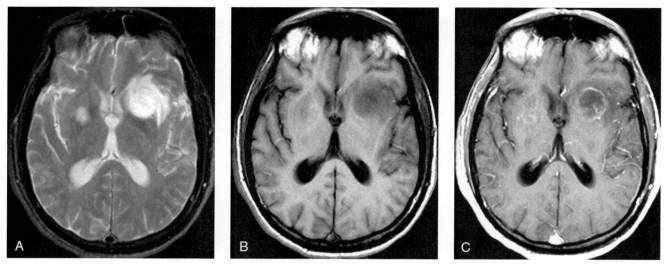

FIGURE 4–30. Toxoplasmosis. Bilateral high-signal-intensity abnormalities are noted in the basal ganglia on the T_2-weighted scan (*A*). Comparison of pre- (*B*) and postcontrast (*C*) T_1-weighted scans reveals faint rim enhancement indicative of active disease. Cerebral edema, depicted as high signal intensity on the T_2-weighted scan and low signal intensity on the T_1-weighted scan, is noted surrounding the larger lesion, specifically extending beyond the thin rim of enhancement defined on the postcontrast scan. The presence of multiple nodular or ring-enhancing basal ganglia (or gray-white matter junction) lesions in the immunocompromised patient suggests the diagnosis of toxoplasmosis, which is the most common intracranial opportunistic infection in AIDS. Other considerations include metastatic disease and lymphoma.

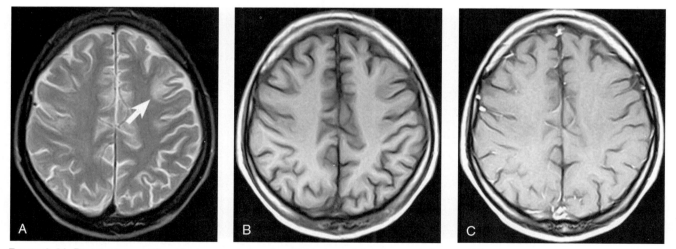

FIGURE 4–31. Progressive multifocal leukoencephalopathy (PML). A small focal area of abnormal high-signal-intensity white matter (*arrow*) is noted in the left frontal lobe on the T_2-weighted scan (*A*). *B*, The precontrast T_1-weighted scan reveals subtle abnormal low signal intensity in the corresponding region. There is no abnormal enhancement on the postcontrast T_1-weighted scan (*C*). Focal areas of abnormal white matter with high signal intensity on T_2-weighted scans, often in an asymmetric distribution, are characteristic of PML. Lesions most often involve the periventricular and subcortical white matter in the parieto-occipital or frontal lobes.

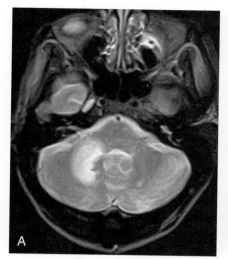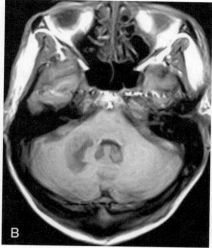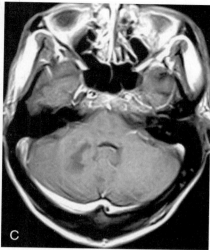

FIGURE 4–32. Progressive multifocal leukoencephalopathy (PML). Although less common, infratentorial white matter lesions also occur in PML. In the case illustrated, a large lesion confined to the white matter of the right cerebellar hemisphere and right middle cerebellar peduncle is seen with abnormal high signal intensity on the T_2-weighted scan (A) and abnormal low signal intensity (without enhancement) on pre- (B) and postcontrast (C) T_1-weighted scans. In a published study of 47 patients, 15 had posterior fossa lesions, and disease was limited to the posterior fossa in 2. In PML, as illustrated with this case, lesions typically lack mass effect and do not demonstrate contrast enhancement.

The result is a focal or diffuse encephalitis. Scattered intracranial calcifications and atrophy are seen in chronic disease. Toxoplasmosis is also the most common intracranial opportunistic infection in AIDS. The disease can be due to reactivation of latent infection or fulminant acquired infection. Toxoplasmosis lesions in the brain demonstrate nodular or ring enhancement postcontrast on T_1-weighed scans, with surrounding cerebral edema clearly depicted on T_2-weighed scans (Fig. 4–30). A common presentation is that of multiple small lesions smaller than 2 cm in diameter. Common locations include the basal ganglia and gray-white matter junction in the cerebral hemispheres. Lymphoma in AIDS, in distinction, is often a single lesion larger than 3 cm in diameter. Central necrosis, with irregular rim enhancement, is also not uncommon in lymphoma in the immunocompromised patient.

Progressive multifocal leukoencephalopathy is a viral demyelinating disease seen in immunocompromised patients, in particular AIDS. Disease progression is rapid; death occurs by 6 months in many cases. On MRI, focal areas of abnormal white matter are seen with high signal intensity on T_2-weighted scans. Involvement is often asymmetric (comparing the two hemispheres) and distant from the ventricular system (Fig. 4–31). Lesions may be at first round or oval. These subsequently enlarge, becoming confluent. Mass effect is minimal or absent. There can be both cerebral and cerebellar (Fig. 4–32) involvement.

5 Brain: Congenital Disease

Magnetic resonance imaging (MRI) is the imaging modality of choice for the study of congenital brain disease. Here, T_1-weighted scans play a dominant role. T_1-weighted scans provide excellent information regarding structural lesions and disorders of white matter. For structural lesions, acquisition of images in multiple planes is important. T_1-weighted and T_2-weighted scans both chronicle the normal myelination process, making possible early diagnosis of the leukodystrophies. The role of T_2-weighted scans is limited, as is the role of contrast enhancement. These only occasionally contribute information about structural defects and significant associated sequelae. Contrast enhancement is, however, important in the evaluation of associated tumors, as may occur with the neurocutaneous syndromes.

NORMAL VARIANTS (VENTRICULAR SYSTEM)
Cavum Septum Pellucidum

The septum pellucidum is a thin, translucent plate consisting of two laminae (leaves) lying in the midline between the frontal horns of the lateral ventricles. The septum pellucidum links the hippocampus to the hypothalamus. Abnormalities of the septum pellucidum may have subtle associated neuropsychiatric symptoms. The cavum septum pellucidum is a normal embryologic space. It is present in all fetuses and premature infants. By 3 months of age, it is seen in only 15%. Persistence into adulthood can occur and is considered a normal variant (Fig. 5–1). When the distance between the leaves is large (greater than 1 cm), obstruction can occur to cerebrospinal fluid (CSF) flow at the foramen of Monro.

Cavum Septum Vergae

The cavum septum vergae is a normal embryologic cavity, like the cavum septum pellucidum. It is essentially a posterior extension of the cavum septum pellucidum. The cavum septum vergae is that part of the midline cavity posterior to the columns of the fornix. It ends at the splenium of the corpus callosum. The cavum septum vergae begins to disappear at 6 months gestational age. In the adult, it is considered a normal variant.

Cavum Velum Interpositum

Cavum velum interpositi are much less common than cavum septum pellucidum or vergae. In this variant,

there is separation of the crura of the fornix between the thalami and above the third ventricle. A cavum septum vergae lies superior to the internal cerebral veins. The latter lie within a cavum velum interpositum.

CRANIOVERTEBRAL ANOMALIES
Basilar Invagination (Impression)

In this bony craniovertebral junction anomaly, the odontoid is high in position relative to the foramen magnum. A more specific definition is that the tip of the odontoid lies more than 5 mm above Chamberlain's line. The latter extends from the posterior edge of hard palate to the posterior lip of the foramen magnum. The dens can compress or displace the medulla (Fig. 5–2).

Basilar invagination can be the result of a primary bone anomaly. In this circumstance, it is often associated with assimilation of the posterior arch of C1 to the occiput. Basilar invagination can also be secondary to other diseases. These include osteoporosis, osteomalacia, Paget's disease, fibrous dysplasia, achondroplasia, and osteogenesis imperfecta. Platybasia may also be present. In platybasia, there is a flattened relationship between the anterior and middle cranial fossae, with the angle formed greater than 140 degrees. Patients with basilar invagination can present clinically with headache, neurologic deficits, and symptoms from vertebrobasilar artery compression.

CHIARI MALFORMATIONS

Chiari type I and II malformations are commonly encountered in clinical practice. The anatomic features of these conditions are well delineated by MRI. Because Chiari type I malformations may present with clinical symptoms suggesting demyelination or neoplastic disease, MRI is the usual mode of examination. Chiari type I malformations are also one of the more common congenital abnormalities encountered in asymptomatic patients. Requests for imaging are frequent with Chiari type II malformations because of the associated spinal anomalies and their sequelae. For the Chiari malformations, MRI is the easiest and most accurate method of diagnosis because of the anatomic detail visualized within the posterior fossa and upper cervical canal.

Chiari Type I Malformation

The primary feature of Chiari type I malformation is the abnormal cerebellar tonsil position and morphology.

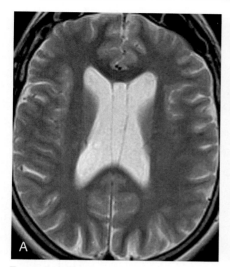
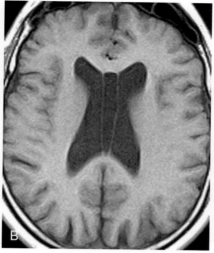
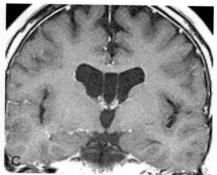

FIGURE 5–1. Cavum septum pellucidum and vergae. T_2- (*A*) and T_1-weighted (*B*) axial images demonstrate separation of the leaves of the septum pellucidum. Fluid, with cerebrospinal fluid (CSF) signal intensity, fills the intervening space. The central CSF space extends posteriorly to the splenium of the corpus callosum (with the posterior portion being the cavum septum vergae). The coronal T_1-weighted image (*C*) is anterior to the columns of the fornix, thus depicting the cavum septum pellucidum component.

There is downward and posterior herniation of the cervicomedullary junction with a variable amount of tissue below the foramen magnum (Fig. 5–3). The tonsils are wedge shaped. The cisterna magna is small or absent. Two thirds of cases with Chiari type I have downward displacement of the tonsils inferior to C1. In one fourth, the herniation reaches the C3 level. Associated anomalies include hydrosyringomyelia (typically cervical), with variable extent, and hydrocephalus. The primary features of Chiari type I that separate it from Chiari type II are the normal position of the fourth ventricle, absence of supratentorial structural anomalies, and lack of an associated myelomeningocele.

Chiari type I may also be associated with bony anomalies involving the skull base and cervical spine. These anomalies include basilar impression, fusion of C1 to the occiput, fusion of C2 and C3, Klippel-Feil deformity, and spine bifida occulta.

Chiari Type II Malformation

Chiari type II refers to a cerebral dysgenesis associated with a neural tube closure abnormality, specifically a myelomeningocele. There is a myelomeningocele in nearly 100% of cases. Myelomeningoceles are the extreme form of spinal dysraphism. There is a midline defect of the posterior bony elements of the vertebral body, usually in the lumbosacral region. Although the muscle, fascia, and skin are split along the midline, the meninges typically remain intact. The incidence of this sporadically appearing syndrome is 0.3%. Chiari type III refers to a very rare dysgenesis, with Chiari type II features and a low occipital or high cervical encephalocele.

Common infratentorial structural changes in Chiari type II include the following (Fig. 5–4). There may be downward displacement of the cervical spinal cord. The brainstem may be elongated, with the medulla inferiorly displaced into the cervical canal. In extreme cases, the displaced medulla may fold over on itself behind the cervical spinal cord, forming a kink. The fourth ventricle is typically inferiorly displaced and may be at or below the foramen magnum. The cerebellum may protrude through the foramen magnum to create a cerebellar peg with compression of the inferior vermis. There may

FIGURE 5–2. Basilar invagination. T_2- (*A*) and T_1-weighted (*B*) sagittal images reveal the odontoid process to be abnormally high in position, lying within the foramen magnum. The odontoid tip, which lies 1 cm above Chamberlain's line, compresses and flattens the medulla.

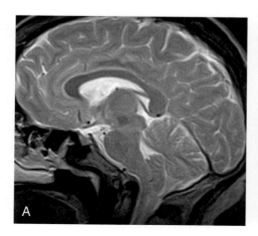
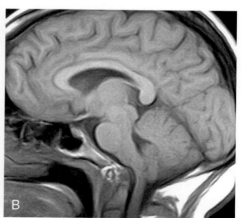

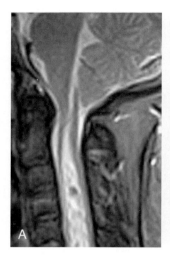
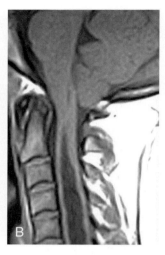
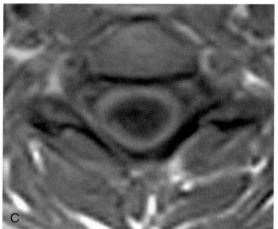

FIGURE 5–3. Chiari type I malformation with associated cervical syrinx. T_2- (A) and T_1-weighted (B) sagittal images reveal the tonsils to be wedge shaped in contour and displaced 5 mm below the foramen magnum. Within the spinal cord, beginning at the level of C2 and extending inferiorly, there is a cavity with the signal intensity characteristics of cerebrospinal fluid. C, The axial T_1-weighted image demonstrates the syrinx to be central in position within the cord.

be forward displacement of the cerebellar hemispheres, enveloping the brainstem. These may touch anteriorly, in front of the pons, in rare cases. In many cases, the folia of the superior cerebellum have an abnormal configuration, with an exaggerated craniocaudal orientation. The tentorial incisura is wide, creating the visual effect of a towering cerebellum with enlarged supracerebellar CSF spaces. The clivus and petrous ridges may have an altered contour.

There are multiple common midbrain and supratentorial structural changes in Chiari type II. The colliculi are typically fused, creating a beaked or bulbous tectum. The massa intermedia may be large. Hydrocephalus is common, with inferiorly pointing frontal horns, large atria, and a prominent suprapineal recess of the third ventricle. Interdigitating gyri are common, accompanying fenestration or partial absence of the falx. The gyri are often thin and numerous, an appearance termed stenogyria. This is not to be confused with polymicrogy-

ria, a finding not seen in Chiari type II and one in which the gross appearance is that of a smooth brain. There is agenesis of the corpus callosum in about one third of all cases. Also common is an abnormal interhemispheric CSF space, of variable size and configuration. Hydrosyringomyelia, which may be cervical or lumbar in location, is seen in about half of all cases.

OTHER ANOMALIES OF THE POSTERIOR FOSSA
Dandy-Walker Malformation

The Dandy-Walker malformation is characterized by absence of the inferior vermis (Fig. 5–5). The fourth ventricle is large and communicates freely with a large cystlike structure, posterior in location. The posterior fossa is usually expanded, with elevation of the torcular. CSF flow dynamics may be abnormal because of obstruction at the foramen of Magendie or Luschka. However, not all cases have obstruction at autopsy, and in vivo demonstration of foraminal patency is difficult.

These structural anomalies are thought to be due to an embryologic dysgenesis and not to a permanent obstructive process. Hydrocephalus is usually present and is highly variable in severity. The severity of hydrocephalus is the most important prognostic factor. Other cerebral anomalies associated with Dandy-Walker malformation are agenesis of the corpus callosum, cortical heterotopias, polymicrogyria, and brainstem lipomas.

In a few patients, the CSF collection is smaller, without posterior fossa expansion. In this Dandy-Walker variant, the torcular is in normal position. The foramen of Magendie is patent, and there are normal CSF dynamics.

Arachnoid Cyst

With a retrocerebellar arachnoid cyst, the inferior vermis is intact and the CSF space anterior to the brainstem small because of mass effect. These features differentiate a retrocerebellar cyst from the Dandy-Walker malformation. However, as with the latter, the torcular may be elevated. The presence of mass effect is used to differentiate a retrocerebellar arachnoid cyst from a prominent cisterna magna.

Other characteristic locations for arachnoid cysts include the middle cranial fossa (the most common), brain convexity (Fig. 5–6), and perimesencephalic cistern. Hypogenesis of the temporal lobe is a common finding in middle cranial fossa arachnoid cysts. Arachnoid cysts are benign CSF-filled lesions. They should be CSF signal intensity on all pulse sequences and lack contrast enhancement. Most arachnoid cysts are congenital in origin. An arachnoid cyst may also form after head trauma, leptomeningitis, and subarachnoid hemorrhage. Although frequently asymptomatic, arachnoid cysts can be symptomatic as a result of mass effect.

Cerebellar Hypoplasia

Cerebellar hypoplasia is characterized by absence of cerebellar or vermian tissue. In its place is a passive CSF

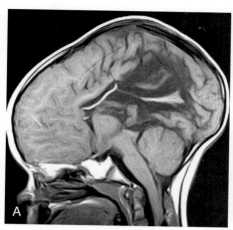
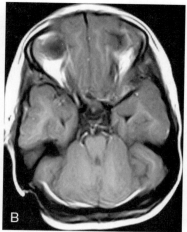
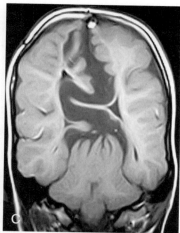

FIGURE 5–4. Chiari type II malformation. *A,* The midline sagittal T$_1$-weighted image demonstrates elongation and inferior displacement of the fourth ventricle, a beak-shaped tectum, and a large massa intermedia. The corpus callosum is thin anteriorly and absent posteriorly. At the level of the fourth ventricle on the axial T$_1$-weighted scan (*B*), the cerebellar hemispheres are displaced anteriorly, partially surrounding the pons. *C,* The coronal T$_1$-weighted scan demonstrates abnormally wide margins of the tentorial incisura, a towering cerebellum, abnormal orientation of the cerebellar folia, an enlarged interhemispheric fissure, and interdigitation of gyri (with absence of the falx).

FIGURE 5–5. Dandy-Walker malformation. On the midline sagittal T$_1$-weighted scan (*A*), the posterior fossa is noted to be enlarged, containing principally cerebrospinal fluid. The inferior cerebellar vermis is absent and the torcular herophili elevated. There is scalloping of the inner table of the occipital bone. Communication between the fluid posteriorly and the fourth ventricle is confirmed on the axial T$_2$-weighted scan (*B*).

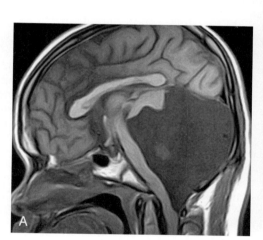
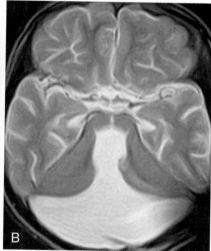

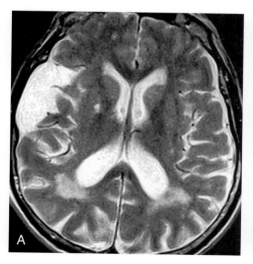
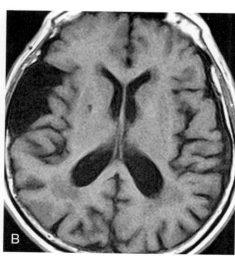

FIGURE 5–6. Arachnoid cyst. A large mass with cerebrospinal fluid (CSF) signal intensity is noted over the right brain convexity on T$_2$- (*A*) and T$_1$-weighted (*B*) images. There was no abnormal contrast enhancement (not shown). Long-standing mass effect is evident, with scalloping of the adjacent calvarium.

space. Usually only the most anterior portions of the cerebellar hemispheres are present. The cerebellar hemispheric remnants may be asymmetric. The cerebellar peduncles and brainstem are hypoplastic. The posterior fossa is small, with a low torcular.

DISORDERS OF CEREBRAL HEMISPHERIC ORGANIZATION
Agenesis of the Corpus Callosum

Agenesis of the corpus callosum is a relatively common congenital anomaly. Agenesis may be partial or complete. The hippocampal and anterior commissures may also be absent. The posterior commissure is typically intact. The corpus callosum is composed of four parts. Progressing anteriorly to posteriorly, the rostrum, genu, body, and splenium can be identified. These structures form embryologically from anterior to posterior. This temporal sequence of formation explains the consistent absence of the more posterior elements in partial agenesis.

Multiple features are associated with agenesis of the corpus callosum (Fig. 5–7). The third ventricle is large and high in location. In the coronal plane, the frontal horns are concave medially. White matter bundles (of Probst) run along the medial wall of the lateral ventricle. The lateral ventricles are widely separated and parallel. The gyri radiate in a medial direction because of the absent cingulate gyrus. The anterior commissure, if present, may be enlarged and dysplastic. The ventricular atria may be rounded because of the absence of the splenium and portions of the forceps major. There may be a wandering anterior cerebral artery. Heterotopic gray matter may be present.

Agenesis of the corpus callosum is easy to identify on MRI scans after the age of 2 years. In neonates, however, myelination is not complete, and agenesis is difficult to diagnose. At this age, the normal corpus callosum is very thin and difficult to visualize. However, if the sulci on the medial surface of the brain radiate directly from the lateral ventricle, the diagnosis may be suggested even in the neonate. Eighty percent of cases of agenesis have other associated findings. The most common anomalies associated with agenesis are Chiari type II malformation, Dandy-Walker malformation, holoprosencephaly, neuronal migration abnormalities, encephaloceles, and interhemispheric cysts.

Lipoma

The incidence of intracranial lipomas is 0.1%. The most common location is midline within the interhemispheric fissure near the corpus callosum (Fig. 5–8) Other common sites include the quadrigeminal plate cistern, tuber cinereum, and cerebellopontine angle. Less common sites include the base of the cerebrum, the cerebellum, the brainstem, cranial nerve roots, ventral aspect of the midbrain, and choroid plexus of the lateral ventricles. Intracranial lipomas arise from the pia and envelop adjacent neural structures. MRI will demonstrate a fat intensity mass. If associated with agenesis of the corpus callosum, the lesion is most often situated in the midline where the genu of the absent callosum would lie. Approximately 50% of interhemispheric lipomas have associated hypoplasia of the corpus callosum. Calcifications may be present but are not readily identified on MRI.

Holoprosencephaly

In utero failure of hemispheric or thalamic separation leads to holoprosencephaly. Half of all cases have chromosomal abnormalities. The incidence is 0.01%. Holoprosencephaly is classically divided into three types by grade of severity. From most to least severe, these are alobar, semilobar, and lobar holoprosencephaly.

Absence of the falx and interhemispheric fissure, fused thalami (with absence of the third ventricle), and a horseshoe-shaped monoventricle characterize the alobar form. The superior sagittal, inferior sagittal, and straight sinuses are absent along with the internal cerebral veins. The roof of the third ventricle may balloon out posteriorly, giving the appearance of a large dorsal "cyst."

Semilobar holoprosencephaly is characterized by partial formation of the interhemispheric fissure and falx (Fig. 5–9). There is rudimentary differentiation of the occipital and temporal lobes and respective ventricular

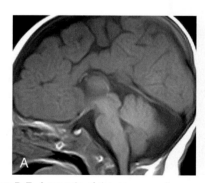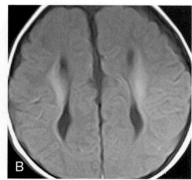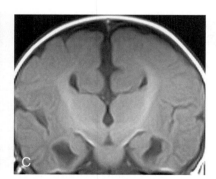

FIGURE 5–7. Agenesis of the corpus callosum. *A*, The midline sagittal T$_1$-weighted image shows a small, dysplastic genu. The remainder of the corpus callosum is absent. Adjacent to the genu, the cingulate gyrus has a normal orientation. Posteriorly, where the corpus callosum is absent, the cerebral gyri have an abnormal radiating appearance. *B*, The axial T$_1$-weighted image reveals the lateral ventricles to be widely separated and oriented parallel to each other. On the T$_1$-weighted coronal image (*C*), the lateral ventricles have an abnormal crescent-like appearance (with indentation medially).

FIGURE 5–8. Interhemispheric lipoma. Axial (*A*) and coronal (*B*) T₁-weighted images reveal a midline high-signal-intensity mass immediately superior to the corpus callosum. The lesion was isointense with fat on all pulse sequences, and there was no abnormal contrast enhancement.

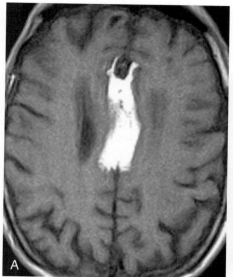

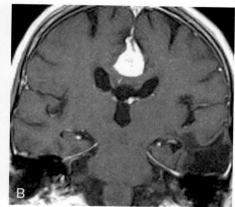

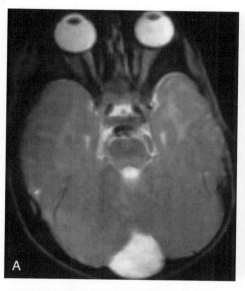

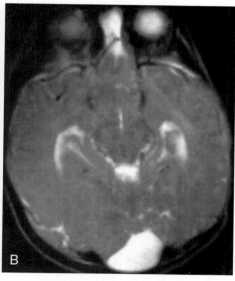

FIGURE 5–9. Semilobar holoprosencephaly. A 9-month-old infant presented with microcephaly and developmental delay. Axial T₂-weighted images demonstrate hypotelorism (*A*), rudimentary formation of the temporal horns (*B*), a small third ventricle with fusion of more anterior structures (*C*), and preservation of the corpus callosum posteriorly (*D*) (*arrow*). The falx is absent anteriorly. There are no identifiable frontal horns. Incidentally noted is a large retrocerebellar cyst.

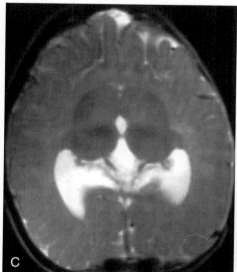

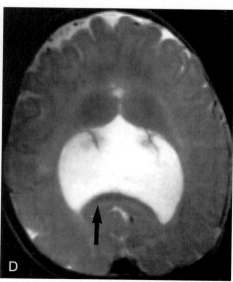

horns. A rudimentary corpus callosum is present. There is cleavage of the thalami to form a third ventricle.

A nearly complete interhemispheric fissure and falx characterize lobar holoprosencephaly. Only a small area of the frontal lobe is fused. There are well-formed occipital and temporal lobes. The thalami, third ventricle, and corpus callosum appear normal or nearly normal.

Septo-Optic Dysplasia

In septo-optic dysplasia, the septum pellucidum is abnormal and there is hypoplasia of the optic nerves (Fig. 5–10). The abnormality of the septum varies from mild dysplasia to complete absence. Half of all patients with septo-optic dysplasia also have schizencephaly. Septo-optic dysplasia is not a single homogeneous entity. Clinical symptoms include blindness, seizures, hypothalamic-pituitary dysfunction, developmental delay, and growth retardation.

NEURONAL MIGRATION ANOMALIES

The neuronal migration anomalies are a varied group of entities caused by abnormal migration of the embryologic neuroblasts, which are arrested along their normal course from the ventricular germinal matrix to the cortical periphery. The primitive neuroblasts normally ascend along radial glial cells during the third and fifth gestational months. If this cellular migration is prevented, abnormal cortical structures result. The entities included in this group are agyria and pachygyria, polymicrogyria, schizencephaly, gray matter heterotopia, and unilateral megaloencephaly.

Agyria and Pachygyria

Agyria and pachygyria represent a spectrum of cortical malformations, with agyria being the most severe form.

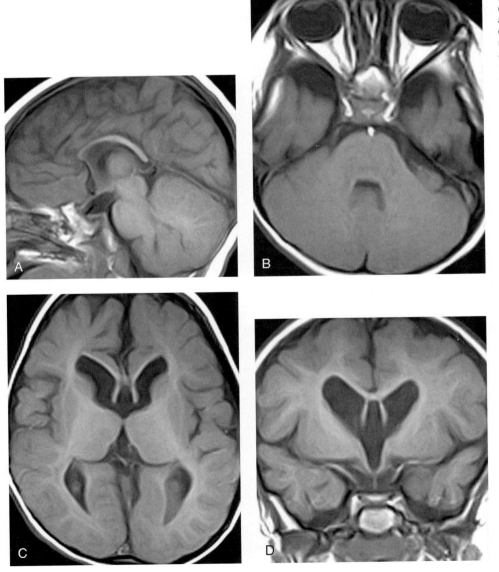

FIGURE 5–10. Septo-optic dysplasia. On sagittal (*A*) and axial (*B*) T₁-weighted images, the optic chiasm and optic nerves are noted to be hypoplastic. Axial (*C*) and coronal (*D*) T₁- weighted images reveal the leaves of the septum pellucidum to be incompletely formed and widely separated. Only the anterior portion of each leaf is present.

FIGURE 5–11. Pachygyria. *A–C*, Axial T₁-weighted images demonstrate a decreased number of cortical gyri that are also too broad. The gyri are abnormal bilaterally, and the gray matter is too thick. *D*, The coronal T₁-weighted image demonstrates abnormal broad gyri in the parietal and superior temporal lobes. However, the inferior gyri of the temporal lobes are normal. Pachygyria may be focal and unilateral but is most commonly a diffuse, bilateral abnormality with relative sparing of the temporal lobes.

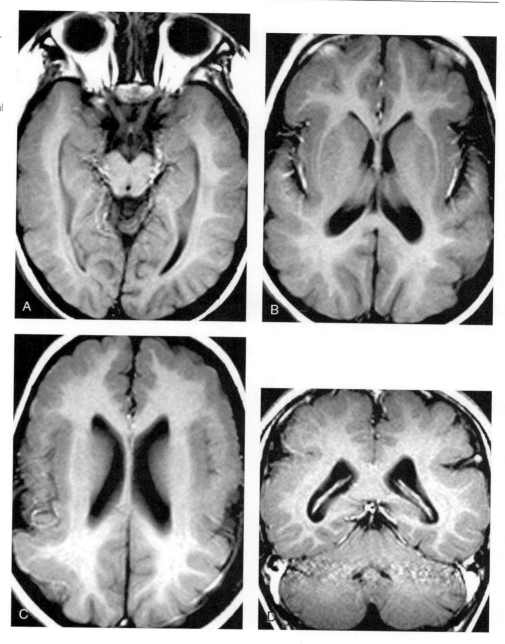

Lissencephalia is a term often used for agyria when gyral formation is very rudimentary, creating the appearance of a "smooth brain." Agyria and pachygyria describe regions of cortical brain that have diminished gyral formation, creating thick, broad gyri (Fig. 5–11). The ratio of the gray matter to white matter is reversed. Thus, the gray matter cortex is broad. The corpus callosum is thin. The brainstem is small because of failure of corticospinal tract formation. On T₂-weighted images, there is a band of increased signal intensity in the peripheral cortex. It is theorized that normal migration is impaired here at the cell-sparse layer.

Polymicrogyria

On imaging in polymicrogyria, the cortex is thick, gyri are not detectable, and the underlying white matter is decreased in quantity (Fig. 5–12). The number of cerebral convolutions is much greater than normal; however, this feature can only be identified histologically. Polymicrogyria is also characterized by an abnormal cellular histology, with the cortex composed of four layers instead of the normal six. Polymicrogyria is to be differentiated from stenogyria. In the latter, the gyri are thin and too numerous but visible on imaging. The cortex in stenogyria has a normal number of cellular layers.

Schizencephaly

Schizencephaly is a disorder of cell migration within a segment of the brain, creating a cleft lined by gray matter traversing the hemisphere from the cortex to the ventricles (Fig. 5–13). The cleft may be unilateral or bilateral. Bilateral clefts are associated with severe clini-

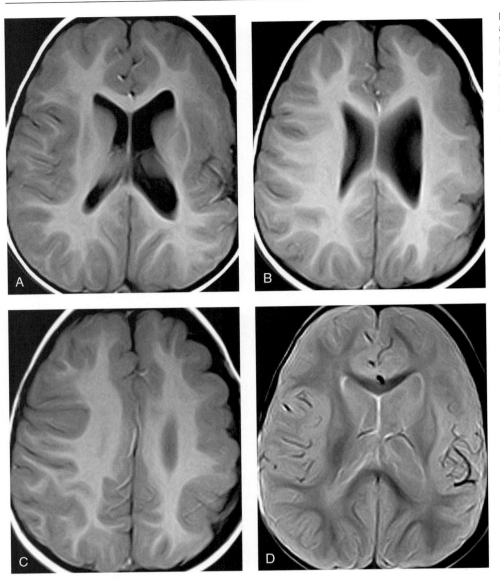

FIGURE 5–12. Polymicrogyria. On axial T₁-weighted images (*A–C*), the gyri in the distribution of the left middle cerebral artery are noted to be abnormally broad and diminished in number. The cortical gray matter is also too thick. The left lateral ventricle is mildly enlarged and the quantity of white matter on the left diminished. Anomalous venous drainage of the abnormal cortex is also often seen in polymicrogyria. This can be noted in the present case by comparing *A* and *D*, the latter a scan with intermediate T₂-weighting, which together show a network of vessels feeding a large abnormal vein within a deep sulcus.

cal impairment. Covering the cleft is a "pial-ependymal" seam, representing fusion of the pial lining of the brain and the ventricular ependyma. The clefts are situated at the precentral or postcentral gyri. Abnormal gyral patterns surround the clefts, including stenogyria and gray matter heterotopia. The clefts may be gaping or "open" or the clefts may be "closed," with only a gray matter seam extending from the peripheral cortex to the ventricular level. The identification of gray matter lining the cleft permits differentiation from porencephaly and other acquired destructive lesions. This differentiation is important because siblings of patients with schizencephaly have an increased incidence of brain anomalies.

Heterotopic Gray Matter

Heterotopic gray matter represents collections of neurons of varying size in aberrant locations (Fig. 5–14). These collections may be found anywhere between the ependyma and the cortex. Heterotopic gray matter may be an isolated asymptomatic lesion or may be associated with other anomalies, such as Chiari type II or neuronal migration anomalies. Sequences that provide high gray-white matter contrast, such as heavily T₁-weighted inversion recovery scans, best delineate these lesions.

Unilateral Megalencephaly

Unilateral megalencephaly is a rare anomaly of the brain characterized by overgrowth of part or all of a cerebral hemisphere, with distorted, thickened cortex and ipsilateral ventricular dilatation. Abnormal signal intensity within the centrum semiovale represents areas of decreased myelination. Because of the intractable seizures associated with this disorder, all areas of abnormal tissue should be delineated to permit surgical resection if possible.

NEUROCUTANEOUS SYNDROMES (PHAKOMATOSES)

The neurocutaneous syndromes refer to a group of disorders that are dysplasias of tissues primarily derived

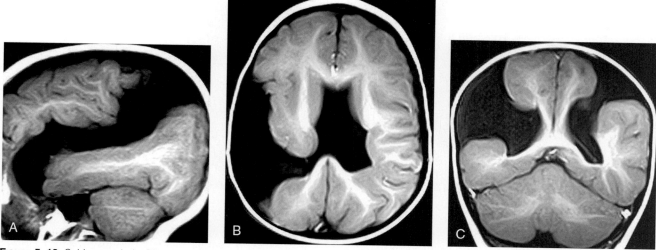

FIGURE 5–13. Schizencephaly. Bilateral cerebrospinal fluid-filled clefts are noted on sagittal (*A*), axial (*B*), and coronal T$_1$-weighted images (*C*). The clefts are lined by gray matter and traverse the brain from the cortex to the ventricular system. Schizencephaly is associated with absence of the septum pellucidum, also noted in this case. Clinical symptoms in this 9-month-old infant included decreased movement of the left arm and leg and a generalized increase in limb tone; the latter suggests bilateral brain involvement.

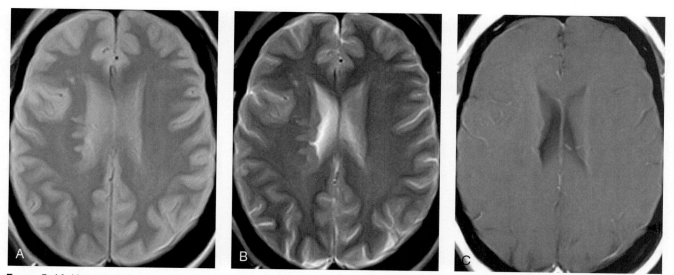

FIGURE 5–14. Heterotopic gray matter. Abnormal soft tissue, isointense with gray matter on all pulse sequences, is seen adjacent to the posterior right lateral ventricle on proton density (*A*), T$_2$-weighted (*B*), and T$_1$-weighted (*C*) images. The lesions project into the ventricle as small nodules. There is no abnormal contrast enhancement (*C*). Most patients present clinically with seizures, as this one did. Late-onset, mild symptoms are characteristic for isolated anomalies.

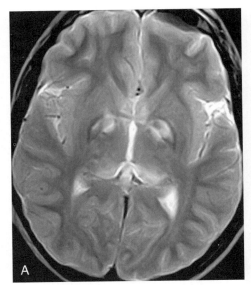
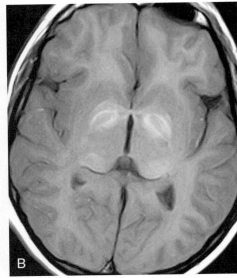

FIGURE 5–15. Neurofibromatosis 1. There is symmetric abnormal hyperintensity in the globus pallidus and posterior limb of the internal capsule on both T_2- (*A*) and T_1-weighted (*B*) axial images. There is no mass effect. This patient also had abnormal hyperintensity in the cerebellar white matter bilaterally (not shown).

from the embryonic ectoderm. These congenital disorders may also affect the embryonic mesoderm and endoderm. The more common syndromes in this group are neurofibromatosis (von Recklinghausen's disease), tuberous sclerosis, von Hippel-Lindau disease, and Sturge-Weber syndrome.

Neurofibromatosis

Neurofibromatosis (NF) is an autosomal-dominant disorder of neuroectodermal and mesodermal tissues in which the Schwann cell is the primary abnormal element. The incidence of NF is approximately 1 in 3000 births. Two main subtypes exist. NF1 is the classic von Recklinghausen's neurofibromatosis with multiple central nervous system (CNS), cutaneous, and osseous lesions. Most patients with NF1 have high signal intensity lesions in the brain on T_2-weighted imaging. These abnormalities are most often seen in the basal ganglia (specifically the globus pallidus), brainstem, and cerebellar white matter. The pathologic basis and clinical consequence of such abnormalities are unknown, although these lesions most likely represent hamartomas or heterotopias. Abnormal hyperintense foci on T_1-weighted scans involving the globus pallidus and internal capsule bilaterally (usually symmetrically) with extension across the anterior commissure have also been described. The same lesions appear smaller and less prominent on T_2-weighted scans. There is typically no associated mass effect or abnormal contrast enhancement (Fig. 5–15). Optic nerve gliomas are the most frequent intracranial tumor associated with NF1. Less common, but seen in 10% to 15% of patients, is a primary glioma. NF2, which is much less common than NF1, is characterized by bilateral acoustic neuromas (Fig. 5–16). Cranial nerve tumors, cranial and spinal meningiomas, paraspinal neu-

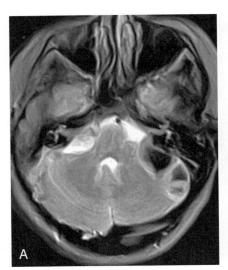
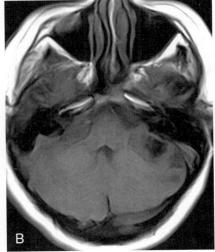
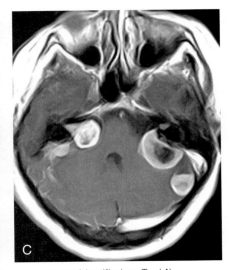

FIGURE 5–16. Neurofibromatosis 2. Bilateral acoustic neuromas, with prominent contrast enhancement, are identified on T_2- (*A*), precontrast T_1-, (*B*), and postcontrast T_1-weighted (*C*) images. Two additional enhancing lesions are seen postcontrast, both adjacent to the dura, compatible with meningiomas. Dense calcification is the cause of the central hypointensity of several lesions.

rofibromas, and spinal cord ependymomas are often seen in NF2.

Tuberous Sclerosis

Tuberous sclerosis is an autosomal-dominant disorder with hamartomatous lesions of multiple organs. Seizures, mental retardation, and facial adenoma sebaceum define the classic clinical triad. On MRI, the combination of parenchymal lesions and subependymal nodules is pathognomonic. Rarely, a subependymal nodule may form a giant cell astrocytoma. These usually arise at the foramen of Monro and can be identified as an enlarging, enhancing mass. The subependymal nodules lie along the ventricular wall and have decreased signal intensity on T_2-weighted scans. The parenchymal lesions involve both gray and white matter and have increased signal intensity on T_2-weighted scans (Fig. 5–17). In some instances, involvement is limited to the subcortical white matter of an expanded gyrus, a "gyral core." Involve-

ment of two adjacent gyri in this fashion may spare the intervening cortex lining the sulcus, forming a "sulcal island." The classic renal lesion is an angiomyolipoma, diagnosed by identification of fat within a renal mass.

Von Hippel-Lindau Disease

Von Hippel-Lindau disease or retinocerebral angiomatosis is an autosomal-dominant disorder of the vascular elements within multiple organ systems. Hemangiomas and hemangioblastomas are found in the CNS, primarily in the cerebellum. The most common presentation is that of a cystic lesion with a highly vascularized mural tumor nodule. Noncystic, solid lesions do occur but are rare.

On angiography, characteristic findings include a densely staining nodule or an abnormal tangle of vessels. Both may have enlarged feeding arteries and draining veins. Malignant tumors may also involve the retina, kidney, adrenal gland, and pancreas. The retinal lesions

FIGURE 5–17. Tuberous sclerosis. A 19-month-old infant presented with seizures and mental retardation. Multiple high-signal-intensity lesions are seen on the T_2-weighted images (*A* and *B*). These involve both gray and white matter. In several instances, the abnormality appears confined to the subcortical white matter core of an expanded gyrus (a "gyral core" lesion). Involvement of two adjacent gyri in this fashion, with sparing of normal intervening cortex lining a sulcus (a "sulcal island"), can also be seen. The parenchymal lesions are of low signal intensity, but in general less well-seen, on T_1-weighted images (*C* and *D*). There are multiple subependymal nodules, best seen on the T_1-weighted scan (*C*).

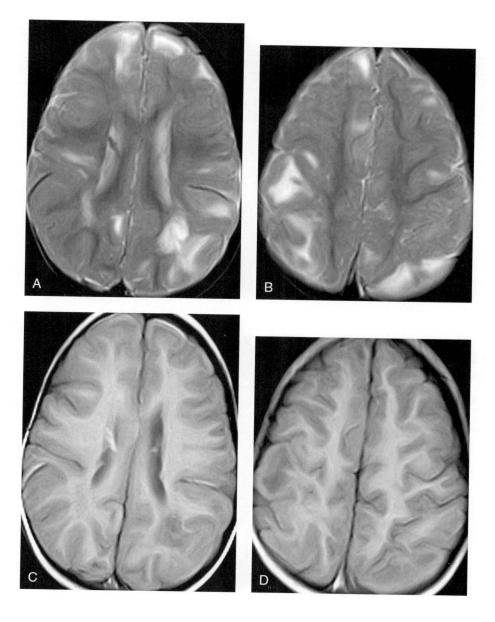

are hemangioblastomas, but the malignancies involving the kidney and pancreas are carcinomas. The rare associated adrenal tumors are pheochromocytomas.

Sturge-Weber Syndrome

Sturge-Weber syndrome or encephalotrigeminal angiomatosis is a sporadic disorder characterized by a facial cutaneous vascular nevus within the first and second divisions of the trigeminal nerve and an ipsilateral leptomeningeal angiomatosis involving the parietal and occipital lobes. The cutaneous lesion is a capillary angioma. The leptomeningeal lesion contains thin-walled venous structures confined to the pia mater. Diagnosis is readily made on the basis of focal atrophy and prominent leptomeningeal contrast enhancement (Fig. 5–18). Patchy, parenchymal increased signal intensity is also seen on T_2-weighted scans. The T_2 changes correspond to gliosis and demyelination, presumably caused by ischemic damage from the overlying angiomatous lesion. The gyriform calcifications seen on computed tomography and plain x-ray film are often not well identified on MRI.

NORMAL MYELINATION

Of all radiologic modalities, MRI is the best for the assessment of myelination. MRI provides an excellent evaluation of the progression of normal myelination,

delays in myelination, and changes caused by the dysmyelinating diseases. Changes of normal myelination follow a well-documented course on both T_1-weighted and T_2-weighted scans. In the newborn, the signal intensity relationship between gray and white matter is in general reversed compared with the adult because of the lack of myelination. This pattern is seen on both T_1- and T_2-weighted scans. On T_1-weighted scans, peripheral gray matter is higher signal intensity than underlying white matter, the opposite of the adult pattern. These differences, and the changes that occur with age, are important to consider in clinical scan interpretation.

Myelination begins in the brainstem and progresses to the cerebellum and cerebral hemispheres. The order of myelination is central to peripheral, inferior to superior, and posterior to anterior. T_1-weighted scans are particularly useful to assess myelination in the first 9 months of life. With normal myelination, white matter becomes higher signal intensity on T_1-weighted scans as a result of increasing cholesterol and protein content. T_2-weighted scans are more useful to assess myelination after 6 months of age. The time to repetition (TR) for a T_2-weighted scan in the infant, however, needs to be longer than that typically used in adults. A TR of 4000 ms is sufficient. On T_2-weighted scans, white matter becomes lower signal intensity as it myelinates. This change is due to the myelin becoming progressively hydrophobic, with lower water content, as it matures. Myelination on T_1-weighted scans precedes that on T_2-

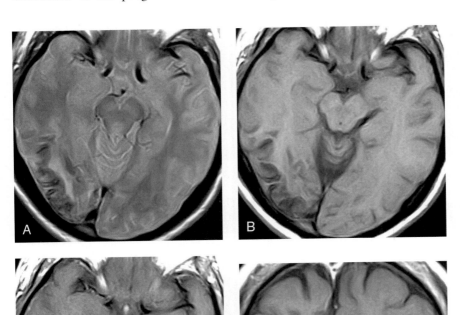

FIGURE 5–18. Sturge-Weber syndrome. There is abnormal low signal intensity in a gyriform pattern in the posterior parietal lobe on precontrast T_2- (A) and T_1-weighted (B) scans. This is most compatible with dense calcification. Axial (C) and coronal (D) postcontrast T_1-weighted scans reveal prominent leptomeningeal enhancement. Mild atrophy is also present in the involved region.

FIGURE 5–19. Normal myelination in a neonate. A portion of the posterior limb of the internal capsule is low signal intensity on the T₂-weighted scan (*A*) and high signal intensity on the T₁-weighted scan (*B*) consistent with normal myelination. Peripheral white matter (nonmyelinated) is high signal intensity on the T₂-weighted scan and low signal intensity on the T₁-weighted scan, the reverse of the normal adult pattern.

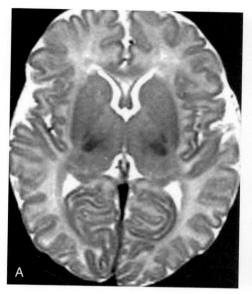
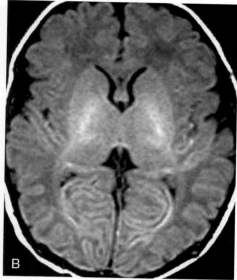

weighted scans as a result of the different components evaluated.

In the newborn, the dorsal pons, superior and inferior cerebellar peduncles, posterior limb of the internal capsule, and ventral lateral thalamus demonstrate partial myelination (Fig. 5–19). These structures will have increased signal intensity on T_1-weighted scans and decreased signal intensity on T_2-weighted scans. The corpus callosum is not yet myelinated and will be very thin.

At 6 months of age, the cerebellum, posterior limb and genu of the internal capsule, occipital lobe, and posterior centrum semiovale are normally myelinated on T_1-weighted scans (Fig. 5–20). The corpus callosum is still thin but now partially myelinated (high signal intensity on T_1-weighted scans). The genu myelinates slightly later than the splenium at 8 months of age as opposed to 6 months. On T_2-weighted scans, only the posterior limb of the internal capsule demonstrates low signal intensity, indicative of myelination.

At 1 year of age, the adult pattern of myelination (for deep and peripheral white matter) is present on T_1-weighted scans. Peripheral arborization continues up to 2 years of age, with visual thinning of the gray matter mantle. At 1 year of age on T_2-weighted scans, the deep white matter (internal capsule, corpus callosum, and corona radiata) will appear mature, with low signal intensity (Fig. 5–21). However, the white matter of the frontal, temporal, parietal, and occipital lobes as well as the peripheral (subcortical) white matter will not appear mature. These structures will be isointense to gray matter on T_2-weighted scans.

At 2 years of age, deep and superficial white matter of the frontal, temporal, parietal, and occipital lobes are low signal intensity, like the adult, on T_2-weighted scans (Fig. 5–22). The signal intensity of these white matter structures may not, however, be as low as the internal capsule. This is achieved by 3 years of age. The deep white matter of the parietal lobes, surrounding the ventricular trigones, is the last region to completely myelinate. This process is referred to as terminal myelinization. Mild hyperintensity in this region on T_2-weighted

scans may persist up to 10 years of age. Histologically, however, myelination proceeds into late adolescence.

In addition to myelination patterns, other features of immaturity can be observed. The relative ventricular size and width of the extra-axial cerebral spaces may appear differently in the neonate and in the older child. The normal ventricle-to-brain ratio in the neonatal period, as measured at the frontal horns, should be approximately one third of the width of the brain. The extra-axial spaces are less variable. The normal width over the convexities should be 4 mm.

DYSMYELINATING DISEASE

Dysmyelination is defined as the improper laying down or subsequent breakdown of myelin. The dysmyelinating diseases are genetically determined and appear early in life. MRI is extremely sensitive to white matter disease of all types. Thus, it is the imaging modality of choice for the diagnosis and evaluation of the dysmyelinating diseases. Although not indicated in every patient, contrast enhancement provides definition of areas of active demyelination on the basis of focal blood-brain barrier disruption.

Adrenoleukodystrophy

Patients with adrenoleukodystrophy present with adrenal insufficiency and progressive multifocal demyelination. Although there are many subtypes, childhood adrenoleukodystrophy is the most common. For this specific disease, the defective gene is located in the Xq28 region of X chromosome. There is impaired degradation of saturated very long chain fatty acids. The disease onset is from 5 to 14 years of age, with rapid neurologic deterioration. In most instances, at presentation, there will be involvement of the splenium of the corpus callosum, the fornix, and the parieto-occipital white matter. These structures will have abnormal low signal intensity on T_1-weighted scans and abnormal high signal intensity on T_2-weighted scans (Fig. 5–23). On postcontrast scans,

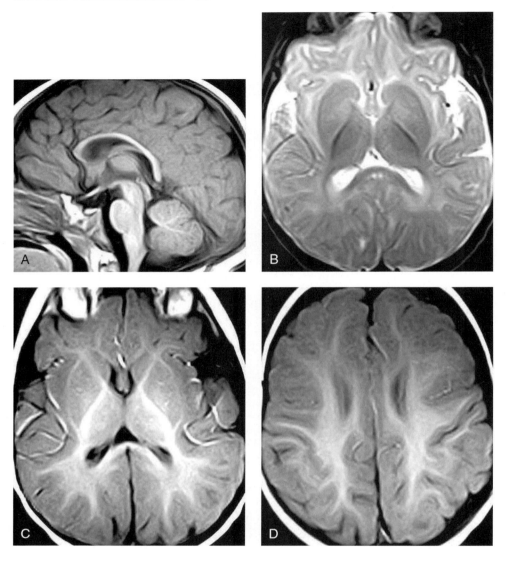

FIGURE 5–20. Normal myelination at 6 months of age. Although the corpus callosum is thin, it is of increased signal intensity on the sagittal T₁-weighted scan (*A*), indicating that it is myelinated. The posterior limb of the internal capsule is low signal intensity, consistent with normal myelination, on the axial T₂-weighted scan (*B*). The genu and posterior limb of the internal capsule are high signal intensity on the axial T₁-weighted scan (*C*). The periatrial and occipital white matter are also high signal intensity (consistent with normal myelination) on *C*, whereas the frontal white matter is close in signal intensity to that of gray matter. The periatrial and occipital white matter still have immature signal intensity on the T₂-weighted scan. At a higher level with T₁-weighting (*D*), it is evident that myelination has progressed further in the posterior portion of the centrum semiovale than the anterior.

FIGURE 5–21. Normal myelination at 1 year of age. On the T₂-weighted scan (*A*), the deep white matter (internal capsule, corpus callosum) appears normally myelinated, with low signal intensity. Peripheral subcortical white matter is not yet mature (as judged by the T₂-weighted scan), having signal intensity isointense to gray matter. The T₁-weighted scan (*B*) looks much like that of an adult, with high signal intensity in both deep and peripheral white matter.

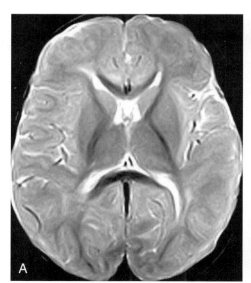

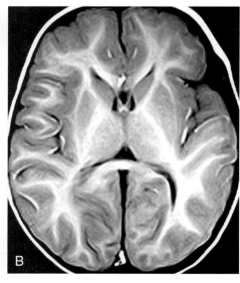

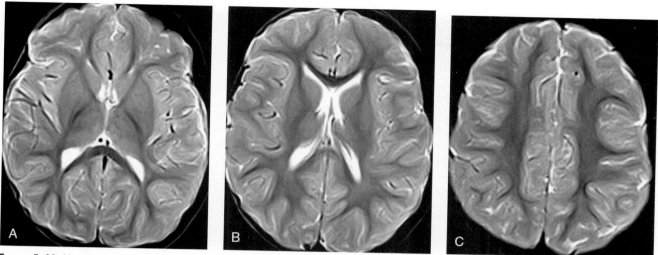

FIGURE 5–22. Normal myelination at 2 years of age. Deep and peripheral white matter have low signal intensity on T$_2$-weighted scans (A–C) consistent with normal myelinization. The signal intensity of white matter surrounding the ventricular trigones is not as low, reflecting terminal myelinization.

FIGURE 5–23. Adrenoleukodystrophy. The patient is a 15-year-old with impaired vision, hearing loss, and intellectual decline. A and B, Sagittal T$_1$-weighted scans reveal abnormal hypointensity in the splenium of the corpus callosum and parieto-occipital white matter. C and D, Axial T$_2$-weighted scans demonstrate abnormal hyperintensity in the corresponding areas.

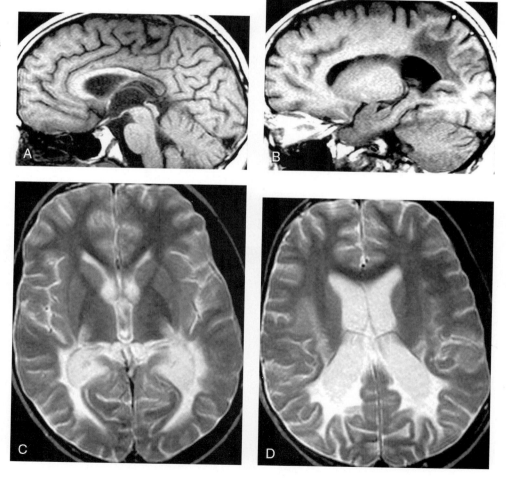

mild enhancement may be noted along the anterior margin (leading edge) of the involved white matter. If followed temporally, the disease can be seen to progress in anatomic involvement from posterior to anterior. Atypical patterns of white matter disease also occur, with frontal, cerebellar, and asymmetric involvement described.

Canavan's Disease

Canavan's disease presents clinically during the first 6 months of life. There is macrocephaly, which is helpful in differential diagnosis. The only other leukodystrophy with macrocephaly is Alexander's disease. Other clinical findings include hypotonia, developmental regression, and cortical blindness. Canavan's disease is autosomal recessive; enzyme tests reveal a deficiency of aspartoacylase. Imaging findings include cortical atrophy, ventriculomegaly, and symmetric abnormal white matter (Fig. 5–24). These findings are not specific for Canavan's disease. Diffuse abnormal white matter, with high signal intensity on T_2-weighted scans, is seen in most of the leukodystrophies.

Leigh's Disease

Leigh's disease presents in the first few years of life. Clinical findings include feeding difficulties, psychomotor retardation, and visual disturbances. Leigh's disease is autosomal recessive; tests reveal cerebral inhibition of adenosine triphosphate-thiamine pyrophosphate phos-

phoryl transferase. Imaging findings include abnormal high signal intensity on T_2-weighted scans in the spinal cord, brainstem, basal ganglia (putamen), and optic pathways (Fig. 5–25).

Hurler's Disease

Hurler's disease is the most common of the mucopolysaccharidoses. Hunter's syndrome, or type II, is the second most common. Both are lysosomal storage diseases; this group of congenital enzyme deficiencies includes two main types: the sphingolipidoses and the mucopolysaccharidoses. The sphingolipidoses include the gangliosidoses, including Tay-Sachs disease, as well as Krabbe's disease, Fabry's disease, Gaucher's disease, Niemann-Pick disease, and Farber's disease. The mucopolysaccharidoses include Hurler's disease, Hunter's syndrome, Sanfilippo's syndrome, Morquio's disease, Scheie's syndrome, and Maroteaux-Lamy syndrome. The mucopolysaccharidoses all display coarse facial features ("gargoylism") and have both skeletal and multiple organ involvement.

Patients with Hurler's disease present clinically with mental retardation, deafness, short stature, corneal clouding, and coarse facial features. Death is usually by the teenage years. Enzyme tests in Hurler's disease reveal a deficiency of alpha-L-iduronidase. Imaging findings include ventriculomegaly, cerebral atrophy, a J-shaped sella, cavitated white matter lesions, and diffuse

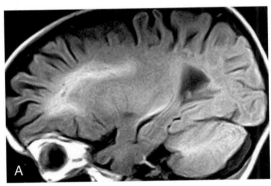

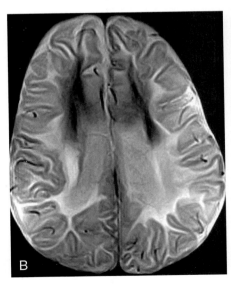

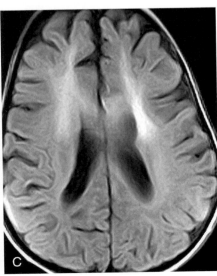

FIGURE 5–24. Canavan's disease. The patient is a 4-year-old child who is blind and has macrocephaly, progressive weakness, and severe learning disabilities. Sagittal T_1- (*A*), axial T_2- (*B*), and axial T_1-weighted (*C*) images reveal cortical atrophy and ventriculomegaly. Anteriorly, the central white matter may be of normal signal intensity. However, both posteriorly and peripherally, the signal intensity of white matter is abnormal for age (hyperintense on T_2- and hypointense on T_1-weighted scans relative to gray matter).

FIGURE 5–25. Leigh's disease. On T$_2$-weighted scans, there is abnormal hyperintensity in both the brainstem (*A*) and the optic radiations (*B*) (adjacent to the ventricular trigones). The corresponding T$_1$-weighted scans (not shown) were normal.

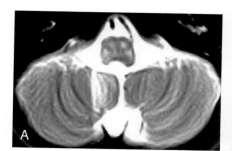

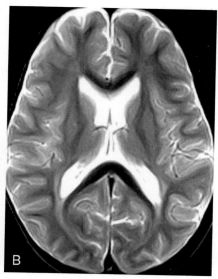

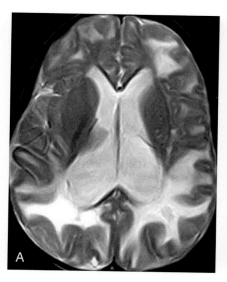

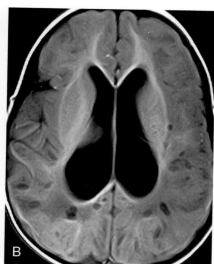

FIGURE 5–26. Hurler's disease. This 2-year-old child demonstrates diffuse abnormal white matter hyperintensity on the T$_2$-weighted scan (*A*). Best demonstrated on the T$_1$- weighted scan (*B*) are numerous small holes, principally in white matter, containing cerebrospinal fluid. Moderate ventriculomegaly is also noted.

FIGURE 5–27. GM$_1$ gangliosidosis. This 11-month-old infant has diffuse abnormal white matter hyperintensity on the T$_2$-weighted scan (*A*). The T$_1$-weighted scan (*B*) is also grossly abnormal, with diffuse white matter hypointensity. The pattern of involvement is nonspecific, other than suggesting an inherited metabolic storage disease. There is normal myelination, by signal intensity, of only the posterior limb of the internal capsule.

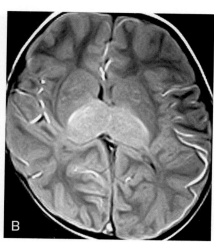

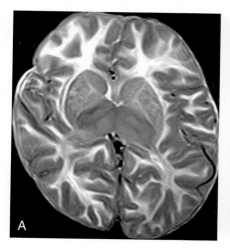

white matter high signal intensity on T_2-weighted scans (Fig. 5–26).

Other Inherited Metabolic Storage Diseases

The inherited metabolic storage diseases share a common imaging appearance, particularly in end-stage disease. In most instances, there is cerebral atrophy and diffuse white matter abnormality (Fig. 5–27). The appearance of adrenoleukodystrophy and Leigh's disease can be distinct. Otherwise, however, MRI is not able to differentiate between the many types of dysmyelinating disease.

Cervical Spine

6

NORMAL CERVICAL SPINE

There are seven cervical vertebral bodies and eight cervical nerves. C1 is called the atlas and is a bony ring. C2 is called the axis and features the dens anteriorly, which extends superiorly like a thumb. From C3 to C7, the size of the vertebral body progressively increases. There are bilateral superior projections (referred to as the uncinate processes) from C3 to C7, which indent the disk and vertebral body above (posterolaterally), forming the uncovertebral joints. The transverse foramen lies within the transverse processes of each cervical vertebral body and contains the vertebral artery. There is a slight increase in spinal cord size from C4 through C6. The neural foramina course anterolaterally at a 45-degree angle with a slight inferior course, oblique to the sagittal and axial imaging planes. The epidural venous plexus is prominent in the cervical region; epidural fat is sparse (the opposite of the lumbar region). In regard to dermatomes, the hand is innervated by C6 (thumb), C7 (middle finger), and C8 (little finger).

On T_1-weighted spin echo imaging, the vertebral body marrow, which is primarily fat, has high signal intensity. The cord and disks have intermediate signal intensity. On high signal-to-noise (SNR) and spatial resolution images, gray and white matter within the cord can be distinguished on the basis of signal intensity. In the cord, the gray matter is central and the white matter peripheral. Cerebrospinal fluid (CSF) is of low signal intensity. On sagittal images, the neural foramina are poorly visualized because of their oblique orientation. Advantages of T_1-weighted spin echo imaging include the ability to acquire scans with high spatial resolution and SNR in a relatively short scan time. T_1-weighted scans are used to visualize structural abnormalities, marrow infiltration, degenerative disease, and contrast enhancement (using a gadolinium chelate).

On T_2-weighted spin echo imaging, CSF and hydrated disks are high signal intensity. The cord and soft tissues are intermediate signal intensity. Fat, including the vertebral body marrow, is intermediate to low signal intensity. Fast spin echo (FSE) techniques, using repeated 180-degree radiofrequency pulses, have for the most part replaced conventional T_2-weighted spin echo techniques. The use of fast spin echo technique results in a much shorter scan time and less sensitivity to motion artifacts (especially CSF pulsation). T_2-weighted scans are used to detect spinal cord abnormalities, including edema, gliosis, demyelination, and neoplasia,

and to evaluate the thecal sac dimensions, looking for canal compromise).

Gradient echo imaging is still used in the cervical spine, particularly in the axial plane. Scans are acquired with a low flip angle, resulting in T_2-weighting. On such scans, CSF and normal intervertebral disks are high signal intensity, the cord intermediate signal intensity, and the marrow low signal intensity (as a result of magnetic susceptibility effects). Gray and white matter within the cord are usually well differentiated on the basis of signal intensity. Myelographic-like sagittal and axial images can be acquired, with diagnostic utility for the detection of degenerative disease (disk herniation, canal compression, and foraminal stenosis) and the evaluation of intrinsic cord abnormalities in the axial plane (multiple sclerosis, tumors, edema, and hemorrhage). Canal and foraminal stenoses are typically exaggerated on gradient echo imaging as a result of magnetic susceptibility effects.

Three major arteries supply the spinal cord and lie along its surface. One is anterior (the anterior spinal artery, which supplies 70% of the cord) and two are posterior (the posterior spinal arteries, which together supply 30% of the cord). In the cervical region, several radicular arteries supply the anterior spinal artery. In the thoracolumbar region, the artery of Adamkiewicz, which arises from a lower intercostal or upper lumbar artery, supplies the anterior spinal artery.

Magnetic resonance imaging (MRI) has the capability of providing flexion and extension views in the cervical spine. These scans can be of substantial clinical value. Flexion and extension views are typically acquired with some sort of rapid imaging technique, of which today there is a plethora. A very simple scheme, which can be used for rapid image acquisition on most scanners, is to acquire the T_1-weighted scan with a reduced number of phase-encoding steps and the T_2-weighted scan with FSE technique. Depending on the available coils, the range of possible motion may be limited. Flexion and extension views have substantial use in the demonstration of spinal cord compression not visualized in the neutral position (e.g., with rheumatoid arthritis) and in the evaluation of potential instability. The latter can be an important diagnostic question both after trauma and in chronic inflammatory disease (particularly at the occipitoatlantal and atlantoaxial levels).

Intravenous administration of a gadolinium chelate (the most common type of contrast agent currently used in MRI) produces enhancement of the normal venous plexus on cervical spine exams. The external vertebral

117

plexus consists of a network of veins along the anterior vertebral body, laminae, and spinous, transverse, and articular processes. The internal vertebral plexus consists of a network of veins lying within the epidural space both anteriorly and posteriorly. The internal plexus is more important in regard to the interpretation of MRI scans. The anterior part of this plexus is larger (than that posteriorly), with longitudinal veins lying on each side of the posterior longitudinal ligament. The anterior plexus tapers at the disk space level. Displacement and engorgement of the anterior plexus often accompany disk herniation. All of the plexus drain via intervertebral veins that accompany the spinal nerves within the foramina.

In regard to the reading of MRI scans of the cervical spine, there is a need for a consistent, thorough approach to scan interpretation. All structures, including the contents of the thecal sac, the bony vertebral column, and the surrounding soft tissues, should be consciously examined. The cerebellar tonsils, thyroid, facet joints (looking specifically for perched facets), and surrounding soft tissues (looking specifically for lymphadenopathy) deserve particular attention because disease is common and often overlooked in these areas.

SPINAL STENOSIS
Congenital

Congenital stenosis in the cervical spine is caused by short pedicles. There may be an underlying primary disease, such as achondroplasia or Down syndrome. Cervical spinal stenosis causes myelopathic symptoms, which include extremity weakness, gait abnormalities, reflex changes, and muscular atrophy. Relative spinal stenosis is defined as a canal less than or equal to 13 mm in diameter (but greater than 10 mm). Patients with this degree of narrowing may be symptomatic. Absolute spinal stenosis is defined as a canal smaller than 10 mm in diameter. Patients with cervical spinal stenosis are predisposed to early, more severe degenerative changes and traumatic spinal cord injury.

Degenerative (Acquired)

Degenerative (also known as acquired) spinal stenosis is caused by advanced degenerative disk disease (Fig. 6–1). Advanced degenerative disk disease is also referred to by the term spondylosis. Factors contributing to narrowing of the spinal canal include decreased disk height with thickening and buckling of intraspinal ligaments, calcification of the posterior longitudinal ligament and ligamentum flavum, disk bulges and herniations, osteophytic spurs (anteriorly), and hypertrophy of facet joints (posteriorly) (Fig. 6–2). Symptom onset is usually in middle age or older patients. This is older than the population affected by disk herniation, although there is considerable overlap. Symptoms are typically myelopathic. These include progressive or intermittent numbness, weakness of the upper extremities, pain, abnormal reflexes, muscle wasting (specifically the interosseous muscles of hand), and a staggering gait. The dimensions of the canal are most accurately measured on axial images. The normal anteroposterior dimension in the cervical region is greater than 13 mm. Patients with a borderline size canal, 10 to 13 mm, may experience symptoms. An anteroposterior dimension of less than 10 mm is considered to be diagnostic of cervical stenosis. The most commonly affected levels are C4-5, C5-6, and C6-7. Multilevel involvement is also very common. On MRI, with mild disease, the ventral subarachnoid space is effaced. With severe disease, there may be cord flattening, impingement, and myelomalacia (edema, gliosis, and cystic changes within the cord).

Neuroforaminal (Uncovertebral Joint) Spurring

The uncovertebral joints, also known as the joints of Luschka, lie along the posterolateral margins of the cervical vertebral bodies. These joints are formed by the uncinate process of the lower vertebral body extending superiorly to articulate with a depression in the inferior end plate of adjacent superior vertebral body. Uncovertebral joints are present from C3 to C7. Thus, degenerative disease of the uncovertebral joints can cause foraminal narrowing from C2-3 to C6-7. As part of the degenerative process, hypertrophic spurs may form around these joints, which then narrow the anteromedial part of the neural foramen. When combined with disk space narrowing, which causes decreased height of the neural foramen), uncovertebral joint spurs can cause nerve root compression (Fig. 6–3). This is a more common cause of radiculopathy in the cervical spine than disk herniation. Because of the anterolateral and slightly inferior course of the neural foramen, oblique images provide the best view of the foramina.

Ossification of the Posterior Longitudinal Ligament

Ossification of the posterior longitudinal ligament is an uncommon cause of acquired spinal stenosis. More common causes include ligamentous and facet joint hypertrophy. Ossification of the posterior longitudinal ligament is more common in the oriental population. Patients are at risk for traumatic spinal cord injury. Multilevel involvement is typical. The ossified posterior longitudinal ligament will be very low signal intensity on both T_1- and T_2-weighted scans but may contain centrally intermediate- to high-signal-intensity soft tissue (fat and marrow).

CONGENITAL DISEASE
Klippel-Feil Syndrome

In the Klippel-Feil syndrome, there is congenital fusion of two or more cervical vertebrae, most commonly C2-3 and C5-6. At the affected levels, the intervertebral disk is absent. About half of all patients with Klippel-Feil syndrome demonstrate the classic triad, which consists of limited neck motion, a short neck, and a low posterior hairline. Common associated anomalies include deafness, congenital heart disease, Sprengel's deformity (elevation and rotation of the scapula), and uro-

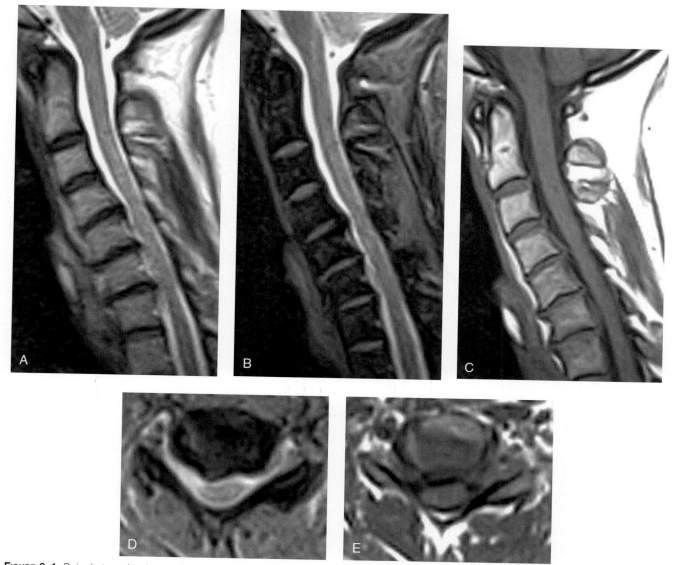

FIGURE 6–1. Spinal stenosis, degenerative (acquired) in origin. *A*, On the sagittal fast spin echo T_2-weighted scan, there is encroachment anteriorly on the thecal sac by disk bulges and osteophytic spurs at the C4–5, C5–6, and C6–7 levels. In degenerative spinal stenosis of the cervical spine, these are the most commonly affected levels. Multilevel involvement, as in this case, is also common. The same findings are apparent on the sagittal gradient echo T_2-weighted scan (*B*). The latter scan is easily identified by the low signal intensity of vertebral body marrow, which is due to magnetic susceptibility effects. The osteophytic spurs are well visualized on the sagittal T_1-weighted scan (*C*), although the encroachment on the thecal sac is less evident. On axial imaging, the asymmetry of the canal compromise in this patient is clearly seen, together with the cord flattening and deformity. As with imaging in the sagittal plane, on axial imaging (*D*) the T_2-weighted scan depicts the interface between soft tissue and cerebrospinal fluid better than the T_1-weighted scan (*E*).

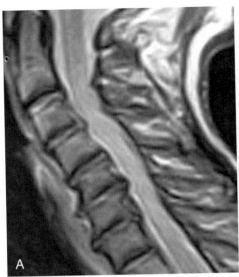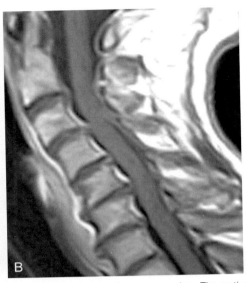

FIGURE 6–2. Degenerative stenosis of the cervical spinal canal, with both anterior and posterior compression. The patient is a 69-year-old woman with neck pain and intermittent numbness and weakness in both arms. *A*, The sagittal T_2-weighted scan reveals canal compromise at the C2–3 through C6–7 disk space levels. Disk bulges and osteophytic spurs cause compression anteriorly on the thecal sac at the C3–4 level and below. At both C2–3 and C3–4, facet hypertrophy causes posterior compression. The subarachnoid space is obliterated at multiple levels, with accompanying cord deformity (flattening). There is mild reversal of the normal cervical lordosis in the lower cervical spine. *B*, The postcontrast T_1-weighted image demonstrates thin curvilinear high signal intensity (enhancing epidural venous plexus) along the posterior margins of the vertebrae. With contrast enhancement, the true canal dimensions are better visualized. The failure to clearly visualize epidural soft tissue is one reason that precontrast T_1-weighted scans are generally less useful than T_2-weighted scans in imaging cervical degenerative disease (spondylosis). Disk space narrowing is identified at the C4–5 through the C6–7 levels on the T_1-weighted scan. The disk bulges and spurs are also clearly seen, as on the T_2-weighted scan.

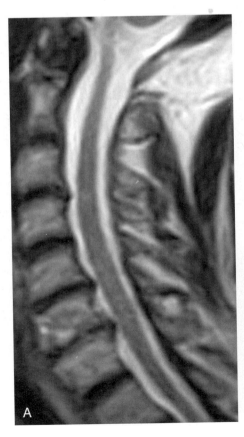

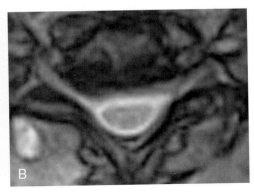

FIGURE 6–3. Neuroforaminal narrowing caused by uncovertebral joint bony spurs. The patient is 54 years old and presents with neck and bilateral arm pain. *A*, The midline sagittal T_2-weighted scan reveals disk bulges and osteophytic spurs at C3–4, C5–6, and C6–7 with effacement of the ventral subarachnoid space at each level. Because of their oblique orientation, the neural foramina are not well visualized in the cervical spine on sagittal images. Although the foramina would be best depicted on oblique scans, axial scans are used in most clinical practices for their assessment. *B*, The axial gradient echo T_2-weighted scan in this case at the C6–7 level reveals narrowing of the right neural foramen as a result of hypertrophic changes and sclerosis (with accompanying bony spurring) of the right C6–7 uncovertebral joint.

logic abnormalities. Other less frequently associated anomalies include syringomyelia and diastematomyelia. There are three types, defined on the basis of the extent and location of vertebral fusions. In type I, there is extensive cervical and thoracic fusion. In type II, the most common (Fig. 6–4), there are one or two cervical fusions; there may also be associated hemivertebrae and occipitoatlantal fusion. Type III is defined as type I or II with additional lower thoracic or lumbar fusions.

Clinically, patients with Klippel-Feil syndrome are often asymptomatic from a neurologic point of view. They can, however, have cord or nerve root compression. Patients with Klippel-Feil syndrome are predisposed to spinal cord injury after minor trauma. Patients may have hypermobility (and thus instability) between the unfused segments.

Abnormalities Involving the Cerebellar Tonsils

Ectopia

The position of the cerebellar tonsils is best evaluated on sagittal images. Mild inferior displacement (ectopia) can be seen in asymptomatic normal individuals. In the majority of normal individuals, the tonsils lie above the foramen magnum. The tonsils may, however, lie as far as 5 mm below the foramen magnum and still be normal. In individuals with tonsillar ectopia, the tonsils retain their normal globular configuration.

Chiari Type I

In the Chiari type I malformation, the cerebellar tonsils are low lying and pointed or wedge shaped (Fig. 6–5).

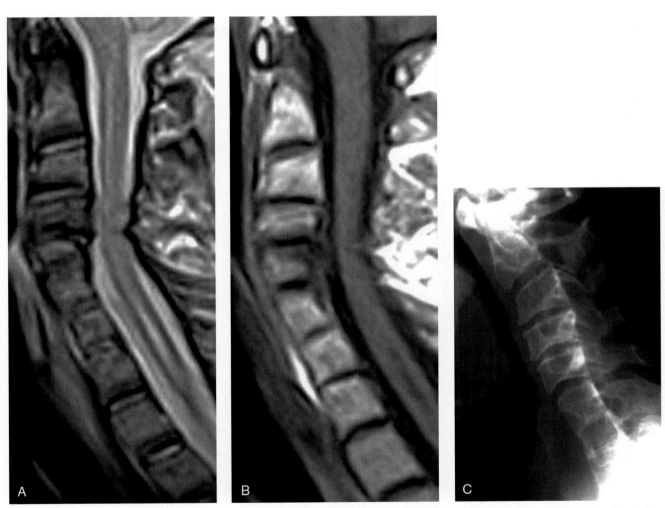

FIGURE 6–4. Klippel-Feil syndrome. A 51-year-old presented with diffuse neck pain and otherwise no neurologic findings referable to the cervical spine. Midline sagittal T_2- (A) and T_1-weighted (B) scans reveal marked degenerative disease at the C4–5 level. More importantly, there is an abnormal shape to vertebral bodies C6, C7, and T1 (height greater than width) and decreased height to the C6–7 and C7–T1 disk spaces. The shape of these vertebral bodies, together with the absence of normal disk material, raises the question of fusion. A syrinx is noted on the sagittal T_2-weighted exam and confirmed on T_1-weighted exam. Cervical spinal stenosis extends from C3 to C5 as a result of degenerative disease, best seen on the T_2-weighted exam. The lateral cervical spine x-ray film (C) obtained in flexion confirms the fusion of C6–T1, forming a block vertebra. In Klippel-Feil syndrome, there is fusion of two or more cervical vertebral bodies, most commonly C2 and C3 or C5 and C6. With the advent of magnetic resonance imaging, associated cord abnormalities, including syringomyelia and diastematomyelia, have been reported. Patients with Klippel-Feil syndrome are predisposed to spinal cord injury.

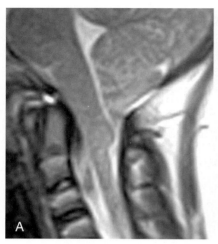
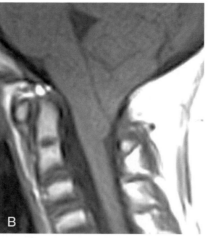
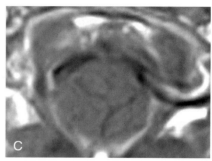

FIGURE 6–5. Chiari type I malformation. The patient is an 11-year-old with severe scoliosis. Fast spin echo T$_2$-weighted (*A*) and spin echo T$_1$-weighted (*B*) midline sagittal images reveal that the cerebellar tonsils are abnormally low in position (these extend 11 mm below the foramen magnum). The tonsils have also lost their usual globular configuration and are pointed (or wedge shaped) in appearance. Because of the patient's scoliosis, the lower cervical spine is seen in a parasagittal plane. The fourth ventricle is normal in shape and position, an important negative finding. *C,* The T$_1$-weighted axial view at the level of the arch of C1 confirms the abnormally low position of the cerebellar tonsils, which are wedged posteriorly and laterally. These compress and deform the spinal cord (anteriorly) at the cervicomedullary junction.

Associated findings include syringomyelia (Fig. 6–6) and craniovertebral junction abnormalities (basilar impression, occipitalization of the atlas, and Klippel-Feil syndrome). The fourth ventricle will be in normal position, an important differentiating feature from the Chiari type II malformation. As with all congenital malformations of the brain, the Chiari type I malformation is best evaluated by MRI.

Clinical findings are variable. Most patients are asymptomatic. When symptomatic, clinical findings in-

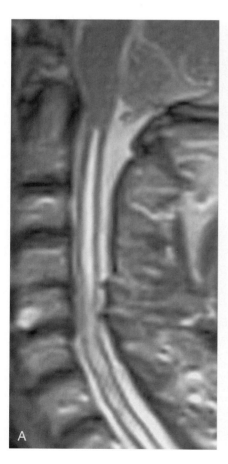
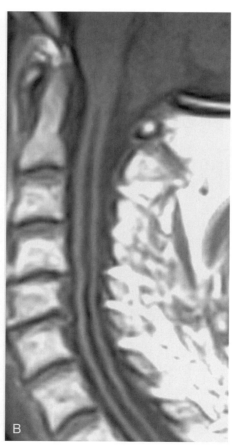

FIGURE 6–6. Chiari type I malformation with hydrosyringomyelia. This 69-year-old woman presented with left arm weakness and atrophy of the left trapezius muscle. On both the fast spin echo T$_2$-weighted (*A*) and the spin echo T$_1$-weighted (*B*) midline sagittal images, the cerebellar tonsils are noted to be low in position, extending 8 mm below the foramen magnum. The cerebellar tonsils also have an abnormal wedge-shaped configuration. An extensive syrinx is present within the cervical and upper thoracic spinal cord. Small bony spurs are incidentally noted at C4–5 and C5–6. The syrinx (containing cerebrospinal fluid) is depicted with high signal intensity on the T$_2$-weighted scan and low signal intensity on the T$_1$-weighted scan.

clude those related to brainstem compression (headache, cranial nerve deficits, nystagmus, and ataxia) or a cervical syrinx (extremity weakness, hyperreflexia, and central cord syndrome). In rare cases, a syrinx can extend into the medulla (syringobulbia). Symptoms in these patients include hemifacial numbness, facial pain, vertigo, dysphagia, and loss of taste. Symptomatic patients may benefit from decompression of the foramen magnum or shunting of the syrinx.

Chiari Type II

The Chiari type II malformation is the most common major congenital malformation of the posterior fossa. It is nearly always associated with hydrocephalus and a myelomeningocele. Findings in the brain include low insertion of the tentorium cerebelli (small posterior fossa), hypoplastic tentorium cerebelli (large incisura), towering cerebellum, extension of the cerebellum around the brainstem (laterally and anteriorly), a flattened pons with scalloping of the clivus and petrous bones, a prominent prepontine CSF space, an elongated midbrain, a small elongated slitlike fourth ventricle (10% of cases have a "ballooned" or trapped fourth ventricle), fusion of the colliculi (beaking of the quadrigeminal plate/tectum), fenestration of the falx (with interdigitation of cerebral gyri), agenesis of the corpus callosum, and a large massa intermedia. Findings in the spine (Fig. 6–7) include displacement of the brainstem and hypoplastic cerebellum into the upper cervical canal, cervicomedullary kinking (the medulla and cervical cord overlap), an enlarged foramen magnum and upper cervical canal, a small C1 ring with compression of the displaced brainstem and tonsils and vermis, a bifid C1 arch, posterior arch defects (C3-C7) and syringomyelia. The latter can occur in any location, more commonly in the low cervical and thoracic regions.

Chiari Type III

The Chiari type III malformation is quite rare. Findings are similar to a Chiari type II but with the addition of a cervico-occipital encephalocele. There is an osseous defect of occiput and upper cervical spine, with cerebellar herniation into the encephalocele.

Basilar Invagination

Patients in whom the tip of the odontoid process is 5 or more mm above Chamberlain's line (which is drawn from posterior margin of the hard palate to the posterior lip of the foramen magnum) are said to have basilar invagination. This anatomic variant can be primary or secondary (acquired) in type. The primary type is often associated with fusion of the atlas and occiput (occipitalization or assimilation). The secondary or acquired type is also called basilar impression. Acquired basilar invagination can be seen with osteomalacia, osteoporosis, fibrous dysplasia, Paget's disease, achondroplasia, and osteogenesis imperfecta. Platybasia can accompany basilar invagination. The normal angle formed by the clivus and floor of anterior cranial fossa measures 125 to 140 degrees. Platybasia is defined as an angle greater than 140 degrees.

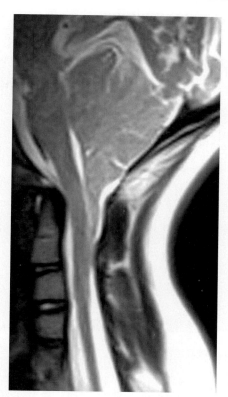

FIGURE 6–7. Chiari type II malformation. On the midline sagittal T₂-weighted image, a complex congenital abnormality involving the brainstem and cerebellum is clearly depicted. The cerebellar tonsils are elongated and extend down to the C2–3 level. The fourth ventricle is slitlike. The insertion of the tentorium is low, making for a small posterior fossa. The colliculi are fused, forming a "beaked" tectum. All are common features of the Chiari type II malformation.

Os Odontoideum

Both congenital and acquired causes have been described for os odontoideum. In this structural anomaly, a corticate ovoid ossicle is present, distinct from the body of C2 (Fig. 6–8). Os odontoideum must be distinguished from a fracture of the dens, the latter being not uncommon after major trauma. Familial cases and associated congenital abnormalities support the existence of congenital lesions. Reports of development of this abnormality after trauma support the existence of acquired lesions. In a patient with os odontoideum, the anterior arch of C1 will also be enlarged and have a convex posterior margin.

Neurofibromatosis

There are two major types of neurofibromatosis (NF). Both are autosomal dominant, but type 1 (NF1) is much more common. The abnormality has been localized to chromosome 17 in NF1 and to chromosome 22 in NF2.

Distinctive physical exam findings in NF1 include café au lait spots and iris hamartomas (Lisch nodules). Findings on MRI of the spine include scoliosis, a patulous dural sac, lateral meningoceles, and neurofibromas of the exiting nerve roots. Findings on MRI of the spine in NF2 include intradural extramedullary lesions

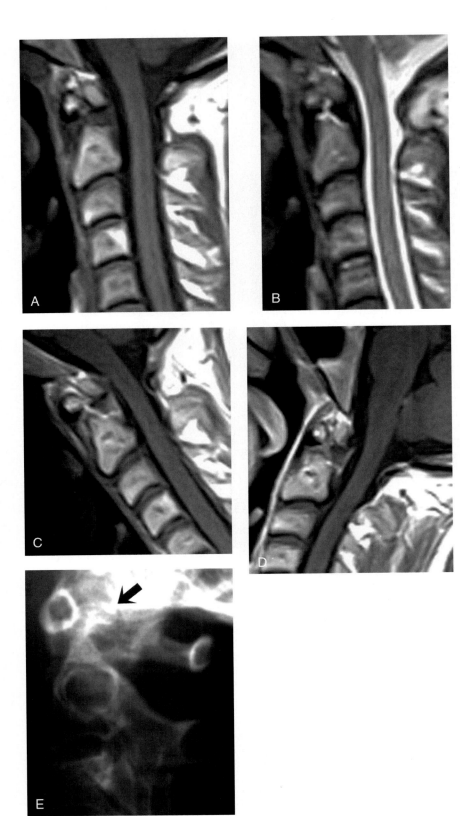

FIGURE 6–8. Os odontoideum, with stable fibrous union. This 46-year-old is being seen for neck pain after a car accident. *A,* On the sagittal T$_1$-weighted scan, the tip of the dens appears separate from the base. There is intervening intermediate signal intensity soft tissue. The marrow signal intensities of both the tip and the base are normal. The anterior arch of C1 is large and has a convex, not concave, posterior margin. *B,* On the sagittal fast spin echo T$_2$-weighted scan, no soft-tissue edema is noted. The cervical canal is normal in caliber. T$_1$-weighted sagittal images obtained in flexion (*C*) and extension (*D*) reveal no change in the distance between the tip of the dens and the anterior arch of C1. No cord compression is noted. The normal marrow and soft-tissue signal intensity seen on magnetic resonance imaging makes acute trauma very unlikely, with substantial edema otherwise anticipated. *E,* The lateral radiograph confirms the nonunion of the superior dens with its base. The superior fragment (*arrow*) is well corticated.

(neurofibromas and meningiomas) and intramedullary lesions (ependymomas and low-grade astrocytomas) (Fig. 6–9). The presence of bilateral acoustic neuromas on imaging of the head is considered pathognomonic of NF2. These patients may also have schwannomas, meningiomas, gliomas, and hamartomas of the brain. Peripheral nerve lesions, either solitary or involving multiple nerves in plexiform manner, are considered hallmarks of NF, but these are less commonly seen on MRI because of the focus of the exam being the brain or spine.

INFECTION AND INFLAMMATORY DISEASE
Epidural Abscess

Causes for an epidural abscess include hematogenous spread, direct extension, and penetrating trauma. *Staphylococcus aureus* is the most common organism. On MRI, thickened inflamed soft tissue is seen initially, which progresses to a frank abscess with a liquid center (Fig. 6–10). Depending on the stage of disease, the enhance-

FIGURE 6–9. Neurofibromatosis 2. *A,* The midline sagittal T$_2$-weighted image reveals two intramedullary lesions (likely either ependymomas or low-grade astrocytomas) with abnormal high signal intensity. One lesion is at the level of C3 and the other at the cervicomedullary junction. A third lesion, at C2, was better seen on adjacent slices. *B,* The midline sagittal T$_1$-weighted image reveals an extramedullary mass with soft tissue signal intensity along the posterior margin of the thecal sac anterior to the posterior arch of the C1. The mass causes mild deformity of the upper cervical cord. *C,* On the postcontrast sagittal T$_1$-weighted image, two foci of abnormal intramedullary enhancement are seen (corresponding to the abnormalities noted on the T$_2$-weighted scan): one within the cervical spinal cord and one at the cervicomedullary junction. The cord shows mild enlargement at the lesion sites. An intradural extramedullary enhancing mass (a meningioma) with a broad base abutting the dura is also seen along the posterior thecal sac just below the margin of the foramen magnum. *D,* An axial contrast-enhanced T$_1$-weighted image through the posterior fossa reveals bilateral (enhancing) acoustic schwannomas. Other images through the brain (not shown) demonstrated multiple meningiomas.

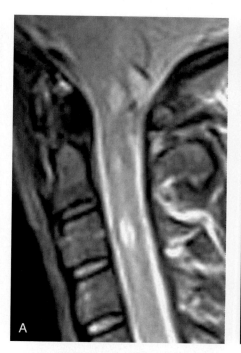
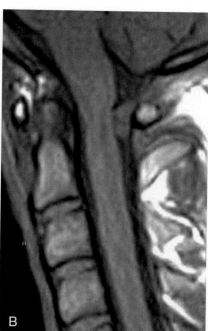
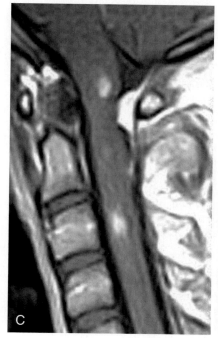
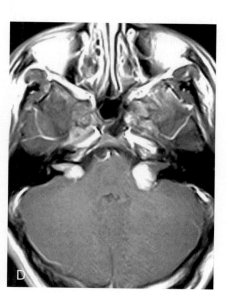

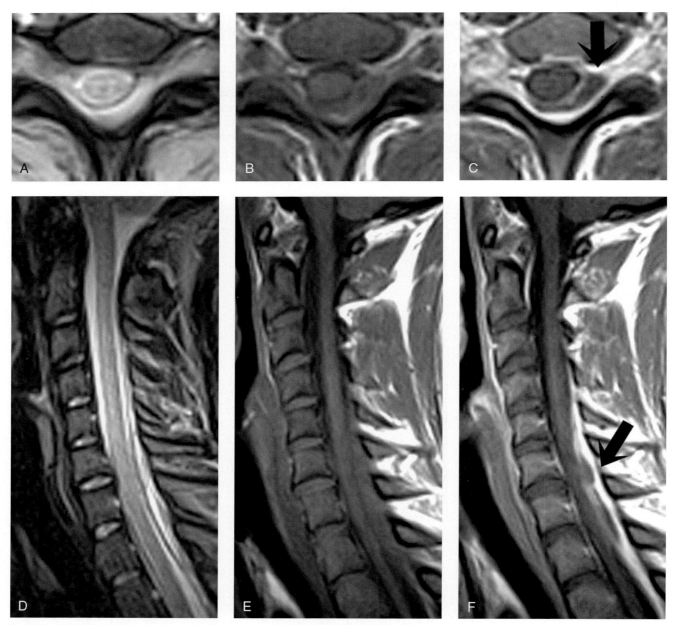

FIGURE 6–10. Epidural abscess. A cervical epidural catheter had previously been placed (now removed) for management of chronic left upper extremity pain. *A*, The T₂-weighted axial scan reveals anterior displacement of the thecal sac. *B*, The T₁-weighted scan raises the question of a posterior soft tissue mass. *C*, Postcontrast, an epidural fluid collection (*arrow*) is noted, with prominent enhancement of surrounding soft tissue. These findings are confirmed on the sagittal T₂- (*D*), T₁- (*E*), and postcontrast T₁-weighted (*F*) scans. Contrast use permits identification of the fluid pocket, with surrounding inflammatory change (*F, arrow*), indicating the diagnosis of infection.

ment on MRI after contrast administration can be homogeneous or rimlike with central low signal intensity (pus). An epidural abscess may cause cord compression as a result of the presence of inflammation, granulation tissue, or pus.

Sarcoidosis

Sarcoidosis is a noncaseating granulomatous disease of unknown cause. The CNS is involved clinically in 5% of patients. The basal leptomeninges and floor of the third ventricle are the most common sites of involvement. Spinal cord involvement is much less common.

MRI findings in sarcoidosis of the spine include fusiform cord enlargement, nodular parenchymal enhancement (broad based along the cord surface), and thin pial enhancement. Treatment is with steroids. Follow-up scans may demonstrate a return to normal appearance.

Rheumatoid Arthritis

Rheumatoid arthritis is a synovitis. This disease can involve any synovium-lined joint. In the axial skeleton, the upper cervical spine is most commonly involved, usually at the articulation of the atlas and dens (Fig. 6–11). Imaging findings include increased distance between

FIGURE 6–11. Rheumatoid arthritis with atlantoaxial subluxation. A 72-year-old woman with advanced rheumatoid arthritis presented clinically with neck and left arm pain. *A*, The sagittal T$_2$-weighted image reveals abnormal high signal intensity (resulting from fluid and inflammation) between the anterior arch of C1 and the dens. Areas of low signal intensity consistent with fibrosis and chronic reactive changes are also present. *B*, The sagittal precontrast T$_1$-weighted image demonstrates a large soft tissue mass predominantly anterior to the odontoid process. The cortex of the dens is mildly irregular. Enhancements of a portion of the abnormal soft tissue is seen on the postcontrast sagittal T$_1$-weighted image (*C*). The distance between the dens and the anterior arch of C1 is normal on the axial gradient echo image obtained in neutral position (*D*). *E*, The axial gradient echo image obtained in flexion demonstrates increased space measuring 8 mm between the dens and C1 consistent with atlantoaxial subluxation. The upper cervical cord is compressed between the dens and the posterior arch of C1. Atlantoaxial subluxation was confirmed on a lateral plain radiograph of the cervical spine (not shown). The distance between the anterior arch of C1 and the dens measured 11 mm.

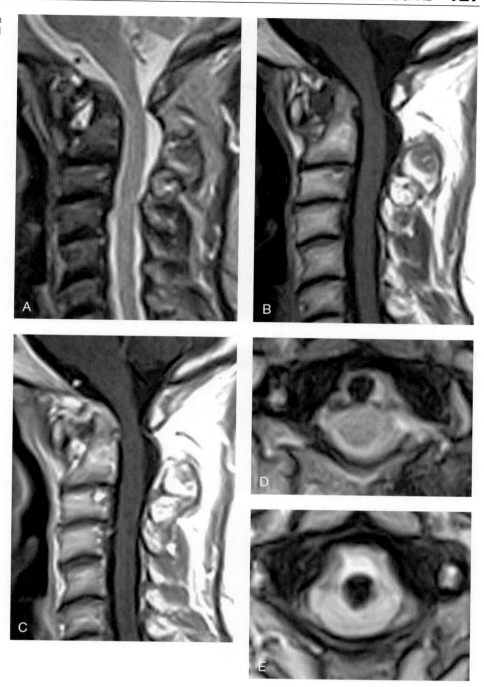

the atlas and dens (with instability), erosion of the dens (by surrounding inflammatory pannus), a retrodental soft tissue mass (resulting from involvement of the transverse ligament), and settling of the skull on the atlas. Rheumatoid arthritis, with involvement of the atlas and dens, can lead to cord compression.

BENIGN FOCAL LESIONS
Osteochondroma

An osteochondroma, also known as an osteocartilaginous exostosis, is a bony excrescence, with a cartilaginous covered cortex and a medullary cavity contiguous with the parent bone. Osteochondromas are rare in the spine. However, when present, the cervical spine is the most common location (half of all cases). The lesion is typically located in a spinous or transverse process.

Aneurysmal Bone Cyst

Aneurysmal bone cysts are benign, nonneoplastic lesions. This lesion is typically osteolytic, multiloculated, expansile, and highly vascular. Aneurysmal bone cysts often contain blood degradation products. Eighty percent are seen in patients younger than 20 years. Twenty percent of all lesions are seen in the spine; the cervical and thoracic spine are the most common locations. Most spinal lesions occur in the posterior elements.

Eosinophilic Granuloma

Eosinophilic granuloma is a benign, nonneoplastic disease. The preferred terminology for this disease is Langerhans' cell (eosinophilic) granulomatosis. Lesions may be solitary or multiple and are typically lytic without surrounding sclerosis. Eosinophilic granuloma is the classic cause of vertebra plana (a single collapsed vertebral body).

Cavernous Angioma

Cavernous angioma is one of the four general types of vascular malformations; the other three are capillary telangiectasia, venous angioma, and arteriovenous malformation. Cavernous angiomas are angiographically occult. They are thus grouped together with capillary telangiectasias, which most commonly are solitary, occur in the pons, and are clinically silent, under the term occult cerebrovascular malformations. Cavernous angiomas occur throughout the CNS and are multiple in one third of all cases. Eighty percent are familial. The majority of cavernous angiomas are clinically silent; the most common clinical presentation is seizure.

The typical cavernous angioma is small and smoothly marginated on imaging studies (Fig. 6–12). The border or rim of the lesion is markedly hypointense on T_2-weighted scans as a result of hemosiderin and ferritin deposition within macrophages after hemorrhage. Centrally, a cavernous angioma contains a honeycomb of vascular spaces separated by fibrous stands, which appears as a mixture of high and low signal intensity on T_2-weighted scans.

NEOPLASTIC DISEASE

Astrocytoma

Astrocytomas are the most common intramedullary tumor in the cervical region. This tumor type has a lower incidence in the distal spinal cord, the opposite of ependymomas. The peak incidence for spinal cord astrocytomas is the third and fourth decades. The tumor grade tends to be lower than for brain astrocytomas.

On imaging, an astrocytoma causes fusiform enlargement of the spinal cord (Fig. 6–13). Typically, a long segment of cord is involved (several vertebral segments in length) along with nearly the complete cross-section of the cord. Abnormal high signal intensity on T_2-weighted scans reflects both tumor and edema. Enhancement postcontrast is common with cord astrocytomas but is not seen in all cases. This is one entity in which the addition of delayed scans (obtained 30 to 60 minutes after contrast administration) improves the detection of abnormal enhancement. Cord enlargement, limited to one or two levels, favors the diagnosis of an ependymoma over an astrocytoma. Contrast administration is mandatory in the MRI examination of postoperative cases for tumor recurrence (Fig. 6–14). Postsurgical changes can be difficult to distinguish from recurrent

tumor without contrast administration, and recurrent tumor almost invariably enhances regardless of whether the primary lesion did so. Cord ischemia or infarction (in the subacute time frame) should be kept in mind in terms of differential diagnosis for an enhancing cord lesion of substantial craniocaudal extent (Fig. 6–15).

Hemangioblastoma/Von Hippel-Lindau Disease

Hemangioblastomas of the spinal cord can be solid, with surrounding cord edema, or cystic, with an enhancing mural nodule. If the lesion is cystic, the fluid contents, although similar, will be differentiable from CSF on some pulse sequences. Hemangioblastomas are highly vascular lesions and thus enhance prominently on MRI. Their appearance on x-ray angiography is distinctive because of the tumor blush and enlarged feeding arteries and draining veins. Hemangioblastomas are most frequently found in the posterior fossa. They are much less common in the cord, but when in this location have an equal incidence in the cervical and thoracic spine. Spinal cord hemangioblastomas can be solitary or multiple, the latter pathognomonic of von Hippel-Lindau disease.

Von Hippel-Lindau disease is an autosomal-dominant syndrome. Features of this disease outside the CNS include renal cell carcinoma, pheochromocytoma, and cysts of the kidney and pancreas. In regard to neurologic disease, these patients present with hemangioblastomas of the cerebellum or spinal cord (Fig. 6–16).

Meningioma

Of all intraspinal tumors, meningiomas represent 25% and are second in incidence to neurinomas. Meningiomas are usually solitary lesions. The peak age incidence is 45 years. Meningiomas are histologically benign and slow growing and cause symptoms because of cord and nerve root compression. On MRI, spinal meningiomas look much like meningiomas of the brain, often demonstrating a broad dural base and consistently displaying intense enhancement. One percent to 3% of all meningiomas occur at the foramen magnum (Fig. 6–17). Of extramedullary lesions in this location, three quarters are meningiomas and one quarter neurofibromas.

Metastases to Bone

Vertebral metastases are a major source of morbidity in cancer patients. The spinal column is involved in up to 40% of patients dying of metastatic disease. Bone expansion, pathologic fractures, and cord compression are not uncommon. Plain x-ray films are insensitive for lesion detection; at least 50% of the bone needs to be destroyed in order for the lesion to be seen. Bone scans have high sensitivity but low specificity. Reasons for false-positive results on bone scan include infection, trauma, and degenerative disease. Computed tomography (CT) is typically limited in the extent of coverage and offers poor soft tissue contrast. With myelography, cord compression can be evaluated, but lesions are inferred (not directly visualized). MRI offers high sensitivity and specificity, excellent anatomic coverage, and

Text continued on page 134

FIGURE 6–12. Cavernous angioma. The patient is a 34-year-old woman with right and left hand, arm, and neck pain and numbness. On T$_2$-weighted scans using fast spin echo (*A*) and gradient echo (*B*) technique, a high-signal-intensity abnormality is noted within the cord at the T1 level, with a circumferential rim of hypointensity. The lesion is well marginated from surrounding tissue. Although the central high-signal-intensity portion of the lesion is clearly seen on the fast T$_2$ scan, the rim of hypointensity is much less evident. Gradient echo scans, because of their sensitivity to susceptibility effects, clearly depict the presence of hemosiderin and ferritin. Fast T$_2$-weighted scans are inferior in this regard because of the acquisition of closely spaced spin echoes and thus relative insensitivity to susceptibility effects. The lesion is not well seen on the sagittal noncontrast T$_1$-weighted image (*C*). *D,* The axial gradient echo scan demonstrates the central hyperintense fluid collection (methemoglobin), together with the smooth peripheral rim of hypointensity (hemosiderin/ferritin). A second lesion with similar characteristics was present within the medulla (not shown).

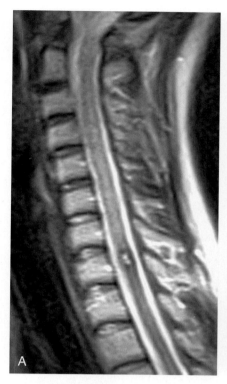

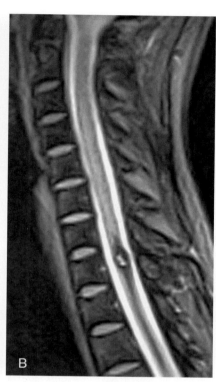

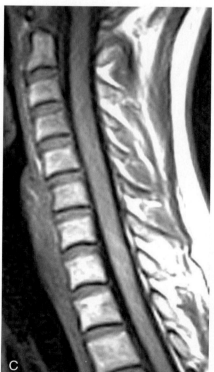

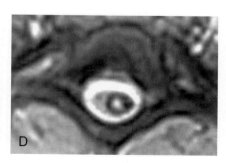

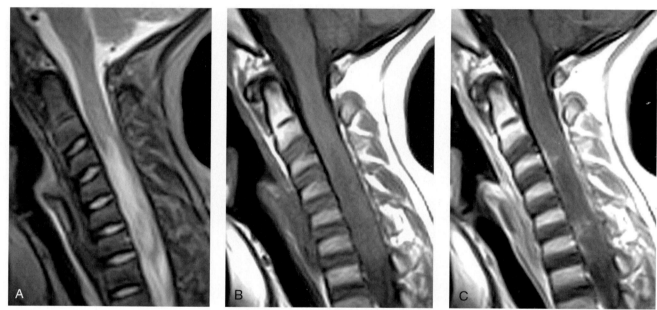

FIGURE 6–13. Cervical cord astrocytoma. A 10-year-old presented with arm weakness. *A,* On the precontrast T$_2$-weighted sagittal scan, a hyperintense cord lesion is noted, which extends from C3 to C7. *B,* The precontrast T$_1$-weighted scan reveals marked cord enlargement. *C,* Postcontrast, there is mottled abnormal enhancement within portions of the lesion. Although not all cord astrocytomas demonstrate enhancement postcontrast on magnetic resonance imaging, this finding, when present, improves differential diagnosis and provides guidance for biopsy. Administration of contrast is particularly important in the presence of a syrinx if a neoplastic origin is in question.

FIGURE 6–14. Recurrent astrocytoma. The magnetic resonance imaging (MRI) exam was performed several years after an extensive laminectomy for resection of a spinal cord astrocytoma. Examining the sagittal precontrast T_2- (*A*) and T_1-weighted (*B*) scans, a syrinx cavity is noted, which expands the cord and extends from C2 to T2. The signal intensity characteristics of the syrinx differ from that of cerebrospinal fluid, suggesting a neoplastic origin. On the sagittal (*C*) and axial (*D*) postcontrast T_1-weighted scans, there is abnormal enhancement of a large soft tissue nidus within the syrinx at the C5–6 level. This finding was new from the prior MRI exam and represents recurrent tumor. Postcontrast scans in the spine are particularly valuable for detecting recurrent intramedullary neoplastic disease. Such lesions are often difficult to detect without contrast administration because of the distortion of normal structures and the isointensity of the lesion with surrounding soft tissue.

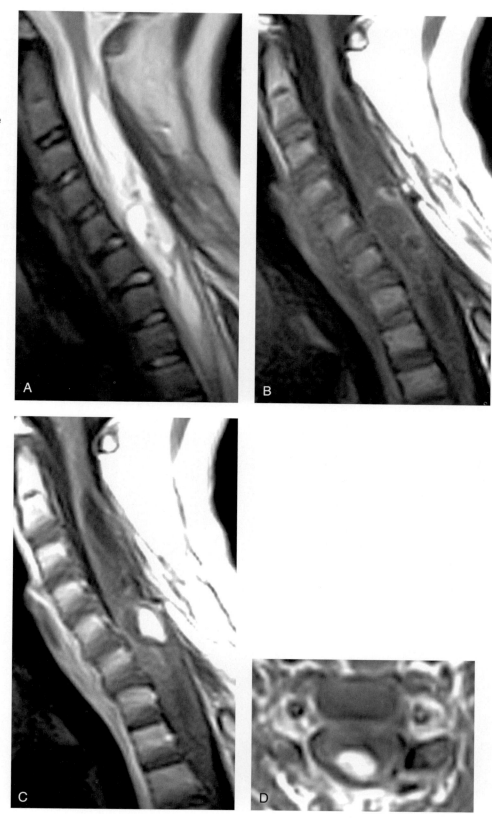

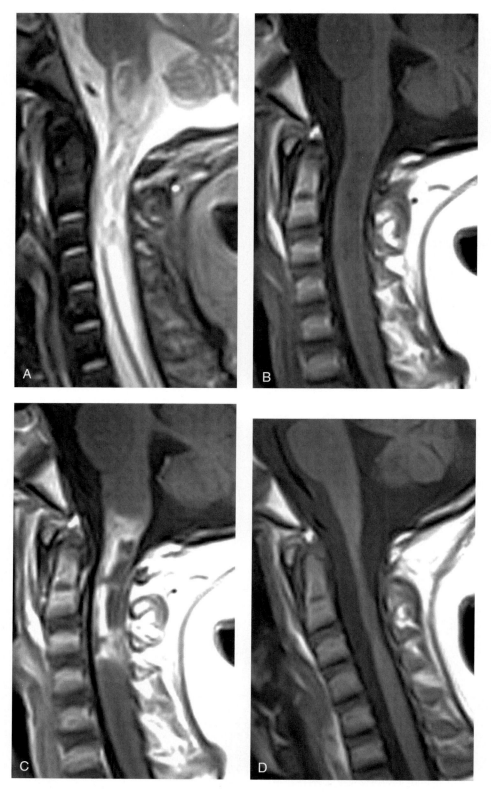

FIGURE 6–15. Cord ischemia (resulting from therapeutic radiation). This 7-year-old became quadriplegic after spinal axis radiation for acute lymphocytic leukemia. Biopsy revealed gliosis. A cervical spine magnetic resonance imaging (MRI) scan obtained before treatment was normal. *A,* On the sagittal T_2-weighted scan, there is abnormal hyperintensity within the cervical cord and lower brainstem. Enlargement of the upper cervical cord is best visualized on the precontrast T_1-weighted scan (*B*). Comparison of pre- (*B*) and postcontrast (*C*) sagittal T_1-weighted scans reveals marked abnormal enhancement within the upper cervical cord. The MRI exam was repeated 5 months later with a sagittal T_1-weighted scan (*D*). At that time, only atrophy of the upper cervical cord was noted. There was no abnormal contrast enhancement.

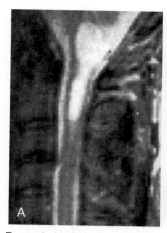
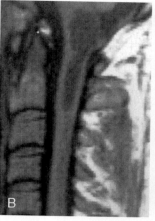
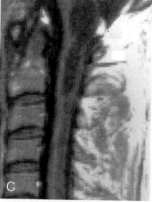
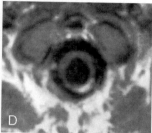

FIGURE 6–16. Spinal cord hemangioblastoma. A 42-year-old with known von Hippel-Lindau disease presented clinically with increasing gait disturbance. A cord syrinx is noted, with high signal intensity on the T_2-weighted scan (*A*) and low signal intensity on the T_1-weighted scan (*B*), which extends from the medulla to C2–3. There is secondary expansion of the spinal cord. No abnormal soft tissue mass is noted precontrast. The cerebellar tonsil is globular in shape and normal in position, ruling out a Chiari type I malformation. After contrast administration (*C*, sagittal; *D*, axial), an enhancing nodule is identified along the posterior wall of the upper portion of the syrinx. Hemangioblastomas are relatively rare benign epithelial tumors. In von Hippel-Lindau disease (with which there is an association), these tumors may be multiple.

FIGURE 6–17. Foramen magnum meningioma. On the precontrast T_2- (*A*) and T_1-weighted (*B*) axial images, a mass is seen at the level of the foramen magnum. There is substantial deformity of the medulla. Axial (*C*) and coronal (*D*) postcontrast images demonstrate intense lesion enhancement (*D*, arrow). The dural-based origin of the lesion, questioned on the basis of precontrast scans, is confirmed postcontrast.

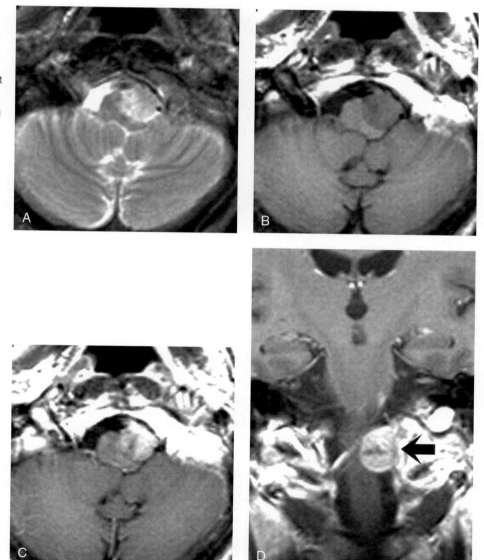

excellent soft tissue lesion detection. MRI is universally accepted as the modality of choice for the detection and assessment of metastases involving the spinal column.

High cervical vertebral metastases, in particular, can be a cause of great morbidity (Fig. 6–18). Sensory and motor deficits from such lesions can be extensive. Cranial neuropathies can occur as a result of spread to the skull base. Compression of the cervical cord above C3 can lead to death by respiratory embarrassment. In regard to tumor type, involvement of cervical spine and skull base by squamous cell carcinoma of neck is not uncommon. This tumor generally spreads by local invasion. Cervical vertebral metastases also commonly arise from a distant primary, with prostate, lung, and breast carcinoma common causes.

Metastases to a vertebra, regardless of location, appear

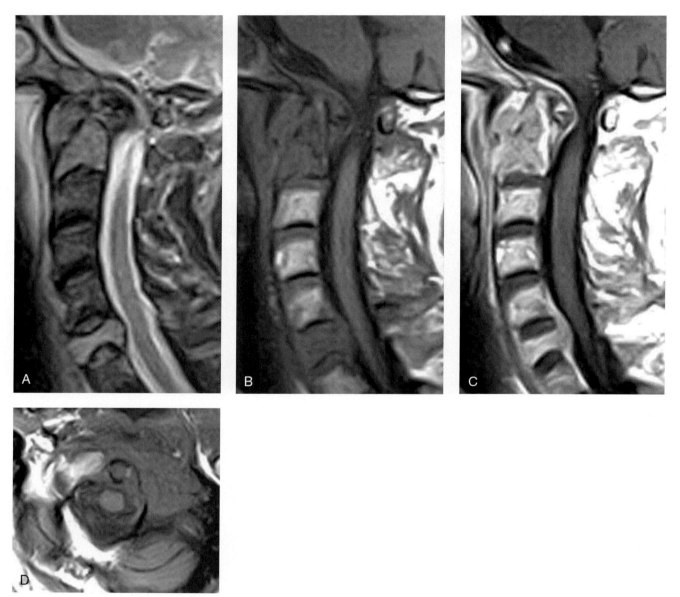

FIGURE 6–18. Cervical bony metastases with skull base involvement causing basilar impression. The 61-year-old patient had extensive laryngeal carcinoma and presented with increasing neck pain. Sagittal images just to the left of midline reveal abnormal signal intensity within the C1, C2, and C6 vertebral bodies, high on T$_2$-weighted scans (*A*) and low on T$_1$-weighted scans (*B*). The clivus is also involved. At both C1 and C6, there is anterior compromise of the thecal space resulting from the expansile nature of the lesions. Sagittal images more off to the side (not shown) revealed contiguity of the vertebral lesions with the patient's extensive laryngeal squamous cell carcinoma. The tip of the dens lies within the foramen magnum 1 cm superior to Chamberlain's line. *C*, Postcontrast, the affected vertebrae and skull base enhance to isointensity with normal marrow. Thus, it is difficult postcontrast to identify the marrow replacement by neoplastic disease on the basis of signal intensity alone. Epidural extension of the abnormality at C6, however, is more clearly depicted. *D*, A precontrast T$_1$-weighted axial image at the C1 level confirms the abnormal low signal intensity within the dens and much of the anterior arch of C1. The abnormal soft tissue that infiltrates the arch of C1 on the left involves as well the adjacent occipital condyle. Abnormal soft tissue is also present within the anterior spinal canal, but no cord compression is visualized at this level. Causes of basilar impression (acquired basilar invagination) include osteoporosis and osteomalacia, Paget's disease, and achondroplasia. However, any disease that produces abnormal bone softening, such as metastases, may lead to basilar impression.

on MRI as low signal intensity lesions on T_1-weighted scans because of the replacement of normal high signal intensity fatty marrow. Metastases are often high signal intensity on T_2-weighted scans. The appearance on T_2-weighted scans is, however, variable. Blastic metastases are often low signal intensity on T_2-weighted scans. Thus, most MRI sites use precontrast T_1-weighted scans for detection of vertebral metastases. After intravenous contrast administration, vertebral metastases often enhance to isointensity with normal surrounding marrow. Postcontrast scans, particularly as commonly used without fat saturation, are poor for detection of lesions within the bones of the spinal column. However, contrast enhancement generally improves the depiction of the epidural soft tissue extent of metastatic disease.

Leptomeningeal and Spinal Cord Metastases

Five percent of all metastatic disease to the CNS will have intramedullary spinal metastases (metastasis to the spinal cord itself). The thoracic cord is most often involved. Bronchogenic carcinoma is the most common primary. On imaging, spinal cord metastases have a central enhancing focus with surrounding cord edema, an appearance expected from the imaging of brain metastases.

Leptomeningeal metastases in the cervical region can present on imaging as soft tissue nodules within the thecal sac (Fig. 6–19), irregularity of the cord surface contour (tumor adherent to or encasing the cord) (Fig.

FIGURE 6–19. Leptomeningeal metastases from pineoblastoma. Two years before the current exam, this 9-year-old boy presented with persistent headaches and vomiting. Imaging revealed obstructive hydrocephalus, with a mass in the pineal region which proved (by subtotal resection) to be a pineoblastoma. The patient subsequently received brain and spinal axis radiation as well as chemotherapy. At this time, he presents with intractable vomiting, ataxia, and back pain. A bulky soft tissue mass is noted at the C1–2 level on sagittal T_2- (A) and T_1-weighted (B) scans, causing marked cord compression. The T_2-weighted scan identifies an additional lesion at the C6 level, which is poorly seen on the T_1-weighted exam. A portion of the larger lesion at C1–2 is of low signal intensity on the T_2-weighted scan, suggesting tumoral hemorrhage. In the midthoracic region, multiple additional soft tissue masses were seen within the thecal sac (not shown). These were immediately adjacent to the cord and produced an irregular surface contour (C, D). Head magnetic resonance imaging obtained 2 weeks later reveals intracranial metastases. Two low signal intensity foci (arrows) can be identified precontrast on the T_2-weighted exam (C). At least two enhancing lesions (arrows) are identified postcontrast on the T_1-weighted exam (D). Pineoblastomas are primitive tumors of pinealocyte origin (as opposed to the more differentiated pineocytomas) that present in the first decade of life and are more common in males. Dissemination via the cerebrospinal fluid (CSF) is common. Another pediatric tumor with a propensity for early CSF spread is medulloblastoma.

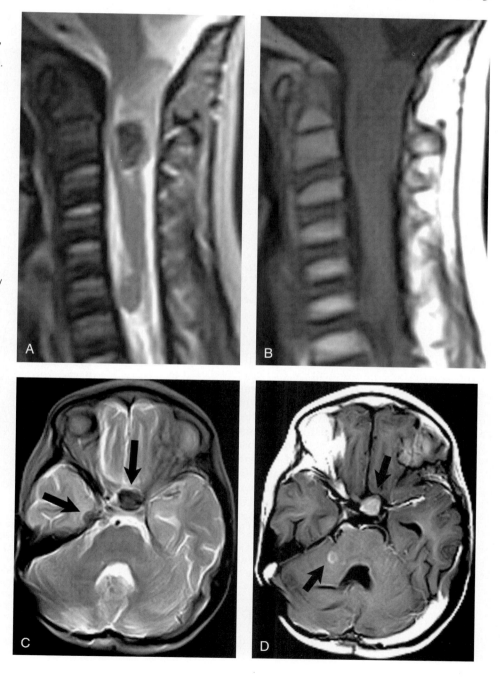

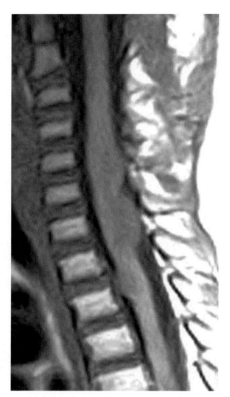

FIGURE 6–20. Leptomeningeal ("drop") metastases from medulloblastoma. The patient is a 4-year-old who had headaches for 9 months and now presents with diminished coordination. Head magnetic resonance imaging (not shown) revealed a midline enhancing posterior fossa mass with obstructive hydrocephalus. On the midline sagittal T$_1$-weighted cervical image, multiple large soft tissue nodules are noted adjacent to the cervical cord. These demonstrated only very slight enhancement postcontrast (not shown). The posterior fossa mass was resected, followed by whole brain and spinal axis radiation. The follow-up scan 2 months later (not shown) revealed a normal thecal sac and spinal cord.

6–20), or thin coating of the spinal cord (especially the dorsal aspect). Diffuse subarachnoid spread of tumor can cause coating and encasement (with deformity) of the spinal cord, leading to an appearance on gross exam resembling "icing." Most leptomeningeal metastatic disease enhances postcontrast on MRI; contrast administration is highly recommended for diagnosis. The entire spinal axis (cervical, thoracic, and lumbar) should be studied to rule out leptomeningeal metastases, with attention to the lumbar region (because of the effect of gravity). MRI, performed with and without contrast enhancement, has been consistently demonstrated in published studies to be superior to CT myelography for the detection of leptomeningeal metastases. This is particularly true for small tumor nodules and coating of the spinal cord by tumor. CT myelography is also not sensitive to intramedullary tumor involvement.

RADIATION THERAPY

The changes encountered with radiation therapy can at times be readily identified because of the confinement to the treatment area or port. After therapeutic radiation, there is uniform fatty replacement of bone marrow. This occurs as early as 2 weeks after initiation of therapy, with temporal progression. Imaging in the sagittal plane with T$_1$-weighted scans is recommended. Vertebral bodies within the port will have substantially higher signal intensity on such scans (Fig. 6–21), assuming that the choice of time to echo and time to repetition has been made appropriately to obtain moderate to heavy T$_1$-weighting.

HYDROSYRINGOMYELIA

According to terminology developed for histopathology, syringomyelia is defined as an abnormal cavity within

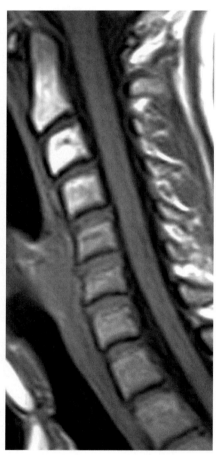

FIGURE 6–21. Radiation therapy changes with fatty replacement of bone marrow. The patient is a 45-year-old woman with a clinical history of radical neck dissection and radiation therapy for squamous cell carcinoma of the mouth. The midline sagittal T$_1$-weighted image demonstrates diffuse homogeneous high signal intensity throughout the marrow spaces of the C2–4 vertebral bodies. The high signal intensity in the marrow spaces shows an abrupt transition to the normal marrow signal intensity of the adjacent lower cervical vertebral bodies. Detection of this change was aided by comparison with the previous exam (not shown) and inspection of the relative signal intensity of the cord, disk spaces, and marrow. The increase in marrow signal intensity and uniformity of signal is due to radiation therapy with resultant replacement of normal red marrow by fat.

FIGURE 6–22. Hydrosyringomyelia. Sagittal (*A*) and axial (*B*) T_2-weighted images demonstrate apparent dilatation of the central canal of the spinal cord over a two-vertebral-body segment in the lower cervical spine. The abnormality is equally well seen on sagittal (*C*) and axial (*D*) T_1-weighted images. The signal intensity of this centrally located fluid cavity is that of cerebrospinal fluid on all scans, being high signal intensity on T_2-weighted images and low signal intensity on T_1-weighted images. The patient's symptoms were unrelated to this incidental finding.

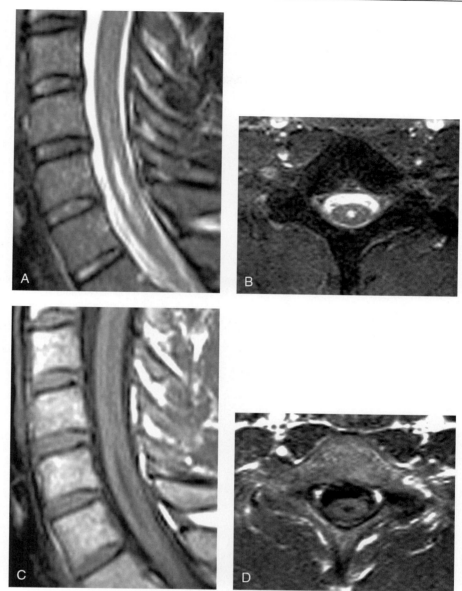

the spinal cord that is separate from but may communicate with the central canal. This is to be differentiated from hydromyelia, which is a dilatation of the central canal, lined by ependymal cells. These two entities are indistinguishable on imaging. Thus, the term hydrosyringomyelia should be used (Fig. 6–22). On imaging, hydrosyringomyelia is seen as a longitudinally oriented fluid cavity (with CSF signal intensity on all pulse sequences) within the spinal cord.

Of special note in the cervical spine is syringobulbia, which is simply extension of a syrinx into the brainstem (Fig. 6–23). This lesion is caused by obstruction of CSF flow at the foramen magnum, usually because of the presence of a Chiari type II malformation. Extension of the syrinx superiorly to involve the brainstem, with a tubular or saccular configuration, is thought to be the result of episodes of increased intra-abdominal pressure (as a result of coughing or sneezing). Symptoms of syringobulbia include facial pain and numbness, dysphagia, vertigo, loss of taste, and respiratory problems (in severe cases).

On MRI, the sagittal plane is typically used to define the extent of a syrinx. Imaging in the axial plane is often helpful to visualize small syrinxes and to confirm intermediate size lesions. Hydrosyringomyelia has many causes, including trauma (with development of the syrinx over years after the event), neoplasm, arachnoiditis, surgery, and developmental abnormalities such as the Chiari malformations.

Clinical symptoms of a cervical syrinx include progressive upper extremity weakness, muscle wasting, decreased upper extremity reflexes, and loss of pain and temperature sensation (with preservation of light touch and proprioception). A syrinx that enlarges in the posttraumatic patient can cause clinically significant neurologic deterioration. Large symptomatic syrinxes are treated surgically by shunting into the subarachnoid, pleural, or peritoneal spaces (Fig. 6–24).

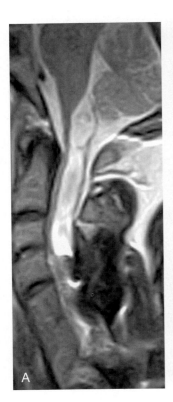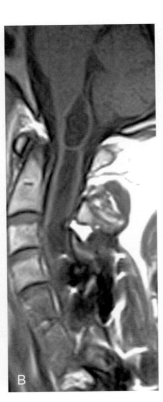

FIGURE 6–23. Syringobulbia. This 31-year-old is status postcervical fusion 8 years ago for multiple fractures. *A*, The T_2-weighted midline sagittal image reveals postoperative changes at C5–6. The C5 and C6 vertebral bodies have been surgically fused, with loss of the normal intervening disk space. A large amount of metallic artifact is present in the region of the posterior elements compatible with known stainless steel fixation wires. A fluid collection, which is noted to be septated on the T_1-weighted image (*B*), is identified within the spinal cord above the site of fusion, extending superiorly to near the inferior extent of the fourth ventricle. The abnormality (a posttraumatic syrinx) is isointense with cerebrospinal fluid with on T_1- and T_2-weighted images.

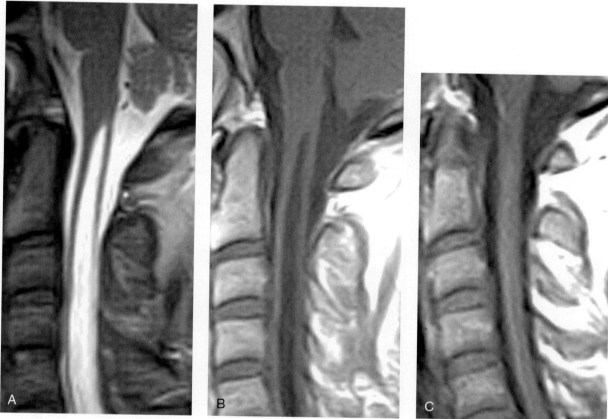

FIGURE 6–24. Posttraumatic hydrosyringomyelia with interval shunting and collapse. This 44-year-old man suffered a fracture of T9 that was treated by laminectomy and fusion 12 years ago. The patient now presents with delayed, progressive neurologic deficits. *A* and *B*, The preoperative study demonstrates fluid signal extending down the central portion of the spinal cord from the cervicomedullary junction through the visualized lower cervical region. This is seen as high signal intensity within the cord on the sagittal T_2-weighted image (*A*) and low signal intensity on the postcontrast T_1-weighted image (*B*). No abnormal enhancement is noted. The lesion is a posttraumatic syrinx secondary to a severe wedge compression fracture of T9 (not shown). The spinal cord is expanded with effacement of the surrounding subarachnoid space. The patient underwent a thoracic laminectomy with placement of a syringoperitoneal shunt. *C*, The postoperative sagittal T_1-weighted image of the cervical spine demonstrates collapse of the syrinx. The spinal cord is mildly atrophic, with cerebrospinal fluid now present surrounding the cord. Postoperatively, the patient's muscle strength and sensation improved.

TRAUMA

In flexion injuries, anterior wedging of the vertebral body and vertebral body fractures occur. In severe flexion injury, there can be disruption of the posterior longitudinal ligament and interspinous ligaments, facet distraction, and anteroposterior subluxation. In extension injuries, posterior element fractures occur. In severe extension injury, there can be rupture of the anterior longitudinal ligament and subluxation. Axial loading injuries (with vertical compression from diving or jumping accidents) produce vertebral body compression (burst) fractures and lateral element fractures. Rotation injuries, although rarely isolated and usually occurring with flexion-extension injury, produce lateral mass fractures and facet subluxations. High-resolution CT with multiplanar reconstruction is commonly used in acute trauma and best evaluates bony lesions. MRI is best in regard to the evaluation of the cord and soft tissues.

Cord hemorrhage after spinal cord injury carries in general a poor prognosis (Fig. 6–25). Cord edema, in the absence of hemorrhage, carries a much better prognosis, often with substantial neurologic recovery. Several patterns of acute spinal cord injury have been described on T$_2$-weighted MRI scans. Type I injury has central hypointensity with a thin rim of hyperintensity (deoxyhemoglobin centrally with methemoglobin at the periphery) and carries a very poor prognosis, with little neurologic recovery anticipated. Type II injury has uniform hyperintensity as a result of spinal cord edema and carries an excellent prognosis, with substantial, often complete, neurologic recovery (Fig. 6–26). Type III injury has an isointense center with a thick rim of hyperintensity, representing a combination of hemorrhage and edema, and follows a variable course; some recovery of function is anticipated.

Myelomalacic changes in the spinal cord after trauma follow a well-known sequence. Early on there is cord edema, with compression and stasis within venules and blood-cord barrier disruption. In this early stage, the area of injury in the cord is high signal intensity on T$_2$-weighted scans because of the presence of vasogenic edema. With progression of time, cystic necrosis occurs within the central gray matter. This has high signal intensity on T$_2$-weighted scans and low signal intensity on T$_1$-weighted scans. In the chronic stage, progressive cystic degeneration centrally may lead to a syrinx. The presence and extent of a syrinx is often best defined on axial T$_1$ images; visualization on sagittal images suffers from partial volume imaging. Cord atrophy may also develop in the chronic period. Cord atrophy is defined by a cord diameter of less than 6 mm in the cervical region and less than 5 mm in the thoracic region.

In the imaging of spine trauma, as previously stated,

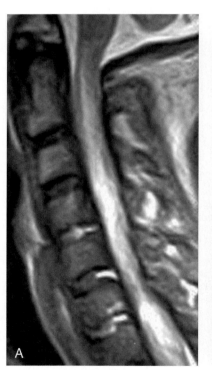 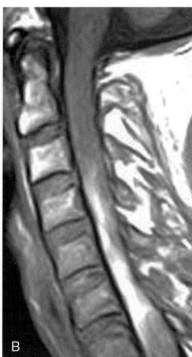 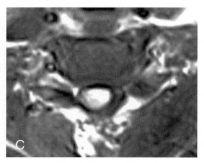

FIGURE 6–25. Traumatic spinal cord injury, with cord hemorrhage (and edema) and canal compromise. The 34-year-old patient was an unrestrained passenger in a single-vehicle motor accident. *A,* On the midline sagittal T$_2$-weighted image, there is abnormal high signal intensity within the cord extending from the tip of the dens to below the C7 level. There is compromise of the spinal canal posteriorly at the C5 and C6 levels. Abnormal high signal intensity is noted within the C4–5, C5–6, and C6–7 intervertebral disks, suggesting fluid accumulation or edema (secondary to trauma). *B,* On the corresponding T$_1$-weighted sagittal image, there is abnormal hyperintensity within the cord from C4 to C6, corresponding to methemoglobin. Posterior compromise of the spinal canal is again noted. *C,* On the single axial T$_1$-weighted image, the posterior soft tissues are asymmetric, suggesting additional injury, and the lamina on the left appears fractured. Lamina fractures were noted on computed tomography (not shown) at both the C5 and C6 levels on the left. The patient, who was quadriplegic after the accident, died 2 weeks later of multisystem failure.

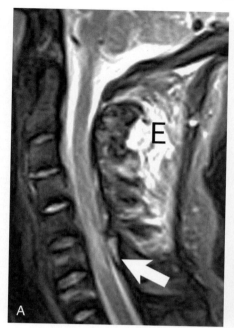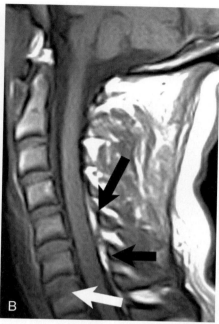

FIGURE 6–26. Cord contusion with a small posterior epidural hematoma. The patient is a 25-year-old man who 12 hours earlier was involved in a motor vehicle accident and now complains of bilateral upper extremity and shoulder pain. *A,* On the T_2-weighted exam, abnormal high signal intensity is identified within the cord from C5 to C6 consistent with edema (E) (cord contusion). There is obliteration from C4 to C6 of the cerebrospinal fluid space that normally surrounds the cord. Posteriorly in the epidural space, abnormal soft tissue (with mixed high and low signal intensity) is identified (*A, white arrow*), causing thecal sac compression. *B,* The sagittal T_1-weighted exam at first glance appears unremarkable, with perhaps only subtle loss of definition of the superior end plate of C7 (*white arrow*). Examining closely the epidural space at the C5 and C6 levels, abnormal high signal intensity corresponding to methemoglobin is identified (*B, black arrows*). Without comparison to the T_2-weighted scan, this small extradural hematoma might have been mistaken for normal epidural fat. High signal intensity is identified on the T_2-weighted image within the bodies of C6 and C7 as a result of microfractures and resultant marrow edema. This finding is consistent with the poor visualization of the superior end plate of C7 (*B*), which suggests gross bony damage. Extensive high signal intensity in the soft tissues posteriorly on the T_2-weighted exam indicates substantial soft tissue and ligamentous injury.

CT is superior for the demonstration of osseous injury. CT is preferred (over MRI) for the evaluation of posterior element fractures and canal narrowing resulting from retropulsed fragments. MRI is preferred for evaluation of the spinal cord in trauma. MRI is superior for the demonstration of cord injury and cord compression by soft tissue, such as a traumatic disk herniation (Fig. 6–27). Traumatic disk herniations most commonly occur in the cervical spine as opposed to the thoracic or lumbar spine. The incidence of disease increases with the severity of trauma. A traumatic disk herniation is common with hyperextension injury, specifically at C5-6 (Fig. 6–28). In whiplash injuries (acceleration hyperextension), acute posterolateral disk herniations are primarily seen. Symptoms include immediate neck and arm pain. In patients with cervical fractures, a disk herniation is most common at the level immediately below the fracture. Cord compression can be due to a traumatic disk herniation, bone fractures or dislocations, or, not to be forgotten, an epidural hematoma (Fig. 6–29). T_2-weighted images are important for the demonstration of marrow edema (vertebral body microfractures) and soft tissue injury.

A number of specific osseous injuries occur with some frequency after cervical trauma, and several carry colorful names. Atlanto-occipital dislocation is often fatal. Diagnosis is made on sagittal images (or a lateral x-ray film); the normal distance between the dens and the anterior margin of foramen magnum is no more than 12.5 mm. Jefferson's fracture is a burst fracture involving both the anterior and posterior arches of C1 (the atlas). Unless the transverse ligament is disrupted, the patient will be neurologically intact. This can be an unstable fracture. A fracture of the dens (Fig. 6–30) can occur with either hyperflexion or hyperextension. Dens fractures are classified by the anatomic location of the fracture line. Type I fracture involves the upper dens. Type II fracture involves the junction of the dens and the body. This is the most common type of injury and has the highest rate of nonunion. Type III extends into the C2 body. It is important to note that transverse fractures, such as those that occur in the dens, can be inapparent on axial images. Hangman's fracture, which is hyperextension injury, is a fracture or fracture dislocation at the level of C2 and C3 that extends through the pedicles of C2. The clay shoveler's fracture is a flexion injury, with avulsion of the spinous process, usually C6 or C7.

Injury to the cervical spine can be the result of abnormal flexion (or extension), rotation, or a combination of flexion and rotation. Bilateral facet fractures or dislocation are the result of flexion injury. Unilateral facet fractures are the result of flexion plus rotation (Fig. 6–31). Vertebral body compression fractures result from flexion injury. Injury to the posterior musculature and

Text continued on page 146

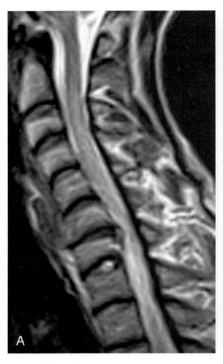

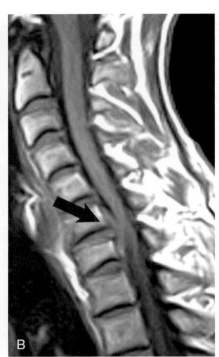

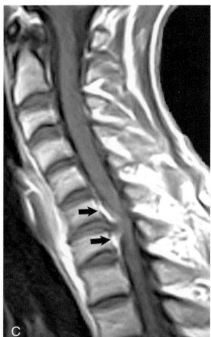

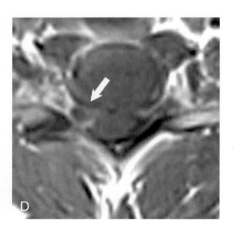

FIGURE 6–27. Posttraumatic right foraminal disk herniation at C6–7. This 36-year-old presented with severe right arm and neck pain after a "whiplash" injury. *A,* The T$_2$-weighted sagittal image, just to the right of midline, reveals a prominent extradural defect at the C6–7 level. *B,* On the corresponding T$_1$-weighted sagittal image, the abnormal soft tissue is noted to be contiguous with the C6–7 disk (*arrow*) but also extends well above and below the level of the disk. After contrast administration (*C*), it is evident that the soft tissue above and below the disk space level corresponds to dilated epidural venous plexus (which enhances postcontrast, *arrows*). *D,* A postinfusion axial image at the C6–7 level confirms the disk herniation (*arrow*), which fills the right C6–7 neural foramen. Mild mass effect on the right side of the spinal cord is also noted.

FIGURE 6–28. Traumatic disk herniation (C5–6), with cord contusion and hemorrhage. This 30-year-old was an unrestrained driver in a motor vehicle accident. *A*, On the T_2-weighted scan, abnormal soft tissue (isointense with disk material) is noted posterior to the C5–6 disk space. Abnormal high signal intensity (consistent with edema) is also noted within the spinal cord, extending for at least two anatomic levels (C5–C6). *B*, On the T_1-weighted scan, the abnormal soft tissue is again noted, abutting the spinal cord. The lesion is contiguous with the disk and has similar signal intensity. *C* and *D*, Two sagittal gradient echo images are also presented. The first scan (*C*) is along the midline, in the same anatomic position as the T_1- and T_2-weighted images. The traumatic disk herniation, contiguous with the C5–6 disk and of similar signal intensity, is again noted. This causes mild mass effect on the thecal sac. Cord edema is also confirmed. On the adjacent cut (*D*), slightly off the midline, the lesion is larger in size but remains contiguous with the disk space. Abnormal hypointensity is noted within the cord at the C5–6 level, consistent with hemorrhage (deoxyhemoglobin). A C5 pedicle fracture was noted on computed tomography (not shown). The patient was left with C5 quadriplegia on the right and C7 on the left. Drug screen was positive for cannabinoids and benzodiazepines.

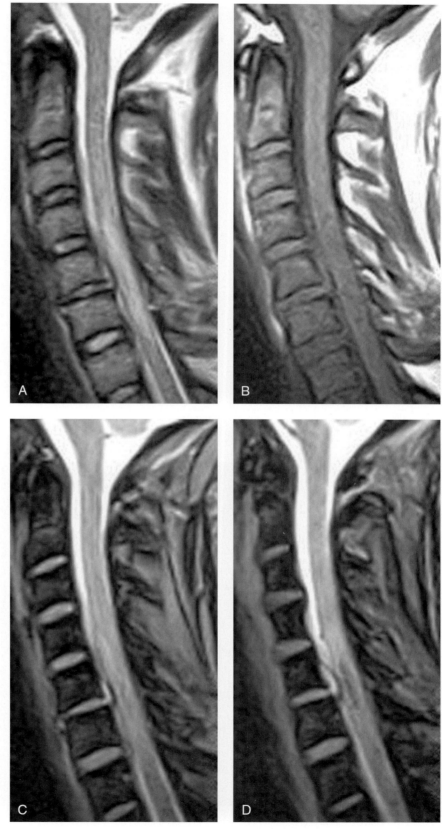

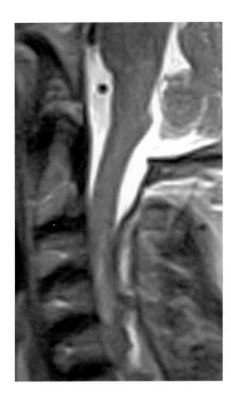

FIGURE 6–29. Posttraumatic epidural hematoma. On the midline sagittal T_2-weighted image, the cord is displaced anteriorly because of a large high signal intensity (methemoglobin) epidural fluid collection. This hematoma extends from C3 to C5 (and possibly below), obliterating the normal cerebrospinal fluid space. High signal intensity is seen within the cord, corresponding to edema, at the C3 and C4 levels.

FIGURE 6–30. Type II dens fracture. The patient is a 19-year-old woman who is being scanned 1 month after an unrestrained motor vehicle accident. Sagittal T_2- (*A*) and postcontrast T_1-weighted (*B*) images demonstrate a fracture through the base of the dens. Mild anterior slippage of the superior fracture fragment relative to the C3 vertebral body is also present. A small amount of enhancing granulation tissue or venous plexus is identified posterior to the dens on the T_1-weighted scan. No evidence for cord compression or contusion is seen. The dens fracture and the offset of the C2 and C3 vertebral bodies were confirmed on a lateral x-ray film of the cervical spine (not shown).

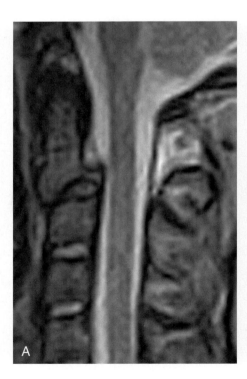

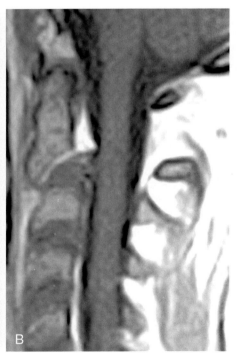

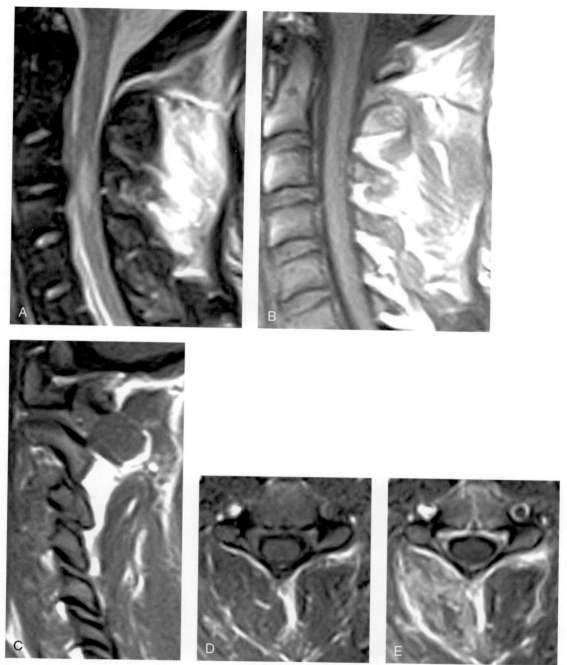

FIGURE 6–31. Flexion-rotation injury of the cervical spine. The patient is a 28-year-old man with central cord syndrome who is being imaged 3 days after a motor vehicle accident. *A,* The midline sagittal T_2-weighted image demonstrates mild increased signal intensity within the C3 and C4 vertebral bodies suggestive of microfractures. Increased signal is present within the spinal cord at the C3–4 level consistent with edema and cord contusion. There is also abnormal high signal intensity within the posterior musculature, as a result of edema. *B,* The corresponding precontrast T_1-weighted image demonstrates a small central disk herniation at the C3–4 level with resultant canal compromise. No abnormal signal intensity is present in the cord to suggest hemorrhage. The vertebral bodies are grossly normal in height and alignment. *C,* The precontrast T_1-weighted parasagittal image reveals discontinuity and deformity of the left C3 pedicle consistent with a fracture. The pre- (*D*) and postcontrast (*E*) T_1-weighted axial images demonstrate asymmetric abnormal enhancement within the injured right paraspinous muscles. Plain cervical spine films (not shown) revealed a fracture-dislocation of C3–4 with approximately 3 mm anterior slippage of C3 on C4. No vertebral fracture was detected. Computed tomography (not shown) revealed a linear fracture through the left pedicle at C3. Mild anterior slippage of C3 on C4 was present with 20% compromise of the spinal canal but no direct impingement on the spinal cord. Traction was applied before the magnetic resonance imaging exam accounting for the normal alignment on this study.

ligaments occurs with flexion. Unilateral involvement suggests a rotational component.

Perched Facet

Plain x-rays films may be suboptimal for evaluation of the lower cervical spine. On CT, misalignment of the facets may be inapparent unless sagittal reconstructions are performed. In distinction, MRI, with direct sagittal imaging, clearly delineates vertebral and facet alignment. It is incumbent on the radiologist to examine closely the alignment of the facets on all cervical spine MRI exams (Fig. 6–32). Perched or locked facets are not uncommonly missed in the setting of acute trauma; continued pain brings the patient back for further evaluation weeks to months later.

Brachial Plexus Injury

Injury to the brachial plexus can lead to a posttraumatic neuroma, fibrosis, or meningocele (with or without nerve root avulsion). On MRI, meningoceles caused by brachial plexus injury are clearly seen. The lesion will follow the course of the nerve root in the foramen and manifest CSF signal intensity on all pulse sequences

(Fig. 6–33). Nerve root avulsions per se are best evaluated by myelography.

DISK HERNIATION

The cervical spine is most mobile at the C4-5, 5-6, and 6-7 levels. Thus, these are also the levels at which most disk herniations occur. Prior surgery with fusion at one level places the level above and below at increased risk for herniation. Cervical disk herniations are most commonly seen in the third and fourth decades of life. MRI and postmyelographic CT have equivalent sensitivity in the detection of acute cervical disk herniations; CT is better for demonstrating accompanying bony degenerative disease.

Clinical symptoms of a cervical disk herniation depend on its location. Large central herniations cause myelopathic symptoms (Fig. 6–34). Posterolateral or foraminal herniations can compress the exiting nerve root and cause radicular symptoms (Fig. 6–35).

Thin-section (less than 2 to 3 mm) images should be acquired in both the sagittal and axial planes on MRI when a disk herniation is suspected. T_1-weighted spin echo and T_2-weighted fast spin echo images are typically

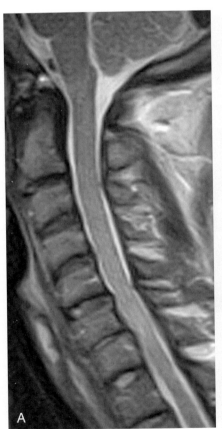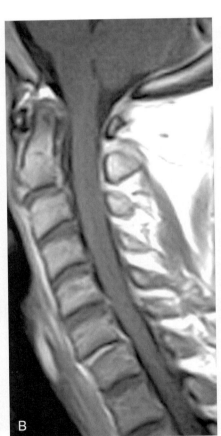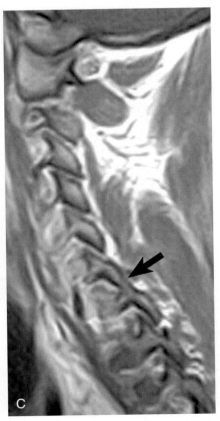

FIGURE 6–32. C2 teardrop fracture and unilateral perched facet at C6–7. The patient presented 6 months after a motor vehicle accident with persistent left arm pain. Midline sagittal T_2- (*A*) and T_1-weighted (*B*) images demonstrate a teardrop fracture at the base (anteriorly) of C2, which had been noted on previous diagnostic exams. Mild anterior slippage of C6 on C7 is also apparent. The T_1-weighted sagittal image (*C*) to the left of midline reveals a facet dislocation at C6–7 (*arrow*). The alignment of the facets on the right was normal (not shown).

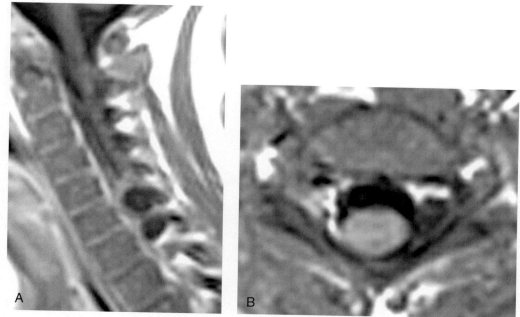

FIGURE 6–33. Meningocele secondary to birth trauma. The patient is a 15-month-old infant with left upper extremity spasticity since birth. *A,* The T_1-weighted left parasagittal image of the cervical spine reveals two low signal intensity extradural fluid collections within the C6–7 and C7–T1 neural foramina, respectively. These two abnormalities remained isointense with cerebrospinal fluid on T_2-weighted scans (not shown). *B,* An axial T_1-weighted spin echo scan confirms, at one level, the extradural location of the lesion and association with the exiting nerve root sleeve.

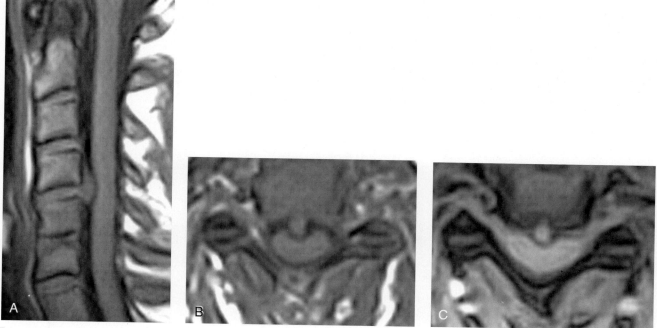

FIGURE 6–34. Large central disk herniation at C4–5. The 42-year-old patient presented with recurrent neck pain. The clinical history is significant for a prior diskectomy and fusion at C5–6. *A,* The T_1-weighted midline sagittal image reveals a prominent anterior extradural soft tissue mass contiguous with and posterior to the C4–5 intervertebral disk. The abnormality is of relatively low signal intensity, similar to the intervertebral disks, on this T_1-weighted scan. On T_2-weighted images (not shown), the abnormality remained isointense to disk material. The C5–6 disk space is narrowed and indistinct, compatible with the prior anterior diskectomy and fusion. *B,* A T_1-weighted axial view through the C4–5 disk confirms the extradural soft tissue mass, with resultant central cord compression. The lesion is again noted to be contiguous with and isointense to the C4–5 disk. *C,* The corresponding axial gradient echo scan depicts this central disk herniation as high signal intensity.

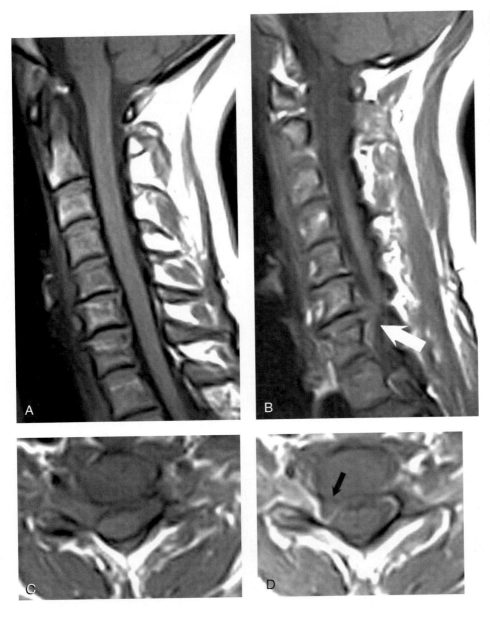

FIGURE 6–35. Right foraminal disk herniation at C6–7. This 49-year-old patient presents with excruciating right arm pain. *A,* A midline T_1-weighted sagittal image demonstrates small spurs and end plate degenerative changes at the C5–6 and C6–7 levels. *B,* A T_1-weighted sagittal image to the right of midline demonstrates abnormal soft tissue (*white arrow*) extending posterior to the vertebral bodies at the C6–7 level. This abnormality was isointense to disk material and contiguous with the C6–7 disk on both this image and the corresponding T_2-weighted scan (not shown). *C,* An axial T_1-weighted image at the C6–7 level does not clearly demonstrate the abnormality. However, the spinal cord does appear mildly shifted to the left. *D,* After contrast administration, the soft tissue abnormality (*black arrow*) is highlighted by the enhancement of the epidural venous plexus within the neural foramen. The disk herniation fills the right neural foramen at the C6–7 level.

acquired in the sagittal plane. T$_2$-weighted gradient echo images are of high value in the axial plane. On the latter, a thin rim of low signal intensity often outlines the high-signal-intensity disk herniation (along its posterior aspect). The low-signal-intensity rim corresponds to the dura and posterior longitudinal ligament. An acute disk herniation is seen on sagittal and axial images as an anterior epidural soft tissue mass. The abnormal soft tissue will be contiguous with the disk space unless a disk fragment is present. The signal intensity of the herniated material is similar to the native disk on both T$_1$- and T$_2$-weighted scans. A decade ago, postcontrast T$_1$-weighted images were also commonly acquired. These can be very useful in diagnosis, but cost constraints led to their elimination in most clinical practices for the study of cervical disk disease. On postcontrast T$_1$-weighted scans, the dilated epidural venous plexus surrounding a disk herniation will enhance, outlining the disk material and improving visualization of the

neural foramina (Fig. 6–36). Without contrast administration, the epidural venous plexus is isointense with and cannot be distinguished from disk material on T$_1$-weighted scans.

A "hard" disk is the result of a long-standing herniation (Fig. 6–37). A chronic disk herniation is covered above and below by bony spurs from the end plates. These form as a result of bone remodeling; elevation of the periosteum by the disk herniation leads to bone deposition at the site. Myelopathic symptoms are more common with chronic disk herniations as opposed to radicular symptoms, which are more common with acute disk herniations. Damage to the blood–spinal cord barrier, on the basis of chronic repetitive trauma at the level, can lead to enhancement within the cord at the level of a hard disk herniation (see Fig. 6–37). This is rarely visualized in current clinical practice because of the nonuse of contrast in the setting of chronic degenerative disease.

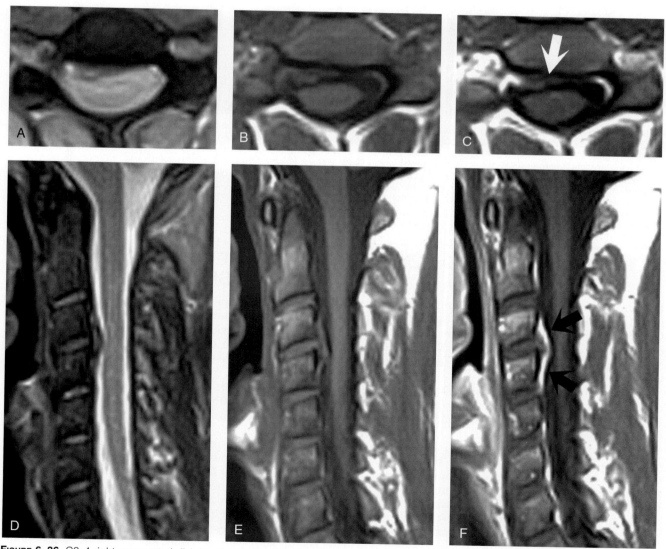

FIGURE 6–36. C3–4 right paracentral disk herniation. This 35-year-old patient presents with neck and right arm pain after a motor vehicle accident. Precontrast axial and sagittal T$_2$- (*A* and *D*), and T$_1$-weighted (*B* and *E*) scans reveal abnormal soft tissue at the C3–4 disk level anterior and to the right of the thecal sac, causing mild cord deformity. The lesion is difficult to separate from the contents of the right neural foramen. Postcontrast (*C* and *F*), the disk herniation itself (*white arrow*) can be differentiated from dilated epidural venous plexus (*black arrows*) because of prominent enhancement of the latter. There is no foraminal component.

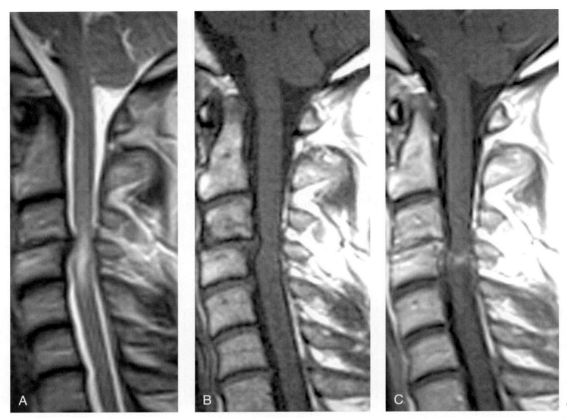

FIGURE 6–37. Early compressive myelomalacia secondary to a large "hard" disk herniation at C3–4. This 44-year-old presented clinically with increasing pain and numbness in the upper extremities. *A,* On the midline fast spin echo T$_2$-weighted sagittal image, abnormal increased signal intensity (likely a combination of edema and gliosis) is seen within the cord, extending from mid C3 to C4–5. At the C4–5 level, prominent osteophytes obliterate the cerebrospinal fluid space anterior to the cord. Mild retrolisthesis of C3 on C4 is identified on the midline sagittal T$_1$-weighted image (*B*). The C3–4 intervertebral disk is narrowed, and abnormal soft tissue extends posterior to the disk, causing deformity of the cervical cord. *C,* The corresponding postcontrast T$_1$-weighted image reveals prominent enhancement within the flattened cervical cord. Abnormal enhancement resulting from de novo scar and dilated epidural venous plexus is also apparent about the C3–4 disk.

HYPERTROPHIC END PLATE SPURS

Hypertrophic end plate spurs (osteophytes) are a common finding on MRI of the cervical spine (Fig. 6–38). Careful image inspection is necessary to distinguish these from a disk herniation. In most instances, spurs are asymptomatic. Imaging findings do not correlate well with clinical symptoms.

End plate spurs are the long-term result of a disk bulge or herniation. During healing, bone is laid down on elevated ligamentous attachments, resulting a bony spur. On MRI, these osteophytes can and should be distinguished from an acute disk herniation. T$_2$-weighted gradient echo images are very useful in this regard. Disk material is high signal intensity, and spurs are very low signal intensity. The high-signal-intensity CSF also tends to well outline these spurs. If large osteophytes are present along the anterior margin of the vertebral bodies at the levels in question, it is also likely that the compromise of the thecal sac posterior to the vertebral body is due to degenerative disease as opposed to an acute disk herniation. On postcontrast T$_1$-weighted spin echo images, enhancement of the epidural venous plexus may outline the low signal intensity of the spur.

SURGERY FOR CERVICAL SPONDYLOSIS

Damage to the spinal cord in cervical spondylosis is the result of ischemia from chronic compression. The aim of surgery is to prevent further deterioration. An anterior surgical approach is used for one- to two-level stenosis (Figs. 6–39 and 6–40), and is the most common neurosurgical procedure in cervical disk disease. The disk is resected (using an anterior approach) and a bone graft placed between the two adjacent vertebral bodies to achieve a stable fusion. Portions of the adjacent vertebral bodies may or may not be removed. The signal intensity characteristics of the graft are variable. After more than 2 years, continuous marrow signal intensity is typically seen at the site of fusion, with no evidence of bone graft or native disk. There is a propensity over the long term for new disk herniations to develop above and below the site of fusion. The posterior approach, which is less common, involves a laminectomy and is used for congenital narrowing or extensive contiguous disease (multiple levels). MRI can be diagnostic in postoperative cases despite the presence of substantial metal hardware. Artifacts from metal will be greatest in general on gradient echo scans (because of the lack of a 180-degree

Text continued on page 155

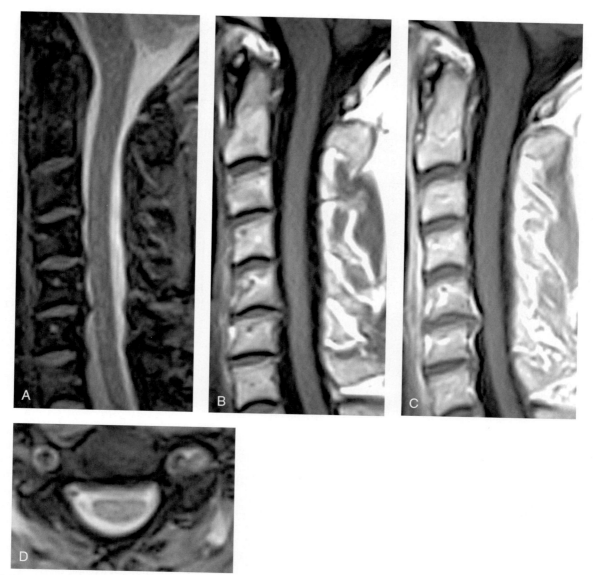

FIGURE 6–38. Hypertrophic osteophytic end plate spurs. A 57-year-old woman presented with right-sided neck and arm pain. Midline sagittal T₂-weighted gradient echo (*A*) and T₁-weighted spin echo images before (*B*) and after (*C*) contrast administration demonstrate a ventral extradural defect along the anterior margin of the thecal sac at the C5–6 level. *A,* The sagittal T₂-weighted gradient echo image demonstrates, in addition to the low signal intensity spurs at C5–6, smaller spurs at C4–5 and C6–7 that partially efface the ventral subarachnoid space. *B,* The precontrast sagittal T₁-weighted image shows pointed extensions of bone marrow signal intensity along the posterior end plates adjacent to the C5–6 disk. *C,* Postcontrast, enhancement of dilated venous plexus is noted immediately above and below the C5–6 level. Mild irregularities of the posterior margin of the vertebral end plate are present on the axial T₂-weighted gradient echo image (*D*). The signal intensity of these projections is very low, indicative of cortical bone. These findings are consistent with osteophytes extending from the posterior vertebral end plates.

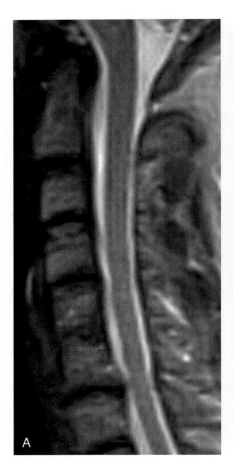
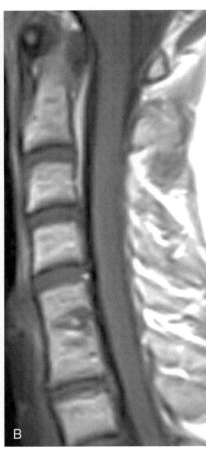

FIGURE 6–39. Normal late appearance of anterior cervical diskectomy and fusion. The patient has continued left arm pain 4 months after anterior diskectomy and fusion for a C5–6 disk herniation. *A*, On the midline sagittal T$_2$-weighted image, the C5–6 intervertebral disk is not seen. Small spurs with mild compromise of the thecal sac are noted at the levels above and below (C4–5 and C6–7). *B*, The sagittal T$_1$-weighted image (obtained after contrast administration) demonstrates fusion of the C5 and C6 vertebral bodies. Mild decreased signal intensity is evident within the central portion of the fusion. The alignment of the cervical spine is normal.

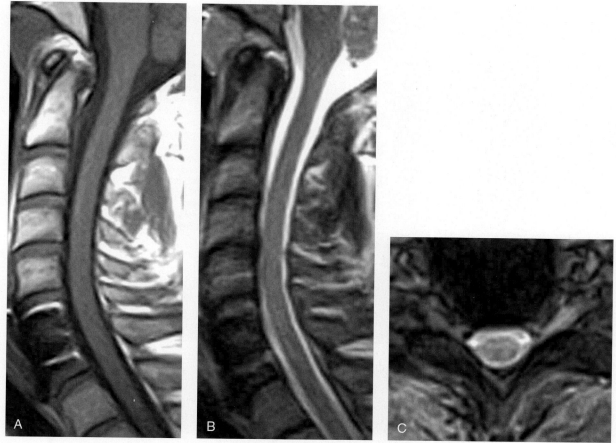

FIGURE 6–40. Normal appearance after anterior diskectomy and titanium plate fusion at C6–7. This 48-year-old patient presented clinically with continued neck pain after surgery for a C6–7 disk herniation. *A*, The T_1-weighted midline sagittal image reveals prominent metallic artifact anterior to and within the C6 and C7 vertebral bodies. The alignment of the cervical vertebral bodies is normal. No significant canal stenosis is present. The artifact is again present, but less apparent, on the fast spin echo T_2-weighted sagittal image (*B*). A small osteophyte causes effacement of the ventral subarachnoid space at C4–5. *C*, On the axial gradient echo image at C6–7, the metal artifact is more extensive, with artifactual mild effacement of the anterior thecal sac. A lateral radiograph of the cervical spine (not shown) demonstrated a metallic plate and three screws that fused the C6 and C7 vertebral bodies.

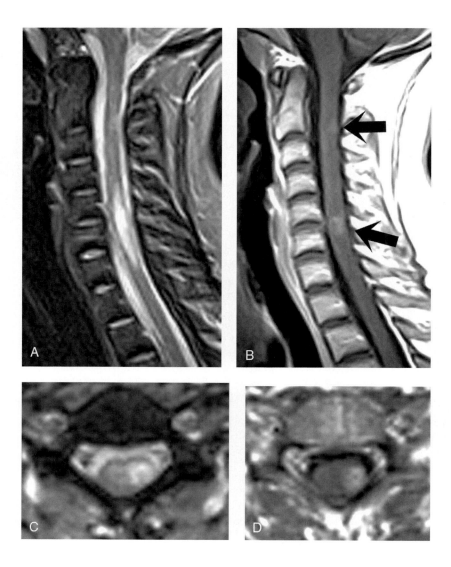

FIGURE 6–41. Multiple sclerosis, with active spinal cord plaques. The patient is a 28-year-old white woman with new onset 2 months ago of numbness below the waist, now involving the left arm. Several episodes of blurred vision in one eye have also occurred during the past 2 years. *A,* On the T_2-weighted midline sagittal scan, two intramedullary lesions are noted, at C2–3 and C5–6, with the latter larger and exhibiting a flamelike pattern of edema extending superiorly and inferiorly. *B,* On the postcontrast T_1-weighted midline sagittal scan, faint lesion enhancement (*arrows*) is identified at both levels. Axial T_2-weighted gradient echo (*C*) and postcontrast T_1-weighted spin echo (*D*) scans confirm the lower lesion, which is eccentrically located, causes focal cord enlargement, and demonstrates prominent enhancement.

FIGURE 6–42. Multiple sclerosis (MS) (inactive or chronic disease). The patient is a 52-year-old white man with long-standing neurologic problems. He ambulates with a cane. Bowel function is intact; however, there is bladder incontinence. Heavily T_2-weighted midline sagittal images of the cervical (*A*) and thoracic (*B*) spine are presented. A single hyperintense intrinsic cord abnormality is noted in the cervical spine at the C2 level, suggesting cord atrophy. Two thoracic cord lesions are also seen, both somewhat elongated in appearance. Incidental note is made of an osteophyte situated between the two thoracic cord lesions, causing anterior compression of the thecal sac. The lesions (all chronic MS plaques) do not cause cord enlargement, and there was no abnormal contrast enhancement (not shown).

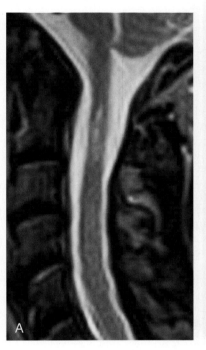

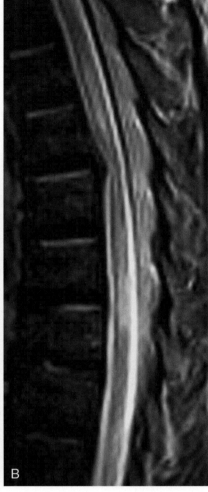

refocusing pulse), moderate on spin echo scans, and least on fast spin echo scans (as a result of the short interecho interval). High signal intensity within the cord postoperatively on T_2-weighted scans is seen occasionally and can be due to gliosis (present preoperatively) or postoperative complications (such as cord contusion and infarction).

MULTIPLE SCLEROSIS

Spinal cord multiple sclerosis (MS) plaques are best detected on T_2-weighted scans. Short segments of the cord are typically involved and demonstrate abnormal high signal intensity. Focal cord enlargement is seen with acute lesions as a result of the presence of edema. Symptomatic (active) lesions may or may not demonstrate substantial surrounding edema but will consistently enhance postcontrast (Fig. 6–41). Edema, if present, can extend in a flamelike pattern above and below the lesion. Lesions are haphazard in distribution both in cross-section and longitudinally, disregarding anatomic boundaries. MS plaques tend to be elliptical in shape, with greatest dimension along the length of the cord. Cord atrophy, which can be focal or generalized, is seen

in long-standing disease (Fig. 6–42). Not all patients with spinal cord lesions will demonstrate characteristic brain lesions on MRI. The histologic appearance of spinal cord MS plaques is that of multifocal sharply marginated areas of demyelination.

Clinically, MS is characterized by recurrent focal neurologic attacks, progressive deterioration, and ultimately permanent neurologic dysfunction. Symptoms include decreased vibration and position sense, weakness of one or more extremities, and disorders of micturition (urination). Differential diagnosis, based on the results of MRI of the spinal cord, includes transverse myelitis. The presence of multiple cord lesions, combined with characteristic brain lesions, favors the diagnosis of MS.

ACUTE TRANSVERSE MYELITIS

In acute transverse myelitis, a section of the cord demonstrates fusiform enlargement and abnormal high signal intensity on T_2-weighted scans. The area involved usually extends over several vertebral segments. Clinical symptoms include a sudden loss of sensory and motor function in a segmental distribution. The pathogenesis is unknown. Possible causes include viral, vascular, and autoimmune disease.

7

Thoracic Spine

NORMAL THORACIC SPINE

There are normally 12 thoracic vertebral bodies. The ribs articulate with the vertebrae both at the disk and at the transverse process. However, the latter articulation occurs only for T1 through T10. On sagittal magnetic resonance imaging (MRI) scans, the exit foramina for the basivertebral veins can be clearly identified posteriorly within the midvertebral body. Epidural fat is prominent posterior to the thecal sac.

The thoracic spine presents several unique problems in regard to MRI, necessitating attention to imaging technique to obtain a high-quality exam. A coronal saturation pulse (or presaturation slab) is routinely used to eliminate motion artifacts from the chest wall and heart. This saturation pulse is used in both sagittal and axial imaging of the thoracic spine. A maximum slice thickness of 3 mm is recommended regardless of imaging plane. Thoracic disk herniations, in particular, are often small and not well visualized when thicker sections are acquired. With conventional T_2-weighted spin echo techniques, focal signal loss within the cerebrospinal fluid (CSF) is common. This is due to the strong pulsatile nature of CSF in the thoracic region, which is also present in the cervical spine. Fast spin echo T_2-weighted scans suffer substantially less from this problem and are routinely used for sagittal imaging. However, axial T_2-weighted scans suffer from CSF flow artifacts regardless of specific technique (conventional or fast). Thus, gradient echo T_2-weighted scans are routinely used for axial imaging in the thoracic spine.

Although not strictly "normal," one finding (indicative of a prior diagnostic exam) that can still be seen in older patients deserves comment: the presence of residual Pantopaque (iophendylate) from a myelogram performed before 1990. Pantopaque was an early contrast agent used for myelography. It is no longer used in part because of the high incidence of arachnoiditis after the exam. Pantopaque is an oily, non-water-soluble substance. It was not uncommon for a small amount to be left within the thecal sac after completion of a myelogram. This persists indefinitely. Currently, on MRI, Pantopaque is still occasionally seen in older patients either free within the thecal sac or trapped within a root sleeve or scar. It is easily recognized because of its appearance on MRI (typically a small globule) with high signal intensity on T_1-weighted scans and low signal intensity on T_2-weighted scans. Correlation with conventional x-ray films is recommended because Pantopaque is extremely x-ray dense.

CONGENITAL OR DEVELOPMENTAL ABNORMALITY

Butterfly vertebrae have concave superior and inferior end plates with a central osseous defect. In some instances, this is an incidental finding of no clinical significance. However, butterfly vertebrae can be associated with congenital abnormalities such as diastematomyelia, necessitating close review of images.

A lateral meningocele is produced by a protrusion (laterally) of the dura and arachnoid through an enlarged neural foramen. The adjacent pedicles and lamina may be thinned, and the dorsal surface of the vertebral body scalloped. The vast majority of lateral meningoceles (85%) are seen in neurofibromatosis. Thoracic paraspinal masses, when present in neurofibromatosis, are more likely to be meningoceles than neurofibromas. Most lateral meningoceles are right sided, occur in a single foramen, and are seen in the upper thoracic spine (T3-7). Lateral meningoceles are typically asymptomatic. They are easily characterized and diagnosed by MRI, with CSF signal intensity on all pulse sequences.

Neuroenteric cysts are an embryologic remnant. During early embryonic development, a temporary structure (the canal of Kovalevsky) connects the amnion and the primitive yolk sac. Persistence of this canal after embryologic development leads to a fistula from gut, through the vertebral bodies and spinal cord, to the dorsal skin. Persistence of only a portion of the canal is believed to be the origin of mesenteric cysts, enteric diverticula, neuroenteric cysts, diastematomyelia, and spina bifida. Neuroenteric cysts are by definition enteric lined cysts that lie within the spinal canal. There can also be a component outside the canal. Neuroenteric cysts are usually ventral in location to the spinal cord and are most frequently seen at the cervicothoracic junction and conus medullaris. There are frequently associated vertebral body anomalies. The imaging appearance on MRI is varied depending on the blood and protein content, viscosity, and pulsatility. Included in the differential diagnosis is an arachnoid cyst. However, arachnoid cysts are isointense to CSF on all pulse sequences and not associated with vertebral body anomalies.

Epidural lipomatosis is the result of excessive fat deposition in the epidural space. It is seen in morbid obesity, chronic steroid use, and Cushing's disease. Sixty percent of cases occur in the thoracic spine and 40% in the lumbar spine. In extreme cases, patients can be symptomatic; pain and weakness result from compression of the thecal sac by overabundant fat.

INFECTION
Osteomyelitis

Vertebral osteomyelitis is often insidious; nonspecific symptoms make diagnosis difficult. Delay in treatment, however, dramatically increases morbidity. In children, osteomyelitis occurs after hematogenous spread of bacteria to the vascularized intervertebral disk. However, in adults, the infection is the result of hematogenous spread to the more vascular end plate, with the disk itself involved secondarily. Plain x-ray films are frequently unremarkable until late in the disease. MRI is the modality of choice for diagnosis; sensitivity is higher for MRI than for radionuclide scintigraphy. Findings on MRI include abnormal low signal intensity on T_1-weighted scans and high signal intensity on T_2-weighted scans within the vertebral body. These signal abnormalities are due to edema and inflammatory changes. There is typically a paraspinous and epidural soft tissue mass, which enhances after contrast administration. The longer the delay in diagnosis, the greater is the size of the associated abnormal soft tissue. Specific diagnosis is usually possible because of the presence of an irregular very high signal intensity area within the disk space on T_2-weighted scans corresponding to fluid. Involvement of the intervening disk space distinguishes this disease (infection) from vertebral metastases.

Tuberculous Spondylitis

Tuberculous spondylitis follows a more indolent clinical course than pyogenic infection. It is uncommon in the United States except among immigrants (specifically those from Southeast Asia and South America) and immunocompromised patients. From an imaging perspective, abnormal marrow signal intensity is seen within two or more adjacent vertebral bodies, with accompanying cortical bone destruction and abnormal extradural soft tissue. Distinguishing features from pyogenic infection include involvement of three or more levels (50% of cases), "skip" lesions, relative sparing of the disk, and a disproportionately large soft tissue mass. Tuberculous spondylitis often spreads along the anterior longitudinal ligament involving multiple contiguous vertebral bodies. The extradural component is typically prevertebral in location, but can extend into the spinal canal. In long-standing disease, there can be extensive bone destruction, a gibbous deformity (vertebral collapse with anterior wedging), and cord compression (resulting from angulation or the soft tissue mass). Computed tomography (CT) clearly depicts the extensive bone destruction and soft tissue (paraspinous) mass. MRI, however, offers superior depiction of both the vertebral and paravertebral involvement. As medical treatment begins to take effect, there is a return to normal in signal intensity (on

both T_1- and T_2-weighted scans) of the vertebral bodies and a decrease in the abnormal enhancement of paravertebral soft tissue.

AIDS-Related Infection

AIDS-related infections involving the thecal space in the thoracic area may present as polyradiculopathy or myelopathy. The cause is generally viral but can be direct or indirect in nature. Cytomegalovirus, herpes simplex type 2, varicella-zoster, and toxoplasmosis have been implicated and represent "direct" disease as a result of viral infection. "Indirect" effects include postinfectious demyelination and parainfectious vasculitis. The differential diagnosis should include neoplasia and specifically lymphoma.

NEOPLASTIC DISEASE
Metastases to Bone

T_1-weighted scans are generally the most useful for detection of vertebral body metastases because of their high sensitivity to disease and intrinsic high signal to noise ratio (and thus good image quality). Malignant lesions, with increased cellularity, are low signal intensity on T_1-weighted scans and thus quite distinct from the normal high signal intensity marrow (Fig. 7–1). After contrast injection, metastatic lesions usually enhance and are thus less clearly seen unless fat suppression is used. Postcontrast scans can, however, display more effectively the soft tissue extent of disease and canal compromise (Fig. 7–2), although the latter is often also clearly seen on T_2-weighted scans. Lytic and blastic lesions appear distinct from one another; the latter is very low signal intensity on T_1-weighted scans (Fig. 7–3). With tumors that spread via the lymphatics (e.g., carcinoid), it is important to scrutinize the off-midline sagittal images (and axial scans) for retroperitoneal lymphadenopathy.

In regard to sensitivity, it is well established that MRI is overall more sensitive than radionuclide bone scanning for metastatic disease. MRI may detect lesions despite a normal bone scan. Furthermore, radionuclide bone scans suffer from lower specificity. Degenerative changes, infection, and fractures can all cause a false-positive bone scan. MRI better discriminates between benign and malignant processes.

MRI has replaced myelography in most institutions for the assessment of cord compression by epidural metastatic disease as a result of high sensitivity and low morbidity. Myeloma, prostate, and renal cell carcinoma all have a propensity to develop epidural metastatic disease. However, the highest incidence of epidural metastatic disease is with lung carcinoma; this is the most common cause of metastatic disease to the vertebral column. In terms of symptoms, there is a prodromal phase with central back pain at the level of disease involvement. This is followed by a compressive phase with neurologic deficits, which begin with motor impairment (resulting from anterior cord compression). In lesions causing compression of the conus, autonomic dysfunction may occur without sensory or motor defi-

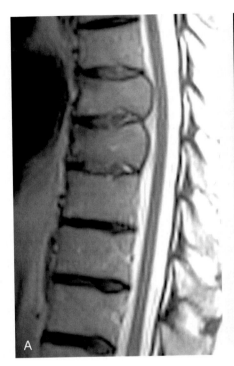
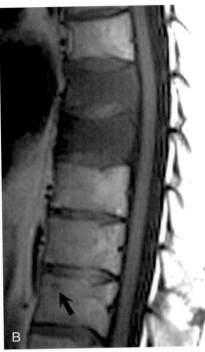

FIGURE 7–1. Metastatic disease (from lung carcinoma), with mild anterior compromise of the thecal sac. *A*, On the sagittal T$_2$-weighted scan, the posterior margins of T7 and T8 bulge in a convex manner posteriorly, encroaching on the spinal canal. The signal intensity of the marrow (of T7 and T8) is misleading on this fast spin echo scan (obtained without fat suppression), appearing isointense with adjacent normal vertebral bodies. Fast T$_2$-weighted spin echo scans should be acquired with fat saturation to improve their sensitivity to bony metastatic disease. *B*, The T$_1$-weighted scan clearly demonstrates the metastatic involvement of T7 and T8. There is replacement of normal marrow in these vertebral bodies by metastatic disease, which demonstrates substantially lower signal intensity. A small focus of metastatic disease (*B, arrow*) is also present in the anterior superior quadrant of T11.

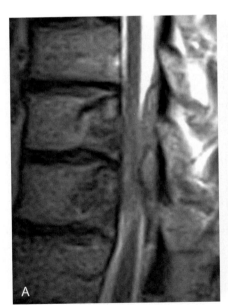
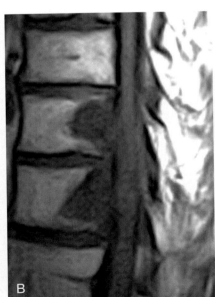
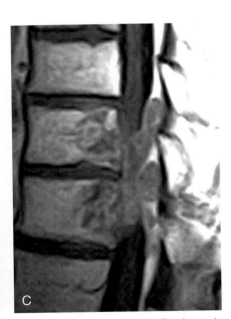

FIGURE 7–2. Vertebral metastatic disease (from lung carcinoma), with epidural extension and severe cord compression. *A*, The fast spin echo T$_2$-weighted midline sagittal image demonstrates compromise of the thecal sac by abnormal soft tissue posteriorly and anteriorly. *B*, The corresponding T$_1$-weighted sagittal scan, although not demonstrating as clearly the interface between cerebrospinal fluid (CSF), cord, and soft tissue, clearly depicts the involvement of the posterior portion of both T10 and T11 by metastatic disease. Both the vertebral and epidural lesions demonstrate inhomogeneous enhancement on the postcontrast T$_1$-weighted sagittal image (*C*). Contrast enhancement decreases the conspicuity of the vertebral body involvement by metastatic disease but improves the visualization of canal compromise by soft tissue.

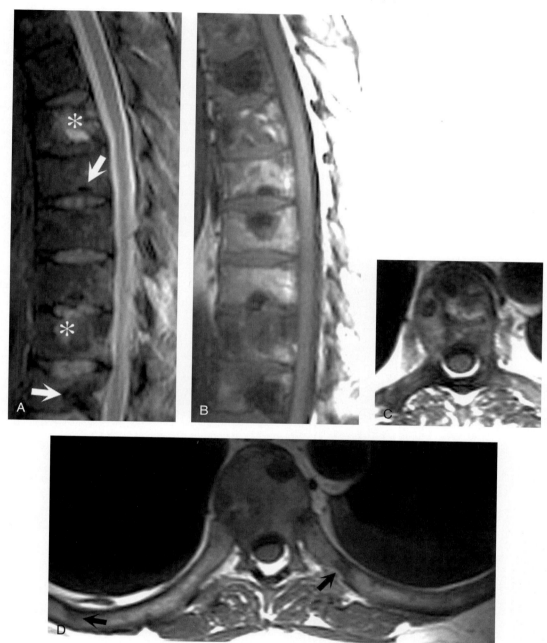

FIGURE 7–3. Metastatic disease (from prostate carcinoma) with both lytic and blastic lesions. Metastatic vertebral lesions most often demonstrate decreased signal intensity on T_1-weighted images and increased signal intensity on T_2-weighted scans. Blastic metastases, however, may remain low signal intensity on T_2-weighted images. *A,* The fast spin echo T_2-weighted scan, obtained with fat suppression, reveals at least two vertebral body lesions with slight high signal intensity (asterisks). Several low signal intensity lesions are also evident (*white arrows*). *B,* The T_1-weighted scan better depicts the widespread extent of metastatic disease; the lytic lesions are seen as gray or intermediate low signal intensity (slightly lower in signal intensity than the intervertebral disks), and the blastic lesions as very low signal intensity (almost black). One of the lesions also contains methemoglobin, with abnormal high signal intensity on the T_1-weighted scan. *C,* The axial section through this lesion reveals abnormal low and high signal intensity. *D,* A lower axial section demonstrates a focal vertebral body lesion, with additional metastases seen in the ribs (*black arrows*). A common mistake in film reading is to examine only the midline sagittal scan for metastatic disease. The entire bony skeleton visualized on the scan should be inspected for the presence of metastatic disease, when clinically suspected.

cits. Compression of the thecal sac and cord can occur from any direction, anterior or posterior (Figs. 7–4 and 7–5) or lateral (Figs. 7–6 and 7–7), necessitating close image inspection and acquisition of two perpendicular planes (typically sagittal and axial).

Leptomeningeal Metastases

Leptomeningeal metastases can be seen with central nervous system (CNS) tumors (including specifically glioblastoma, ependymoma, medulloblastoma, and pineal tumors) as well as with non-CNS tumors (most commonly lung carcinoma, breast carcinoma, melanoma, and lymphoma). The clinical presentation is varied and includes back pain, leg pain, headache, cranial and spinal nerve deficits, and gait disturbance. The gold standard for diagnosis is CSF cytology. However, this may require multiple samples and a large volume of CSF. The diagnosis of leptomeningeal metastases by CT is based on visualization of nodular filling defects within the CSF and clumping of nerve roots. The advent of high-quality contrast-enhanced spine MRI provided a major advance in the imaging diagnosis of leptomeningeal metastases. MRI is markedly more sensitive than CT for the detection of leptomeningeal metastases when intravenous

contrast is used. Small and large enhancing nodules, direct invasion of the cord by metastases, and seeding along the cord surface or exiting nerve roots are all well visualized.

Hematologic Neoplasia

Spinal involvement is seen in lymphoma (Fig. 7–8) in 15% of cases. Paravertebral, vertebral, and epidural lesions all occur. Spinal lymphoma is most commonly caused by local spread from retroperitoneal nodes and is thus paravertebral in location. Isolated epidural lesions do occur as a result of hematogenous spread or spread from epidural lymphatics. Epidural disease in lymphoma frequently results in clinically significant cord compression. The appearance of epidural disease is not specific for lymphoma but merely reflects the characteristics of an epidural soft tissue mass. On T_1-weighted scans, a lymphomatous epidural mass is isointense to slightly hyperintense to the spinal cord and on T_2-weighted scans hyperintense to cord. Contrast enhancement is typically homogeneous. Vertebral involvement is also nonspecific in appearance, sharing that of metastatic disease from many causes with inhomogeneous low signal intensity on T_1-weighted scans and intermediate to high signal intensity on T_2-weighted scans.

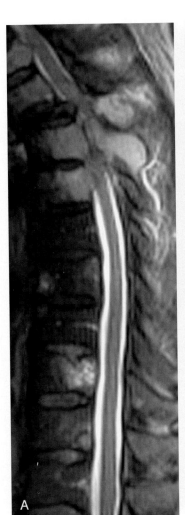
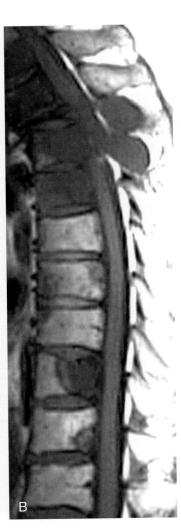

FIGURE 7–4. Cord compression (in the upper thoracic spine) by expansile bony metastatic disease (from lung carcinoma), revealed on an emergency magnetic resonance imaging scan. *A*, The fast spin echo T_2-weighted scan with fat suppression reveals extensive abnormal high-signal-intensity bony metastatic disease involving the vertebral bodies and in the upper thoracic spine the spinous processes (posterior elements) as well. The cerebrospinal fluid space surrounding the cord is obliterated, with compression from abnormal soft tissue both anteriorly and posteriorly. *B*, The T_1-weighted scan clearly depicts the extent of bony metastatic disease but provides a relatively poor view of the canal compromise. Unless intravenous contrast is administered, cord compression is seen best on fast spin echo T_2-weighted scans.

FIGURE 7–5. Cord compression at multiple levels from metastatic colon carcinoma. Just because compression is demonstrated at one level, inspection of the film and the search for other areas of involvement (and possible canal compromise) should not be discontinued. Metastatic disease is typically widespread; therefore, presentation with more than one discrete level of canal compromise is not uncommon. Fast spin echo T$_2$-weighted (A) and conventional T$_1$-weighted (B) sagittal scans show severe canal compromise as a result of metastatic involvement of two adjacent vertebral bodies in the upper thoracic spine. However, not to be overlooked is significant anterior cord compression at a level two bodies higher, best seen on the T$_2$-weighted scan.

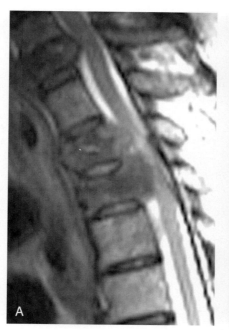
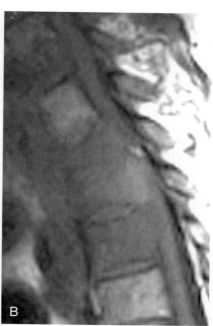

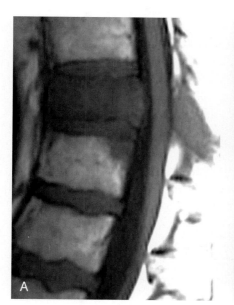
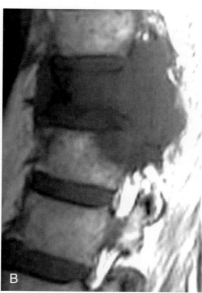

FIGURE 7–6. Lateral cord compression resulting from pedicle involvement by metastatic disease. A, The midline sagittal T$_1$-weighted scan reveals only mild anterior compression of the thecal sac by metastatic disease (which involves both the vertebral body and spinous process). Involvement of the superoposterior quadrant of the adjacent lower vertebral body, with a normal intervening disk space, favors the diagnosis of neoplastic disease as opposed to infection. However, it cannot be concluded from the midline sagittal scan alone that significant canal compromise is not present. Such may occur by involvement of the pedicles laterally, as shown in an adjacent slice (B). Lateral thecal sac compromise was confirmed on the axial scan (not shown).

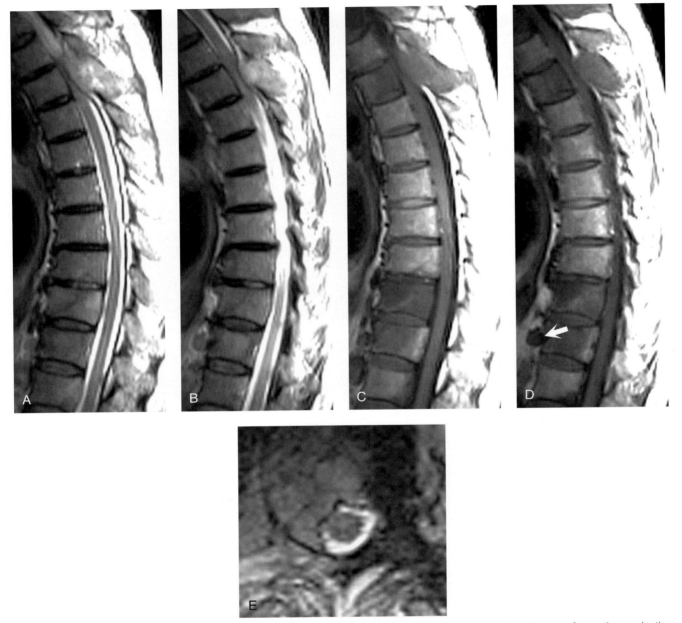

FIGURE 7–7. Metastatic disease from prostate carcinoma, illustrating the importance of both sagittal and axial scans for routine evaluation of canal compromise. On the basis of the sagittal T_2-weighted fast spin echo scans (*A* and *B*), there is significant cord compression (by abnormal posterior soft tissue) at T4 (only). The lack of fat suppression, however, makes assessment of the extent of bony metastatic involvement difficult. The multiplicity of lesions is readily appreciated from the sagittal T_1-weighted scans (*C* and *D*). An enlarged lymph node (*white arrow*), involved by metastatic disease, is also noted anterior to T11. Although the T10 vertebral body is involved in its entirety by metastatic disease, there does not appear to be any substantial canal compromise at this level (on the basis of the sagittal scans alone). However, the axial gradient echo scan at T10 (*E*) demonstrates substantial anterior and lateral compromise of the canal.

FIGURE 7–8. Lymphoma. *A,* The T$_2$-weighted midline sagittal image reveals a large epidural mass at the T8–9 level posterior to and compressing the cord. The lesion is slightly hyperintense to the cord but of lower signal intensity than cerebrospinal fluid (CSF). *B,* The axial postcontrast T$_1$-weighted image reveals moderate homogeneous enhancement of the lesion (*black arrow*), with the cord displaced and compressed anteriorly (and to the right). On the precontrast axial T$_1$-weighted scan (not shown), the cord and mass were isointense and could not be distinguished.

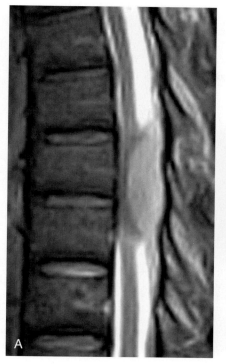

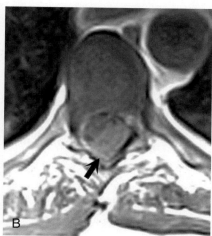

Leukemia is the most common malignancy of childhood and the ninth most common in adults. The disease arises in lymphoid tissue and bone marrow and from a simplistic point of view represents a malignant proliferation of hematopoietic cells. A common symptom is bone pain caused by pressure from rapidly proliferating cells. Bone involvement is most often diffuse but can be focal. The latter is most common in acute myelogenous forms. The CNS serves as a sanctuary for the disease during chemotherapy; thus, the CNS is a frequent site of relapse.

Multiple myeloma is caused by a neoplastic overgrowth of plasma cells. The peak incidence is from 50 to 70 years of age. Vertebral involvement is most common in the thoracic region. MRI is far more sensitive than either plain x-ray films or radionuclide bone scans for disease detection. The most common appearance on MRI is that of diffuse marrow infiltration (Fig. 7–9).

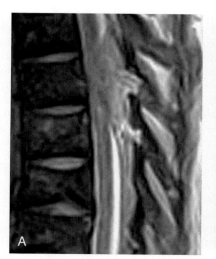

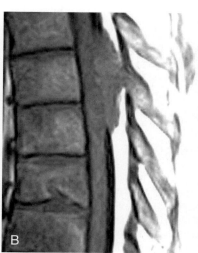

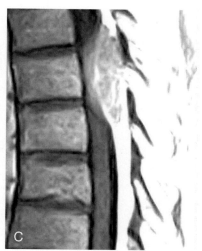

FIGURE 7–9. Multiple myeloma with diffuse marrow involvement and an epidural mass at T6. An epidural soft tissue mass is noted on the midline sagittal T$_2$-weighted scan (*A*). The mass is posterior to the cord, displacing it anteriorly. *B,* The precontrast T$_1$-weighted scan depicts both the mass and the diffuse involvement of vertebral marrow. The latter has abnormal low signal intensity. Diffuse marrow involvement may elude detection if the marrow signal intensity is not compared with a standard, such as that of the normal intervertebral disks. On T$_1$-weighted scans, normal marrow should be hyperintense to the intervertebral disk. The heterogeneity of the marrow signal intensity on both the T$_1$- and T$_2$-weighted scans in this patient confirms the widespread metastatic involvement. *C,* After contrast administration, both the marrow and the epidural mass demonstrate substantial enhancement. The latter improves markedly the depiction of cord compression by the mass.

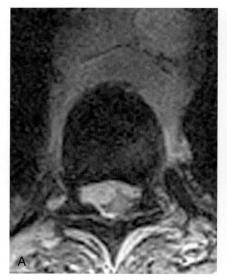
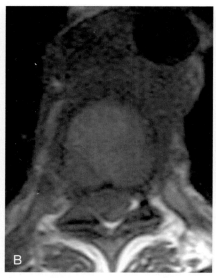
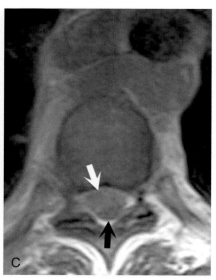

FIGURE 7–10. Multiple myeloma with prevertebral and epidural extent. *A,* On the axial gradient echo T₂-weighted scan, a high-signal-intensity prevertebral soft tissue mass is noted. The mass partially encases the aorta. The cord is displaced posteriorly and compressed by abnormal epidural soft tissue. *B,* On the precontrast T₁-weighted scan, the prevertebral mass is clearly seen, but the epidural mass and cord have similar signal intensity and are difficult to separate. *C,* Postcontrast, both the prevertebral and epidural (*white arrow*) portions of the mass (myeloma) enhance, improving differentiation from the cord (*black arrow*), which lies compressed posteriorly.

Another not uncommon pattern is that of nodular deposits surrounded by normal marrow. As with other hematologic neoplasias, paravertebral and epidural soft tissue masses can also be seen (Fig. 7–10).

Astrocytoma/Ependymoma

The majority of intramedullary spinal cord tumors are either astrocytomas or ependymomas. Astrocytomas are more common in children and ependymomas more common in adults. MRI cannot differentiate an astrocytoma from an ependymoma, although certain imaging features favor one or the other. Involvement of the entire width of the cord, with homogeneous high signal intensity on T₂-weighted scans, favors an astrocytoma (Fig. 7–11). Extensive cord involvement, extending over three or more vertebral segments, also favors an astrocytoma. A small nodular lesion (especially with a cystic component) is more likely to be an ependymoma. Three fourths of all spinal astrocytomas occur in either a cervical or thoracic location.

Neurogenic Tumors (Nerve/Nerve Sheath Origin Tumors)

The majority of paraspinal lesions in the thoracic region are neurogenic tumors. These tumors are also the most common cause of a posterior mediastinal mass. In adults, schwannomas and neurofibromas are most common. These two tumors have similar imaging characteristics. In young children, neuroblastoma is most common.

In the radiologic literature, the term schwannoma has been used interchangeably with neurinoma and neurilemmoma. Schwannomas arise from the Schwann cells of the nerve root sheath. Thus, these lesions are seen, at dissection, to be extrinsic (eccentric) to the nerve root. On MRI, schwannomas are hypo- to isointense on T₁-weighted images to the cord and hyperintense on T₂-weighted images (Fig. 7–12). On the latter type of scan, schwannomas are also often heterogeneous in appearance; high-signal-intensity areas correspond to small cysts. Enhancement is typically heterogeneous and often more intense peripherally.

Neurofibromas are distinguished from schwannomas by the presence of abundant connective tissue and nerve cells. Neurofibromas enlarge the nerve itself. Neurofibromas are usually associated with neurofibromatosis, even when solitary. Homogeneous contrast enhancement makes the diagnosis of a neurofibroma more likely than that of a schwannoma.

Three related but different tumors–neuroblastoma, ganglioneuroblastoma, and ganglioneuroma–are thought to arise from primitive sympathetic neuroblasts (the embryonic neural crest). These are differentiated histologically by the degree of cellular maturation. On imaging, the three tumor types are indistinguishable. Neuroblastoma is a malignant tumor composed of undifferentiated neuroblasts. Most neuroblastomas arise in the adrenals and the remainder along the sympathetic chain. The clinical prognosis is worse with increasing age of presentation. The prognosis, however, is better with spinal lesions as opposed to abdominal or pelvic lesions. Extradural extension is common with paravertebral lesions. Ganglioneuroblastoma is also a malignant tumor but contains mature ganglion cells in addition to undifferentiated neuroblasts. Ganglioneuroma (Fig. 7–13) is a benign tumor that contains mature ganglion cells. Ganglioneuromas are more common in adolescents and young adults.

Meningioma

One third of all spinal meningiomas occur in the cervical region and two thirds in the thoracic region. There is a

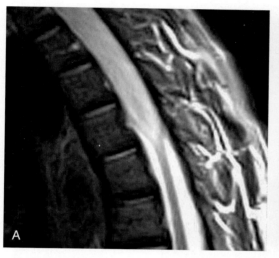

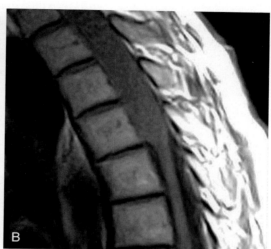

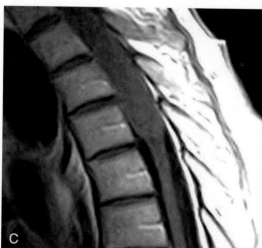

FIGURE 7–11. Astrocytoma. Sagittal T_2- (*A*) and T_1-weighted (*B*) scans reveal abnormal expansion of the lower cervical and upper thoracic spinal cord. The area involved spans more than three vertebral segments. The lesion is higher in signal intensity than normal cord on the T_2-weighted scan and slightly lower in signal intensity than normal cord on the T_1-weighted scan. *C,* Postcontrast there is no enhancement of the mass, which is again demonstrated to be intramedullary in location, expanding the cord to fill the spinal canal.

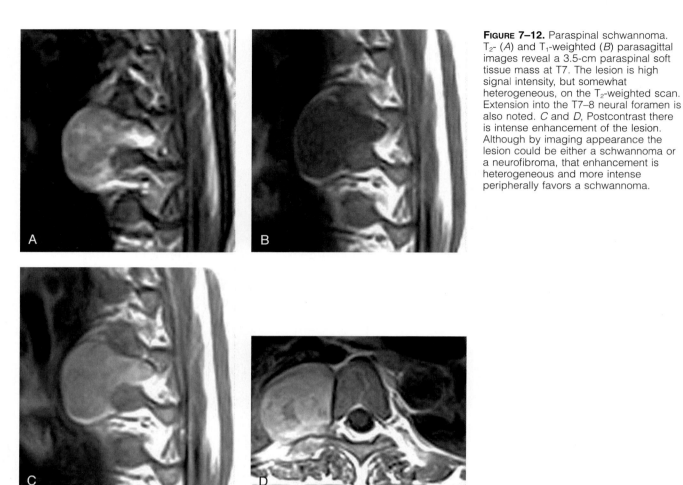

FIGURE 7–12. Paraspinal schwannoma. T_2- (*A*) and T_1-weighted (*B*) parasagittal images reveal a 3.5-cm paraspinal soft tissue mass at T7. The lesion is high signal intensity, but somewhat heterogeneous, on the T_2-weighted scan. Extension into the T7–8 neural foramen is also noted. *C* and *D*, Postcontrast there is intense enhancement of the lesion. Although by imaging appearance the lesion could be either a schwannoma or a neurofibroma, that enhancement is heterogeneous and more intense peripherally favors a schwannoma.

FIGURE 7–13. Ganglioneuroma. *A*, On the T_2-weighted sagittal image to the right of midline, a large paraspinal soft tissue mass is noted. The patient is a 2-year-old child who presented with respiratory distress. The mass extends into and widens the T5–6 neural foramen. *B*, On the axial postcontrast T_1-weighted image, the mass is noted to enhance. However, the epidural portion enhances more intensely than the remainder of the lesion (the large paravertebral portion). The thoracic spinal cord is severely compressed and displaced to the patient's left.

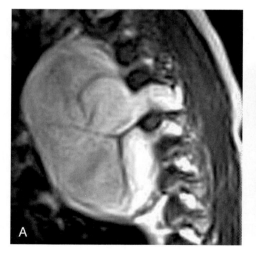

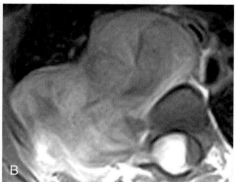

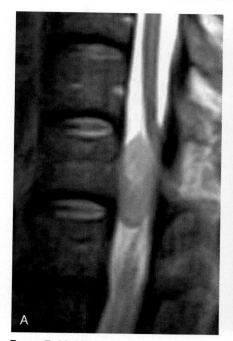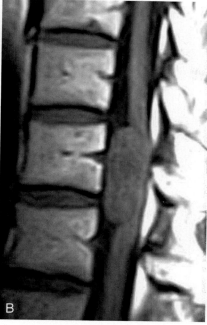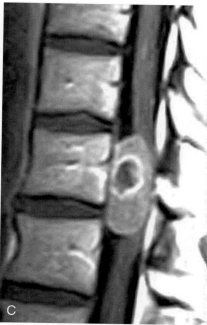

FIGURE 7–14. Meningioma. On precontrast T_2- (*A*) and T_1-weighted (*B*) sagittal scans, a mass is noted within the thecal sac, outlined by cerebrospinal fluid. The flattening and displacement of the cord favor an intradural extramedullary location. Intense enhancement postcontrast (*C*) improves demarcation of the lesion and places a meningioma first on the list of differential diagnoses. This 48-year-old woman presented with paraplegia and progressive back pain. The lesion was surgically removed.

3:1 female-male incidence. Spinal meningiomas are most often intradural in location but may be extradural. Complete removal can be achieved surgically in 95% of cases. Microsurgical technique is important to minimize neurologic deficits. Despite "complete" removal, 5% recur.

Meningiomas are isointense to the spinal cord on both T_1- and T_2-weighted scans. This tumor displays marked contrast enhancement, which can improve lesion identification and demarcation (Fig. 7–14). The capping of a meningioma inferiorly and superiorly by CSF is characteristic and demonstrates the lesion to be intradural and extramedullary in location (by far the most common location). On plain film and CT, dense calcification is common.

VASCULAR AND HEMATOPOIETIC DISEASE (NON-NEOPLASTIC)
Arteriovenous Malformation and Fistula

An arteriovenous malformation (AVM) is defined as a nidus of pathologic vessels between enlarged feeding arteries and draining veins. This is to be differentiated from an arteriovenous fistula (AVF), in which the arteries drain directly into enlarged veins. Within this group of lesions, three types are described in the spine: dural AVF (the most common), intramedullary AVM, and intradural extramedullary AVF.

Dural AVFs occur along the dorsal aspect of the lower cord and conus (Fig. 7–15). These feature a single transdural arterial feeder. Dural AVFs are found in elderly men and present with progressive neurologic deficits resulting from venous stasis and infarction.

Intramedullary AVMs occur in young patients and are one cause of intramedullary hemorrhage. They are typically dorsal in location and occur most often in the cervicomedullary region. Multiple feeding vessels lead to a compact vascular plexus, which drains into a tortuous venous plexus surrounding the cord. Intramedullary AVMs present with acute hemorrhagic stroke. The imaging appearance on MRI is that of multiple flow voids within the cord together with enlarged extramedullary feeding vessels (typically anterior to the cord).

Intradural extramedullary AVFs occur in the third to sixth decades. The most common presentation is that of a lesion at the level of the conus but anterior to the cord with supply by the anterior spinal artery. Intradural extramedullary AVFs present with progressive neurologic deficits.

MRI is an important technique for the initial diagnosis of a spinal AVM or AVF. Abnormal large vessels are identified as filling defects on conventional two-dimensional scans. These are best appreciated within the cord on T_1-weighted images and within the CSF space on T_2-weighted images (see Fig. 7–15). Small lesions are clearly seen postcontrast because of the enhancement of the large draining veins. Associate cord findings include hemorrhage, edema, and myelomalacia. An important pitfall on image interpretation is that CSF flow artifacts may mimic an AVM on T_2-weighted scans. These artifacts can be prominent on conventional spin echo T_2-weighted scans but may on occasion also be present on fast spin echo scans. On x-ray myelography, filling defects may be seen as a result of enlarged vessels

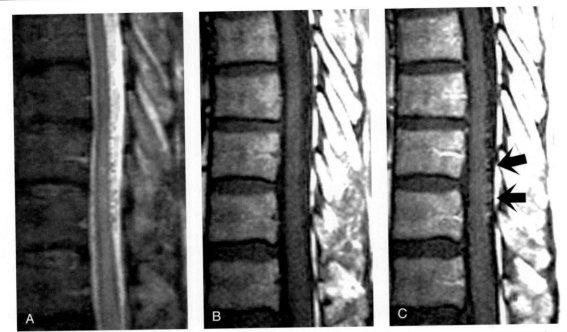

FIGURE 7–15. Dural spinal arteriovenous fistula. *A*, On the sagittal T$_2$-weighted scan, the question of abnormal hyperintensity within the lower cord and conus is raised. Immediately posterior to the cord, multiple small serpiginous signal voids are identified, spanning at least two vertebral segments. *B*, The precontrast T$_1$-weighted scan is normal. *C*, Postcontrast, abnormal enhancement (*arrows*) is noted along the dorsal aspect of the cord, confirming the presence of enlarged draining veins. The diagnosis was confirmed surgically. By enhancement of slow flow within dilated veins, contrast administration improves visualization of spinal arteriovenous malformations and fistulas.

and cord atrophy detected, if present. X-ray angiography is used for definitive diagnosis. Selective vessel catheterization, assessing feeding vessels and venous drainage, is performed after initial intra-aortic injection. Spinal AVMs and AVFs are also clearly visualized by contrast-enhanced magnetic resonance angiography, which may with future refinements replace x-ray angiography.

Spinal Cord Ischemia/Infarction

There are many causes for spinal cord ischemia and infarction, including atherosclerosis, vasculitis, embolism, infection, radiation, trauma, and surgery (specifically after abdominal aortic aneurysm resection). Infarction and ischemia typically involve the central gray matter of the cord. Anatomically, the lower thoracic cord and conus are most commonly involved. The artery of Adamkiewicz, typically arising from the 9th to 12th intercostal artery, supplies this region. Blood flow is highest to this section of the cord, given the abundance of gray matter and its higher metabolic need. Thus, it is this region of the cord that is most vulnerable to hypoperfusion.

MRI is, without question, the imaging modality of choice for the diagnosis of spinal cord ischemia and infarction. The extent of abnormality as visualized by MRI correlates well with clinical findings and prognosis. The area involved can be minimal (e.g., just the anterior horns). In severe cases, the entire cord is involved in cross-section. In intermediate cases, both the anterior and posterior horns are involved together with the adjacent central white matter. On T$_2$-weighted scans, abnor-

mal high signal intensity is noted in the involved region (Fig. 7–16), corresponding to vasogenic edema in acute and subacute disease. On T$_1$-weighted scans, cord enlargement may be the only finding. Abnormal contrast enhancement of the cord can be present as a result of disruption of blood-cord barrier (secondary to ischemia). There may be associated marrow changes also resulting from ischemia. Differential diagnostic considerations include multiple sclerosis (MS), transverse myelitis, and neoplasia. Recognition of the vascular distribution, both in craniocaudal extent and cross-section, aids in differentiation of spinal cord ischemia/infarction from other disease processes.

Hemorrhage

Subarachnoid hemorrhage may be secondary to a spinal aneurysm or AVM or may originate from a cerebral source. With acute hemorrhage, a moderate increase in the signal intensity of CSF on T$_1$-weighted scans may be observed, obscuring the cord and nerve roots. With subacute hemorrhage, high signal intensity is seen on T$_1$-weighted scans because of the presence of methemoglobin.

Epidural and subdural hemorrhage has many causes, including lumbar puncture, trauma, bleeding diatheses, anticoagulant therapy, vascular malformations, vasculitis, and pregnancy. The signal intensity on MRI is dependent largely on the stage of hemorrhage and dilution by CSF. It can be difficult to identify whether a hemorrhage is epidural or subdural in location. When abnormal high signal intensity is seen in the epidural or subdural space,

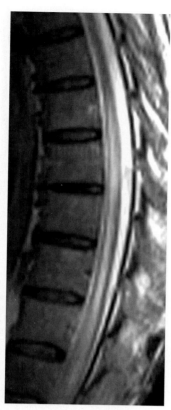

FIGURE 7–16. Spinal cord infarction. The mid- and lower thoracic cord is slightly expanded and has abnormal high signal intensity. These findings correspond to vasogenic edema. Infarcts can be limited to a few vertebral segments or can be very extensive as in this case. With sufficient time, cord atrophy will occur, although the abnormal high signal intensity on T_2-weighted scans can persist (as a result of gliosis).

two other disease processes should be considered in the differential diagnosis. Angiolipomas are rare benign tumors composed of lipocytes and abnormal blood vessels. The latter cause hyperintensity on T_2-weighted scans on the basis of slow flow. These tumors are usually epidural in location and occur in the midthoracic region. Angiolipomas can cause bone erosion, pathologic fractures, and cord compression. The other consideration should be extradural lipomatosis, although with this disease process the abnormal soft tissue should be readily identifiable as fat (by inspection of both T_1- and T_2-weighted scans).

Extramedullary Hematopoiesis

Extramedullary hematopoiesis is a compensatory response to insufficient red blood cell production by bone marrow. It is seen in thalassemia, hereditary spherocytosis, and myelosclerosis. Favored sites of involvement include the spleen, liver, and lymph nodes. Thoracic involvement is rare and usually asymptomatic. Thoracic involvement is seen on imaging as a paraspinal mass resulting from extrusion of proliferating marrow from vertebral bodies into a subperiosteal location. Intraspinal lesions can occur as a result of extrusion of bone marrow or development of marrow from embryonic hematopoi-

etic rests. Intraspinal involvement can cause cord compression. The appearance on MRI of thoracic extramedullary hematopoiesis is that of multiple, smoothly marginated, paraspinal masses without bone erosion (Fig. 7–17). The masses have the signal intensity of marrow on all pulse sequences. The differential diagnosis should include lymphoma and metastatic disease.

TRAUMA

Burst fractures are the most common traumatic bone injury encountered in the thoracic spine. Burst fractures are caused by an axial loading injury. Vertical compression forces the nucleus pulposus into the vertebral body, with radial displacement of fragments. Burst fractures are most common from T9 to L5. The injury is typically limited to one vertebral body, but associated injuries are common. Neurologic deficits occur as a result of the retropulsed fragments. CT is often used for initial evaluation. MRI detects associated cord (edema and hemorrhage) and ligamentous injuries, which are not clearly seen by CT.

DEGENERATIVE DISK AND BONY DISEASE

In the thoracic spine, disk herniations are most common at the lower four interspaces, where the spine is more mobile. Thoracic disk herniations are less common than either cervical or lumbar herniations. The clinical presentation is often not clear-cut. Symptoms include back pain, paresthesias, and motor weakness. On high-quality MRI images, small thoracic disk herniations are clearly seen (Fig. 7–18). MRI also clearly demonstrates mass effect on the cord, when present, and contour deformities of the cord. As with cervical disk herniations, part of the abnormality may actually represent dilated epidural venous plexus. On contrast-enhanced images, the dilated, engorged epidural venous plexus above and below the herniated disk (Fig. 7–19) is readily identified.

In addition to dedicated thoracic spine images, a high-quality large field of view localizer should be acquired, on which the dens can be identified, to define the level of disk herniation correctly. The use of MRI markers can assist in correct level identification. Commonly used markers include vitamin E capsules (an oily vitamin that has high signal intensity on T_1-weighted scans) or oil (such as Johnson's baby oil) in a strip of intravenous tubing.

ABNORMAL ALIGNMENT

Scoliosis is defined as a lateral curvature of the spine. Ninety percent of cases are idiopathic with no underlying cause. Idiopathic thoracic scoliosis is more common in females, and the thoracic curvature is typically convex to right (with an **S**-shaped curve). Progression beyond 50 degrees necessitates surgery.

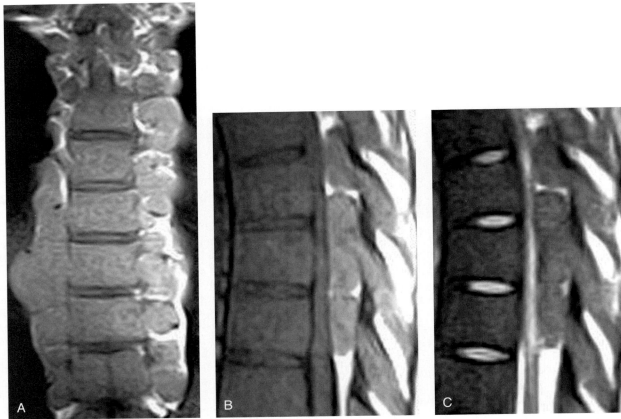

FIGURE 7–17. Extramedullary hematopoiesis with severe cord compression. The patient is 32 years of age with thalassemia and presents clinically with progressive paraplegia. *A,* The T_1-weighted coronal image demonstrates large bilateral lobulated paraspinal masses in the upper and midthoracic regions. *B,* On the T_1-weighted midline sagittal view, large intraspinal masses with resultant severe cord compression are identified at the T6 to T8 levels. The soft tissue masses lie within the same space as the thoracic epidural fat. Also noted is a generalized decrease in signal intensity of the thoracic vertebral bodies. *C,* The corresponding fast spin echo T_2-weighted sagittal image confirms the abnormal intraspinal soft tissue masses. The lesions remain relatively low in signal intensity on the T_2-weighted scan. Abnormally increased signal intensity compatible with edema or gliosis is identified within the compressed thoracic spinal cord. On postcontrast scans (not shown), there was mild, homogeneous enhancement of the paraspinal and the intraspinal lesions.

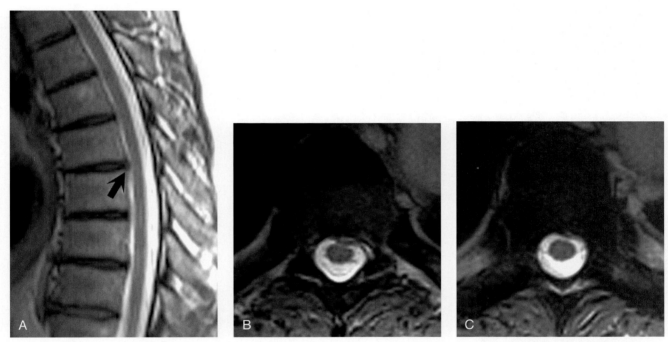

FIGURE 7–18. Thoracic disk herniation. *A,* The midline sagittal fast T$_2$-weighted scan reveals mild anterior indentation of the thecal sac (*arrow*) at a midthoracic level. *B* and *C,* Axial gradient echo T$_2$-weighted scans reveal small left paracentral disk herniations at this level and two levels below. It cannot be determined, however, whether these lesions are acute or chronic in nature. Attention to detail and high-quality images are necessary to diagnose thoracic disk herniations because these are often very small in size (despite being clinically symptomatic).

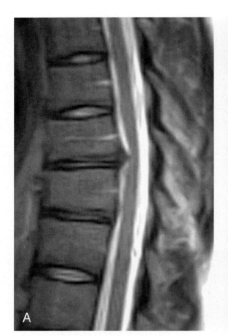

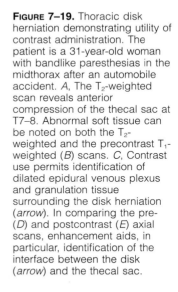

FIGURE 7–19. Thoracic disk herniation demonstrating utility of contrast administration. The patient is a 31-year-old woman with bandlike paresthesias in the midthorax after an automobile accident. *A*, The T$_2$-weighted scan reveals anterior compression of the thecal sac at T7–8. Abnormal soft tissue can be noted on both the T$_2$-weighted and the precontrast T$_1$-weighted (*B*) scans. *C*, Contrast use permits identification of dilated epidural venous plexus and granulation tissue surrounding the disk herniation (*arrow*). In comparing the pre- (*D*) and postcontrast (*E*) axial scans, enhancement aids, in particular, identification of the interface between the disk (*arrow*) and the thecal sac.

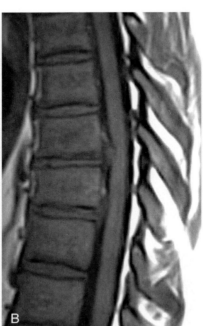

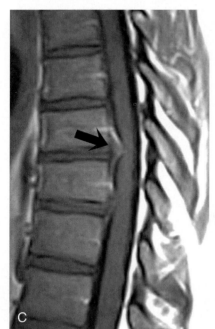

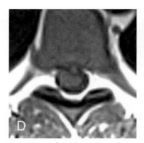

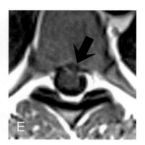

Ten percent of thoracic scoliosis can be attributed to congenital, neuromuscular, or posttraumatic causes. In the congenital category are both vertebral anomalies (butterfly vertebral body and hemivertebra) and abnormalities of the cord. The latter include Chiari malformations, hydrosyringomyelia, diastematomyelia, and spinal cord neoplasm. Cerebral palsy is the primary neuromuscular cause and leads to a C-shaped curve. Posttraumatic causes include fractures, old osteomyelitis, surgery, and radiation therapy. MRI is the imaging modality of choice for study of atypical or progressive scoliosis. In a patient with scoliosis, coronal images are particularly useful in conjunction with sagittal images. Plain x-ray films are used for quantitation of the curvature (degree) and monitoring of progression.

MULTIPLE SCLEROSIS

MS lesions of the thoracic cord are clearly seen on high-quality MRI images, with no difference in appearance than that described for the cervical spine. In acute disease, there can be focal cord swelling, edema (limited to a focal region in both cross-section and craniocaudal extent and best seen on T_2-weighted images), and abnormal contrast enhancement (as a result of blood-spinal cord barrier disruption seen on contrast enhanced T_1-weighted images). Chronic lesions can be identified on T_2-weighted scans because of focal cord atrophy and gliosis (Fig. 7–20).

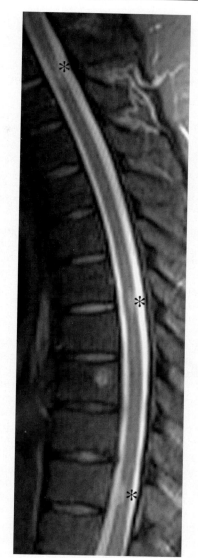

FIGURE 7–20. Multiple sclerosis (inactive disease). Three short-segment high-signal-intensity lesions (*asterisks*) are noted within the thoracic cord on a fast spin echo T_2-weighted scan. Cord atrophy is noticeable at the level of the highest lesion, determining it to be chronic in nature (with the abnormal signal equating to gliosis). Neither of the lower lesions causes cord expansion, making it unlikely that either represents active disease. The lack of contrast enhancement (images not shown) confirmed the chronic nature of disease in this patient.

8

Lumbar Spine

NORMAL LUMBAR SPINE

The lumbar spine consists of five lumbar segments (vertebral bodies), five (fused) sacral segments, and the coccyx. Each intervertebral disk is composed of a central gelatinous core (the nucleus pulposus, which is high signal intensity on T_2-weighted images) surrounded by dense fibrous tissue (the annulus fibrosus, which is low signal intensity on T_2-weighted images). The bony elements of the lumbar spine include the pedicles, transverse processes, articular pillars (pars interarticularis, superior and inferior articular facets), laminae, spinous processes, and vertebral bodies. The facet joints are diarthrodial (synovial lined) and richly innervated. On axial imaging, the superior articular facet forms a "cap" anterolaterally with the inferior articular facet posteromedial and connecting to the lamina. The ligamentum flavum extends from the anterior aspect of the upper lamina to the posterior aspect of the lower lamina. The epidural venous plexus is prominent in the lumbar spine. In regard to important dermatomes (for clinical diagnosis with a disk herniation), L4 innervates the medial big toe, L5 the midfoot, and S1 the little toe.

In the sagittal plane, the conus can be seen to terminate between L1 and L2. The posterior longitudinal ligament lies immediately posterior to the vertebral bodies and anterior to the thecal sac. Normal dimensions for the posterior longitudinal ligament are 1-mm thickness (anteroposterior) and 5-mm width (left to right). The facet joints of the upper lumbar spine are oriented in the sagittal plane. Those of the lower lumbar spine are oriented more in the coronal plane. On off-midline sagittal (parasagittal) images, the dorsal root ganglion (and ventral root) can be seen within the superior portion of the neural foramen. Parasagittal images are used to evaluate foraminal stenosis. In regard to the margins of the foramen, the disk and vertebral body lie anteriorly, the pedicles superiorly and inferiorly, and the facet joints posteriorly. On axial imaging, the margins of the bony (spinal) canal consist of the vertebral body anteriorly, the pedicles laterally, and the lamina posteriorly.

On T_1-weighted spin echo images, normally hydrated (nondegenerated) disks are slightly hypointense to vertebral marrow. The normal ligamentum flavum is clearly seen, with intermediate signal intensity. Slice thickness should be no greater than 4 mm in the sagittal plane and 3 mm in the axial plane. It is important that a coronal saturation slab be placed anteriorly to decrease artifacts (from the motion of structures anterior to the

spine), which would otherwise degrade the images. Saturation of anterior structures is equally important on T_2-weighted images in the lumbar spine (and on both types of scans in the cervical and thoracic regions as well). The disks are best visualized in the axial plane when the slices are angled to be parallel to each disk space. Fast spin echo has replaced conventional spin echo technique for T_2-weighted imaging of the lumbar spine, and such scans are clinically valuable in both the sagittal and axial planes. Fat saturation is advocated (for fast spin echo T_2-weighted scans), and when used normally, hydrated (nondegenerated) disks will be markedly hyperintense to vertebral marrow. In the sagittal plane in adults, a central horizontal band of low signal intensity is typically noted (the "intranuclear cleft") within the intervertebral disk as a result of fibrous transformation.

Surface coils are used to image the lumbar spine. Today these are often an integral part of the patient table. The signal received from the body falls with distance from the surface coil. This situation is quite different from that with cylindrical coils (such as those used for imaging the head), which are specifically designed to achieve homogeneous signal intensity across the entire field of view. Because of the use of a surface coil in lumbar imaging, superficially located structures (close to the coil) will have artifactual high signal intensity. In routine clinical practice, the window and center for the image are chosen to adequately display the spinal canal; thus, posterior structures (soft tissue) are obscured (because of marked hyperintensity). If it is important to view the posterior soft tissues (e.g., to rule out an abscess after surgery), then the images should be rewindowed specifically for these structures. On some magnetic resonance image (MRI) scanners, the images can be normalized with postprocessing software. The aim is to attenuate signal from tissues close to the coil and thus provide more homogeneous signal intensity across the field of view.

The injection of contrast media (specifically, a gadolinium chelate) plays an important role in lumbar imaging, primarily because of the large population of postsurgical diskectomy patients presenting with recurrent pain. Normal enhancing structures include the epidural venous plexus (also known as Batson's plexus), the basivertebral vein, and the dorsal root ganglion. The capillaries of the epidural venous plexus have nonfenestrated endothelium, which confines the contrast to the intravascular space. The basivertebral vein is commonly visualized on midline postcontrast sagittal images, running from the center of the vertebral body posteriorly. The

174

endothelium of the dorsal root ganglion is fenestrated, like that in muscle and marrow, permitting contrast to enter the interstitial space. Enhancement of the dorsal root ganglion is only moderate in degree. The most common indication for contrast use in the lumbar spine is for the differentiation of scar from disk in the postoperative patient. On scans obtained within 20 minutes after contrast injection, scar enhances whereas recurrent (or residual) disk herniation does not. On precontrast scans, scar and disk material have similar signal intensity; differentiation is not possible. Contrast injection can also be beneficial in the more general population with low back pain but without previous surgery. Contrast use improves definition of the disk-thecal sac interface, permits identification of the epidural venous plexus and (de novo) scar, and improves visualization of the neural foramina. Contrast injection is recommended in patients with a high clinical suspicion of intradural or soft tissue extradural involvement by neoplastic disease. Disease involving the spinal cord (in particular neoplasia, ischemia, and demyelinating disease) is often better evaluated with the addition of postcontrast scans. Contrast use is mandatory when infection is suspected because extensive, active disease can be missed on precontrast scans.

The lumbar spine undergoes a marked change in appearance on MRI during the first year of life. Changes occur more gradually thereafter, with distinct differences in appearance between the young adult and the elderly. There is absence of the normal adult lumbar lordosis in the infant. Before 1 month of age, the ossification center within the vertebral body has low signal intensity on both T_1- and T_2-weighted scans. A distinct band with slight high signal intensity on T_1-weighted images within the ossification center corresponds to the basivertebral venous plexus. The cartilaginous end plate has higher signal intensity on T_1-weighted scans than paraspinous muscle and has high signal intensity on T_2-weighted scans. The disk itself is thin, isointense on T_1-weighted images to paraspinous muscle, and very high signal intensity on T_2-weighted images. The anteroposterior dimension of the ossification centers is less than that of the intervertebral disks.

From 1 to 6 months of age, the ossification center has low to intermediate signal intensity on T_1-weighted images and is isointense with the end plates. On T_2-weighted scans, the cartilaginous end plates have higher signal intensity than muscle or the ossification center. The intervertebral disk is low signal intensity on T_1-weighted scans and high signal intensity on T_2-weighted scans.

By 7 months of age, the spine attains a more adult appearance. The ossification center is more rectangular and is now hyperintense to muscle on T_1-weighted scans. On both T_1- and T_2-weighted scans, the signal intensity of the cartilaginous end plate is similar to that of the ossification center. The intervertebral disk is low signal intensity on T_1-weighted scans (isointense to muscle) and high signal intensity on T_2-weighted scans.

The vertebral body contains both red and yellow marrow; the relative proportion of the two determines the signal intensity on MRI. Red (hematologically active) marrow has lower signal intensity on T_1-weighted scans than yellow (fatty) marrow. The change in signal intensity from the infant to the young adult to the elderly reflects the conversion from red to yellow marrow. With increasing age, both diffuse and focal replacement of red marrow by yellow marrow occurs. Focal changes (focal "fat") are more common near the end plates perhaps because of decreased vascularity and earlier marrow conversion in this location.

At birth, the conus should terminate above the L3-4 level. Termination below this level is abnormal regardless of age. By 2 months of age, the conus should lie in the adult location: L2-3 or above. The conus lies, on average, at the L1-2 level in children and adults.

CONGENITAL DISEASE (INCLUDING STRUCTURAL ANOMALIES)
Transitional Vertebrae

Transitional vertebrae are common at the lumbosacral junction (occurring in 4% to 8% of the population). By definition, there is articulation or fusion of an enlarged transverse process of the lowest lumbar segment to the sacrum. The articulation or fusion can be unilateral or bilateral. On sagittal images, the body of a transitional segment may be square (normal configuration for lumbar), wedge shaped (like the sacral segments), or intermediate in shape. The presence of a transitional vertebra on MRI is readily apparent if one is aware of the following key. Because numbering of the lumbar vertebrae is critical in patients being examined for possible disk surgery, close attention should be paid to the curve formed by the anterior margin of the lumbar vertebral bodies and sacrum. There should be a smooth curve with the apex anteriorly encompassing the lumbar vertebrae. This should then reverse at L5-S1 to a smooth curve with the apex posteriorly encompassing the sacral segments. Any variation from these two smooth curves indicates the presence of a transitional vertebra; plain film correlation is necessary to determine whether the body in question is lumbarized or sacralized. Transitional vertebrae are a known cause of back pain. There is decreased mobility at the affected level and increased mobility and stress at the interspace immediately above.

Spina Bifida Occulta (Occult Spinal Dysraphism)

In spina bifida occulta, skin covers a developmental anomaly involving incomplete midline closure. On physical exam, there is no visible neural tissue or mass. Spinal bifida occulta includes diastematomyelia, dermal sinus tracts, fibrous bands, dermoids, neurenteric cysts, and lipomas. This class of congenital malformations is distinct (separate) from meningoceles and myelomeningoceles. Spina bifida occulta is not associated with the Chiari type II malformation.

Caudal Regression (Sacral Agenesis)

In caudal regression, there is absence of sacrococcygeal vertebrae with or without lumbar involvement. The

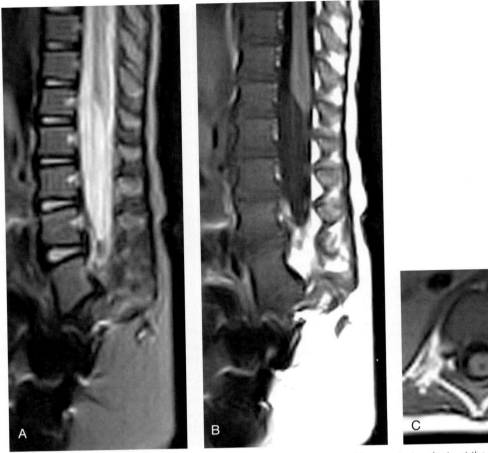

FIGURE 8–1. Sacral agenesis. *A,* On the midline sagittal T$_2$-weighted scan, the cord is seen to terminate at the L1-2 level. The L5 vertebral body is dysplastic. Only a portion of S1 is present (the remainder of the sacrum is absent). *B,* On the midline sagittal T$_1$-weighted scan, the contour of the cord terminus is noted to be unusual, with the cord ending in a wedge shape (the dorsal aspect extends further caudally). There is abnormal signal intensity centrally within the cord, low signal intensity on the T$_1$-weighted scan, and high signal intensity on the T$_2$-weighted scan, suggesting a small syrinx. *C,* The axial T$_1$-weighted scan just above the level of the cord terminus confirms the presence of a dilated central canal (hydromyelia). This 21-month-old infant presented with lower extremity sensory and motor deficits.

level of regression is below L1 in most cases. Agenesis is limited to the sacrum in about half of all cases (Fig. 8–1). Associated anomalies include cord tethering, renal dysplasia, pulmonary hypoplasia, and neuromuscular weakness or paralysis. Caudal regression is associated with maternal diabetes. On MRI, a wedge-shaped cord terminus is seen in about half of patients, with the dorsal aspect extending further caudally than the ventral aspect. MRI clearly depicts the level of regression, presence of stenosis (in the area of vertebral absence), and associated structural anomalies.

Myelomeningocele

Spina bifida is defined as incomplete closure of the posterior bony elements. The contents of the spinal canal can extend through this defect (with tethering of the cord). A meningocele contains dura and arachnoid. Neurologic deficits are uncommon with a simple meningocele. A myelomeningocele contains neural tissue within the expanded posterior subarachnoid space (Fig. 8–2). On intrauterine ultrasonography, the neural arch is open and the posterior elements are flared. There is

an associated Chiari type II malformation in almost all cases. MRI is usually obtained postoperatively. A wide dysraphic defect is typically seen, together with a cerebrospinal fluid (CSF)-filled sac covered by skin. There is often retethering of the cord. MRI is the modality of choice for evaluation of the soft tissue elements in suspected spinal dysraphism.

Anterior Sacral Meningocele

In an anterior sacral meningocele, there is protrusion of the dura and leptomeninges anteriorly through a defect in sacrum. On plain film, the lesion is recognized because of semicircular erosion of the sacrum (the "scimitar sign"). On MRI, the abnormal fluid collection will have CSF signal intensity on all pulse sequences. Myelography may not be diagnostic because the pedicle connecting the cyst and the thecal sac can be obstructed by adhesions and thus the cyst not filled with contrast.

Diastematomyelia

In diastematomyelia, the spinal cord is split into two hemicords, each invested by pia (Fig. 8–3). Each

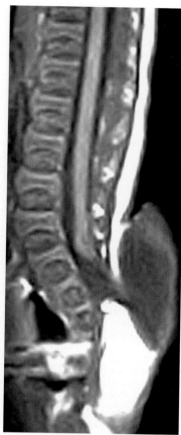

FIGURE 8–2. Meningomyelocele with tethered cord. The midline sagittal T$_1$-weighted scan reveals a sac filled with cerebrospinal fluid located posteriorly in the lower lumbar region. The sac communicates with the normal thecal space. The spinal cord extends at least to the lumbosacral junction. The posterior bony elements are dysraphic from L4 to S1. Abundant fatty tissue is present immediately below the defect. Note also the distinct signal intensity and configuration of the vertebral bodies and intervertebral disks, normal for the patient's age. This newborn presented with a normal neurologic exam and a low lumbosacral mass covered by skin. At the time of surgery for repair of this defect, a single nerve (not seen on magnetic resonance imaging or computed tomography) was identified within the fluid-filled sac.

hemicord contains a central canal and has both dorsal and ventral horns. In 60% of cases, the hemicords are contained within one subarachnoid space and dural sac. In 40% of cases, separate sacs with a fibrous band or an osteocartilaginous spur is nearly always present at the most inferior aspect of the cleft. Gradient echo scans are more sensitive than T$_2$-weighted scans, which are likewise more sensitive than T$_1$-weighted scans, for detecting the spur. In 85% of cases, the cleft occurs between T9 and S1. In 50% of cases, the cleft is lumbar in location. Associated anomalies include vertebral segmentation anomalies, spina bifida (which is nearly always present), orthopedic foot problems such as clubfoot (half of patients), and hydromyelia. Associated vertebral segmentation anomalies, which are common, include fusion (block vertebrae), hemivertebrae, and butterfly vertebrae. Patients with diastematomyelia often present clinically with nonspecific symptoms. Symptoms may be re-

lated to cord tethering. Cutaneous stigmas (hairy patches, nevi, and lipomas) are seen in more than 50% of cases. On MRI it is critical to obtain axial scans; coronal scans are also useful. With sagittal scans alone, the split cord can be overlooked.

Lipomyelomeningocele

A lipomyelomeningocele is differentiated from a myelomeningocele (a protrusion of the membranes and cord through a defect in the vertebral column) by the presence of a lipoma and an intact overlying skin layer. The lipoma is firmly attached to the dorsal surface of the neural placode (cord terminus), which then herniates through the dysraphic spinal canal. The lipoma merges with and is indistinguishable from subcutaneous fat. The distal cord is tethered by the lipoma. Lipomyelomeningoceles occur in the lumbosacral region. They make up 20% of skin-covered lumbosacral masses and 50% of occult spinal dysraphisms.

Associated anomalies include butterfly vertebrae (and other vertebral segmentation anomalies), sacral anomalies, scoliosis, and maldevelopment of the feet. Patients with lipomyelomeningoceles typically present clinically before 6 months of age with a fluctuant subcutaneous mass. Neurologic symptoms include lower extremity weakness, sensory loss, urinary incontinence, and gait disturbance. Symptoms are usually progressive if corrective surgery is not performed. Occasionally, lipomyelomeningoceles go undetected until adulthood because the lesion is covered with skin.

Dorsal Dermal Sinus

A dorsal dermal sinus is a midline epithelium-lined tract that extends from the skin inward for a variable distance. More than 50% occur in the lumbosacral region (Fig. 8–4). The tract can terminate in the posterior soft tissue, at the dura, or within the thecal sac. Cord tethering is common. On the skin surface, there may be a hairy nevus, hyperpigmented patch, or capillary angioma. Half of all patients have an associated dermoid or epidermoid tumor at the tract termination. Patients present clinically in two different ways: either with infection or with symptoms of cord compression (by a tumor mass). On MRI, if an infection is present, intravenous contrast enhancement improves delineation of the sinus tract, particularly the intraspinal portion.

Tethered Cord

A tethered cord is a congenital anomaly in which the conus is held at an abnormally low position. Causes include a short (tight) filum terminale, an intradural lumbosacral lipoma (Fig. 8–5), diastematomyelia, and a delayed consequence of myelomeningocele repair. With a tight filum, the age of presentation is variable. Adults present frequently with radiculopathy. The normal filum should be 2 mm or less in diameter. Caution should be exercised when interpreting postoperative cases (after myelomeningocele repair) because not all patients with evidence of tethering on imaging are symptomatic.

Clinical symptoms are due to cord ischemia caused

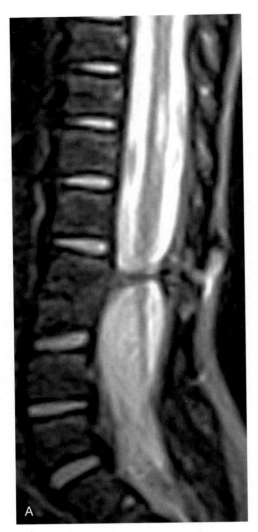

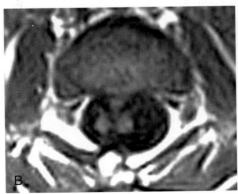

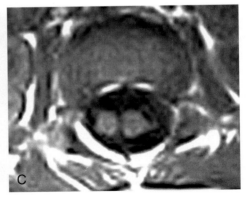

FIGURE 8–3. Diastematomyelia. *A,* The midline sagittal T_2-weighted scan demonstrates a segmentation anomaly (block vertebrae) at L2-3. A low-signal-intensity band spans the thecal sac at the L2-3 level. A central region of high signal intensity, consistent with a small syrinx (hydromyelia), is present within the lower thoracic spinal cord. *B,* The T_1-weighted axial image at the L2 level reveals splitting of the spinal cord by the previously noted band or spur. Bony dysraphism is noted posteriorly. *C,* An additional T_1-weighted axial image at a slightly higher level more clearly depicts the separation of the cord into two hemicords. This 18-month-old infant presented clinically with lower extremity spasticity.

FIGURE 8–4. Dorsal dermal sinus. Sagittal T$_2$- (*A*) and T$_1$-weighted (*B*) images of the lumbar spine reveal a sinus tract (*A, arrows*) coursing from the skin to the thecal sac. This abnormality is less apparent on the T$_1$-weighted scan because of the high signal intensity of fat posteriorly, accentuated by the proximity to the surface coil. The conus lies at L2. A portion of tract (*arrow*) is also visualized on the axial T$_1$-weighted image (*C*).

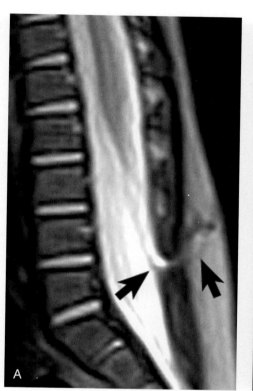
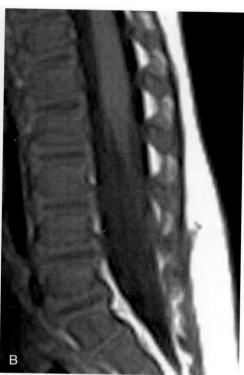
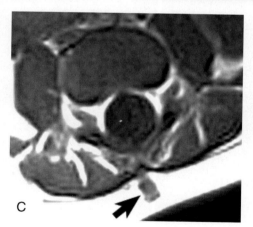

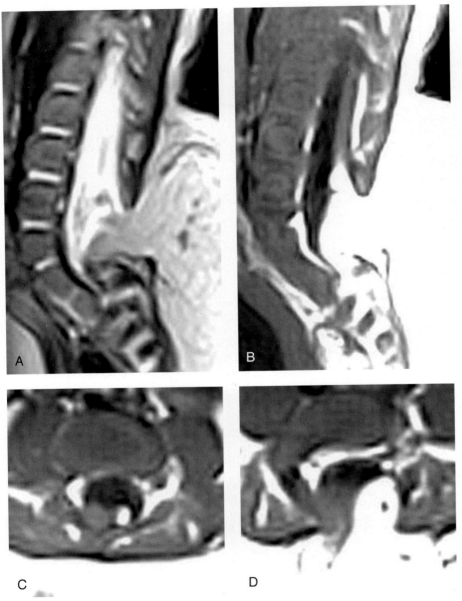

FIGURE 8–5. Tethered spinal cord with lipomyelomeningocele. *A,* The midline sagittal T$_2$-weighted scan demonstrates spinal dysraphism at L4-5, a capacious lumbar thecal sac, and a large abnormal fat pad posteriorly. *B,* The corresponding T$_1$-weighted scan reveals the cord to be low lying and tethered to a lipoma at the L4-5 level. *C,* On axial imaging, the low lying cord is seen in cross-section with a separate, but adjacent, intrathecal lipoma. *D,* On a lower axial section, the cord is tethered posteriorly and attached to a large lipoma that extends into both the thecal sac and the posterior soft tissues. This 2-month-old infant presented at birth with a posterior lumbar mass that subsequently increased in size. Motion and strength of the lower extremities were normal.

by traction. The typical patient is a young child with progressive neurologic dysfunction. Symptoms include gait difficulty, motor and sensory loss in the lower extremities, and bladder dysfunction. On imaging, the cord is seen to extend without change in caliber to the lumbosacral region, where it is tethered posteriorly. Also commonly present is a lipoma and dysraphism of the posterior spinal elements. Hydromyelia may be present as well. When small, this is usually not symptomatic. T_1-weighted scans in all three orthogonal planes are important for depiction of the abnormal anatomy. The axial plane is superior to the sagittal plane for determination of the level of the conus. On sagittal images, differentiation between the conus and cauda equina can be difficult. For the diagnosis of retethering, the presence of adhesions is a good criterion.

The aim of surgical therapy is to untether the cord and thus arrest symptom progression. Early diagnosis and surgery can prevent urinary incontinence. The associated lipoma is typically removed as completely as possible, with attention to release of the tether. The use of synthetic dural grafts decreases the incidence of retethering. After surgery, the level of the cord termination does not change.

A terminal myelocystocele is a rare congenital cystic dilatation of the caudal central spinal canal with an associated posterior bony defect. There is a trumpet-like flaring of the distal central canal, which is a pia-lined CSF space and may be larger than the accompanying surrounding meningocele. Associated anomalies of the gastrointestinal tract, genitourinary tract, and vertebral bodies are common.

Spinal Meningeal Cysts

Spinal meningeal cysts are diverticula of the meningeal sac, nerve root sheath, or arachnoid. Most cysts are congenital in origin. There are three types. Type I cysts are extradural in location and do not contain nerve roots. This group includes arachnoid cysts and sacral meningoceles. Type II cysts are extradural in location and contain nerve roots. This group includes spinal nerve root diverticula and Tarlov cysts. The latter are not infrequently seen in clinical practice. More correctly known as Tarlov perineural cysts, these lesions are simply nerve root sleeve cysts (focal dilatation of the nerve root sleeves). The nerves may be in the cyst or in the wall. The cyst communicates freely with the thecal sac (Fig. 8–6). Type III cysts are intradural in location and are simply intradural arachnoid cysts.

Spinal meningeal cysts are usually asymptomatic. These lesions are common in the sacral area. The cysts are frequently large, multiple, and bilateral. They can cause erosion and scalloping of the vertebral body, pedicle, and foramen. On MRI, the cysts are CSF signal intensity on all pulse sequences.

Lumbosacral Nerve Root Anomalies

Lumbosacral nerve root anomalies occur in 1% to 3% of the population. These usually involve the L5 and S1 roots unilaterally. There are three types of lumbosacral nerve root anomalies. The first, type I, is a simple conjoined root (Fig. 8–7). This is the most common anomaly. Two roots arise from a single root sleeve but exit separately (in the appropriate foramina). In type II, two roots exit through a single foramen (and there may be one foramen without a root). In type III, an anastomotic root connects two adjacent roots. Lumbosacral nerve root anomalies are asymptomatic. However, it is important to recognize their presence and report this in the dictation. For lumbar disk surgery to be successful, in the presence of a nerve root anomaly, adequate decompression is required. On computed tomography (CT) without intrathecal contrast, a nerve root anomaly can be mistaken for a herniated disk.

Fatty Filum Terminale

The normal filum terminale runs from the tip of the conus to the end of the thecal sac, inserting on the first coccygeal segment. As previously noted, the normal filum is 2 mm or less in diameter at the L5-S1 level. One percent to 5% of the population have a small amount of fat within the filum. This is usually an incidental finding; however, it can be associated with cord tethering.

Achondroplasia

Achondroplasia is an autosomal-dominant disorder of enchondral bone formation. In this disease, there is premature synostosis (bony ankylosis) of ossification centers of the vertebral bodies. In childhood, cervical changes may dominate the presentation, with canal narrowing and constriction at the foramen magnum. Classic findings in the lumbar spine include thick, short pedicles, an interpediculate distance that decreases from L1 to L5, canal stenosis (with a predisposition to disk herniation), and accentuated lumbar lordosis (horizontal sacrum).

SPINAL STENOSIS
Congenital

In congenital spinal stenosis, both the anteroposterior and transverse dimensions of the canal are decreased. The pedicles are typically short and thick with a decreased interpediculate distance. The spinal canal tapers in the lumbar region (Fig. 8–8). This is the opposite of normal, in which the canal is usually equal in size to or greater (in anteroposterior dimension) than that in the thoracic region. The lateral recesses and neural foramina may also be narrowed. The lower limit of normal for the anteroposterior canal dimension is 11.5 mm, and the normal lateral recess should be 5 mm. The L4-5 level is the most common site for canal stenosis and tends to be the most severely affected level when the canal is diffusely narrowed. Congenital spinal stenosis predisposes the patient to early degenerative disk disease. Clinical presentation typically includes myelopathic symptoms. Radicular symptoms may be present as a result of nerve root impingement.

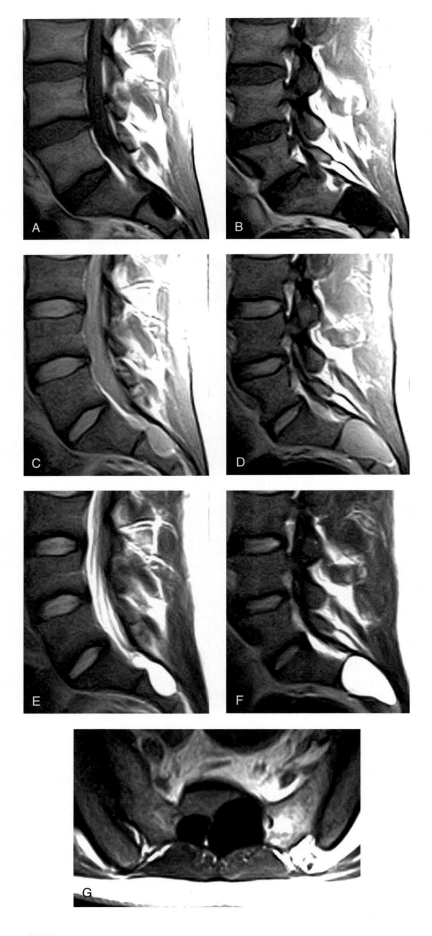

FIGURE 8–6. Tarlov cysts. *A* and *B*, Precontrast T$_1$-weighted sagittal images reveal two oval areas of low signal intensity posterior to the S1 and S2 vertebral bodies, both to the right and left of midline. There is erosion and scalloping of the adjacent sacral segments. On the proton density (*C* and *D*) and heavily T$_2$-weighted (*E* and *F*) sagittal images, the signal intensity of these cysts follows that of cerebrospinal fluid. Chemical shift artifact is noted at the interface between the lesions and the adjacent fatty marrow of the sacrum. There was no abnormal contrast enhancement (images not shown). *G*, The axial T$_1$-weighted image through S2 reveals both cysts, which occupy (albeit markedly enlarged) the expected location of the nerve root sleeves.

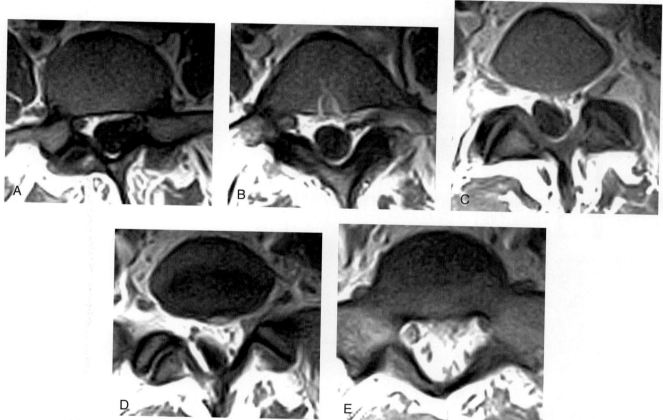

FIGURE 8–7. Conjoined nerve root. *A–E,* Axial postcontrast T$_1$-weighted scans are depicted from the middle of the L5 vertebral body to the middle of S1. On the first scan, the right L5 nerve root has already exited from the thecal sac (and is normal). A large abnormal nerve root sleeve is seen on the left, having not yet separated from the sac. On the next scan, two separate nerve roots are noted adjacent to one another on the left. On the third scan, at the level of the L5-S1 foramen, a nerve root (S1) is identified on the left medial to the enhancing dorsal root ganglion of L5. On the last two scans, the left S1 nerve root is seen to remain within the bony canal to descend to a position more symmetrical and normal relative to the right S1 nerve root.

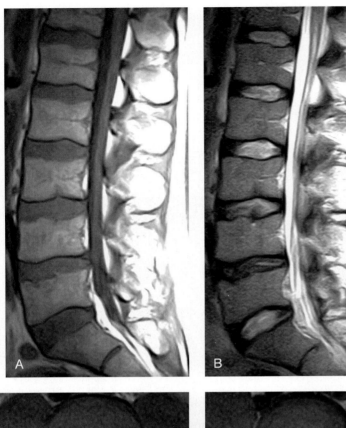

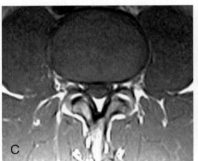
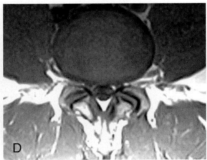

FIGURE 8–8. Congenital spinal stenosis. *A,* The midline sagittal T_1-weighted scan demonstrates tapering of the spinal canal from the T12-L1 level through the lower lumbar spine. This is most prominent at the L3-4 and L4-5 levels. These findings are confirmed on the sagittal fast spin echo T_2-weighted scan (*B*). Diminished signal intensity consistent with disk degeneration is also seen at L3-4 and L4-5. Small posterior spurs are present, further compromising the anteroposterior dimension of the canal. Axial T_1-weighted images at the L3-4 (*C*) and L4-5 (*D*) levels show narrowing of the canal with deformity of the thecal sac and crowding of the nerve roots. The anteroposterior dimension of the sac measured 9 at both levels. The lateral recesses are also narrowed bilaterally at the L3-4 and L4-5 levels, resulting in minimal space for the passage of the nerve roots. This 35-year-old patient presented with low back pain and left leg pain and numbness.

Degenerative (Acquired)

There are three types of degenerative spinal stenosis: central, lateral recess, and foraminal. The lateral recess is the space between the posterior margin of the vertebral body and the anterior margin of the superior facet. Its anatomic boundaries include the thecal sac medially and the pedicle laterally. The lateral recess is normally larger than 5 mm in diameter. Patients with a lateral recess smaller than 3 mm in diameter are usually symptomatic.

Ligamentum flavum hypertrophy is one cause of degenerative spinal stenosis. The ligamentum flavum is a paired, thick, fibroelastic band. The normal thickness is 3 mm in the lumbar spine. The ligamentum flavum connects the lamina of adjacent vertebral bodies and is situated posterolaterally in the canal. It extends from the anteroinferior aspect of the superior lamina to the posterosuperior aspect of the inferior lamina. Anterolaterally, the ligamentum flavum is contiguous with the capsule of the facet joint. With degenerative spine disease, the ligamentum flavum becomes fibrotic, visibly

thickened (Fig. 8-9), and buckled. It narrows the posterolateral canal and thus the lateral recess. It may also narrow the central canal and/or the neural foramina.

Facet joint hypertrophy is another cause of degenerative spinal stenosis (Fig. 8–10). Hypertrophy of the superior articular facet is a primary cause of lateral recess stenosis. Failure to recognize lateral recess stenosis is a major cause of persistent symptoms after lumbar diskectomy.

A third cause of degenerative spinal stenosis is neural foraminal degenerative disease. The neural foramen is bounded by the pedicles superiorly and inferiorly, the vertebral body and disk anteriorly, and the facets posteriorly. In the lumbar spine, the nerve root exits from the lateral recess and enters the neural foramen. Stenosis of the neural foramen is most common at L4-5 and L5-S1. Degenerative disease of the disk, end plates, and posterior elements (facets) all contribute to foraminal stenosis (Fig. 8–11). The most common cause is hypertrophy of the superior facet. The stenosis is accentuated if the disk is narrowed. Foraminal stenosis causes radicular symptoms as a result of nerve root compression. Pain

FIGURE 8–9. Spinal stenosis with marked thickening of the ligamentum flavum. *A,* The sagittal T₁-weighted scan just to the right of midline demonstrates narrowing of the thecal sac at L4-5, with indentation posteriorly by intermediate-signal-intensity soft tissue: the thickened ligamentum flavum (*arrow*). Less marked findings are present on the midline sagittal T₁-weighted scan (*B*). These two sagittal images also reveal disk degeneration at L4-5 with disk space narrowing, a disk bulge with associated spurs, end plate irregularities, and adjacent degenerative end plate disease. *C,* The axial T₁-weighted image at the L4-5 disk level demonstrates severe central stenosis of the spinal canal. The thecal sac is very small and triangular in shape, narrowed anteriorly by the disk bulge and spurs and posteriorly by the markedly thickened ligamentum flavum (extending along the posterolateral margins of the thecal sac). The thickened ligaments (measuring 6 mm in cross-section) and facet hypertrophy have obliterated the lateral recesses. A tiny amount of epidural fat is seen in the posterior canal.

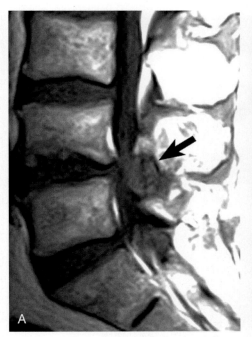
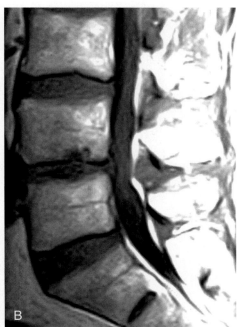
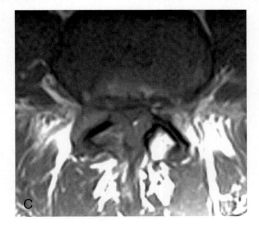

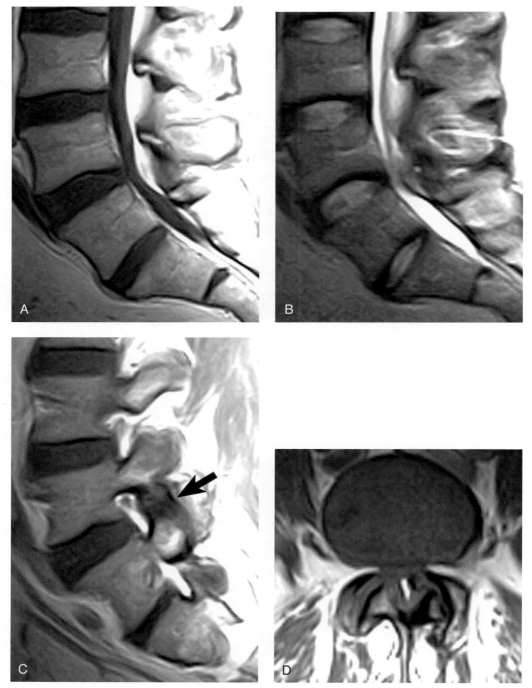

FIGURE 8–10. Severe spinal stenosis and lateral recess stenosis at L4-5 resulting from facet joint hypertrophy. *A,* The midline sagittal postcontrast T$_1$-weighted image reveals prominent narrowing of the lumbar canal at the L4-5 level. The canal stenosis is also well seen on the fast spin echo T$_2$-weighted sagittal image (*B*). *C,* A T$_1$-weighted sagittal image in the plane of the left lumbar facet joints reveals hypertrophy and sclerosis of the L4-5 facet (*arrow*). The neural foramen remains patent at this level. A similar appearance was present at the right facet joint of L4-5 (not shown). *D,* A T$_1$-weighted axial image at the L4-5 level confirms the marked facet hypertrophic changes, left greater than right. The superior articulating facet of L5 is particularly affected. The facet hypertrophy results in bilateral lateral recess stenosis, more severe on the left, where the lateral recess is less than 3 mm in width. Sclerosis of the facet joints is also apparent. The spinal canal is narrowed, measuring 11 mm in anteroposterior dimension. Even more striking is the degree of narrowing of the thecal sac, which measures 4 mm in anteroposterior diameter.

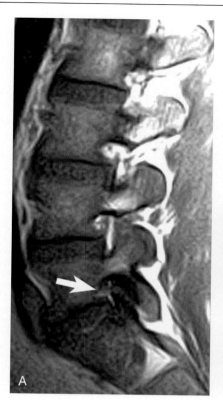

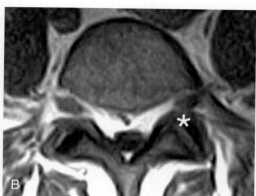

FIGURE 8–11. Degenerative foraminal stenosis on the left at L5-S1. *A,* The T$_1$-weighted sagittal image to the left of midline reveals a small neural foramen at L5-S1 (*arrow*), which is moderately narrowed secondary to degenerative spurs and hypertrophic facet disease. Only a minimal amount of fat is seen about the exiting L5 nerve root. The more normal keyhole appearance of the fat-filled neural foramina is present at L3-4 and L4-5. *B,* The T$_1$-weighted axial image at the inferior L5 level displays the L5 dorsal root ganglia bilaterally. The right dorsal root ganglion is surrounded by fat. The left ganglion is contacted posteriorly by the hypertrophied superior articulating facet of S1 (*) and anteriorly by an osteophyte arising from the L5 vertebral body.

can also originate from the degenerated facet joints, which are richly innervated. The neural foramen is best imaged in the lumbar spine in the sagittal plane. Stenosis is easily visualized as a result of obliteration of the normal fat that surrounds the nerve root in the foramen.

The clinical presentation for degenerative spinal stenosis is that of chronic pain in the lower back and buttocks. There may be paresthesias (abnormal sensation) or pain in the posterolateral leg. Standing and walking aggravate the pain, and resting (sitting or lying down) relieves it. This is the opposite of clinical symptoms for an acute disk herniation, in which the pain is aggravated by sitting. Neurologic deficits are minimal with degenerative spinal stenosis. The pathogenesis is nerve root ischemia.

INFECTION AND INFLAMMATORY DISEASE
Disk Space Infection

Disk space infection can be either hematogenous (Fig. 8–12) or postoperative (Fig. 8–13) in origin. In children, with hematogenous seeding, the disk serves as the initial site of infection (because it is richly vascularized). In adults, the initial site of infection (with hematogenous seeding) is the vertebral body (subchondral portion) or soft tissue. Patients with postoperative disk space infection present clinically with severe back pain 1 to 4 weeks after surgery. Disk space infection is seen in 1% to 3% of all back surgery patients. *Staphylococcus aureus* is the most common organism. Delays in diagnosis are com-

mon. Fever, wound infection, and elevation of white blood cell count are seen in only a minority of patients.

On lumbar spine x-ray films, disk space narrowing, poorly defined end plates, and sclerosis of the adjacent vertebrae may be seen. On CT, disk space narrowing, cortical bone loss (from the end plate), and abnormal paraspinous soft tissue may be seen. All are late changes. Radionuclide bone scans are sensitive but nonspecific in disk space infection.

On MRI, the disk itself will be narrow and irregular but with high signal intensity on T$_2$-weighted scans. The adjacent vertebral end plates will also demonstrate high signal intensity on T$_2$-weighted scans as a result of edema (with low signal intensity on T$_1$-weighted scans). The edema within the adjacent vertebrae forms a horizontal band involving one third to one half of the vertebral body. This appearance can be confused with degenerative type I end plate changes. The signal intensity and irregularity of the disk permit differentiation. After intravenous contrast administration, the end plates and disk space enhance. Pockets of nonenhancing fluid, representing pus, are commonly seen within the disk space. The vertebral end plates will be indistinct. Also common is a paraspinous soft tissue mass, which enhances postcontrast. MRI is both sensitive and specific for the diagnosis of disk space infection. With adequate treatment, the edema within the adjacent vertebral bodies and the size of the paraspinous soft tissue mass will both gradually decrease.

Arachnoiditis

In arachnoiditis, there is clumping and thickening of nerve roots on the imaging exam regardless of modality.

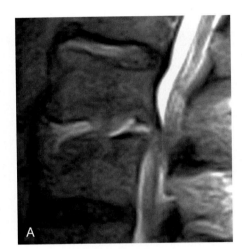

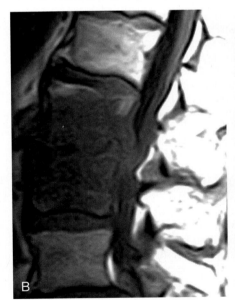

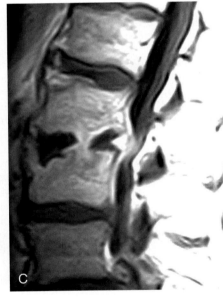

FIGURE 8–12. Hematogenous diskitis. *A,* On the T$_2$-weighted scan, the L2-3 disk is high signal intensity (which by itself could be normal), yet irregular in contour. There is absence of the normal intranuclear cleft. The thecal sac is narrowed at the L2-3 level. *B,* On the precontrast T$_1$-weighted scan, both the L2 and L3 vertebral bodies are of abnormal low signal intensity. There is loss of definition between the L2-3 disk and the adjacent vertebral end plates. *C,* On the postcontrast T$_1$-weighted scan, there is enhancement of the L2 and L3 marrow space, with irregular enhancement along the disk margin and residual low-signal-intensity (nonenhancing) soft tissue within the disk space. The latter corresponds in position to the high signal intensity noted on the T$_2$-weighted scan and represents inflammatory exudates. The basis for thecal sac narrowing is now evident, with abnormal paraspinal enhancing the soft tissue. In the adult patient, noniatrogenic disk space infection is usually the result of hematogenous seeding to the soft tissue or to the subchondral portion of the vertebral body.

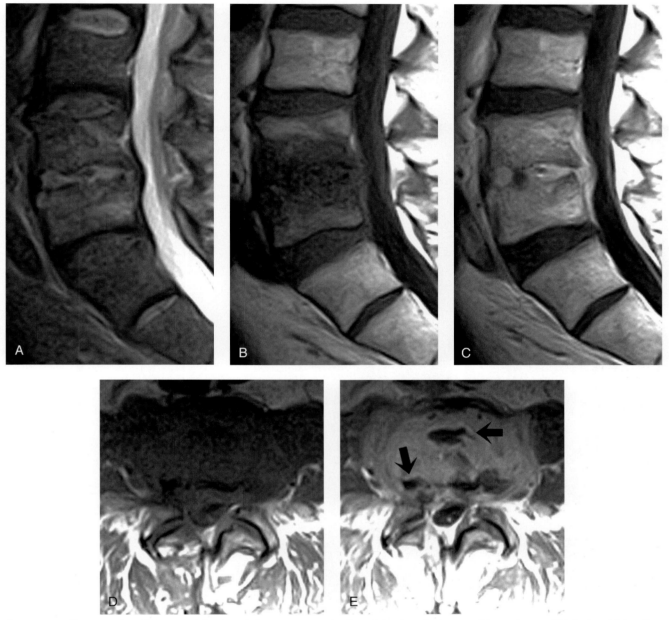

FIGURE 8–13. Postoperative disk space infection. *A,* Precontrast on the T_2-weighted sagittal scan, diffuse abnormal high signal intensity (SI) is noted within the marrow of the L4 and L5 vertebral bodies. The disk is reduced in height, irregular, and of abnormal high SI. *B,* On the precontrast T_1-weighted scan, the L4-5 disk is difficult to identify. Also noted is abnormal low SI within the lower half of L4 and the upper half of L5, paralleling the disk. *C,* Postcontrast, abnormal enhancement of the disk space is noted, together with a soft tissue mass that compresses the thecal sac. Comparison of pre- (*D*) and postcontrast (*E*) T_1-weighted axial scans at the disk level reveals a paraspinous mass with enhancement. There is abnormal enhancement of the disk as well, permitting identification of fluid pockets that remain low SI (*arrows*).

Inflammation initially elicits only a minimal cellular response, which then progresses to collagenous adhesions. The pathogenesis includes infection, which is uncommon today, previous surgery, hemorrhage within the thecal sac, and prior myelography with Pantopaque.

CT findings in arachnoiditis, which are seen with moderate involvement, include nodular or cordlike intradural masses and nerve roots that are adherent to the dura. On myelography, with mild involvement, there can be blunting of the nerve root sleeves, fusion of nerve roots, and irregularity of the thecal sac margin. With moderate involvement, there can be obliteration of the nerve root sleeves, multisegmental fusion of nerve roots, adhesions, scarring of the thecal sac, and loculation of intrathecal contrast.

The nerve roots and abnormalities thereof are clearly seen on MRI. Several common patterns of nerve root involvement in arachnoiditis are subsequently described. In mild disease, nerve roots can be clumped and lie centrally within the sac (Fig. 8–14). Alternatively, individual nerve roots may be adherent to the periphery of the sac. With severe disease, abnormal soft tissue can fill the majority of the thecal sac, with no discernible individual nerve roots. With acute infection (viral or bacterial meningitis), the nerve roots themselves enhance (Fig. 8–15). Care should be exercised in the diag-

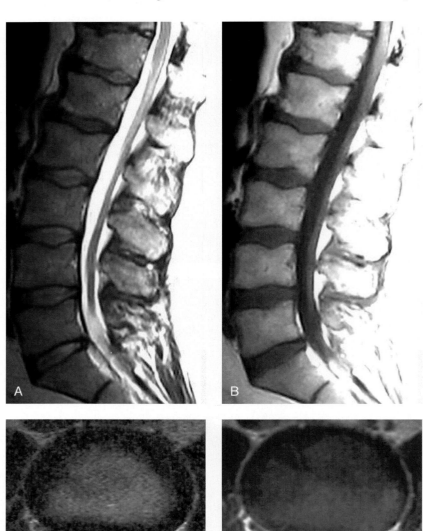

FIGURE 8–14. Arachnoiditis. Midline sagittal T$_2$- (*A*) and T$_1$-weighted (*B*) images suggest clumping of nerve roots along the posterior margin of the thecal sac. No individual nerve roots are visualized; rather a single thick strand is seen. The clumping of nerve roots is confirmed on the axial T$_2$- (*C*) and T$_1$-weighted (*D*) images.

FIGURE 8–15. Spinal meningitis with progression to arachnoiditis. Postcontrast sagittal (*A*) and axial (*B*) images reveal prominent enhancement (*white arrows*) of the lumbar nerve roots. These also appear mildly thickened but retain their usual position within the dependent portion of the thecal sac. The patient returned for follow-up after 1 month of antibiotic therapy. Her back pain remained severe at this time. *C,* The postcontrast T$_1$-weighted sagittal image reveals persistent enhancement of the lumbar nerve roots. The nerve roots now lie anteriorly within the thecal sac. *D,* A postcontrast axial image at L3-4 demonstrates the enhancing nerve roots to be clumped anteriorly. Cultures in this patient revealed *Staphylococcus aureus* as the causative organism.

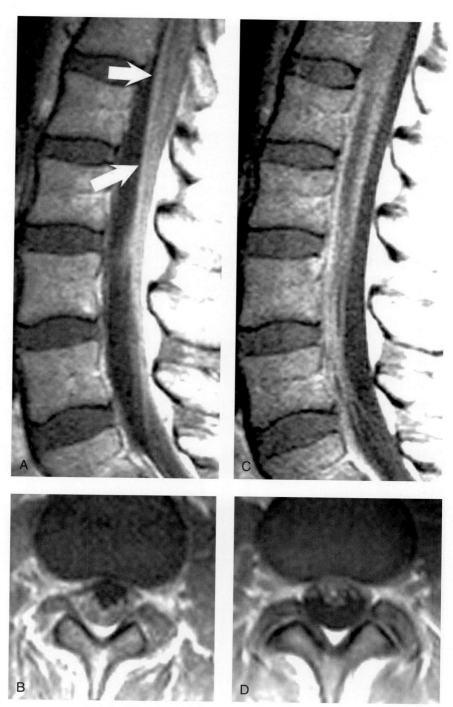

nosis of arachnoiditis when spinal stenosis is present. Spinal stenosis can lead to a false impression of nerve root clumping.

NEOPLASTIC DISEASE
Benign Neoplasms of Bone

Vertebral Body Hemangioma

Vertebral body hemangiomas are a common incidental finding on MRI. This benign neoplasm can be found, on autopsy, in more than 10% of the population. Solitary lesions are most common, although multiple lesions are not uncommon. The size is variable, ranging from small to large, involving the entire vertebral body. Posterior extension can cause canal compromise. A large lesion can weaken the vertebral body and lead to fracture. Histologically, vertebral hemangiomas are composed of a mixture of adipose and angiomatous tissue with prominent bony trabeculae. The coarse vertical trabeculation can be seen on plain film and CT, which also depict the lesion as generally lucent. On MRI, vertebral hemangiomas are classically high signal intensity on both T_1- and T_2-weighted scans (Fig. 8–16). Also commonly noted is a reticular pattern of low signal intensity (prominent vertically) corresponding to the thickened trabeculae. The major differential diagnosis on MRI is that of focal fat (within the vertebral bodies). The latter is a common finding, particularly with increasing age. Focal fat deposition will be seen to follow the signal intensity of fat on all pulse sequences.

Osteoid Osteoma

Osteoid osteoma is a common benign skeletal neoplasm found most often in young patients. The lesion consists of a central nidus of osteoid, woven bone, and fibrovascular tissue, with an overall diameter of less than 2 cm. Osteoid osteomas are sharply demarcated from surrounding bone with variable surrounding sclerosis. The classic clinical presentation is that of pain, which is relieved by aspirin. Ten percent of osteoid osteomas occur in the spine. Here the most common location is in the neural arch of a lumbar vertebra. Scoliosis is common. On CT, sclerosis will be seen surrounding a small lytic lesion. CT may also demonstrate the nidus to be calcified. Bone scintigraphy is useful for diagnosis; focal activity is seen on both immediate and delayed scans. On MRI, the nidus is low signal intensity on T_1-weighted images. The nidus is commonly surrounded by extensive edema, which can involve the adjacent soft tissue in addition to the bone.

Giant Cell Tumor

In the lumbar spine, the most common location of a giant cell tumor is the sacrum. Patients with this tumor, predominantly female, typically present at between 20 and 40 years of age. Vertebral lesions carry a better prognosis than giant cell tumors elsewhere in the body, with a low rate recurrence after resection. Giant cell tumors are lytic and expansile lesions, but they rarely cross the periosteum. On MRI, a giant cell tumor is typically lobular, with intermediate signal intensity on T_1-weighted scans and mixed signal intensity on T_2-weighted scans. High signal intensity on T_2-weighted scans corresponds to hemorrhagic and cystic foci. A low-signal-intensity rim is seen on both T_1- and T_2-weighted scans as a result of dense sclerosis at the tumor margin. Giant cell tumors are quite vascular and demonstrate contrast enhancement. The differential diagnosis includes osteoblastoma (more common in the posterior

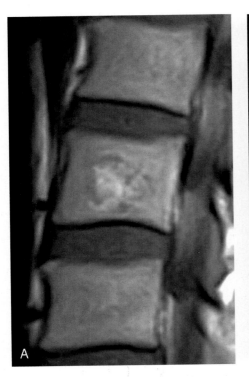
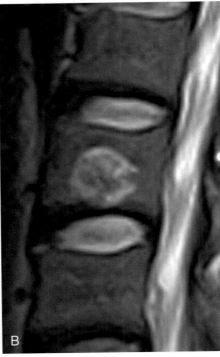

FIGURE 8–16. Vertebral hemangioma. A round, mottled area of increased signal intensity is seen in the central portion of the L3 vertebral body on the sagittal T_1-weighted image (*A*). The postcontrast T_1-weighted image (not shown) revealed mild enhancement. The lesion also exhibits high signal intensity on the sagittal T_2-weighted image (*B*). Mottled signal intensity is demonstrated with interspersed areas of very low signal intensity on all imaging sequences corresponding to prominent trabeculae.

A   B

elements, less lobular), aneurysmal bone cyst (younger age group), and metastatic disease.

Malignant Neoplasms of Bone

Lumbar Metastases

The vertebral column is the most common site of skeletal metastatic disease. Lung cancer is the most common cause. Other causes include breast cancer, prostatic carcinoma, renal cell carcinoma, and hematologic malignancies. Most cases of epidural compression of the cord or cauda equina are due to vertebral metastases, with either bony collapse or posterior extension. In most such patients, the compression is at only one level.

Most patients with lumbar metastatic disease present clinically with back pain. Motor impairment can occur and usually precedes sensory deficits. Radiculopathy is uncommon. However, compression of a single nerve root can occur (with epidural tumor extension), mimicking a disk herniation. Plain x-ray films are notoriously insensitive to metastatic disease. The classic finding was that of an absent pedicle. This led to the misimpression that vertebral metastatic disease most often originated in the pedicle. The advent of MRI showed this clearly not to be true but rather simply that pedicle lesions were better seen by plain film than lesions in other locations. In the past, myelography was, but is no longer, the modality of choice for examination of the patient with a suspected compressive lesion. Myelography carries a high risk in patients with a block. Neurologic deterioration is seen after the exam in up to 25% of patients. Lesions above a block are also missed by myelography.

MRI is the modality of choice for detecting and assessing vertebral metastatic disease. MRI is more sensitive (as well as more specific) than bone scintigraphy for detecting vertebral metastases. We now know, because of MRI, that the vertebral body is nearly always the initial site of involvement. Sagittal scans provide screening of the area of interest. These should be supplemented with axial scans in areas where canal compromise is questioned. Imaging of the entire spine in the body coil is not recommended for screening because smaller metastases and even compressive lesions in some instances will be missed. Bony metastatic lesions are low signal intensity on (precontrast) T_1-weighted scans, which are used by most practices for lesion detection (Fig. 8–17). Epidural extension is also well seen on MRI; axial scans play an important role here as well (Fig. 8–18). It is important to compare the signal intensity of the disk and the vertebral body (on sagittal images) in order not to miss diffuse metastatic disease. On T_1-weighted scans, normal marrow should always be higher in signal intensity than the intervertebral disk. If the marrow is isointense with the disk or lower signal intensity, then the marrow is diffusely abnormal and widespread metastatic disease is likely (although other causes should be considered, including hematologic abnormalities).

Fast short time inversion recovery (STIR) scans are used in some practices as the primary scan for detection of vertebral metastases. These scans, although more mo-tion sensitive, can be slightly superior to T_1-weighted spin echo scans for lesion detection. Although STIR images are predominantly T_1-weighted, the gray scale is reversed compared with spin echo images, and metastases appear as hyperintense vertebral body lesions. On spin echo T_1-weighted scans, contrast administration is not helpful for detecting bone metastases. Most metastases enhance postcontrast to near isointensity with normal marrow, decreasing their conspicuity. Contrast enhancement is, however, useful for improved depiction of epidural and soft tissue extent of metastatic disease and for the detection of leptomeningeal metastases (Fig. 8–19). T_2-weighted scans are not of great use in the evaluation of metastatic disease to the vertebral column, although they are routinely acquired (Fig. 8–20). Many bony metastases will have abnormal high signal intensity on T_2-weighted scans, but many will also be isointense. Osteoblastic metastases, which are common with prostate carcinoma, deserve special comment. These are typically low signal intensity on both T_1- and T_2-weighted scans. When both osteoblastic and lytic lesions are present, it is commonly observed that the blastic lesions are substantially lower in signal intensity on T_1-weighted scans than the lytic lesions. Metastatic lesions in lung and breast carcinoma are typically lytic but may be osteoblastic when treated. Bony sclerosis is seen, of course, on plain film with osteoblastic metastases.

Chordoma

Chordomas are locally invasive, destructive, lytic, lobular, slow-growing lesions. Calcification is seen on x-ray exams in half. A mixture of solid and cystic components is common. In regard to location, 50% occur in the sacrum or coccyx, 35% at the skull base (clivus), and 15% in the vertebral body.

Plasma Cell Myeloma

The term plasma cell myeloma is used to describe a malignant disease of plasma cells that includes both multiple myeloma and plasmacytoma. A plasmacytoma is a solitary lesion of bone. Laboratory blood studies may be positive or negative. Additional lesions can develop with time. The spine and pelvis are the most common locations for a plasmacytoma. This lesion is osteolytic and expansile.

Intraspinal Neoplasms

Intradural Lipoma

Lipomas within the thecal sac lie on the benign end of the spectrum that includes lipomyelomeningocele. A dorsal spinal defect, if present, is minimal. Developmentally, there is premature separation of cutaneus ectoderm from neuroectoderm, with mesenchyma entering the neural tube and later differentiating into fat. Lipomas compose 1% of all intraspinal tumors. Most lie along the dorsal aspect of the spinal cord. On MRI, lipomas will have fat signal intensity on all pulse sequences. At high field (1.5 T and above), chemical shift artifact is commonly observed at the interface between fat and CSF along the frequency encoding direction. Nerve

Text continued on page 198

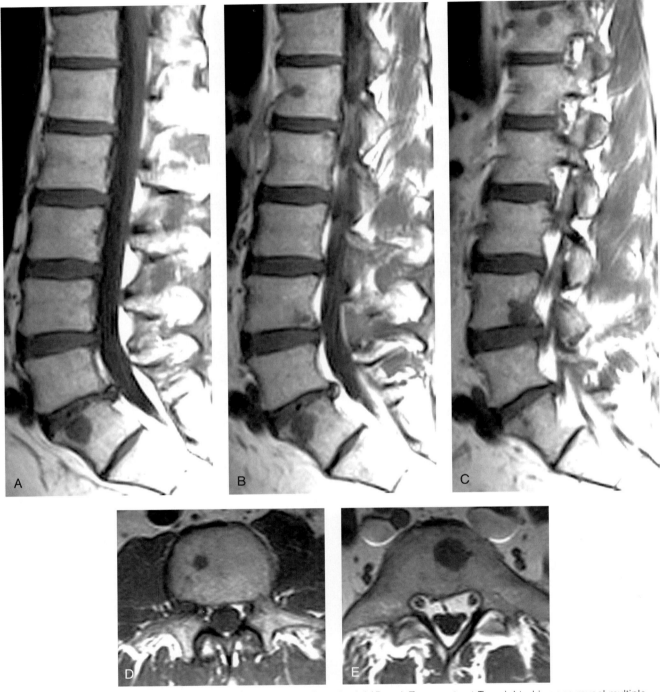

FIGURE 8–17. Lumbar vertebral metastatic disease. Sagittal (*A–C*) and axial (*D* and *E*) precontrast T$_1$-weighted images reveal multiple low-signal-intensity vertebral body lesions. These involve T12, L1, L4, and S1. The metastases are in general round and well demarcated, occasionally extending to the cortex of the vertebral body. Incidental note is made of a lumbarized S1 vertebral body.

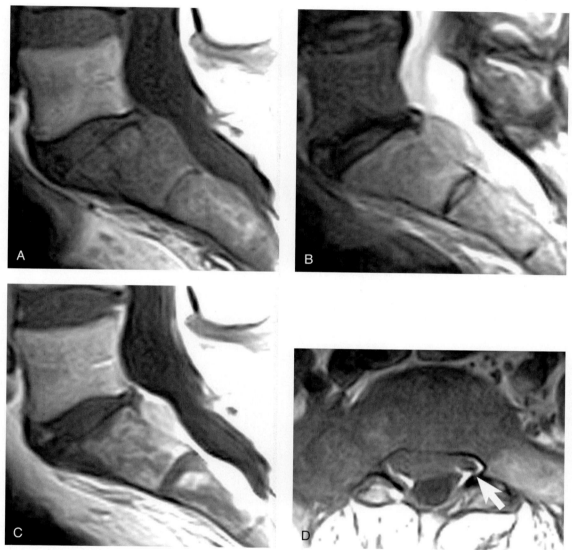

FIGURE 8–18. Sacral metastases with epidural tumor causing right S1 nerve root compression. *A,* The T_1-weighted midline sagittal image demonstrates abnormally decreased signal intensity throughout the sacrum, most prominent at the S1 level. Epidural soft tissue involvement is apparent posterior to both S1 and S2. These abnormalities are increased signal intensity on the corresponding T_2-weighted sagittal image (*B*). Irregular enhancement of the sacrum is apparent on the postcontrast T_1-weighted sagittal image (*C*). The epidural disease demonstrates homogeneous enhancement. *D,* A precontrast T_1-weighted axial image at the S1 level confirms the abnormal low signal intensity within the sacrum. The epidural soft tissue mass distorts the thecal sac and severely compresses the right S1 nerve root. The normal left S1 nerve root (*arrow*) is unaffected. Expansion of the right sacral ala with paraspinal extension is also apparent. This 79-year-old patient with lung cancer presented clinically with a right S1 radiculopathy.

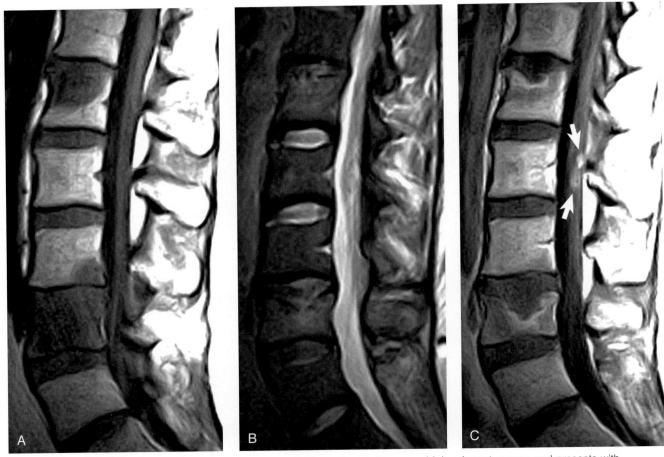

FIGURE 8–19. Vertebral body and leptomeningeal metastases. The patient is 35 years old, has breast cancer, and presents with increasing pain and numbness in the legs. *A,* On the precontrast T_1-weighted midline sagittal scan, vertebral body metastases with low signal intensity relative to normal marrow are noted in L1, L3, and L4. The vertebral body lesions are less apparent on the corresponding T_2-weighted scan (*B*). The lesions in L1 and L4 do demonstrate slight hyperintensity relative to normal marrow. Posterior within the thecal sac, a questionable area of abnormal hyperintensity is noted at the L2 level. *C,* Postcontrast on the T_1-weighted scan, the vertebral body lesions demonstrate enhancement to near isointensity with normal marrow. Partial collapse of L4 is now evident. Critical for prognosis and treatment is, however, the identification of two enhancing nodules (*small arrows*) within the thecal sac, consistent with leptomeningeal tumor spread.

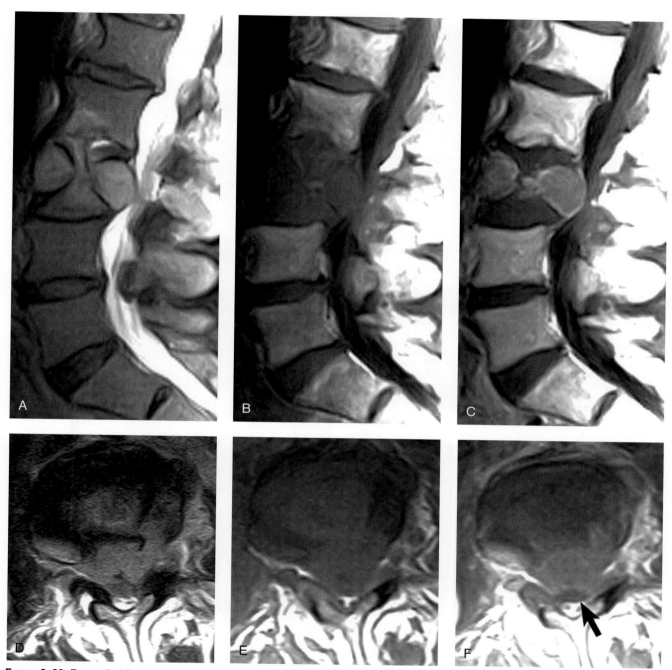

FIGURE 8–20. Expansile L3 vertebral body metastasis. *A,* The T₂-weighted scan reveals abnormal high signal intensity within the L3 vertebral body. This vertebral body also has an abnormal configuration, consistent with a compression fracture. The posterior margin has a convex outward curvature, compressing the thecal sac. The L3 vertebral body is low signal intensity on the precontrast T₁-weighted sagittal scan (*B*) and enhances postcontrast (*C*). Of the axial scans—T₂-weighted (*D*), precontrast T₁-weighted, (*E*), and postcontrast T₁-weighted (*F*)—the postcontrast scan best delineates the thecal sac (*arrow*), which is severely compressed. The patient, who had nonsquamous cell lung carcinoma, presented clinically with pain radiating into the right lower extremity.

roots can in some cases be identified coursing through the lesion (Fig. 8–21).

Care should be exercised in the diagnosis of a lipoma. The lesion should be of the exact same signal intensity as that of fat on all pulse sequences. The presence of septations, a slight difference in signal intensity from fat, or contrast enhancement make it very unlikely that a fatty lesion is a lipoma (Fig. 8–22).

Dermoid and Epidermoid

Dermoids and epidermoids are two of the "pearly" tumors, so named for their gross appearance. Both are ectodermal inclusion cysts, containing squamous epithelium, keratin, and cholesterol. Dermoids are differentiated by the presence of dermal appendages (hair and sebaceous glands). In the spine, most dermoids and epidermoids occur in the lumbosacral region. Dermoids are more common. The lesion can be either intra- or extramedullary in location. Dermoids and epidermoids

are well-defined, rounded lesions. A portion of the tumor may be cystic, containing desquamated epithelium and, in the case of dermoids, sebaceous gland secretions. Frequently associated anomalies include dermal sinus and spinal dysraphism.

Teratoma

Teratomas are rare in the spinal canal, except for the sacrococcygeal form. The latter is the most common presacral mass in a child. Sacrococcygeal teratomas can undergo malignant transformation. Teratomas by definition are composed of tissue from all three germinal layers.

Lymphangioma

This is a congenital lesion resulting from obstruction of lymphatic drainage. Seventy-five percent occur in the neck (posterior triangle). In this location, lymphangiomas are more common in children younger than 2 years.

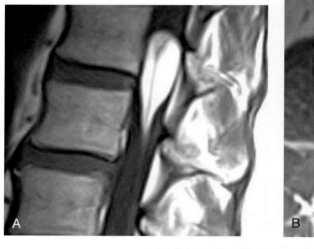
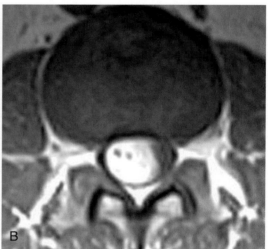
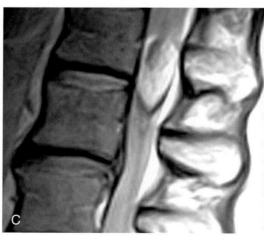

FIGURE 8–21. Intradural lipoma. An intradural, high-signal-intensity soft tissue mass is noted at the L1-2 level on the sagittal T$_1$-weighted scan (*A*). *B*, On the axial T$_1$-weighted scan, nerve roots (with lower signal intensity) are noted to course through the lesion. The mass is isointense with fat on the intermediate T$_2$-weighted scan (*C*). This was also the case on all other pulse sequences. An artifactual low-signal-intensity line is noted at the inferior margin of the mass, at the interface with cerebrospinal fluid. This dark band occurs in the direction of the readout gradient and is caused by chemical shift artifact, with the image being acquired at 1.5 T.

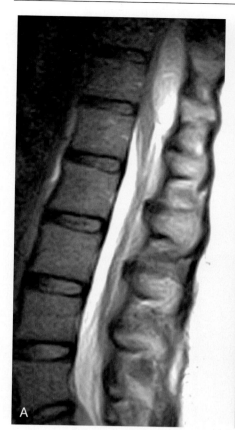 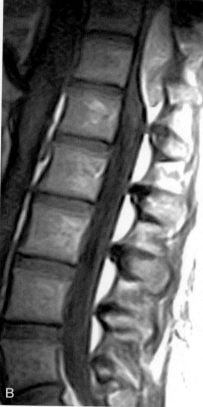 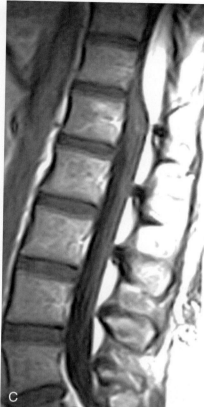

FIGURE 8–22. Angiolipoma. *A,* On the T₂-weighted scan, the conus is displaced anteriorly, but a soft tissue mass is not clearly identified. *B,* The precontrast T₁-weighted scan reveals a posterior epidural mass, extending from T1 to L1, with mixed high signal intensity. *C,* On the postcontrast T₁-weighted scan, the abnormality is noted to enhance to isointensity with fat. Although the lesion is similar in signal intensity to fat, it is heterogeneous and displays abnormal contrast enhancement. These characteristics suggest a neoplastic origin. Angiolipomas are rare benign tumors composed of lipocytes and abnormal blood vessels. These tumors are epidural in location, occur most commonly in the midthoracic region, and can cause cord compression.

Lymphangiomas are typically asymptomatic and treated by surgical resection. These lesions have fluid signal intensity, low on T₁- and high on T₂-weighted scans. Septa and fat may be present between the fluid spaces.

Ependymoma

Ependymomas are slow-growing, well-circumscribed, benign tumors. Complete surgical resection is possible. Ependymomas make up 60% to 70% of all spinal cord tumors. They occur in the third to sixth decades of life. Most arise in the conus, cauda equina, or filum terminale. The cervical cord is the most common site for an intramedullary ependymoma. The clinical presentation is nonspecific and can include motor and sensory deficits and sphincter dysfunction. On MRI, focal cord enlargement limited to two or three levels favors the diagnosis of an ependymoma over an astrocytoma. Virtually all ependymomas enhance strongly after contrast administration (Fig. 8–23).

Neurofibroma and Schwannoma

Neurofibromas (Fig. 8–24) and schwannomas (Fig. 8–25) are the most common of the nerve root sheath tumors. Most are intradural extramedullary in location.

One third are extradural. A foraminal lesion may be mistaken for a herniated disk (Fig. 8–26). Enhancement postcontrast allows differentiation.

It is difficult to differentiate schwannomas and neurofibromas on MRI or, likewise, any imaging exam. Schwannomas are typically solitary and well circumscribed and lie eccentric to the nerve itself (whereas a neurofibroma causes fusiform enlargement of the nerve). Schwannomas tend to be heterogeneous in signal intensity on T₂-weighted scans. Neurofibromas tend to be homogeneous in signal intensity on T₂-weighted scans and may have a target appearance (high signal intensity peripherally, lower signal intensity centrally). Multiplicity of lesions favors the diagnosis of neurofibroma.

Leptomeningeal Metastases

The presence of leptomeningeal metastases portends a poor prognosis. One third of all patients with metastases to the brain or spine will eventually acquire leptomeningeal metastatic disease. Breast and lung carcinomas are the most common visceral neoplasms to spread to the subarachnoid space. In the lumbar region on MRI, leptomeningeal metastases can take on several different appearances. There can be large or small nodules or a

Text continued on page 204

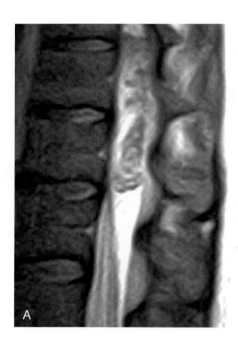

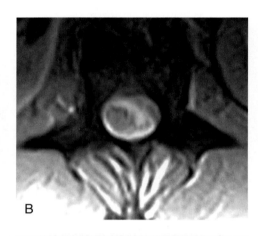

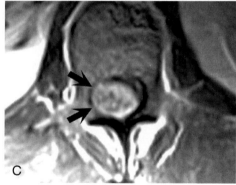

FIGURE 8–23. Mixed papillary ependymoma of the conus medullaris. *A,* On the sagittal T$_2$-weighted scan, an intradural extramedullary soft tissue mass is noted. The spinal cord is displaced anteriorly and flattened. *B,* On the axial T$_2$-weighted scan, the mass is seen posteriorly and to the right, with severe compression of the cord. *C,* On the postcontrast T$_1$-weighted scan, there is heterogeneous enhancement of the mass (*arrows*), greater peripherally and less centrally. The cord itself is thinned and lies anterior and slightly to the left. The patient presented with slowly increasing low back pain and left lower extremity weakness. Virtually all ependymomas demonstrate strong enhancement after intravenous contrast injection on magnetic resonance imaging.

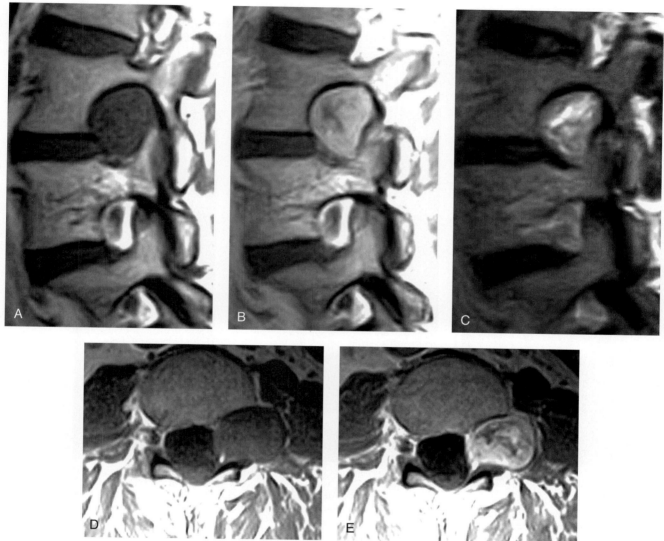

FIGURE 8–24. Neurofibroma. Pre- (*A*) and postcontrast (*B*) sagittal T$_1$-weighted scans reveal a large enhancing soft tissue mass in the left L3-4 neural foramen. The mass is of high signal intensity on the T$_2$-weighted scan (*C*). Comparison of pre- (*D*) and postcontrast (*E*) axial T$_1$-weighted scans reveals a smoothly marginated enhancing lesion, which has expanded the foramen. Contrast enhancement of the mass favors a neural origin and improves lesion demarcation from surrounding soft tissue. Schwannomas tend to enhance in a heterogeneous fashion, often more intense peripherally. Neurofibromas typically demonstrate homogeneous contrast enhancement. The patient is a 66-year-old veteran with neurofibromatosis.

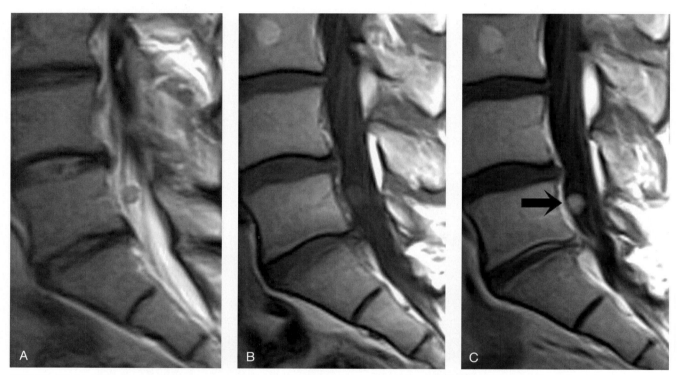

FIGURE 8–25. Lumbar nerve root schwannoma. *A,* On the T₂-weighted scan, a small round lesion with intermediate signal intensity is noted within the thecal sac at the L5 level. The lesion appears to be immediately adjacent to or part of the L5 nerve root. The lesion is nearly isointense with cerebrospinal fluid on the precontrast T₁-weighted scan (*B*) and demonstrates prominent enhancement (*arrow*) postcontrast (*C*). The lesion, a schwannoma, was confirmed on subsequent surgery performed for lumbar disk disease. Incidental note is made of an L3 vertebral body hemangioma.

FIGURE 8–26. Neurofibroma, mimicking a free disk fragment. Parasagittal T$_2$- (*A*) and T$_1$-weighted (*B*) images reveal a soft tissue mass (*B, arrow*) in the left L4-5 neural foramen. The L4 nerve root is not identified. Comparison of pre- (*C*) and postcontrast (*D*) axial T$_1$-weighted scans reveals homogeneous enhancement of the mass (*D, arrow*). Contrast enhancement in this instance provides important information for differential diagnosis, eliminating from consideration a free disk fragment.

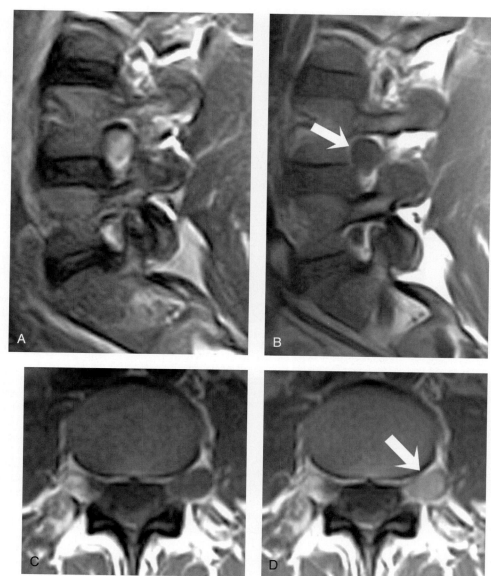

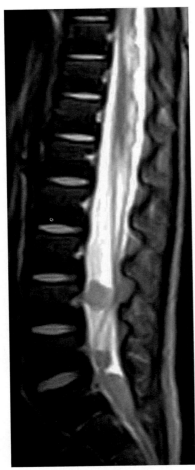

FIGURE 8–27. Leptomeningeal ("drop") metastases from medulloblastoma. The midline sagittal T_2-weighted scan reveals multiple large soft tissue nodules adjacent to the conus, adherent to the cauda equina, and near the termination of the thecal sac. The size and extent of these intrathecal metastases lead to their excellent visualization on the T_2-weighted scan in this instance. The patient, a 4-year-old with metastatic medulloblastoma, presented clinically with diminished coordination.

combination (Fig. 8–27). Alternatively (or concurrently), there can be (smooth) coating of nerve roots and the cord (Fig. 8–28). The nerve roots can also appear "beaded" as a result of nodular metastatic deposits (Fig. 8–29). Intramedullary extension of leptomeningeal metastatic disease, although rare, can occur. Contrast-enhanced MRI is markedly superior to CT myelography for detection. The differential diagnosis should include meningeal infection (in immunosuppressed patients), toxoplasmosis, and sarcoidosis. In the latter disease, cord involvement usually dominates.

EFFECT OF TRAUMA
Flexion Injury

Flexion injuries are seen in motor vehicle accidents when the patient is confined by a lap belt without a shoulder strap. Flexion occurs with the fulcrum centered on the anterior abdominal wall. The principal bony injury is a lumbar spine fracture (Chance fracture). The Chance fracture is a transverse fracture through the body of the vertebra, extending posteriorly through the pedicles and the spinous process. However, fracture of the posterior elements need not be present. This flexion injury is principally a distraction injury with ligamentous disruption. There may be little or no anterior vertebral body compression, and the injury may be unstable.

When the occupant is unrestrained, flexion occurs with the fulcrum centered on the posterior portion of the vertebral body. This results in an anterior body compression fracture. There is accompanying distraction of the posterior elements. This injury is most common at the thoracolumbar junction.

Osteoporotic Compression Fracture

Osteoporotic compression fractures occur in the elderly as a result of insufficiency of bone (senile osteoporosis). They are more common in postmenopausal women. With an acute osteoporotic compression fracture, areas of low signal intensity on T_1-weighted and high signal intensity on T_2-weighted scans, corresponding to edema, will be present within the vertebral body. However, there will also be areas of preserved, normal marrow. Unfortunately, there is little to differentiate an acute benign compression fracture from a pathologic compression fracture. Over the years, value has been placed on many different MRI signs, none of which have proved to be specific. However, with an osteoporotic compression fracture, the edema will eventually resolve (after many months). Chronic osteoporotic fractures can be recognized by their anatomic deformity but demonstrate signal intensity isointense to that of normal marrow.

Pathologic Compression Fracture

Pathologic compression fractures demonstrate low signal intensity on T_1-weighted scans and high signal intensity on T_2-weighted scans. The abnormal signal intensity is principally due not to edema but rather to the presence of neoplastic disease. There may be complete replacement of normal marrow signal intensity within the body, and this may extend into the pedicle. Most patients have multiple lesions in other vertebral bodies (round to oval in appearance), an important differentiating feature from an acute osteoporotic compression fracture. Sagittal T_1-weighted imaging is thus very valuable in screening patients. With the advent of fast spin echo technique, T_2-weighted scans have improved substantially in image quality. Thus, today both T_1- and T_2-weighted scans are typically acquired; axial scans are important in addition to sagittal scans. Although epidural extension and canal compromise are usually well demonstrated on sagittal scans, it is actually the central component that is well visualized. Depiction of abnormal lateral soft tissue and compromise of the canal from either the right or left side is best accomplished with axial scans.

Spondylolysis and Spondylolisthesis

In spondylolysis, there is interruption of the pars interarticularis. This may be unilateral or bilateral. Bilateral

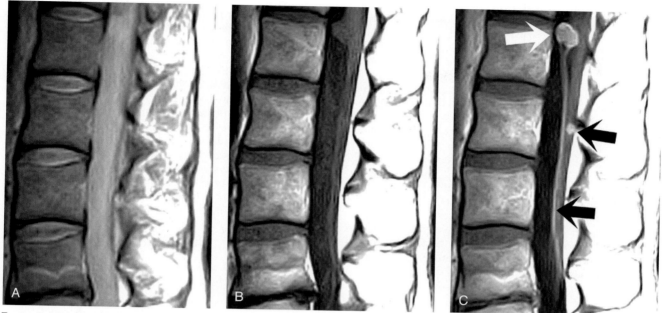

FIGURE 8–28. Leptomeningeal metastases. The presence of an intradural soft tissue mass at T12-L1 is questioned on the basis of precontrast sagittal T$_2$- (*A*) and T$_1$-weighted (*B*) scans. *C*, Postcontrast, the lesion is confirmed because of intense enhancement (*white arrow*). Also noted postcontrast is an enhancing nerve root within the filum terminale and a second smaller mass within the thecal sac at the L2 level (*black arrows*). Leptomeningeal metastases are best identified postcontrast; enhancement in this case permits diagnosis. This elderly individual with lung carcinoma presented 6 months before the current exam with brain metastases.

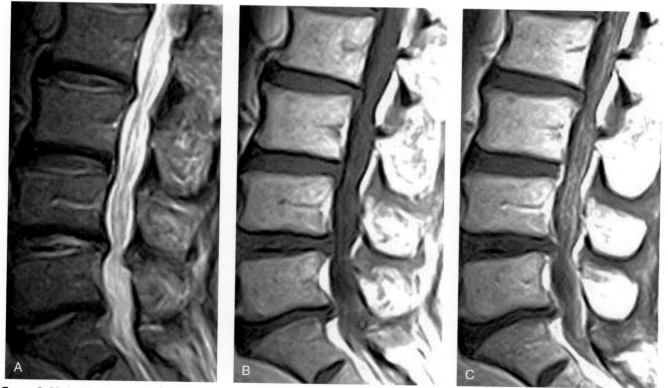

FIGURE 8–29. Leptomeningeal metastases. *A*, On the midline sagittal T$_2$-weighted image, there is diffuse disk degeneration, with narrowing of the thecal sac at multiple levels on the basis of degenerative disease. The lumbar nerves within the thecal sac appear prominent (suggesting nerve root thickening) on both the T$_2$- and precontrast T$_1$-weighted (*B*) images. *C*, Postcontrast, there is striking abnormal enhancement of the cauda equina and lumbar nerves, which now also appear somewhat "beaded." Head computed tomography (not shown) revealed multiple brain metastases. This 83-year-old patient was diagnosed with and treated for small cell carcinoma of the lung 1 year before the current exam. The patient is now admitted with a 2-week history of low back pain, leg weakness, and mental status changes.

involvement allows motion of the posterior elements relative to the adjacent vertebrae. The superior and inferior facets at the involved level can move independently. The superior facet remains attached to the vertebral body. The inferior facet articulates and moves with the more inferior vertebral body. On axial CT, the defects are seen as lucent clefts, oriented in the coronal plane. On axial MRI, the discontinuity of bone may be difficult to visualize. One key to diagnosis is the presence of a "continuous facet" sign from the disk space above to the disk space below. The bony defect is often clearly seen on sagittal MRI.

Spondylolisthesis is defined as forward slippage of one lumbar vertebral body relative to the adjacent lower vertebral body (or sacrum). There are many causes, including trauma, surgery, degenerative disease (of the facet joints), and congenital disease. Spondylolisthesis causes narrowing of the neural foramen, which may cause nerve root impingement. The foramen assumes a more horizontal orientation as seen on sagittal scans.

Spondylolisthesis is graded according to the degree of subluxation. Grade I is up to one fourth of the vertebral body, grade II between one fourth and one half, grade III between one half and three fourths, and grade IV greater than three fourths.

With degenerative spondylolisthesis, the midline sagittal image demonstrates narrowing of the spinal canal (Fig. 8–30). The posterior elements are contiguous with and, therefore, move anteriorly with the displaced vertebral body. When spondylolisthesis occurs in combination with spondylolysis, the canal is typically not narrowed because the posterior elements move independently from the vertebral body (Fig. 8–31). The adjacent posterior elements remain in alignment, and the spinal canal may widen in this situation.

Retrolisthesis

A retrolisthesis is a posterior subluxation of a vertebral body relative to the adjacent lower body. This is caused

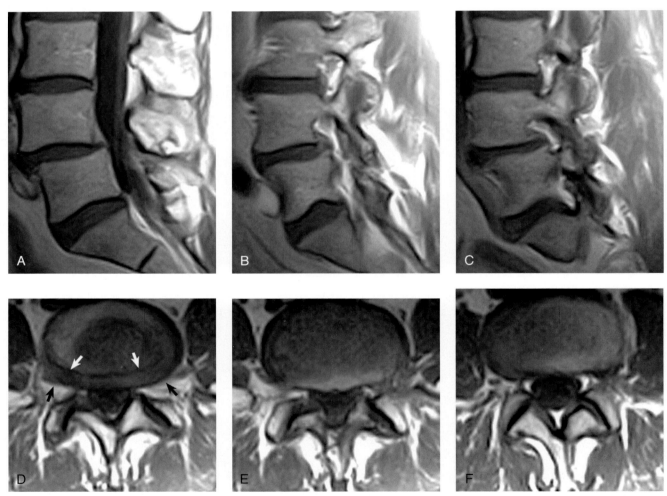

FIGURE 8–30. Spondylolisthesis secondary to degenerative facet changes. *A,* The midline sagittal T$_1$-weighted image demonstrates grade I anterior listhesis of L4 on L5. The right (*B*) and left (*C*) parasagittal T$_1$-weighted images show the pars interarticularis to be intact bilaterally at L4. This excludes spondylolysis as a cause of the spondylolisthesis. These images reveal facet degeneration with irregular, narrowed facet joints. *D,* The axial T$_1$-weighted image through the L4-5 disk again demonstrates the anterior listhesis of L4 on L5. The curvilinear low signal intensity of the posterior L4 body (*small white arrows*) projects 7 mm anterior to the posterior L5 body (*small black arrows*). *E,* The axial T$_1$-weighted image through the L4-5 facets reveals irregularity and narrowing of the facet joints. Compare these to the axial image (*F*) showing normal smooth facets at L3-4.

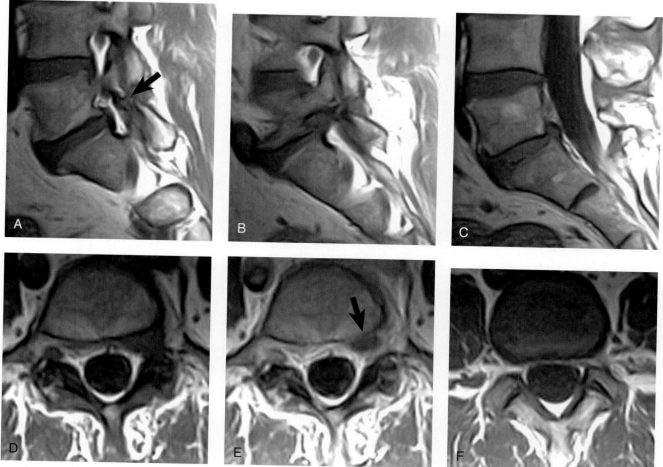

FIGURE 8–31. Bilateral spondylolysis with spondylolisthesis. *A,* A right parasagittal T$_1$-weighted image shows a break (*arrow*) in the right pars interarticularis at the L5 level. The neural foramen is narrowed because of the anterior listhesis. *B,* A left parasagittal section also demonstrates a left L5 pars interarticularis defect. A disk herniation is also present at the L5-S1 level extending into the left neural foramen. *C,* The midline sagittal T$_1$-weighted image shows grade I spondylolisthesis at the L5-S1 level. The axial pre- (*D*) and postcontrast (*E*) T$_1$-weighted images show bilateral irregular pseudarthroses in the posterior ring of L5 corresponding with the pars defects. Mild enhancement of the pseudarthroses is present presumably because of volume averaging with the surrounding soft tissues. The disk herniation is again demonstrated (*arrow*). The axial image at the level of the articular facets at L4-5 (*F*) demonstrates the appearance of the normal facet joints above the pars defects.

by disk degeneration with preservation of the facet joints. A retrolisthesis can occur after surgery or other intervention (Fig. 8–32), with resultant neural foraminal narrowing (and nerve root impingement). This is one cause of the failed back surgery syndrome. Retrolisthesis is most common in the lumbar and cervical spine. In the lumbar spine, L3-4 and L4-5 are the most frequently involved levels. Disk bulges and spurs commonly accompany a retrolisthesis. Central canal stenosis is uncommon, but neural foraminal narrowing is common.

Pseudomeningocele

A pseudomeningocele is an accumulation of CSF (outside the normal confines of the thecal sac) caused by a tear in the dura with (most common) or without a tear in the arachnoid membrane. The connection to the subarachnoid space is variable in size. Pseudomeningoceles can occur after laminectomy. In this instance, they are most common in the cervical spine, particularly after surgery involving the occiput. Pseudomeningoceles are

rare after laminectomy in the lumbar spine, but here they can produce radicular symptoms. A pseudomeningocele will follow CSF signal intensity on all pulse sequences.

Postoperative Lumbar Spine

The recurrence of symptoms after lumbar surgery, which occurs in 10% to 40% of patients, defines the failed back surgery syndrome. Causative factors include recurrent disk herniation, spinal stenosis, arachnoiditis, and epidural fibrosis (scar). MRI plays an extremely valuable role in the evaluation of the patient with recurrent pain after lumbar spine surgery. On postcontrast scans, postoperative scar can be differentiated from a recurrent or residual disk herniation; the distinction is critical for the therapeutic decision making process (Fig. 8–33). This use of intravenous contrast accounts for a substantial amount of the contrast used overall in spine MRI.

In the postoperative back, postcontrast scans should

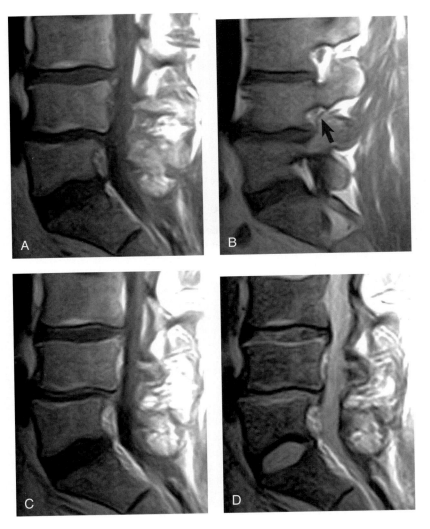

FIGURE 8–32. Retrolisthesis. *A,* The sagittal T_1-weighted image near the midline shows disk space narrowing at L4-5 and mild posterior displacement of the L4 vertebra on L5. A small disk bulge is present at L4-5 with thin, high-signal-intensity type II end plate changes adjacent to the L4-5 and L3-4 disks. *B,* The parasagittal T_1-weighted image through the right neural foramina demonstrates narrowing of the L4-5 bony foramen. The inferior aspect of the foramen is obliterated by the posteriorly displaced L4 vertebra and the associated disk bulge. The right L4 nerve root exits under the L4 pedicle with a small amount of surrounding high signal intensity fat. The superior articular facet of L5 (*arrow*) has moved in an anterior and cephalad direction, obliterating the inferior aspect and narrowing the superior aspect of the neural foramen. *C,* The sagittal T_1-weighted image after intravenous contrast administration confirms the retrolisthesis at L4-5. The malalignment is more easily detected because of enhancement of the epidural venous plexus along the posterior margin of the vertebrae. *D,* The comparable sagittal, intermediate T_2-weighted image again demonstrates the malalignment at L4-5. Decreased T_2 signal intensity in the L3-4 and L4-5 disks is due to disk degeneration at these levels. The patient, 41 years old, presents with recurrent low back and bilateral leg pain after L4-5 disk surgery.

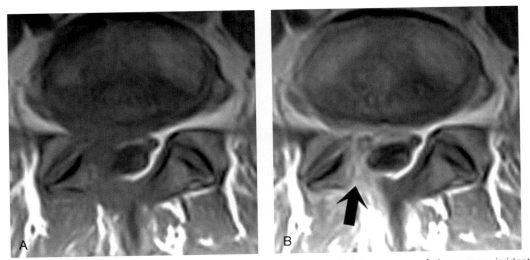

FIGURE 8–33. Postdiskectomy scar tissue. Two months after a right laminectomy and diskectomy, a soft tissue mass is identified anterior and to the right of the thecal sac on the precontrast T_1-weighted axial scan (*A*). *B,* Postcontrast, there is uniform enhancement of this abnormal soft tissue (*arrow*), consistent with scar. The right S1 nerve root can only be identified postcontrast surrounded by scar.

be obtained within 20 minutes after intravenous contrast administration. After this time, there may be diffusion of contrast from enhancing to nonenhancing tissue, making interpretation difficult. Postoperative scar demonstrates homogeneous enhancement as a result of intrinsic vascularity. However, this is not seen consistently until 3 months after surgery. Scar is one cause of persistent pain after lumbar disk surgery and is in general a contraindication to further surgery. Although the presence of a soft tissue mass favors the diagnosis of a recurrent disk, scar can also have this appearance (Fig. 8–34). Thus, noncontrast scans are not reliable for differentiation. In the patient with recurrent pain and postoperative scar, the fibrosis is often extensive and surrounds an exiting nerve root, presumably the basis for symptoms. A recurrent or residual disk herniation (Fig. 8–35) will not show enhancement on MRI scans obtained after contrast administration (assuming, of course, that these are obtained within 20 minutes of injection). Correct diagnosis on MRI mandates the use of thin sections, 3 mm or less, to avoid partial volume effects. A recurrent disk herniation will be seen as a focal, smooth posterior protrusion of nonenhancing soft tissue (contiguous with the native disk). The disk is commonly circumscribed posteriorly by a thin rim of enhancing soft tissue (Fig. 8–36) corresponding to scar (but in minimal amounts with a normal expected finding).

On contrast-enhanced MRI in the postoperative patient, the decompressed nerve may also enhance. This should resolve by 6 months after surgery. The facet joints may enhance presumably because of surgical manipulation. This can persist long term.

ARTHRITIS

Ankylosing spondylitis is an inflammatory disease of unknown etiology. The sacroiliac joints are involved early in the disease course. Erosion of cortical margins with subchondral bony sclerosis is seen first. Joint space widening, due to bony erosion, follows. The end result is fusion (obliteration) of the sacroiliac joints. In the spine, syndesmophytes are the hallmark of ankylosing spondylitis (Fig. 8–37). These slender, vertical ligamentous calcifications extend from the osseous excrescence of one vertebral body to the next. In the spine, the inflammation associated with ankylosing spondylitis occurs at the junction of the annulus fibrosus and the vertebral body. The outer annular fibers become replaced by bone, or syndesmophytes, which eventually bridge adjacent vertebral bodies. In advanced disease, this leads to the appearance on plain film of a "bamboo spine." One significant complication of ankylosing spondylitis is bony fracture after minor trauma. In the cervical spine, this can lead to quadriplegia.

DEGENERATIVE DISEASE

Spondylosis is a term that refers nonspecifically to any lesion of the spine of a degenerative nature (but usually involving specifically bone). Common degenerative processes seen in the lumbar spine include Schmorl's nodes, osteophytes, and end plate sclerosis.

Focal Fat Deposition

Focal fat deposition in the vertebral marrow can occur at any level and is frequently seen in multiple vertebral bodies. These deposits are round and up to 15 mm in diameter. Focal fat deposition is more common in elderly patients. It is seen on MRI in more than 90% of patients older than 50 years. The pathogenesis is focal marrow ischemia, with fatty replacement of hematopoietic marrow. On MRI, focal fat deposition follows the signal intensity of fat on all pulse sequences.

Schmorl's Node

A Schmorl's node represents a prolapse of the nucleus pulposus through the end plate into the medullary space of a vertebral body. The prolapse occurs as a result of axial loading. Schmorl's nodes are typically asymptomatic. On plain film, a focal depression, contiguous with the vertebral end plate, is seen with a sclerotic rim. On MRI, Schmorl's nodes will be of lower signal intensity than marrow on T_1-weighted scans and of higher signal intensity on T_2-weighted scans. There is often surrounding focal end plate changes. Contrast enhancement occurs, often peripheral in location, because of the presence of granulation tissue. Sagittal scans demonstrate the lesion to be immediately adjacent to the disk space and are thus most useful for diagnosis.

Synovial Cyst

In the spine, synovial cysts are associated with degenerative facet disease. When symptomatic, a synovial cyst can present with radicular pain, often sciatic in nature. This can mimic a disk herniation. Large synovial cysts can compress the thecal sac. On CT, the lesion can be hypo- or hyperdense. Synovial cysts may be calcified and are recognized by their location adjacent to a facet joint. On MRI, the signal intensity of the fluid within the cyst is variable; synovial cysts can have any combination of low or high signal intensity on T_1- and T_2-weighted scans. Postcontrast, the cyst capsule and any solid component will demonstrate enhancement (Fig. 8–38). Delayed enhancement of the cyst contents has been observed. Recognition of the relationship to the facet joint is critical for diagnosis.

Degenerative Disk and End Plate Changes

There are many signs of disk degeneration on MRI. There can be loss of disk height. Annular tears, with high signal intensity on T_2-weighted scans, may be seen. However, decreased signal intensity of the disk itself on T_2-weighted scans is the most sensitive indicator of early disk degeneration. This finding is often referred to in clinical dictations as disk dehydration or desiccation and occurs with varying degrees and may early on involve only a part of the disk. The actual cause of the decrease in signal intensity is a decrease in proteoglycans and in the ratio of chondroitin sulfate to keratin sulfate. With the exception of trauma, disk herniation without changes

Text continued on page 214

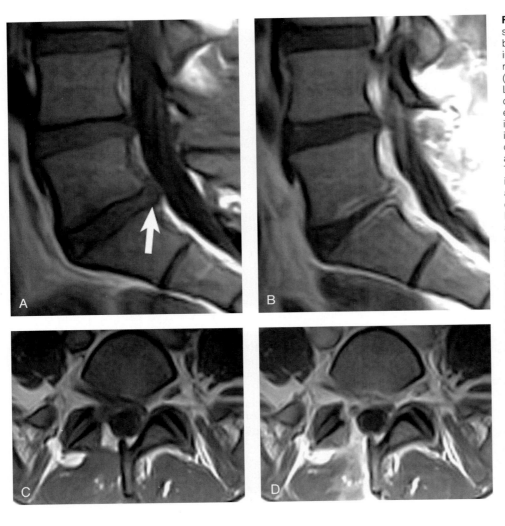

FIGURE 8–34. Differentiation of scar from disk in the postoperative back. *A,* The T_1-weighted sagittal image to the right of midline reveals abnormal soft tissue (*arrow*) projecting posterior to the L5-S1 intervertebral disk. *B,* After contrast administration, this tissue enhances intensely. Enhancement is also apparent both superior and inferior to the L5-S1 intervertebral disk, at the interface with the adjacent vertebral bodies. *C,* A T_1-weighted axial view at the inferior L5 level confirms the abnormal soft tissue in the ventral epidural space. The right laminectomy defect is also apparent. *D,* Postcontrast, the abnormal extradural soft tissue (which is now seen to surround the right S1 nerve root) is noted to enhance. Enhancement within soft tissue posteriorly at the laminectomy site and within the right paraspinal musculature is also noted. The patient presented with continued right leg pain 2 months after diskectomy at L5-S1. The anterior epidural mass in this case, which appears contiguous to the L5-S1 disk, would be suspicious for a recurrent disk herniation on the precontrast scans. The homogeneous enhancement of the abnormality, however, allows confident diagnosis of the lesion as epidural fibrosis (scar).

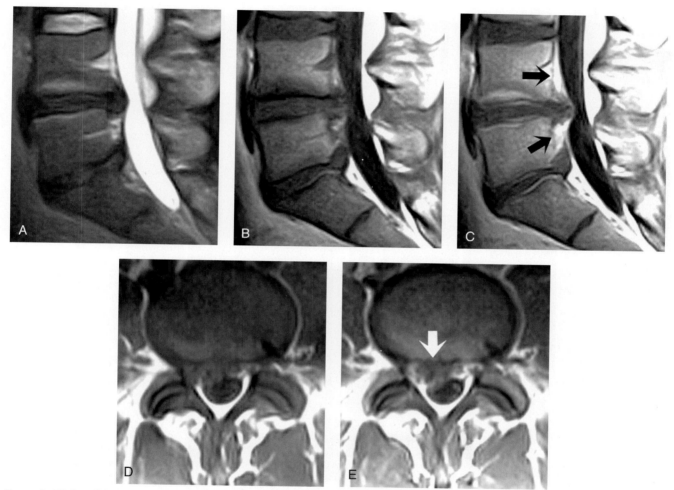

Figure 8–35. Postdiskectomy recurrent disk extrusion. T_2- (*A*) and T_1-weighted (*B*) midline sagittal scans reveal abnormal soft tissue anterior to the thecal sac at the L4-5 and L5-S1 levels. Two previous percutaneous diskectomies had been performed. *C*, Postcontrast, the majority of abnormal soft tissue at each level does not enhance. Enhancing soft tissue (*C, arrows*) above and below the L4-5 disk space level corresponds to a dilated epidural venous plexus. Comparison of pre- (*D*) and postcontrast (*E*) T_1-weighted axial scans at the L4-5 level confirms the presence of a recurrent disk herniation (*arrow*), with a small amount of surrounding enhancing granulation tissue. Lumbar microdiskectomy was subsequently performed.

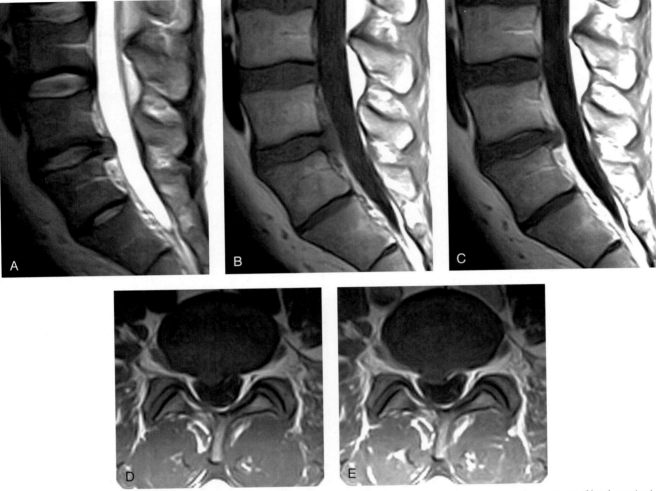

FIGURE 8–36. Pre- and postdiskectomy exams in a patient presenting with a disk extrusion and recurrence after surgery. Also important to the clinical case and surgical approach is the presence of a transitional vertebra. The preoperative exam includes sagittal T$_2$- (*A*), sagittal precontrast T$_1$- (*B*), sagittal postcontrast T$_1$- (*C*), axial precontrast T$_1$- (*D*) and axial postcontrast T$_1$-weighted (*E*) images. The postoperative exam, performed 1 year later, includes the same sequences, specifically sagittal T$_2$- (*F*), sagittal precontrast T$_1$- (*G*), sagittal postcontrast T$_1$- (*H*), axial precontrast T$_1$- (*I*), and axial postcontrast T$_1$-weighted (*J*) images. It should be recognized first that the patient has a transitional vertebra. The level with significant disease is likely to be L4-5, with L5 being sacralized. This was confirmed by reference to plain radiographs. This patient actually had four subsequent magnetic resonance imaging (MRI) exams, with one reader dictating the level as L5-S1 twice and two other readers dictating the level correctly as L4-5 once each. On the preoperative exam, there is a moderate-size right paracentral disk extrusion. Contrast enhancement provides minimal improvement in demarcation of the abnormal disk. On the MRI scan obtained a year later, with intervening surgery, there is a larger recurrent right paracentral disk extrusion. Postcontrast, there is a thin circumferential rim of enhancing scar tissue, which improves differentiation of the disk from adjacent cerebrospinal fluid. The lack of enhancement of the majority of the soft tissue mass confirms that this represents recurrent disk disease. Postoperative changes caused by the right-sided laminectomy are also noted.

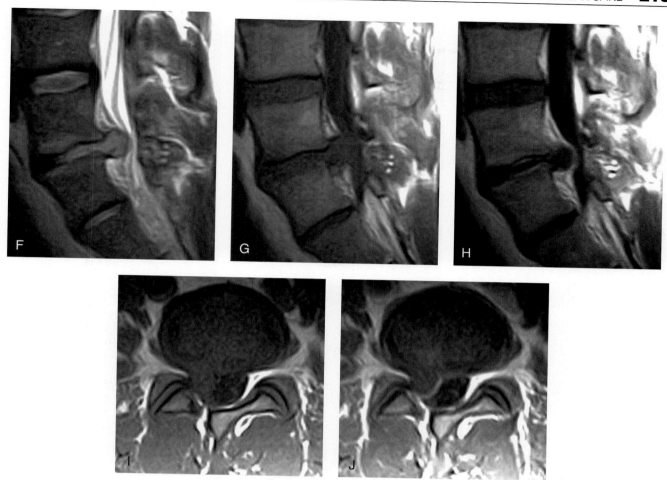

FIGURE 8–36 *Continued. See legend on opposite page*

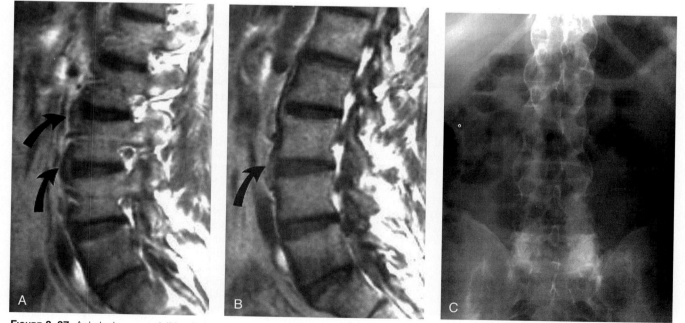

FIGURE 8–37. Ankylosing spondylitis. *A* and *B,* On parasagittal T$_1$-weighted images of the lumbar spine, there are prominent anterior osteophytes (*curved arrows*), which appear to bridge the disk space at several levels. *C,* The anteroposterior plain film of the lumbar spine reveals the sacroiliac joints to be obliterated, with bony bridges (marginal syndesmophytes) connecting adjacent vertebral bodies.

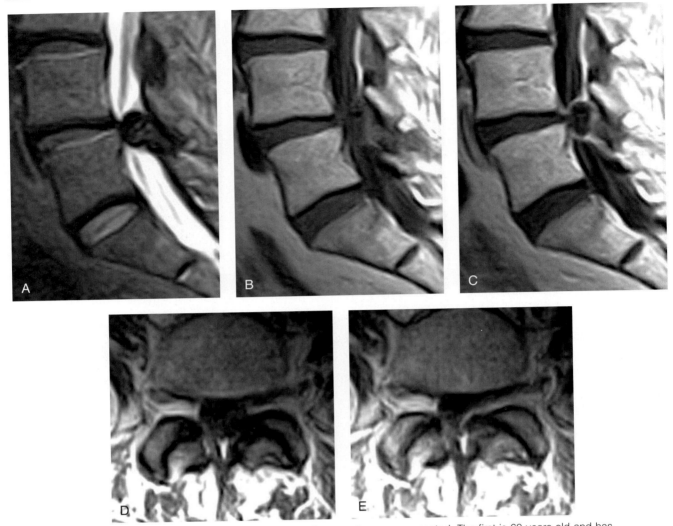

FIGURE 8–38. Synovial cyst. Images from two patients with similar symptoms are presented. The first is 60 years old and has experienced increasing left leg pain and intermittent numbness over the last 6 months. *A,* On the sagittal T_2-weighted scan, a low-signal-intensity abnormality is noted within the bony spinal canal, immediately posterior to the L4-5 intervertebral disk. There is displacement and compression of the thecal sac. *B,* Before contrast administration, the lesion is difficult to identify. *C,* After contrast injection, there is rim enhancement. On this scan, the lesion (a synovial cyst) appears (correctly) to be extradural. Pre- (*D*) and postcontrast (*E*) axial images at the L4-5 level are presented from the second patient's exam. There is facet hypertrophy bilaterally. *D,* Precontrast, the question is raised of a left-sided lesion causing compression posteriorly of the thecal sac. *E,* Postcontrast, there is rim enhancement, which improves the differentiation of the lesion from cerebrospinal fluid within the thecal sac. The lesion appears cystic in nature by signal intensity and enhancement characteristics. The lesion (another synovial cyst) is contiguous with the left facet joint.

of disk degeneration is extremely unusual. This can be very helpful in directing the film reader toward the disk space levels that should be more closely examined (those demonstrating disk desiccation).

A vacuum disk is a degenerated disk with gas (nitrogen) in clefts within the annulus fibrosus and nucleus pulposus. Vacuum disks are more common in the lumbar spine and in elderly patients. On CT, very low density is seen within the disk. On MRI, linear low signal intensity (with the presence of gas resulting in a signal void) is seen on both T_1- and T_2-weighted scans.

Degenerative vertebral body end plate changes are a common finding on MRI of the lumbar spine. A change in signal intensity of the marrow space adjacent to the end plate is by far the most clear indicator of degenerative end plate disease (Fig. 8–39). These changes are

parallel and directly adjacent to the disk space. Such changes typically involve the entirety of both end plates (surrounding a degenerated disk), although involvement of just one end plate (and even just a portion of one) can occur.

Type I end plate changes reflect increased water content and are low signal intensity on T_1-weighted images and high signal intensity on T_2-weighted images. Type I end plate changes enhance after contrast administration, often to isointensity with marrow fat. Type I end plate changes can be mimicked by two other disease entities; differential diagnosis is critical. Metastatic disease can at times resemble type I end plate changes. However, typically, there are multiple additional lesions. Isolated involvement of the end plate by metastatic disease is uncommon. Disk space infection and adjacent osteomy-

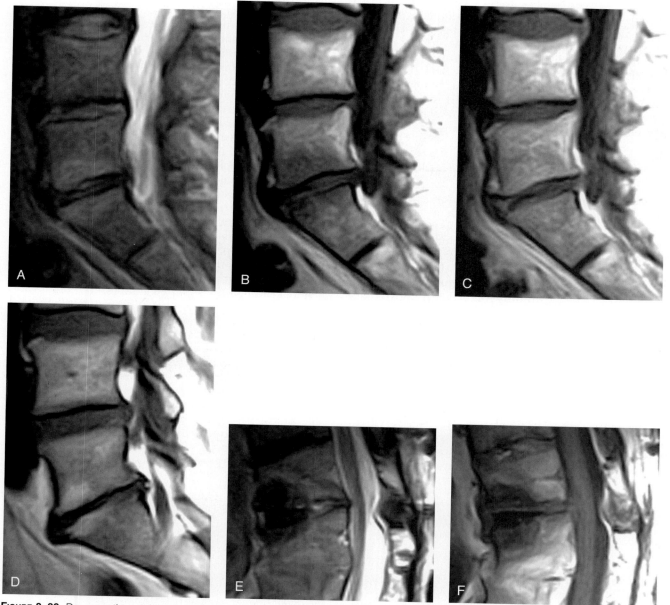

FIGURE 8–39. Degenerative end plate changes. *A–C,* Type I end plate changes histologically show vascular infiltration, fibrosis, and granulation tissue between thickened bony trabeculae. Increased water content results in both T₁ and T₂ lengthening. On magnetic resonance imaging (MRI) the end plates show increased signal intensity on T₂-weighted scans (*A*) and decreased signal intensity on T₁-weighted scans (*B*). The signal is usually parallel to the end plates and directly adjacent to the intervertebral disk. *C,* The affected end plates commonly enhance (to isointensity with normal marrow) after intravenous contrast administration. *D,* Type II end plate changes show fatty infiltration interposed between thickened trabeculae histologically. MRI reveals increased signal intensity on both T₁- (*D*) and T₂-weighted scans (not shown) compared with normal marrow. *E* and *F,* Another end plate pattern, Type III, consists of sclerotic changes. On MRI, the end plates are low signal intensity on both T₂- (*E*) and T₁-weighted (*F*) scans. These areas correspond with sclerosis on plain x-ray films.

elitis can also resemble type I end plate changes. However, with infection, the disk should be grossly abnormal, the demarcation between disk and body lost, and a paraspinous mass often present.

Type II end plate changes reflect fatty infiltration. There is increased signal intensity within the end plate on both T_1- and T_2-weighted scans paralleling fat. The progression of type I to type II has been observed on occasion, leading to the conclusion that type I is an early form of end plate disease, which eventually converts to type II. In clinical cases, type II is by far the most common type of end plate disease observed. Mixed type I and II patterns are also seen. Type III is very rare and corresponds to bony sclerosis, with low signal intensity seen on both T_1- and T_2-weighted scans.

DISK HERNIATION

The strict definition of a disk herniation is the protrusion of degenerated or fragmented disk material into the foramen compressing a nerve root or into the spinal canal compressing the spinal cord or cauda equina. Medicolegal considerations have led many radiologic practices to discard the use of the term disk herniation and adopt a terminology more descriptive of the process and its extent. This terminology, advanced by Michael Modic and others, is described in detail later. It classifies disk disease into four categories: disk bulge, protrusion, extrusion, and free fragment. Tears of the annulus fibrosus are also described; these can be seen on MRI and are no doubt a precursor to more advanced, symptomatic disk disease.

Tears of the annulus fibrosus are classified into three types. Concentric, or type I, is parallel to the curvature of the outer disk. Radial, or type II, involves all the layers of the annulus from the nucleus pulposus to the surface. Transverse, or type III, involves the insertion of Sharpey's fibers into the ring apophysis. Tears of the

annulus fibrosus are high signal intensity on T_2-weighted scans. A tear will also enhance after intravenous gadolinium chelate administration (Fig. 8–40). Contrast enhancement is due to the presence of fibrovascular (granulation) tissue, a result of the body's normal reparative process.

A disk or annular bulge is an extension of the posterior disk beyond the margin of the adjacent vertebral end plates but without focal disk protrusion (Fig. 8–41). The posterior disk margin forms a smooth curvilinear contour. A disk bulge by definition is broad based and circumferential. A disk bulge occurs as a result of laxity of and tears within the annulus fibrosus. It is a sign of early disk degeneration. A disk bulge can, however, narrow the spinal canal and the inferior neural foramen.

A disk protrusion is a herniation of the nucleus through a (small) tear in the annulus but still contained by outer fibers of the annulus. A disk protrusion is differentiated from a bulge by axial imaging, with demonstration of focal extension of disk material beyond the margin of the vertebral end plates (Fig. 8–42). Although disk protrusion and extrusion are distinct entities, differentiated by the degree of rupture of the annulus, this can rarely be appreciated on MRI. In common usage, the term disk protrusion is reserved for a small herniation and disk extrusion for a large herniation of disk material through the ruptured annulus.

A disk extrusion is a herniation of the nucleus through the ruptured annulus with no intact remaining annular fibers. It is important to specify, when interpreting MRI exams, whether a disk extrusion (or protrusion) is central (Fig. 8–43), paracentral (Fig. 8–44), foraminal (Fig. 8–45), or lateral (Fig. 8–46) in location. A disk extrusion, when combined with lateral stenosis, can cause nerve root ischemia with eventual fibrosis, leading to irreversible axonal damage. In an extrusion, the disk material remains in contiguity with the parent disk. This distinction differentiates a disk extrusion from a free fragment. Even without surgery, granulation tissue forms around

Text continued on page 223

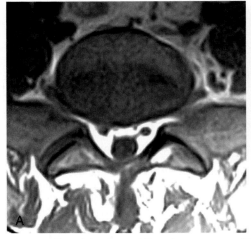 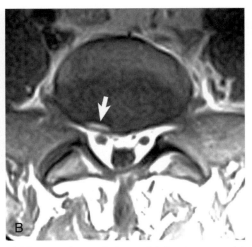

FIGURE 8–40. Annular tear. T_1-weighted pre- (*A*) and postcontrast (*B*) axial images demonstrate a mild, focal, asymmetrical extension of the posterior disk margin. The disk abuts, but does not significantly displace, the right L5 nerve root sleeve. The postcontrast image reveals a curvilinear area of high signal intensity (*arrow*) paralleling the posterior disk margin because of enhancement of a concentric tear in the outer fibers of the annulus fibrosus. A T_2-weighted image was not acquired in this patient in the axial plane. Such an image would have also clearly depicted the tear, with abnormal hyperintensity.

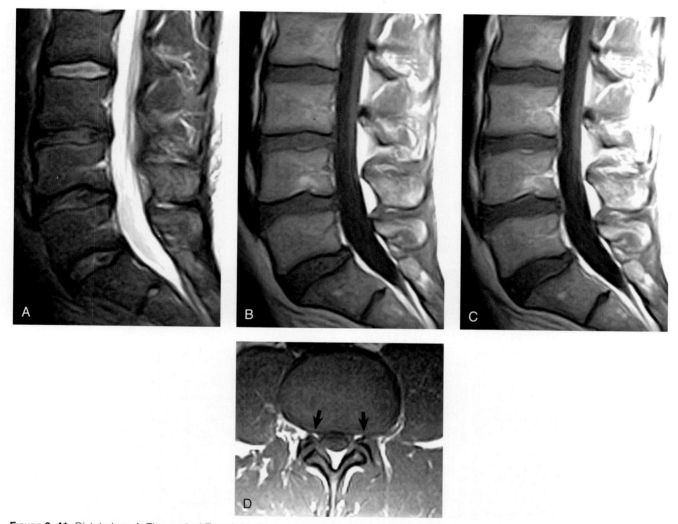

FIGURE 8–41. Disk bulge. *A,* The sagittal T$_2$-weighted image demonstrates decreased signal intensity in the L3-4, L4-5, and L5-S1 disk spaces consistent with disk degeneration. The posterior disk margins extend beyond the adjacent vertebral end plates and indent the anterior thecal sac at these levels. The sagittal pre- (*B*) and postcontrast (*C*) T$_1$-weighted images again show mild posterior extension of disk material from L3-4 through L5-S1. The disk margin is better delineated after the administration of intravenous contrast because of enhancement of the epidural venous plexus. *D,* The axial T$_1$-weighted image through the L3-4 level reveals a generalized disk bulge with mild convexity of the posterior disk margin. The disk material narrows the lateral recesses bilaterally (*arrows*). The posterior disk margin has a smooth curvilinear contour with no focal disk protrusion.

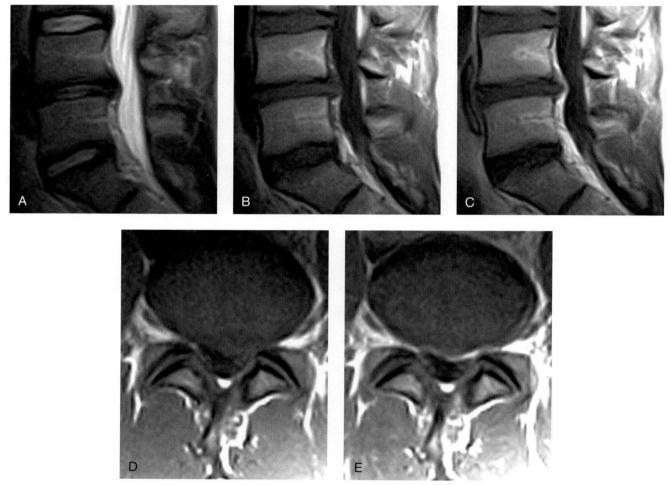

FIGURE 8–42. Disk protrusion. Sagittal precontrast T_2- (*A*) and T_1-weighted (*B*) scans reveal extension of disk material beyond the vertebral end plates at L4-5. *C,* Enhancement of de novo scar and epidural venous plexus postcontrast improves delineation of the disk margin from cerebrospinal fluid on the T_1-weighted scan. Comparison of pre- (*D*) and postcontrast (*E*) axial T_1-weighted scans through the L4-5 disk level reveals the extension of disk material, which is relatively small, to be focal and central in location.

FIGURE 8–43. Central disk extrusion. Midline sagittal precontrast T_2-weighted (*A*) and postcontrast T_1-weighted (*B*) scans demonstrate moderate compression of the thecal sac by posterior extension of disk material at the L4-5 level. Loss of the normal high signal intensity (on the T_2-weighted scan) of the intervertebral disks at L4-5 and L5-S1 is compatible with disk degeneration. Axial pre- (*C*) and postcontrast (*D*) scans at the L4-5 level demonstrate the disk extrusion to be central in location. At high field, with current software, an alternative imaging approach (driven by cost) is to add an axial fast spin echo T_2-weighted scan and not acquire the postcontrast scans.

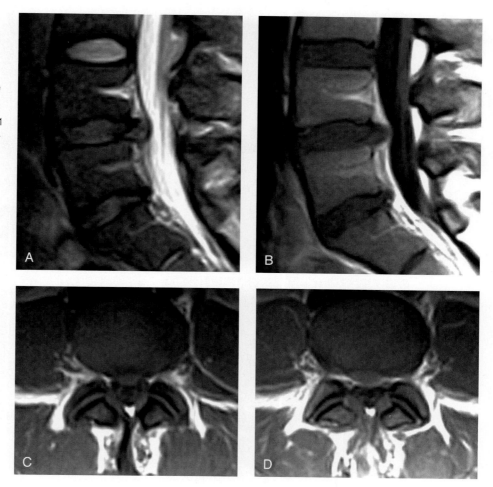

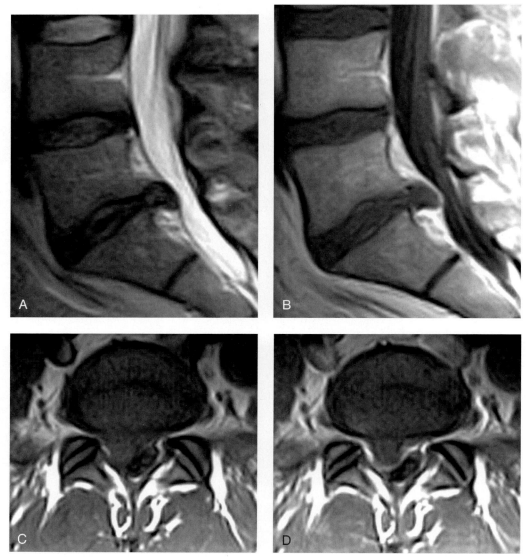

FIGURE 8–44. Right paracentral disk extrusion. Sagittal precontrast T$_2$-weighted (*A*) and postcontrast T$_1$-weighted (*B*) scans, just to the right of midline, demonstrate substantial compression of the thecal sac by disk material at the L5-S1 level. Axial pre- (*C*) and postcontrast (*D*) scans at the L5-S1 level demonstrate this large disk extrusion to be paracentral in location. This 32-year-old patient presented with right leg pain.

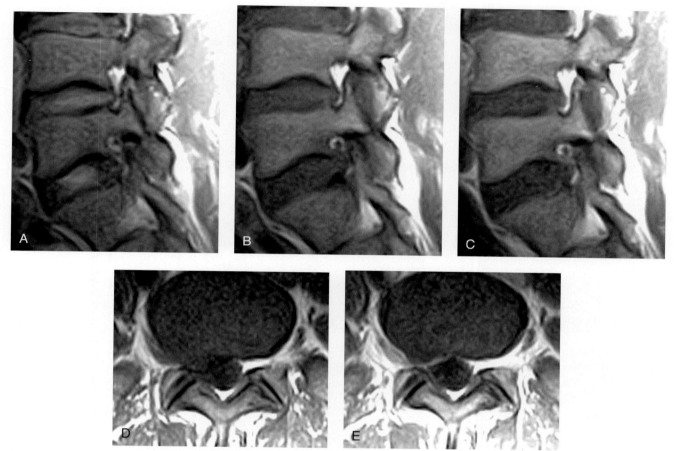

FIGURE 8–45. Foraminal disk extrusion. Parasagittal precontrast T_2- (*A*), precontrast T_1- (*B*), and postcontrast T_1-weighted (*C*) scans reveal extension of disk material into the inferior portion of the foramen at the L5-S1 level. After contrast administration, there is enhancement of a thin line (presumably scar) separating the disk extrusion from the superior portion of the foramen, which contains the L5 nerve root (surrounded by fat). Axial pre- (*D*) and postcontrast (*E*) scans at the L5-S1 level depict very clearly the focal extrusion of disk material within the foramen. The dorsal root ganglion is seen just lateral to the extrusion, with normal enhancement postcontrast. Axial T_2-weighted scans (not shown), although excellent for demonstrating central and paracentral disk disease, are poor for foraminal disease; differentiation of disk material and other foraminal contents is difficult.

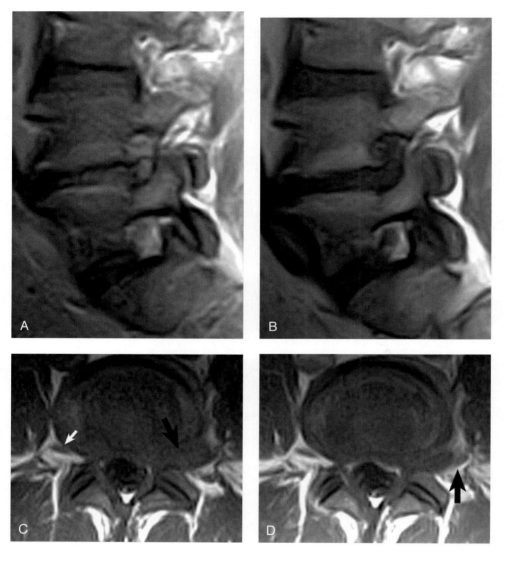

FIGURE 8–46. Lateral disk extrusion. Precontrast sagittal T$_2$-(*A*) and T$_1$-weighted (*B*) scans to the left of midline demonstrate extension of the L4-5 disk posteriorly into the left L4-5 neural foramen. The exiting left L4 nerve root is identified just above the disk extrusion. *C,* The precontrast axial T$_1$-weighted scan reveals a large focal lateral herniation of disk material (*black arrow*). The exiting L4 nerve root (*small white arrow*) is seen on the right but is obscured by the herniated disk material on the left. *D,* The postcontrast T$_1$-weighted axial scan provides clearer delineation of the disk extrusion as a result of enhancement of the epidural venous plexus and foraminal veins. The displaced left L4 nerve root (*D, arrow*) can now be distinguished from the nonenhancing extruded disk. Mass effect on the left side of the thecal sac is also more apparent.

the extruded disk, part of the body's normal reparative process. This tissue enhances postcontrast, forming a thin rim of high signal intensity "wrapping" the extruded disk material on enhanced T_1-weighted exams. This appearance can be confusing to radiologists who have experience principally with nonenhanced MRI scans. Scar in the nonoperated back may potentially assist in recovery by limiting the herniation and with contraction decreasing the degree of compression of neural structures. The neurosurgeons of yesteryear were very familiar with the fact that a substantial reduction in size of a disk herniation could be observed with conservative therapy. Thus, follow-up MRI scans can demonstrate a reduction in size of a disk extrusion without intervening surgery (Fig. 8–47).

Ninety percent of lumbar disk extrusions occur at L4-5 or L5-S1. Of the remainder, most occur at L3-4. Central lesions may cause no symptoms, with the exiting nerve roots unaffected. Paracentral lesions cause symptoms as a result of compression of the exiting nerve root. For example, the S1 nerve root will be compressed by a paracentral L5-S1 disk extrusion. Lateral disk extrusions are the least common because the annulus is thinnest posteriorly. Superior migration of lateral fragments is common. A lateral disk extrusion will compress the ganglion or nerve root within the neural foramen. This causes radiculopathy of the nerve root above the interspace. For example, a lateral disk extrusion at the L3-4 level will compress the L3 nerve. Lateral disk extrusions occur beyond the termination of the nerve root sleeve. Thus, myelography is relatively insensitive to lateral disk disease. Myelographic findings with a disk extrusion include displacement of the contrast-filled sac, elevation, displacement, or amputation of the nerve root sleeve, and nerve root enlargement (as a result of edema). When a nerve is acutely compressed by a disk extrusion, edema of the nerve root in question can occasionally be seen within the thecal sac on MRI (with nerve root enlargement and abnormal high signal intensity on the T_2-weighted exam). Lumbar nerve root

FIGURE 8–47. Resolution of L4-5 paracentral disk protrusion with conservative therapy. Precontrast sagittal (*A*) and postcontrast axial (*B*) T_1-weighted scans from the patient's initial clinical presentation are compared with scans obtained 1 year later (*C* and *D*). At presentation, disk material protrudes posteriorly on the sagittal image at the L4-5 level (*A*). The protrusion (*B*, *arrow*) is well delineated by a thin rim of enhancement on the postcontrast axial scan and is noted to be paracentral in location. On the follow-up exam obtained 1 year later, there is no abnormal posterior extension of disk material on the sagittal scan (*C*). Enhancing scar tissue is noted on the postcontrast axial T_1-weighted scan (*D*) but without compression of the thecal sac.

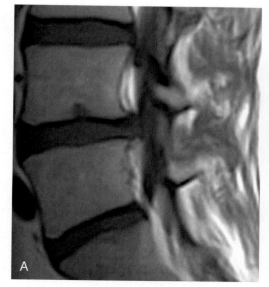
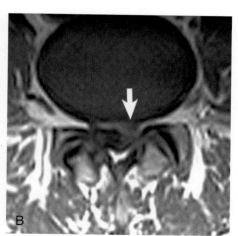
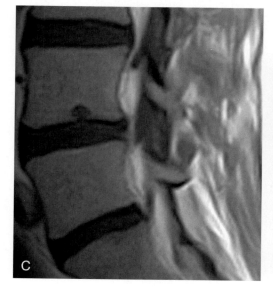
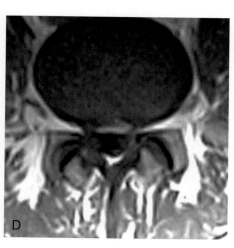

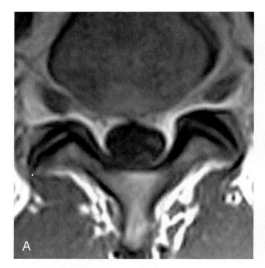
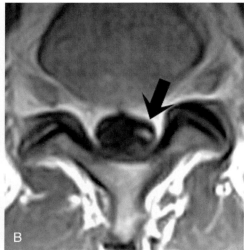

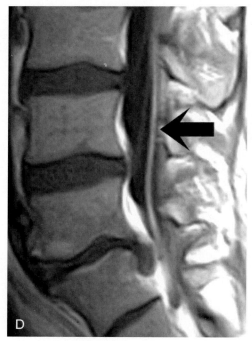

FIGURE 8–48. Enhancing nerve root resulting from compression by a large free fragment. Comparison of pre- (*A*) and postcontrast (*B*) T₁-weighted axial scans at the L5-S1 level reveals intense enhancement of the left S1 nerve root (*arrow*) within the thecal sac. This is confirmed on the postcontrast T₁-weighted sagittal scan (*C, arrow*), which also identifies nerve root compression by a large disk fragment. The patient was referred for a magnetic resonance imaging scan because of recent onset of a left S1 radiculopathy.

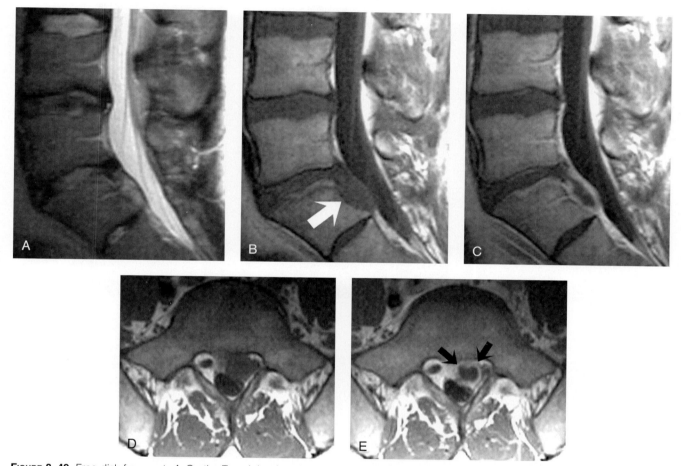

FIGURE 8–49. Free disk fragment. *A,* On the T$_2$-weighted sagittal scan, a soft tissue mass with abnormal high signal intensity is identified posterior to S1. This mass (*white arrow*) is isointense with the remaining disk material at the L5-S1 level on the T$_1$-weighted sagittal scan (*B*). *C,* Postcontrast, the periphery of the mass enhances. Inspection of pre- (*D*) and postcontrast (*E*) axial scans through the S1 vertebral body confirms the presence of a free disk fragment. The fragment is "wrapped" by enhancing scar (*arrows*), deforms the thecal sac, and compresses the left S1 nerve root.

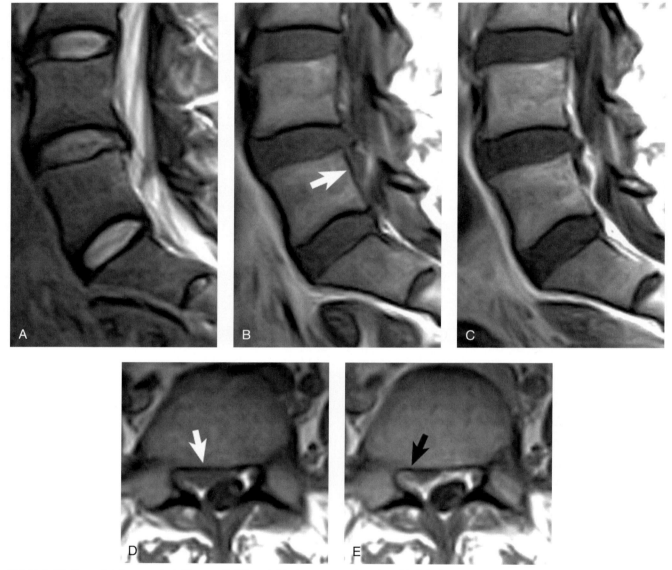

FIGURE 8–50. Free disk fragment. *A,* The sagittal T$_2$-weighted scan reveals only mild disk degeneration at L4-5. *B,* On the precontrast T$_1$-weighted sagittal scan, abnormal soft tissue (*arrow*) is noted partly contiguous with the L4-5 disk but posterior to the L5 vertebral body. *C,* Postcontrast, the lesion (a free fragment) is better delineated because of the surrounding rim of enhancing tissue. Examining the T$_2$-weighted scan in retrospect, the lesion is noted to be of high signal intensity and thus difficult to differentiate from cerebrospinal fluid. The free fragment (*D, white arrow*), which has migrated inferiorly, is well demonstrated on pre- (*D*) and postcontrast (*E*) axial T$_1$-weighted scans, which also reveal compression of the right L5 nerve root (*E, black arrow*). The patient presented 5 days after injury with low back and right leg pain.

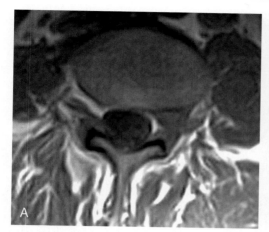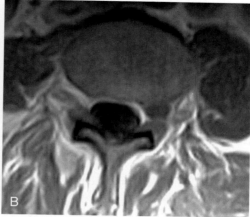

FIGURE 8–51. Free disk fragment within the L4-5 foramen. *A,* Abnormal soft tissue is noted within the left neural foramen on the precontrast axial T_1-weighted scan. *B,* After contrast administration, a thin rim of enhancement better delineates the lesion, which otherwise does not change in signal intensity. Contrast administration in this instance permits the differentiation of a neural origin tumor within the foramen (which would enhance; see Fig. 8–26) from a migrated free fragment (which, as illustrated by this case, does not enhance).

enhancement is not uncommon with acute disk extrusions, although many radiologists are unfamiliar with this appearance. Their unfamiliarity is due to the fact that most screening exams of the lumbar spine for disk disease are performed without contrast enhancement. Lumbar nerve root enhancement occurs as a result of disruption of the blood-nerve root barrier. Its presence supports the clinical significance of a compressive lesion (Fig. 8–48).

With a free fragment or sequestered disk, the herniated disk material is separate from the parent disk. A free fragment may be anterior (contained by) or posterior to the posterior longitudinal ligament. When anterior, a thin midline septum directs the fragment paracentrally away from the midline. Free fragments have characteristic signal intensity on MRI, intermediate to low signal intensity on T_1-weighted scans, and high signal intensity (but less than that of CSF) on T_2-weighted scans (Fig. 8–49). Free fragments can migrate superiorly or inferiorly (Fig. 8–50) within the epidural space or into the neural foramen (Fig. 8–51).

9

Neck, Oropharynx, and Nasopharynx

The technical considerations applicable to head and neck magnetic resonance imaging (MRI) are similar to those involved in non-neurologic imaging of other areas of the body: maximizing the signal-to-noise ratio (SNR) within an acceptable imaging time, optimizing contrast among abnormalities, fat, and muscle, and achieving satisfactory spatial resolution. In addition to the choice of pulse sequence, imaging plane, slice thickness, number of acquisitions, and matrix size, attention should be paid to the choice of imaging coil. The oropharynx and nasopharynx, paranasal sinuses, salivary glands, and facial bones are usually imaged with a standard head coil. However, to maximize SNR, the smallest-diameter cylindrical coil (with the highest SNR) that can be fitted to a given patient's head and that provides an adequate field of view should be used. Superficial structures may be best imaged using a surface coil. Today specialized coils for the head and neck (with both anterior and posterior components) are available for most MRI scanners and should be used to image structures below the face.

As in all of MRI, the choice of pulse sequences is crucial in determining the diagnostic quality of the examination. MRI of the head and neck has been performed almost entirely with spin echo (and fast spin echo) sequences. Use of both heavily T_1-weighted and T_2-weighted sequences is essential in the examination of this region. To attain adequate T_1-weighting, a time to repetition (TR) of less than 600 msec should be used with the shortest time to echo (TE) attainable (5–15 msec). For adequate T_2 weighting, a TR of 2000 to 3000 msec should be used. A TR in the upper part of this range is necessary with higher field (1.5 T) units to achieve comparable T_2-weighting because of the prolongation of T_1 with increasing field strength. As with most of MRI, fast spin echo sequences have generally replaced spin echo scans for acquisition of T_2-weighted images. Fat suppression is commonly used in head and neck imaging, in particular on postcontrast scans to highlight enhancing lesions.

T_1- and T_2-weighted sequences prove complementary in imaging of the head and neck. The short TR, short TE, T_1-weighted scan provides essentially anatomic information and is useful in analyzing the architectural distortion of tissues, disruption of fat planes, mass effect, and adenopathy. The T_2-weighted scan provides higher contrast between pathologic and normal tissues, providing improved localization of the pathologic process. The actual signal characteristics of most pathologic tissues in the head and neck are nonspecific, with the exceptions of cystic and lipomatous lesions.

Optimal slice thickness varies with the abnormality being examined, but a 5-mm thickness (and a 10% to 20% gap between slices) is usually suitable for evaluating this anatomic region. The number of acquisitions and matrix size to be used will vary with the technical capabilities of the scanner and coil. Because T_1-weighted images are usually obtained for anatomic information, the matrix size should be at a minimum 256 × 256, with consideration given to larger matrices or choice of a smaller field of view. With the T_2-weighted scan, fine spatial resolution is relatively less crucial. Scan times should be kept short to minimize image degradation from patient motion. Motion compensation techniques such as gradient moment nulling may be helpful to improve overall image quality.

An initial imaging plane must be chosen that can be used as a localizer for the remainder of the exam. The sagittal plane is usually chosen for the localizer. In general, the axial plane is the most informative single plane, and images in this plane are obtained in most examinations of the oropharynx and nasopharynx, salivary glands, and neck. Images in the coronal and sagittal planes are helpful adjuncts, and at least one of these additional planes is acquired in most exams. The sagittal plane is most helpful in evaluating midline lesions, and the localizer image may be tailored for this purpose by choosing a thin slice thickness and small pixel size (with a sufficiently high number of averages or acquisitions to ensure good image quality). The coronal plane is useful for evaluating laterally located abnormalities and side-to-side symmetry. To facilitate interpretation, both T_1- and T_2-weighted images should be obtained in one of the planes, typically the axial. One or both of the adjunctive planes may then be obtained using a single-pulse sequence.

Intravenous contrast enhancement, using the gadolinium chelates, has a major role in head and neck MRI, as it does in MRI of the head and spine. Contrast use is recommended in exams in which neoplastic involvement or infection is questioned. Normal structures with pronounced vascularity, such as the mucosal lining of the pharynx, exhibit prominent enhancement after intravenous gadolinium chelate administration. One excellent check to make sure that the dose of contrast has not been infiltrated is to inspect the nasal turbinates, which, being highly vascular, exhibit marked enhancement. Inflamed and thickened mucosa, which exhibits prominent enhancement, is clearly demonstrated and differentiated on postcontrast scans from nonenhancing retained secretions, retention cysts, and mucoceles. This differentiation is often also possible on unenhanced T_2-weighted scans and so may not require the use of contrast. As with CT, vascular tumors such as paraganglioma, neural tumors, angiofibroma, chordoma, and carcinoma exhibit prominent enhancement. Postcontrast scans are extremely useful in assessing extension of head and neck tumors into areas that are otherwise difficult to evaluate, such as intracranially, into muscles, and into small fossae and fissures (e.g., the pterygopalatine fossa). Small mucosal and mesenchymal tumors may also be easier to identify after contrast administration.

NOSE AND NASOPHARYNX

MRI has great utility in evaluating mass lesions of the nose and nasopharynx. The indications for an MRI exam of this region are basically fourfold: suspicion of an occult nasopharyngeal carcinoma; documentation of the extent of deep invasion by a known nasopharyngeal carcinoma; evaluation of large, benign lesions; and assessment of a deep, parapharyngeal lesion inaccessible to direct visualization. The ability of MRI to detect metastatic adenopathy is comparable to that of computed tomography (CT). The relationship of tumor to vessels and any intracranial extension can be assessed with a greater degree of accuracy than with contrast-enhanced CT. The multiplanar imaging capabilities of MRI are especially helpful in this regard. In regard to bone invasion, MRI provides a sensitive measure by depicting marrow involvement. However, destruction of cortical bone (such as that of the skull base) is more easily visualized, and best evaluated, by CT.

Nasopharyngeal Carcinoma

The clinical findings that may prompt suspicion of occult squamous cell carcinoma include palpable cervical lymph node metastasis (usually involving the deep cervical chain), nasal obstruction or epistaxis, cranial nerve symptoms (commonly from cranial nerves IX, X, XI, and XII and more unusually II, III, IV, and VI), and unilateral serous otitis media. Rarely, trismus (tonic spasm of the muscles of mastication) may occur after invasion of the pterygoid muscles.

The nasopharynx is a difficult area to examine clinically, and small lesions can easily be missed. Adults usually have a thin layer of adenoidal and mucosal tissue lining the posterior and lateral walls of the nasopharynx just superficial to the longus capitis and colli muscles and the pharyngeal constrictors. This tissue layer is slightly higher in signal intensity than the adjacent muscles on T_1-weighted images and much higher in intensity on T_2-weighted images. The signal characteristics of nasopharyngeal tumors are often similar to those of this band of tissue. Signs of early nasopharyngeal carcinoma include obliteration of the lateral pharyngeal recess (located posterior on axial images and superior on coronal images to the torus tubarius and orifice of the eustachian tube) and infiltration of the fat planes around the lateral tensor and medial levator palatini muscles, which mark the medial boundary of the parapharyngeal space. Subtle asymmetries of the superficial pharyngeal tissue layer are frequently identified in normal patients.

In more advanced cases, an obvious soft tissue mass may be seen in the nasopharynx, with possible extension into the parapharyngeal space fat (Fig. 8-1). Invasion of the skull base, cavernous sinus, foramen ovale, jugular foramen, carotid canal, maxillary, ethmoid, and sphenoid sinuses, nose, pterygopalatine fossa, and orbits should

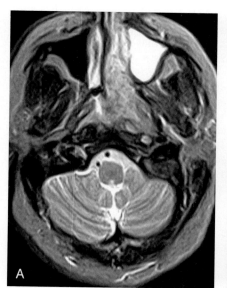
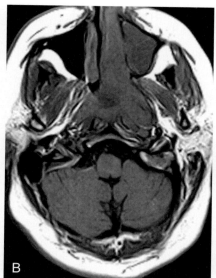
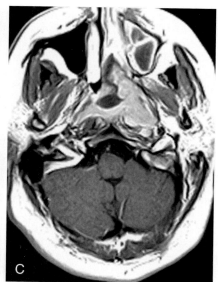

FIGURE 9–1. Squamous cell carcinoma of the nasopharynx. *A,* On the T_2-weighted scan, a large soft tissue mass with intermediate signal intensity is noted in the posterior nasopharynx. The lesion extends anteriorly into the left nasal cavity. Retained secretions, with high signal intensity, are noted in the left maxillary sinus. *B,* On the precontrast T_1-weighted scan, neoplastic tissue, retained secretions, and the normal turbinates are all intermediate signal intensity. *C,* After contrast administration, there is intense enhancement of the turbinates and the mucosal lining of the left maxillary sinus. Neoplastic tissue enhances but to a lesser degree, permitting differentiation.

be assessed in every case. Displacement of the carotid artery and jugular vein is easily evaluated by MRI, especially with sagittal and coronal images. A flow void within vessels, even on a single imaging plane, reliably indicates vascular patency. However, vascular occlusion may at times be difficult to distinguish from flow-related artifacts. If vascular occlusion is suspected, there are many alternative imaging approaches that can resolve this question, including the use of phase images, gradient echo scans, two-dimensional time-of-flight magnetic resonance angiography (MRA), and contrast-enhanced MRA.

Bone destruction can be visualized on MRI, although attention to this aspect of image interpretation is important. Otherwise, significant lesions can be missed. Bone destruction appears as a replacement of the signal void from cortical bone (or cortical bone and air in the case of the petrous portion of the temporal bone) with intermediate- or high-signal-intensity soft tissue. Bone marrow–containing cancellous bone, such as the clivus, exhibits replacement of normal high-signal-intensity marrow fat with intermediate-signal-intensity material on T_1-weighted images. On T_2-weighted images, one may see intermediate- or high-signal-intensity material infiltrating the low-signal-intensity marrow, although T_1-weighted images are better for visualizing most cases of marrow invasion. MRI is usually adequate for assessing bony involvement, although CT may be necessary in some cases for evaluating fine bony detail. There is no doubt that MRI is superior to CT in assessing intracranial extension of tumor.

The nodal groups typically involved by nasopharyngeal carcinoma are the lateral retropharyngeal nodes (the node of Rouvière is the highest of these), the jugular group, including the jugulodigastric node, and the spinal accessory group in the posterior triangle deep to the sternocleidomastoid muscle. Imaging evaluation is especially important in the last group because these nodes are relatively inaccessible to clinical evaluation. Involvement of the upper cervical nodes is common, but mid- and lower cervical node metastases may also occur. Among all head and neck neoplasms, nasopharyngeal carcinoma has the highest incidence of contralateral nodal metastasis (up to 33% of cases). Metastatic lymph nodes tend to be of intermediate signal intensity and inflammatory involvement of high signal intensity on T_2-weighted scans. However, as in other parts of the body, whether a node is involved by tumor cannot be determined solely by its signal characteristics. Reliance must be placed on node size; a diameter of 1.0 to 1.5 cm (and greater) is considered suspicious. Use of size criteria for nodes carries a penalty in sensitivity and specificity. Microscopic involvement is missed, and post-inflammatory nodal enlargement is mistaken for metastatic disease. The larger and more numerous the nodes, the more likely they are to actually represent metastatic involvement. Necrosis within a node of any size, identified as a central area with signal intensity similar to fluid, identifies likely metastatic involvement.

Fluid in obstructed ethmoid and sphenoid sinuses and in the mastoid air cells resulting from obstruction of the eustachian tube can be recognized by its homogeneous appearance and very high intensity on T_2-weighted images (and low intensity on T_1-weighted images). Unusual, malignant lesions, such as esthesioneuroblastoma, lymphoma, rhabdomyosarcoma, and minor salivary gland tumors, cannot be distinguished by their MRI signal characteristics alone. In such cases, anatomic and clinical data, such as the origin of esthesioneuroblastoma in the upper nasal cavity and the occurrence of rhabdomyosarcoma in pediatric patients, are necessary in the differential diagnosis.

Benign Lesions

Inverted papilloma is an aggressive lesion that arises in the nares, expanding the nasal cavity and invading the adjacent maxillary and ethmoid sinuses. These lesions may recur after resection, and there is a known association with squamous cell carcinoma either at presentation or with recurrences. The signal characteristics of this lesion are nonspecific, and CT may help to assess the precise degree of bony destruction.

Nasopharyngeal (juvenile) angiofibroma (Fig. 9–2), the most common benign tumor of the nasopharynx, is seen in young male patients presenting with nasal obstruction or epistaxis. This tumor is thought to arise from the posterolateral wall of the nasal cavity and nasopharynx and may spread extensively via foramina and fissures of the skull base. Extension into the pterygopalatine fossa via the sphenopalatine foramen with anterior bowing of the posterior wall of the maxillary sinus is characteristic. There may be involvement of the sphenoid and ethmoid sinuses, infratemporal fossa, and orbit. Documentation of the extent of this lesion by axial imaging is crucial in management. In particular, intracranial extension greatly complicates surgical management and must be carefully evaluated. MRI is superior to CT in this regard because of the lack of artifact from dental fillings, the availability of high-resolution coronal and sagittal imaging, and the exquisite lesion contrast relative to the brain, extracranial fat, and muscle. This lesion may exhibit characteristic signal voids on MRI. This appearance, in association with clinical findings and typical anatomic involvement, can allow specific diagnosis in some cases by MRI. Nasopharyngeal angiofibromas exhibit marked enhancement after contrast administration, which helps evaluate the full extent of these infiltrating lesions. Noninvasive diagnosis is important because surgeons prefer not to biopsy these highly vascular masses.

Nasal polyps are hyperplastic lesions secondary to allergenic stimuli. They may become large enough to deform the nasal septum. Antrochoanal polyps have a typical appearance, arising in the maxillary antrum and extending into the posterior nasopharyngeal airway. There may be an associated deformity of bone.

A not uncommon benign lesion occurring in the nasopharynx is Tornwaldt's cyst, a well-defined, rounded structure in the midline of the posterior nasopharynx (Fig. 9–3). As is typical for a cystic lesion, Tornwaldt's cyst displays very high, homogeneous signal intensity on T_2-weighted images.

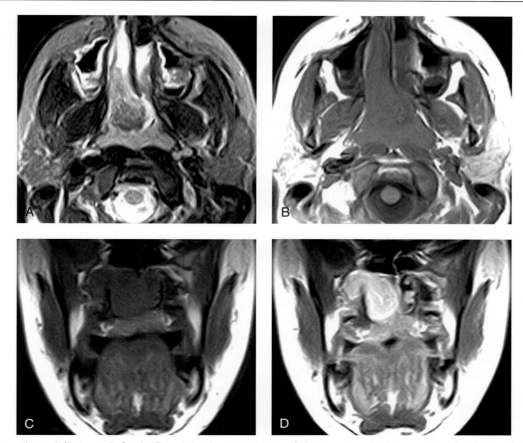

FIGURE 9–2. Juvenile angiofibroma. *A*, On the T_2-weighted scan, a large soft tissue mass with intermediate signal intensity fills the nasal passages and nasopharynx. Inflammatory changes are noted in the maxillary sinuses bilaterally. On precontrast axial (*B*) and coronal (*C*) T_1-weighted scans, the mass is isointense with muscle. *D*, After contrast administration, there is intense lesion enhancement. Abnormal soft tissue expanding the right pterygopalatine fossa is well seen on the postcontrast scan. The borders of the lesion are also best delineated postcontrast.

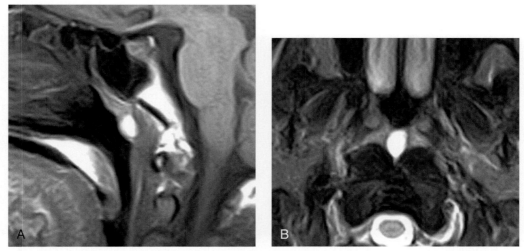

FIGURE 9–3. Tornwaldt's cyst. A small round lesion of increased signal intensity is identified in the midline in the posterior nasopharyngeal recess on the sagittal T_1-weighted image (*A*). No abnormal contrast enhancement was noted (image not shown). *B*, The cyst is hyperintense on the axial T_2-weighted scan. Tornwaldt's cyst is a common incidental finding (4% incidence in autopsy series) occurring in the midline. The cyst arises from the notochordal remnant in the posterior nasopharyngeal vault and is lined by respiratory epithelium. Tornwaldt's cysts are seen on magnetic resonance imaging as oval, well-circumscribed high-signal-intensity masses on T_2-weighted images. These lesions are usually of slightly increased signal intensity on T_1-weighted images, but the signal intensity can vary from hyperintense to hypointense.

Parapharyngeal Space

The parapharyngeal space is marginated by the pharyngobasilar fascia medially, the mandible and pterygoid muscles laterally, the prevertebral fascia posteriorly, and the pterygoid plates anteriorly. It may be further subdivided into prestyloid and poststyloid (or carotid sheath) spaces. Masses in this space may develop insidiously because this is a relatively silent area clinically. The most common lesions of this space include neural tumors (e.g., schwannomas and neurofibromas), paragangliomas (e.g., glomus jugulare and vagale tumors), and benign or malignant salivary gland tumors, which may arise from the deep portion of the parotid gland or from minor salivary glands in the parapharyngeal space. Less common lesions are lymphoma, metastases, congenital second bronchial cleft cysts, and mesenchymal tumors, such as lipoma, liposarcoma, rhabdomyosarcoma, hemangioma, and hemangiopericytoma.

Diagnosis of glomus tumors is aided by knowledge of the typical areas where these tumors occur and their common appearance on MRI (Fig. 9–4). These lesions often exhibit characteristic foci of low signal intensity on both T_1- and T_2-weighted sequences. The signal intensity appearance is likely due to a combination of flow void from vessels and foci of fibrosis. These low-signal areas are easily seen on T_2-weighted images because they contrast with the high signal from the bulk of the tumor and from foci of flow-related enhancement in vessels. Glomus and neural tumors arise within the carotid sheath and tend to displace the carotid artery anteriorly and may displace the internal jugular vein posteriorly. Salivary gland tumors, arising in the prestyloid space, displace the carotid artery and jugular vein posteriorly.

Distinguishing between tumors of parotid and extraparotid origin in the prestyloid space is important for surgery. This may be accomplished by assessing the status of the parapharyngeal fat plane. If the fat plane is displaced medially or obliterated, tumor originating from the deep portion of the parotid is likely. If displaced laterally, clearly separating the lesion from the deep lobe of the parotid gland, an extraparotid origin may be assumed.

Infectious processes may extend into the parapharyngeal space from the petrous bone or tonsils. These are characterized by infiltration of the parapharyngeal tissue planes by intermediate- to high-signal-intensity material on T_2-weighted images. Frank abscess formation may be identified as a localized collection exhibiting the signal characteristics of fluid. Contrast administration (using a gadolinium chelate) is useful when infection is questioned. Abscess formation is simple to recognize postcontrast, with enhancement of a rim of tissue surrounding a nonenhancing necrotic center. In the setting of infection, the extent of surrounding inflammation is also clearly identified by abnormal contrast enhancement.

OROPHARYNX
Squamous Cell Carcinoma

This is the most common oral and oropharyngeal condition referred for MRI evaluation. Oropharyngeal carcinoma may be relatively occult clinically. It can present initially with referred pain distant to the oral cavity (e.g., otalgia) or with metastatic cervical adenopathy. More commonly, the lesion will be diagnosed by the referring clinician in the course of an evaluation of an oral mass or localized pain or by the dentist during a routine oral examination or an examination for ill-fitting dentures. An evaluation of the extent of disease may then be requested. Local submucosal invasion of lesions of the tongue, tongue base, and floor of the mouth may be quite deceiving clinically. MRI can accurately assess the degree of local involvement or midline spread, a very

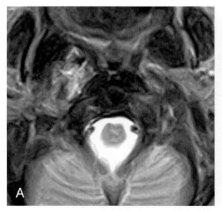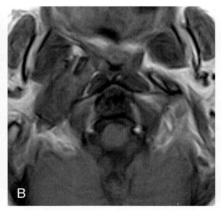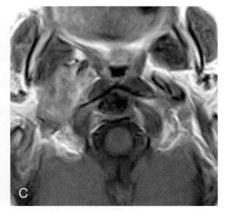

FIGURE 9–4. Carotid body tumor. T_2- (A), precontrast T_1- (B), and postcontrast T_1-weighted (C) images reveal a large lesion in the right carotid sheath at the skull base. The tumor has inhomogeneous signal intensity on both T_2- and T_1-weighted images precontrast (to some extent the characteristic salt-and-pepper appearance) and demonstrates prominent enhancement. Glomus tumors, also called paragangliomas or chemodectomas, are slow growing, usually benign hypervascular neoplasms that arise from neural crest cell derivatives. In the head and neck region, common locations include the middle ear (glomus tympanicum), jugular fossa (glomus jugulare), inferior ganglion of the vagus nerve (glomus vagale), and carotid bifurcation (carotid body tumor). These tumors tend to contain a moderate amount of fibrous stroma separating a few large vascular channels. After contrast administration, enhancement is almost immediate with a slow washout.

important factor in deciding whether a lesion is resectable.

The likelihood of widespread disease depends on the anatomic site of origin of oropharyngeal carcinoma. More than 75% of lesions of the tonsillar regions and base of the tongue and more than 40% of lesions of the retromolar trigone and soft palate exhibit metastatic adenopathy at presentation. Adenopathy most commonly affects the submandibular and high anterior cervical chain, later extending to the middle and lower anterior cervical and posterior triangle nodes. Contralateral adenopathy is commonly seen (20%–30%), with lesions arising in midline structures, such as the soft palate and tongue base. Thus, imaging of oropharyngeal carcinoma has multiple roles similar to those in the nasopharynx: searching for an occult primary lesion, evaluating the extent of local invasion of a lesion diagnosed clinically, evaluating regional nodes, and assessing involvement of adjacent blood vessels.

MRI has a distinct advantage over CT in the evaluation of the oropharynx. The image is not as severely degraded by dental amalgam, although local field distortions may occur. The additional imaging planes offered by MRI can also be very useful in the oral cavity and oropharynx. Lesions of the tongue, floor of the mouth, and palate are often best defined in the coronal plane. The sagittal plane is the least useful for anatomic definition, although it may help in evaluating midline lesions.

The signal characteristics of oropharyngeal carcinoma are nonspecific: low or intermediate signal on T_1-weighted and intermediate or high signal on T_2-weighted images. Both types of images are necessary for complete evaluation. Oropharyngeal carcinoma may exhibit submucosal spread in all directions from the site of the primary tumor, and the precise extent of involvement must be assessed for the purposes of radiation or surgical therapy. Extensive invasion of the tongue is common with lesions of the tongue base and floor of the mouth, and the extent of tongue involvement is especially important for assessing the morbidity of surgical resection. Lesions of the retromolar trigone, palate, tonsil, and posterior oropharynx may extend into the pterygopalatine fossa, pterygoid muscles, and parapharyngeal space. Invasion of adjacent bony structures, such as the mandible, maxilla, and skull base, can be assessed by discontinuity of the cortical signal void and loss of the normal high signal of the marrow fat on T_1-weighted images. The coronal plane is especially helpful in assessing bony involvement of the maxilla and skull base. Superficial tumor, as in the nasopharynx, may be impossible to identify or to differentiate from normal asymmetry, but this is not a serious limitation because it is usually apparent clinically.

Examination of the posttreatment patient is complicated by the resulting architectural distortion and fibrosis. CT has not shown great reliability in distinguishing fibrosis from recurrent tumor; MRI is superior in this regard. On T_2-weighted images, recurrent tumor tends to have high signal intensity, whereas fibrosis is generally isointense with muscle. However, edema, infection, and inflammatory adenopathy may also demonstrate increased signal on T_2-weighted images, reducing the

specificity of this finding. Squamous cell carcinoma does demonstrate contrast enhancement after gadolinium chelate administration. This finding may also aid in distinguishing recurrent or residual tumor from scar. MRI performed 4 months or more after radiation therapy appears to be a reliable tool to differentiate residual tumor from scar tissue. Scar is generally hypointense on T_2-weighted images and does not display enhancement as opposed to residual tumor, which is hyperintense on T_2-weighted images and enhances after administration of a gadolinium chelate. Caution is indicated in image interpretation because signal changes and enhancement, resulting from postradiation changes alone, can persist for months after radiation therapy.

Minor Salivary Gland Tumors

The sublingual glands in the floor of the mouth rarely give rise to tumors, although 80% of those that do occur are malignant. The more common site of origin of oral salivary gland tumors is the minor salivary glands, scattered throughout the mouth and oropharynx but most numerous in the hard and soft palate. Approximately 40% of these tumors are benign (i.e., preponderantly of the benign mixed type), and 60% are malignant (i.e., adenoid cystic carcinoma, adenocarcinoma, and mucoepidermoid carcinoma are the most frequent types). Salivary gland tumors typically present as smooth, rounded masses without ulceration, unlike the ulcerated, exophytic appearance of typical squamous cell carcinomas. Although irregular local extension is characteristic of the malignant tumors, with the adenoid cystic variety typically invading along neural pathways, the benign and malignant types cannot be reliably distinguished on the basis of imaging alone. The MRI signal characteristics of all these tumors are nonspecific. Although these lesions tend to have a higher signal intensity than squamous cell carcinomas on T_2-weighted images, there is a significant amount of overlap, and this differentiation cannot be made reliably on the basis of signal intensity alone.

Miscellaneous Benign Lesions

Benign cystic lesions of the mouth and oropharynx are commonly encountered, and MRI may be requested to evaluate their nature and extent. Cystic lesions may arise as a result of mucus extravasation from salivary ducts, from partial obstruction of salivary ducts with resulting cystic dilatation, from epithelial inclusions (i.e., lymphoepithelial cyst), or from cystic dilatation of thyroglossal duct remnants in the base of the tongue (i.e., thyroglossal duct cyst). All of these lesions may be expected to show the characteristic signs of cysts on MRI: low intensity on T_1-weighted images and high intensity on T_2-weighted images. However, high intensity on T_1-weighted images can be seen if the fluid contents are hemorrhagic or proteinaceous, and very high, homogeneous signal intensity on T_2-weighted images, on which cyst contents should equal the signal intensity of CSF.

A characteristic cystic lesion in the mouth is the ranula, which represents either a mucocele or mucus retention cyst of the sublingual glands (Fig. 9–5). The mucus

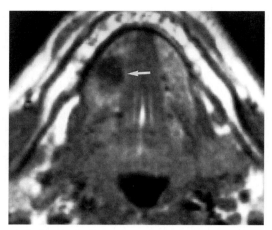

FIGURE 9–5. Ranula (sublingual cyst). A T$_1$-weighted axial image reveals a low-signal-intensity round lesion (*arrow*) in the right sublingual region. The signal intensity was that of fluid on all pulse sequences (images not shown). Ranulas are cystic lesions of the floor of the mouth caused by duct obstruction of a sublingual gland.

retention type, or simple ranula, presents as a smooth, fluctuant mass in the floor of the mouth and may be easily excised or marsupialized. The mucocele type, or plunging ranula, represents mucus extravasation from a sublingual duct and may exhibit extensive spread through the floor of the mouth to the submental area and even to the neck. Surgical treatment in this case is much more difficult, and MRI may help determine the extent of involvement of these lesions.

A variety of miscellaneous benign lesions may be seen. Lingual hemangiomas exhibit the signal characteristics of hemangiomas elsewhere in the body: low or intermediate signal intensity on T$_1$-weighted and very high signal intensity on T$_2$-weighted images (Fig. 9–6). Infections and abscesses in the tonsillar fossa or floor of the mouth show variable low intensity on T$_1$-weighted images and high intensity on T$_2$-weighted images depending on the degree of liquefaction.

MAJOR SALIVARY GLANDS

The major salivary glands include the parotid and submandibular glands. The sublingual glands were discussed with the oropharynx. By far, the leading indication for MRI examination of the major salivary glands is the evaluation of the location and extent of mass lesions. Chronic inflammatory diseases of the salivary glands remain the domain of sialography and, to a lesser extent, CT. Typically, slices 5 mm or less in thickness are obtained through the gland of interest. Although axial images usually supply most of the necessary information, coronal images often help in evaluating the salivary glands and surrounding structures.

Salivary tumors may arise in either the parotid or submandibular glands, although the most common site is the parotid. Three quarters of parotid tumors are benign, but submandibular tumors have an approximately 50% chance of malignancy. The majority of the

benign tumors of the parotid gland and virtually all in the submandibular gland are pleomorphic adenomas (Fig. 9-7). The other significant benign tumor of the parotid is adenolymphoma or Warthin's tumor. Multiplicity of masses favors Warthin's tumor. The unusual, benign mesenchymal masses, lipomas and hemangiomas, exhibit characteristic MRI features as in other areas of the body. Lipomas show very high signal intensity on T$_1$-weighted images and decreased signal on heavily T$_2$-weighted images (isointense with fat). Hemangiomas exhibit very high signal on T$_2$-weighted images, often with a characteristic multiseptated appearance.

The malignant masses include mucoepidermoid carcinoma, adenoid cystic carcinoma, adenocarcinoma, acinic cell tumors, squamous cell carcinoma, and the malignant variant of pleomorphic adenoma, malignant mixed tumors. These tumors are essentially indistinguishable by their MRI characteristics—intermediate intensity on T$_1$-weighted images and high intensity on T$_2$-weighted images—although pleomorphic adenomas are often quite low in signal intensity on T$_1$-weighted sequences.

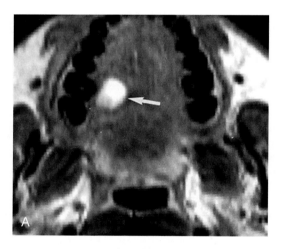

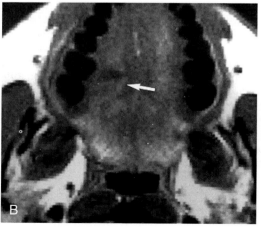

FIGURE 9–6. Hemangioma of the tongue. T$_2$- (*A*) and T$_1$-weighted (*B*) axial images reveal a lesion (*arrows*) lying within the tongue with characteristic very high signal intensity on the T$_2$-weighted exam. Hemangiomas consist of a proliferation of vascular endothelium, and thus vascular spaces, leading to their characteristic high signal intensity on T$_2$-weighted scans and intense enhancement postcontrast.

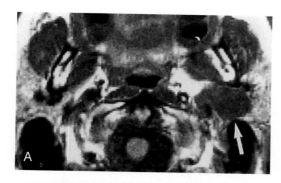

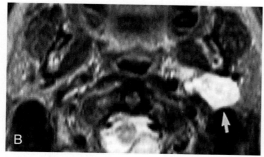

FIGURE 9-7. Pleomorphic adenoma of the deep portion of the left parotid gland. T_1- (*A*) and T_2-weighted (*B*) axial images reveal a parotid lesion (*arrows*) with nonspecific signal intensity characteristics, low on T_1 and high on T_2. The lack of a fat plane separating the tumor from the parotid gland indicates the origin of the lesion to be within the parotid as opposed to the parapharyngeal space.

The contrast of these lesions with the surrounding gland varies with its histologic composition. The relatively greater fat content of the parotid gland gives it higher signal on T_1-weighted images, often making parotid lesions easy to visualize on T_1-weighted images as lower signal intensity masses (similar to muscle) relative to the surrounding gland parenchyma. Contrast enhancement is seen with most primary salivary gland neoplasms.

Marked marginal irregularity and local infiltration favor malignancy, but smooth, regular margins do not ensure benignity. Facial nerve paralysis and pain are ominous signs for malignancy. Metastases, including lymphoma, not uncommonly affect the parotid gland probably because of numerous intraparotid and periparotid lymph nodes. These nodes drain the face and scalp and are commonly affected by squamous cell carcinomas or melanomas arising in these areas. The MRI appearance will be nonspecific, although multiplicity of lesions is characteristic. Warthin's tumor may also be multifocal and bilateral.

In the evaluation of parotid masses, it is crucial to assess whether the lesion involves the superficial or deep portions of the gland and the relationship of the facial nerve to the tumor, because these features dictate the surgical approach. The superficial and deep portions of the gland are separated by the intraparotid facial nerve, which courses anteriorly from the stylomastoid foramen and laterally to the retromandibular vein. Portions of the nerve may be more commonly seen with MRI than with CT, but even if the nerve is not visualized its relationship to a mass may be deduced from its expected

course. Thin cuts angled 30 to 40 degrees caudal to the orbitomeatal line demonstrate the nerve with greater reliability.

Tumors that extend from the superficial to the deep portions of the gland characteristically exhibit a waistlike narrowing as they pass between the styloid process and the mandibular condyle. It is important to assess whether deep masses originate in the parotid gland itself or in the parapharyngeal space. This distinction can usually be easily made on MRI by assessing the direction of displacement of the parapharyngeal fat plane: laterally in the case of parapharyngeal masses and medially in the case of deep parotid lesions. If the fat plane is obliterated, the determination cannot be made, but statistically a parotid origin is likely. The coronal plane often helps in evaluating this fat plane.

Although not a common primary indication for MRI of the salivary glands, inflammatory processes in the glands are important because they share the signal characteristics of tumors. They are usually more diffuse than tumors, but focal areas of inflammation or frank abscesses with irregular margins may mimic malignancy. Ductal ectasia may be seen secondary to ductal stenosis and calculi. Salivary duct calculi can be seen as foci of signal void on MRI but are much more reliably imaged with plain films, CT, or sialography. The parotid gland contains numerous lymph nodes. Normal, small nodes and enlarged, inflammatory nodes are commonly imaged during routine scans of the head and face and should not be mistaken for primary or metastatic tumors. The signal characteristics do not help this distinction, so caution must be exercised when small, nonpalpable masses are seen in or adjacent to the parotid gland. Occasionally, unilaterally or bilaterally hypertrophied masseter muscles are mistaken for parotid masses (on clinical exam). This distinction is easily made with MRI.

PARANASAL SINUSES
Benign Lesions

The high prevalence of incidentally discovered mucosal thickening in the sinuses is immediately evident to anyone beginning to interpret MRI scans of the head and face. This mucosal thickening exhibits very high signal intensity on T_2-weighted images. It may be localized to a portion of one sinus or involve all of the sinuses and tends to be more extensive in pediatric patients. The clinical relevance of this finding is often obscure, and in most of these patients the finding is of no pathologic significance.

Another lesion that is often seen as an incidental finding is a sinus retention cyst (Fig. 9–8). These cysts are usually located in the inferior aspect of the maxillary antrum, exhibit smooth, rounded borders, and have low signal on T_1-weighted images and characteristically very high signal on T_2-weighted images, identical to fluid. Because retention cysts tend to occupy the most inferior portion of the maxillary antrum, the film reader may be misled to believe that there is sinus fluid on the basis of the lower axial cuts. However, on higher axial slices, sinus fluid will exhibit an air-fluid level, and retention

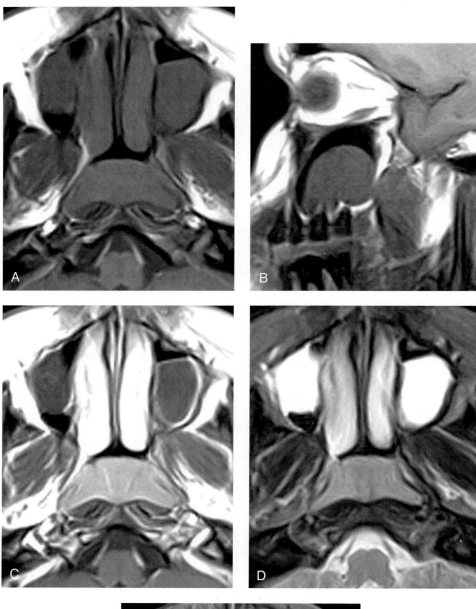

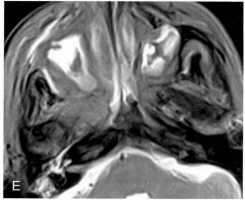

FIGURE 9–8. Large round masses (retention cysts) are identified in the right and left maxillary sinuses on the axial T_1-weighted image (A). B, The parasagittal T_1-weighted image reveals the mass in the left maxillary sinus to be oval in shape with a broad base along the inferior surface of the sinus. Intense peripheral enhancement of the left maxillary sinus mass and subtle peripheral enhancement of the right maxillary sinus mass is seen on the axial T_1-weighted image postcontrast (C). Both masses are hyperintense on the axial T_2-weighted image (D). In clinical practice, incidental sinus disease such as that illustrated is common. It is critical, however, not to be distracted and thus potentially overlook significant accompanying disease. E, A second patient who, on first glance, has bilateral inflammatory sinus disease. Closer inspection of this T_2-weighted image, however, reveals a soft tissue mass (squamous cell carcinoma) with intermediate signal intensity invading the wall of the right maxillary sinus and sphenoid wing.

FIGURE 9–9. Air-fluid level. On sagittal (*A*) and axial precontrast (*B*) T₁-weighted images, abnormal soft tissue is noted in the posterior portion of the left maxillary sinus. There is also inflammatory sinus disease in the right maxillary sinus, which is incidental to the point of this case. The abnormality in the dependent portion of the left maxillary sinus demonstrates marked hyperintensity on the axial T₂-weighted image (*C*). It is important to note that the interface between air anteriorly and the lesion posteriorly is a level horizontal plane, given the patient's positioning in the magnet (supine). That this interface is horizontal, together with the signal characteristics on the T₂-weighted scan, defines the abnormality as an air-fluid level. The peripheral margins of this dependent fluid collection enhance on the axial T₁-weighted image postcontrast (*D*). An important pitfall in image interpretation is that a retention cyst can mimic the appearance of an air-fluid level when viewed in only one plane.

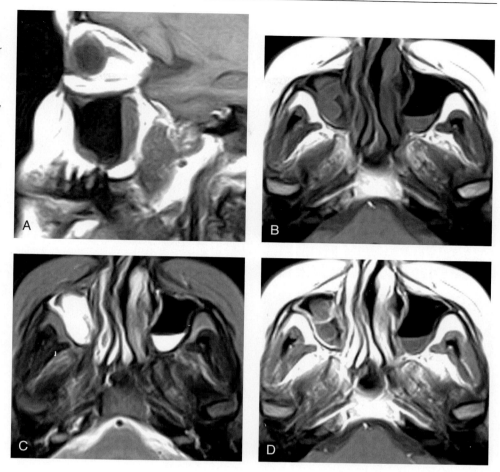

cysts have a rounded upper margin. In questionable cases, sagittal views should resolve the issue (Fig. 9–9). Sinus polyps are a much less common lesion and may be indistinguishable from retention cysts, appearing as smooth, well-defined lesions exhibiting high signal intensity on T₂-weighted images. Mucoperiosteal thickening and inflammation of the mucosal lining enhance markedly after contrast administration (Fig. 9–10). Retained secretions within a cyst or an obstructed sinus do not enhance.

Air-fluid levels, seen in acute sinusitis, are well visualized by MRI, especially on T₂-weighted images, on which the high-signal-intensity fluid exhibits the greatest contrast with air. An exception is sinus hemorrhage. Depending on its age, blood may exhibit the highest signal on T₁-weighted images. This has been reported after trauma and in patients with a blood coagulopathy. The granulomatous diseases that may affect the sinuses, including Wegener's granulomatosis, midline granuloma, sarcoidosis, and tuberculosis, exhibit nonspecific soft tissue signal intensities within the sinuses and may show variable amounts of bone destruction. The degree of bone destruction, however, is more easily appreciated on CT.

Mucoceles (Fig. 9–11) are common cystic expansile lesions involving the paranasal sinuses. Approximately 60% occur in the frontal sinuses and 30% in the ethmoid sinuses; lesions are less common in the maxillary and sphenoid sinuses. The anterior ethmoid air cells are more frequently affected than the posterior ethmoid air cells. Mucoceles are benign slow-growing masses that develop secondary to obstruction of the sinus ostium. They are lined by secretory respiratory columnar epithelium. As the mucosa secretes mucoid fluid, the mass enlarges slowly, expanding and eroding adjacent bony structures. A history of sinus disease, allergies, or trauma is elicited in many of these patients. MRI demonstrates mucoceles as well-defined, expansile paranasal sinus lesions that have variable signal intensity depending on fluid content. Mucoceles can be hyperintense on both T₁- and T₂-weighted sequences, low signal intensity on T₁-weighted sequences, and high signal intensity on T₂-weighted sequences or low signal intensity on both T₁- and T₂-weighted sequences. Increased signal intensity on T₁-weighted images is usually due to the proteinaceous composition of the fluid, although the same appearance can be caused by hemorrhage. As a mucocele ages, the relative water content of the secretions decreases, resulting in increased protein content. Low-signal-intensity mucoceles have been reported with fungal infections, particularly allergic aspergillus sinusitis. The variable signal characteristics of paranasal sinus mucoceles should not lead to confusion if greater emphasis is placed on the morphologic features of these lesions.

The fibro-osseous lesions of the sinuses exhibit decreased signal on both T₁- and T₂-weighted images.

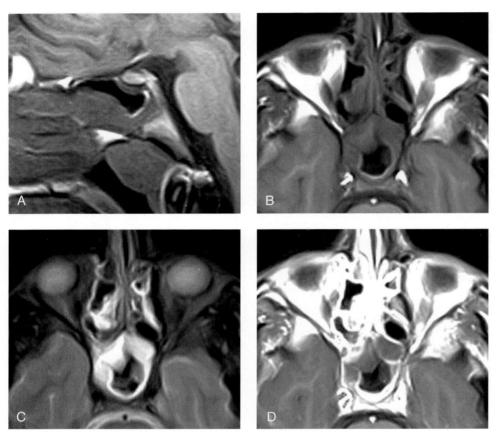

FIGURE 9–10. Mucosal membrane thickening. Abnormal hypointense soft tissue is seen along the periphery of the sphenoid sinus on sagittal (*A*) and axial (*B*) T_1-weighted images. The posterior ethmoid air cells also contain abnormal hypointense soft tissue. This material is of marked hyperintensity on the axial T_2-weighted image (*C*). Enhancement of the abnormal soft tissue is demonstrated on the axial T_1-weighted image postcontrast (*D*). The mucosal thickening is best seen along the posterior wall of the sphenoid sinus; several small retention cysts are noted anteriorly.

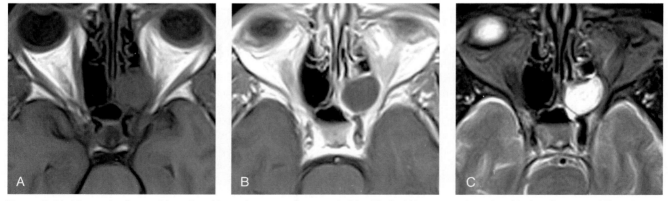

FIGURE 9–11. Mucocele. A round low-signal-intensity expansile mass is identified within a posterior ethmoid air cell on pre- (*A*) and postcontrast (*B*) T_1-weighted images. Peripheral enhancement of this mass is noted postcontrast (*B*). The lesion is of increased signal intensity on the T_2-weighted exam (*C*).

They may have foci of signal void as a result of areas of dense calcification, which is much easier to appreciate on CT. The aggressive benign lesions of the nose and nasopharynx (e.g., inverted papilloma and juvenile angiofibroma) commonly involve the sinuses, especially the maxillary antrum.

Malignant Lesions

The most common malignant lesion of the paranasal sinuses is squamous cell carcinoma. The hallmark of this lesion on all imaging studies is opacification of a sinus, usually the maxillary antrum, by soft tissue with associated bone destruction. The theoretical advantage of CT in delineating bony detail has not proved to be a significant drawback to MRI for sinus carcinoma. With careful evaluation of the signal voids from cortical bone surrounding the sinuses, bone erosion can almost always be evaluated adequately.

MRI has several advantages over CT. It more easily distinguishes tumor from retained secretions within an obstructed sinus (Fig. 9–12). On T_2-weighted images, retained secretions exhibit uniform very high signal intensity, which contrasts with the inhomogeneous, rela-

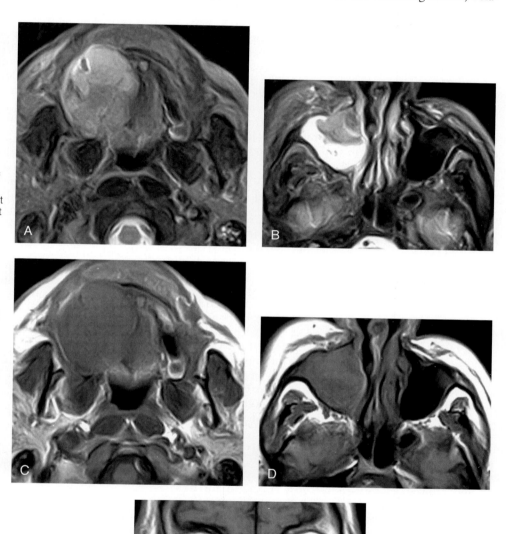

FIGURE 9–12. Squamous cell carcinoma of the maxillary sinus. *A* and *B*, A large soft tissue mass occupies the right maxillary sinus on T_2-weighted scans. *B*, On the more superior section, fluid (with marked hyperintensity) is seen posteriorly within the maxillary sinus; the tumor mass is distinct and anterior. *C* and *D*, On the corresponding T_1-weighted images, the mass is isointense with soft tissue. On the more inferior section (*C*), involvement of the right alveolar ridge can be noted, which is particularly evident by comparison with the normal left side. The posterior wall of the maxillary sinus is expanded but appears intact. By inspection of both axial and coronal (*E*) T_1-weighted images, involvement of both the hard and soft palate can be diagnosed. The coronal image also clearly demonstrates destruction of the floor and medial wall of the maxillary sinus. The symptoms of maxillary sinus carcinoma are similar to those of chronic sinusitis, often resulting in a delay in diagnosis. Common presenting symptoms include tissue swelling, nasal obstruction, nasal discharge, and epistaxis. The great majority of sinonasal tumors have intermediate signal intensity on T_2-weighted images; only approximately 5% are hyperintense. Inflammatory tissue in the sinuses consistently demonstrates marked hyperintensity on T_2-weighted images.

tively lower signal intensity of the tumor. Extension into surrounding spaces, such as the pterygopalatine fossa, infratemporal fossa, parapharyngeal space, and anterior and middle cranial fossae, is more easily evaluated by MRI. Coronal and sagittal T_2-weighted images are especially helpful in evaluating intracranial extension. T_1-weighted images are the most helpful in evaluating extension into fat-containing spaces, such as the pterygopalatine and infratemporal fossae and the parapharyngeal space. Axial images usually suffice in evaluating extension into these regions, but the coronal plane may be useful in assessing parapharyngeal space involvement.

Other rare malignancies of the paranasal sinuses include minor salivary gland tumors, rhabdomyosarcoma, plasmacytoma, and lymphoma. These tumors exhibit nonspecific findings on MRI, and the differential diagnosis depends on the patient's age, presentation, and biopsy. Metastases may also involve the paranasal sinuses. The most common primary carcinoma to metastasize is renal cell carcinoma followed by lung and breast carcinoma. In general, the appearance of these lesions is nonspecific, but highly vascular metastases like renal cell carcinoma may exhibit areas of flow-related signal void.

FACIAL SKELETON

This discussion is limited to the osseous abnormalities of the facial skeleton, with special attention to the mandible and maxilla. Abnormalities of the paranasal sinuses and temporomandibular joints have been discussed in the appropriate sections. MRI can make a significant contribution to the study of abnormalities of the facial skeleton. Despite the ability of CT to define cortical bone precisely, many pathologic processes of bone predominantly affect the medullary cavity, with later destruction or thinning of the cortex. Most of the work on skeletal MRI has been done on the spine and extremities, and this experience has shown MRI to be much more sensitive to medullary abnormalities than CT. In addition, MRI better demonstrates extraosseous soft tissue extension. These principles can be extended to the examination of the facial skeleton.

The multiplanar capabilities of MRI are very useful in evaluating the complex spatial anatomy of the facial skeleton without requiring the patient to assume difficult or uncomfortable positions in the scanner. In addition to a routine initial sagittal scan to serve as a localizer, axial and coronal images are typically obtained. Although the axial images are usually best suited for evaluating the mandible, pathologic processes affecting the maxilla or zygoma may be better appreciated in the coronal plane. This is especially true of the palate, which may be quite difficult to evaluate in the axial plane because of partial volume effects. A slice thickness of 4 to 5 mm is adequate for evaluating most bony abnormalities.

As in other areas of the body, both heavily T_1- and T_2-weighted sequences are essential for evaluating the facial skeleton. Osseous abnormalities are often appreciated as areas of relatively lower signal intensity against the high-signal background of fatty bone marrow on T_1-weighted images. There is typically a reversal of the relative signal intensities of bone marrow and abnormality on T_2-weighted images as a result of the relatively high signal of most pathologic processes. This effect is especially important in children, who typically have a more erythropoietic marrow and in whom the normal bone marrow may be lower in signal intensity on T_1-weighted images, producing less contrast with bone marrow abnormalities. Extraosseous involvement of adjacent facial musculature is also better appreciated on T_2-weighted images, although the status of the surrounding fat planes is more easily seen on T_1-weighted images.

The main pathologic categories of the facial skeleton that can be suitably evaluated with MRI include cystic, neoplastic, and inflammatory lesions. Trauma and congenital abnormalities of the facial skeleton remain the province of radiography and CT, with the exception of frontoethmoidal encephalocele, which is easily evaluated by MRI.

Cystic Lesions

Cystic lesions are especially common in the maxilla and mandible. Those of radiologic interest are of two main types: fissural and odontogenic. Radicular cysts secondary to dental caries rarely require cross-sectional imaging techniques. Fissural cysts (e.g., nasoalveolar cyst, globulomaxillary cyst, and incisive canal cyst) arise in regions of embryonic sutures in the maxilla and mandible. Odontogenic or follicular cysts arise from primordial tooth follicles and may or may not contain a tooth remnant (dentigerous cysts). Occasionally, odontogenic cysts develop a keratinizing epithelial lining, in which case they are referred to as odontogenic keratocysts.

The appearances of these lesions are indistinguishable by MRI. They typically exhibit low or intermediate signal intensity on T_1-weighted images and very high signal intensity on T_2-weighted images. Rarely, these lesions may exhibit high signal intensity on T_1-weighted images as well, possibly caused by high protein content or hemorrhage within the cyst. MRI possesses no definite advantages over CT in evaluating cystic lesions of the maxilla and mandible. In fact, the superior delineation of cortical bone on CT may make it easier to define a continuous, expanded cortical rim, allowing the diagnosis of a nonaggressive lesion.

Neoplastic Lesions

The facial bones are subject to the same osseous neoplasms as bones elsewhere in the body, such as fibrosarcoma, osteosarcoma, chondrosarcoma, lymphoma, myeloma, Ewing's sarcoma, metastatic tumors, eosinophilic granuloma, and giant cell tumor. In addition, the maxilla and mandible are subject to the unique ameloblastoma, a locally invasive tumor. These lesions exhibit the typical signal characteristics of tumors anywhere in the body: intermediate signal on T_1-weighted and increased signal on T_2-weighted images. These tumors typically exhibit the greatest contrast with normal bone marrow on T_1-weighted images. The margins of these lesions vary from well defined with indolent tumors to irregular and infiltrating with aggressive, malignant lesions. The patterns of ossification and calcification within an osseous neoplasm are better appreciated on CT and radiography because of the poor sensitivity of MRI to calcium. Densely calcified and fibrotic areas may be seen as foci of decreased signal on both T_1-weighted and T_2-weighted images.

Inflammatory Lesions

Osteomyelitis, which usually arises from infected teeth, most commonly affects the mandible. It can also be seen in the bony margins of the sinuses, complicating sinusitis. The MRI appearance is nonspecific, with infiltrating, ill-defined low signal on T_1-weighted and high signal on T_2-weighted images. Disruption of cortical bone may be seen, although CT is more sensitive in this regard. However, edema of the surrounding soft tissues is better appreciated on T_2-weighted MRI images than on CT. Contrast enhancement can be extensive in the surrounding soft tissues and can thus assist in differential diagnosis.

NECK

The basic imaging protocol for the neck begins with a sagittal short TR/short TE sequence, which functions as a "scout" image. However, in the case of midline lesions, it may also supply useful additional information. At some clinical sites, with high-field instrumentation, this has been replaced by a fast spin echo T_2-weighted sagittal scan. Axial short TR/short TE and long TR/long TE sequences are then obtained through the area of interest. The slice thickness on axial scans should be 5 mm or less. To provide an additional anatomic perspective, a coronal short TR/short TE sequence may be added.

Lymph Nodes

The lymph nodes of the neck are grouped by location. These include submental, submandibular, anterior jugular (associated with the anterior jugular vein, superficial to the strap muscles), juxtavisceral (associated with the thyroid gland and tracheoesophageal groove), internal jugular, and posterior triangle (spinal accessory). The internal jugular chain is further subdivided into high, middle, and low regions using the levels of the carotid bifurcation and cricoid cartilage as dividing lines. Lymph nodes can be involved by metastatic disease from carcinoma of the head and neck or from distant sites, by lymphoma, or by inflammatory disease.

MRI is as accurate as CT in assessing cervical lymph nodes. Axial T_1-weighted scans, of all planes and sequences, are the most useful for evaluating the cervical nodes. T_1-weighted scans provide high spatial resolution and clear demarcation between the nodes and surrounding fat. Occasionally, coronal scans may provide additional anatomic information. T_2-weighted scans can be helpful in separating nodes from the adjacent musculature; lymph nodes are usually of higher signal intensity.

As with CT, the most reliable criterion for diagnosing pathologic lymph nodes is that of enlargement, a crite-

rion that, unfortunately, has limitations in both sensitivity and specificity. A lymph node diameter of 1.0 cm or greater should be considered pathologic, with the exception of the submandibular and jugulodigastric regions, in which isolated nodes up to 1.5 cm in diameter may be normal. The jugulodigastric nodes are located at the point at which the posterior belly of the digastric muscle crosses the jugular vein, approximately at the junction of the high and middle internal jugular chains. Necrosis of any node, as indicated by fluid density on CT or fluid signal characteristics on MRI, should be considered pathologic. However, whether a particular pathologic node is involved by neoplastic or inflammatory disease cannot be assessed on the basis of imaging characteristics alone. Furthermore, microscopic nodal metastases remain beyond the reach of imaging diagnosis.

Primary head and neck tumors tend to metastasize to the submandibular, internal jugular, and posterior triangle chains. The most commonly involved site is the jugulodigastric node. In general, lesions of the oral cavity tend to spread to the submandibular, submental, and high to middle internal jugular chains, but lesions of the nasopharynx, hypopharynx, and supraglottic larynx may involve nodes at any level along the internal jugular chain and the posterior triangle nodes. Lesions of the tongue base and tonsillar fossa exhibit characteristics more like hypopharyngeal lesions than other lesions of the oral cavity. Nasopharyngeal carcinoma is noteworthy in having an especially high rate of bilateral nodal metastasis (>30%) and of metastatic disease at presentation (up to 90%), and imaging may play an important role in diagnosing the frequently occult primary lesion in the setting of cervical adenopathy.

Larynx and Hypopharynx

Low SNR, together with vascular and respiratory motion artifacts, has limited MRI of the larynx and hypopharynx. Newer coil technology, improved motion compensation techniques, and further decreases in scan time hold promise for improved imaging of this area. The submucosal fat planes throughout the hypopharynx and larynx are clearly depicted on T_1-weighted scans. The anatomic structures of the larynx and hypopharynx, including the epiglottis, laryngeal ventricle, true and false cords, and laryngeal skeleton, are clearly delineated with axial imaging. Additional imaging planes, such as the sagittal for evaluating the epiglottis and coronal for the glottis, can be helpful.

The true cords may be differentiated from the false cords on axial images using the same criteria as with CT. Unlike the false cords, the true cords do not have a submucosal fat plane on T_1-weighted images because they consist entirely of fibrous tissue and the vocalis muscles. The vocal process of the arytenoid cartilages is also a reliable marker of the true cords. The normal anterior commissure is less than 2 mm thick.

The laryngeal skeleton has a variable appearance on MRI images, depending on the state of ossification of the cartilages. In young patients, before significant ossification develops, the laryngeal cartilage exhibits intermediate signal intensity on both T_1-weighted and T_2-weighted scans. As calcification develops, foci of signal void can be seen, and once ossification is complete, a well-defined cortex with fatty marrow can be appreciated. Calcification and ossification of the cartilages occur in an irregular, although more or less symmetrical, pattern, which can make assessment of cartilage destruction problematic.

MRI has shown promise in evaluating squamous cell carcinoma and other lesions of the larynx. As with CT, the primary role of MRI in this disease is assessing submucosal extension before surgery or radiation. Of all scan techniques, T_1-weighted sequences are often the most useful because of the high contrast between the intermediate signal tumor and high signal submucosal fat. In addition, T_1-weighted scans tend to be less degraded by motion artifacts and to have higher SNR. T_1-weighted scans are also more sensitive for detecting enlarged cervical lymph nodes. T_2-weighted images should be obtained as an adjunct because they may help delineate relatively high-signal-intensity tumor from the surrounding normal musculature. Both T_1-weighted and T_2-weighted scans need to be carefully examined to assess involvement of the laryngeal skeleton. Even so, definitive assessment may be impossible in the presence of irregularly calcified or ossified cartilages.

MRI can help in evaluating the postoperative or postradiation patient. On T_2-weighted images, posttreatment fibrosis tends to be very low in signal intensity, with recurrent tumor of intermediate or high signal intensity. Areas of recurrent tumor may exhibit enhancement after contrast administration (using a gadolinium chelate).

Thyroid and Parathyroid

The role of MRI in evaluating parathyroid lesions has been investigated in several reports. Parathyroid adenomas characteristically exhibit high signal intensity on T_2-weighted images. This and their typical location posterior to the lobes of the thyroid gland (or ectopically in the superior anterior mediastinum) allow recognition. They exhibit intermediate signal intensity on T_1-weighted images, allowing differentiation from cystic lesions. Although high-resolution ultrasonography can detect adenomas, it is quite limited for evaluating postoperative patients and those with ectopic parathyroid glands. MRI may make significant contributions in the evaluation of hyperparathyroidism. However, high-resolution MRI scans with excellent SNR is required for the evaluation of these small lesions on T_2-weighted images.

Imaging of the thyroid gland currently is performed with high-resolution ultrasonography and nuclear medicine techniques. These are usually sufficient for the routine evaluation of benign thyroid disease. Nevertheless, benign thyroid lesions are quite common and are often seen on neck images obtained for other indications. The normal thyroid gland is of intermediate signal intensity on T_1-weighted scans and mildly hyperintense on T_2-weighted scans. Thyroid adenomas may exhibit slightly decreased intensity on T_1-weighted sequences and markedly increased intensity on T_2-weighted images. Cystic areas show marked hypointensity on T_1-weighted images and even greater hyperintensity on T_2-weighted images. If hemorrhage is present in the lesion, it may be hyperintense on T_1-weighted sequences. A multinodular goiter is visualized as an enlarged thyroid with lobulated contours and heterogeneous signal intensity on all imaging sequences, depending on the ratio of normal to adenomatous and cystic areas.

Thyroid carcinoma is indistinguishable from benign disease based on signal characteristics alone. Local invasion, nodal metastases, and vascular involvement can be detected. MRI may have a role in evaluating postoperative recurrence because there is evidence that postoperative fibrosis may be detectable based on its low signal intensity on T_2-weighted images compared with the higher signal intensity of recurrent tumor.

Miscellaneous Lesions

The role of MRI in disorders of the neck other than carcinoma and lymphadenopathy has not been widely evaluated. Cystic lesions exhibit typical fluid characteristics—homogeneous, low signal on T_1-weighted and very high signal on T_2-weighted images—allowing easy recognition. Complex cysts, such as those containing hemorrhagic, proteinaceous, or infected fluid, may have unusual signal characteristics, most commonly intermediate or high signal on T_1-weighted images. Branchial cleft cysts, thyroglossal duct cysts, and cystic hygromas may be differentiated by their characteristic locations in the anterior triangle, midline, and posterior triangle, respectively. Cystic hygromas also typically exhibit a more infiltrative growth pattern with multiple septations. Hemangiomas and other mesenchymal tumors show the same MRI appearances as in other areas of the body. Infection demonstrates infiltration of fat and muscle planes with foci of fluid signal intensity corresponding to liquefaction and abscess formation.

The carotid artery and jugular vein are clearly visualized on axial images. Partial volume effects can limit depiction on coronal and sagittal images. The presence of flow void within these vessels on spin echo images is diagnostic of patency, but various flow-related artifacts, such as inflow enhancement and even echo rephasing, may make the interpretation of intraluminal signal problematic. Single-slice gradient echo techniques (two-dimensional time of flight), which produce a bright signal from flowing blood, frequently help in this situation. Arteriovenous malformations can be identified as complexes of vessels with predominant signal voids on spin echo images but with varying degrees of intraluminal signal as a result of foci of thrombosis and flow-related artifact. Gradient echo images clearly demonstrate the patent vessels.

10

Chest

Günther Schneider

BREAST

Since the introduction of magnetic resonance imaging (MRI) in the early 1980s, its use for tissue characterization has been based on measured T_1 and T_2 values using the signal intensity on so called T_1-weighted and T_2-weighted images. The signal intensities and the underlying T_1 and T_2 tissue parameters mainly depend on the content of water as modified by the tissue content, including specifically fibrosis, cells, fluid, or protein content, and thus vary among different tissues. However, these parameters do not correlate with the biological nature of a tumor. There is a significant overlap in T_1 and T_2 characteristics between benign and malignant lesions of the breast; therefore, these fundamental tissue characteristics play no major role in the evaluation of malignant lesions of the breast and in differentiation of breast cancer from other benign lesions. However, unenhanced MRI using T_2-weighted images has been shown to be extremely useful for detecting and evaluating breast implant rupture.

The introduction of contrast-enhanced (CE) MRI was a major breakthrough in the diagnosis of breast tumors, based on the observation that gadolinium (Gd)-DTPA enhances virtually all cancers more than minimal glandular breast tissue. However, although the majority of malignant tumors enhance, significant overlap exists between enhancing benign and malignant tissues. Thus, it is generally recommended to combine CE MRI of the breast with x-ray mammography.

To achieve the necessary image quality in MRI of the breast, the use of a dedicated breast coil is mandatory. Both single-breast coils and newer coils that allow imaging of both breasts exist. The advantages of imaging of both breasts in a double-breast coil include the possibility of detecting multicentric carcinoma, the simultaneous evaluation of bilateral unclear breast diseases, and the additional diagnostic information resulting from the comparison of both breasts.

The slice thickness in imaging of the breast should not exceed 4 mm. The optimal slice thickness seems to be approximately 2 mm with an in-plane resolution of 1 mm or less. To allow direct comparison and subtraction of pre- and postcontrast T_1-weighted images, it is essen-

tial that the patient lie still during the entire examination. Usually the patients are studied in the prone position, which helps to reduce breast motion caused by respiration. Depending on the direction of the phase-encoding gradient, cardiac artifacts that increase after the administration of contrast medium may cross the left breast or both axillae in axial images. Thus, imaging in the sagittal or coronal plane may occasionally be necessary to detect a suspected lesion near the thoracic wall or in the axilla.

Usually a T_2-weighted sequence, either spin echo or fast spin echo, is acquired before the CE studies, because T_2-weighted images allow differentiation of cysts or fibrous fibroadenomas from other well-circumscribed lesions. For the CE T_1-weighted studies, optimally a fast three-dimensional (3D) gradient echo sequence should be used, because these are most sensitive for visualization of paramagnetic contrast medium. To allow later subtraction of CE from nonenhanced images, first an unenhanced T_1-weighted scan of the breast should be performed followed by the injection of a Gd chelate, usually at a dose of 0.1 to 0.2 mmol/kg body weight. Contrast injection should be followed by a flush of at least 20 ml saline to achieve reproducible administration of the entire amount of contrast medium. Immediately after contrast medium injection, serial acquisitions of the T_1-weighted fast 3D gradient echo sequence are performed. The optimal temporal resolution, which is given by the acquisition time of the sequence, is between 1 and 2 minutes. Up to five acquisitions should be performed after the injection of contrast medium.

To eliminate the high signal intensity of fat, which occasionally interferes with the detection of small enhancing lesions, subtraction of the unenhanced images from the CE studies should be performed. This also allows detection of small enhancing lesions. Other techniques that allow elimination of the fat signal include selective fat saturation and selective water excitation. However, with these techniques, signal inhomogeneities may occur because of inhomogeneities of the magnetic field. Thus, the use of image subtraction is a more robust approach for the evaluation of enhancing breast lesions in routine clinical practice.

Imaging studies of the breast in premenopausal patients should be performed between days 6 and 16 of the menstrual cycle because focal or diffuse enhancement within normal tissue as a result of hormonal stimulation outside this time interval may obscure recognition of enhancing lesions or mimic malignant changes. The same observation concerning enhancing lesions is true for postmenopausal patients who are receiving hormone replacement therapy.

In addition to qualitative morphologic information achieved on T_1-weighted CE and subtracted images, quantitative image analysis can be performed. If significant enhancement of a breast lesion is observed, quantitative analysis of the dynamic enhancement may provide important additional information.

Findings indicative of malignancy include morphologic observations, such as irregular contours and enhancement that follows the ducts or starts from the periphery, as well as quantitative observations, such as very fast enhancement in the first sequence after contrast media injection followed by a plateau phase or even a washout. Imaging findings that are more indicative of a benign disease include well-circumscribed contours of an enhancing lesion, diffuse patchy enhancement, typical septations within a well-circumscribed lesion, and a slow rise of enhancement on quantitative analysis.

Candidates for CE MRI of the breast include patients with scarring that is difficult to assess in x-ray mammography or ultrasonography after limited surgery, those with silicon implants, and those who have had limited surgery and irradiation. CE MRI of the breast should be performed no sooner than 6 months after therapeutic procedures. Otherwise, artifacts resulting from surgery or decreased microcirculation from irradiation or chemotherapy may alter the diagnosis. CE MRI should also be used to evaluate patients at high risk for breast carcinoma who have dense breasts, which ultrasonography and x-ray mammography cannot adequately assess, to rule out multifocal or multicentric disease in patients with proven malignancy (Fig. 10-1), to search for a primary tumor if other methods are negative in the detection of a focal breast lesion, and to monitor neoadjuvant therapy. CE MRI of the breast is not recommended for the screening of dense breasts, for differentiation of inflammation and carcinoma, and for differentiation of lesions with microcalcifications detected on x-ray mammography.

Cysts

Ultrasonography remains the principal method for the diagnosis of cysts because it is far more cost effective than MRI. Nevertheless, cysts are often detected incidentally in MRI of the breast performed for other reasons. Histologically, simple cysts present as retained fluid surrounded by a thin wall. On T_1-weighted unenhanced images, simple cysts have low to intermediate signal intensity. However, the signal intensity in T_1-weighted images may vary with the amount of proteinaceous fluid within the cyst, which can increase the signal intensity on T_1-weighted images. In the same way, complicated cysts that contain blood may have increased signal intensity, resulting in a hyperintense appearance

on T_1-weighted images. On T_2-weighted sequences, the signal intensity of the cyst fluid is usually very high, exceeding that of fat. In CE T_1-weighted studies, simple cysts do not show an enhancement. If irregular or nodular enhancement of the cyst wall is evident, cystic necrosis of a malignant tumor, necrosis of a papilloma, and an intracystic carcinoma have to be considered in the differential diagnosis.

Parenchymal Proliferation and Fibrocystic Disease

In x-ray mammography, fibrocystic changes and parenchymal proliferation are characterized by increased density of the breast compared with age-related normal breast tissue. Fibrocystic disease is caused by an increased proliferation of fibrous mesenchymal or glandular tissue and is frequently associated with cysts. Proliferative changes include lobular, ductal, and papillary hyperplastic changes and adenosis. Hormones may play a role in its development, but the exact pathogenesis remains unclear. Parenchymal proliferation and fibrocystic disease may simulate the clinical and radiographic appearance of focal or diffusely growing carcinomas. The increased radiographic density of the breast also impairs mammographic detection of malignancies without microcalcifications. In approximately 5% of the cases in which atypias are present in proliferative changes, a strongly increased risk to develop malignancy exists.

On unenhanced T_1-weighted images fibrocystic disease has low signal intensity, whereas on T_2-weighted images the signal intensity may vary depending on the amount of water present in the tissue. The amount of cystic areas also contributes to an increase of signal intensity on T_2-weighted sequences. If CE MRI is performed during the second or third week of the menstrual cycle, normal breast tissue and nonproliferative dysplasias in middle-aged and older patients show little enhancement. This important imaging finding can be used to exclude malignant disease.

Proliferative dysplasia and adenosis may enhance to a variable degree (Fig. 10-2). In most cases of proliferative dysplasia or adenosis, the enhancement is diffusely distributed with a patchy signal increase within large parts of the breast tissue. In regard to quantitative dynamic analysis, usually a delayed signal intensity increase is observed. In patients with proliferative dysplasia, only absence of enhancement allows exclusion of invasive malignancy with high probability. If diffuse enhancement is present, carcinomas that enhance slowly or diffusely cannot be ruled out. Alternatively, focally enhancing proliferative dysplasia sometimes can mimic malignancy.

Fibroadenoma

Fibroadenomas represent the most common breast tumor. Histologically, these lesions vary from completely fibrosed to adenomatous to myxoid tissue composition. On T_2-weighted images, the signal intensity of fibroadenomas reflects the specific histologic pattern present in an individual fibroadenoma. Whereas fibrous

Text continued on page 250

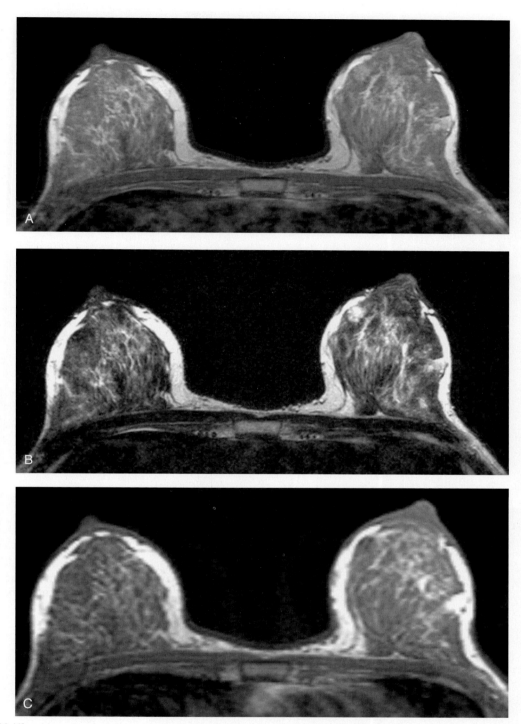

Figure 10–1. Multifocal invasive ductal carcinoma. Proton density (A) and T$_2$-weighted (B) images show a high-signal-intensity (SI) mass in the left breast. Additionally, dense tissue in both breasts consistent with proliferative dysplasia can be noted. In the T$_1$-weighted unenhanced image (C), the mass is low SI.

Illustration continued on following page

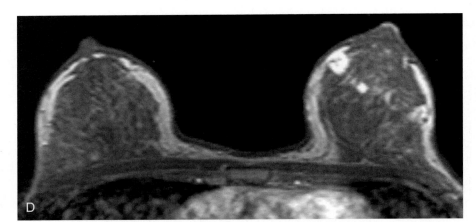

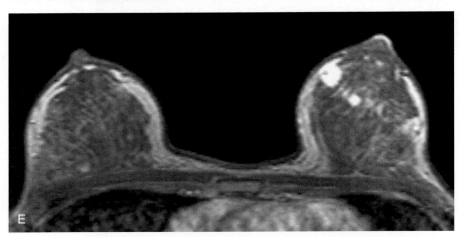

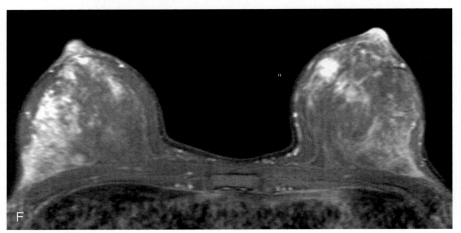

FIGURE 10–1 *Continued.* One minute (*D*) and 5 minutes (*E*) after contrast injection, a strongly enhanced lesion and a more centrally located second tumor are visible. *F,* The T_1-weighted, fat-saturated, contrast-enhanced image also displays both enhancing lesions; however, because of field inhomogeneity, the signal within the field of view is inhomogeneous.

FIGURE 10-1 *Continued. G,* The subtraction image clearly displays both lesions and shows the tumors to be rather well-circumscribed. However, in quantitative assessment of contrast dynamics (*H*), a strong increase of SI in the first minute after contrast administration is noted, and a washout is demonstrated starting 3 minutes after injection.

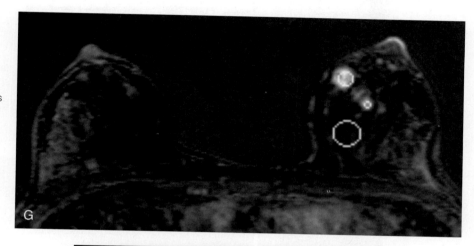

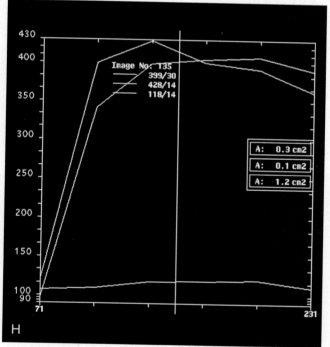

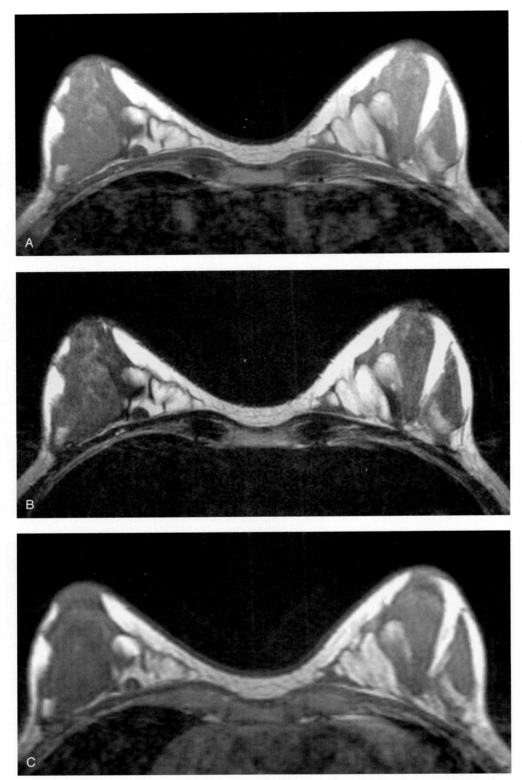

Figure 10–2. Proliferative dysplasia. Unenhanced proton density (*A*), T$_2$-weighted (*B*), and T$_1$-weighted (*C*) images show dense tissue of both breasts with diffuse delayed enhancement on T$_1$-weighted contrast-enhanced

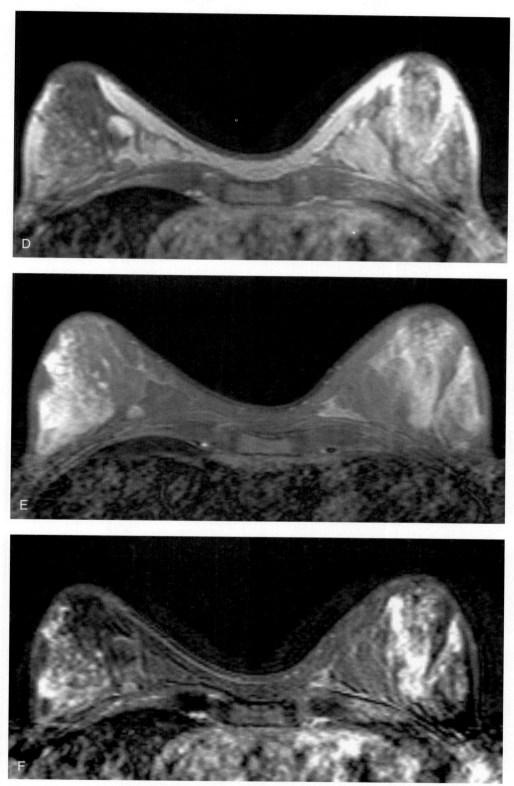

FIGURE 10–2 *Continued.* (*D*) and T$_1$-weighted fat-saturated contrast-enhanced (*E*) images. The enhancement is best appreciated in the subtracted image (*F*), and the increasing enhancement suggests proliferative changes. However, magnetic resonance imaging cannot rule out the presence of malignancy in enhancing breast tissue.

fibroadenomas, which consist of densely packed collagen, have a low signal intensity, adenomatous or myxoid fibroadenomas may have increased signal intensity on T_2-weighted images. Because other well-circumscribed malignancies such as medullary or mucinous carcinomas have similar signal intensity on T_2-weighted images, a distinction between these malignant lesions and adenomatous or myxoid fibroadenomas is not possible. In T_1-weighted images, fibroadenomas usually have low signal intensity. On CE MRI, fibrous fibroadenomas enhance very little. Thus, using the findings on enhanced scans, lesions that have low signal intensity on T_2-weighted images can be distinguished from malignant disease. However, adenomatous or myxoid fibroadenomas do enhance, and although the enhancement is typically delayed, the distinction from malignant lesions is not reliable (Fig. 10-3). On T_2-weighted images, another characteristic finding of a fibroadenoma is a round or oval lobulation in a focal breast lesion. If this lobulation can be demonstrated on T_2-weighted images, a fibroadenoma is very likely.

Breast Cancer

Breast cancer represents the most common malignant tumor in women and is the leading cause of death in women between the age of 40 and 60 years. Whereas in

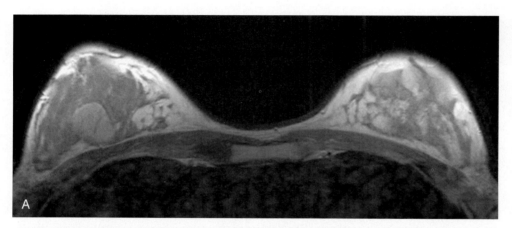

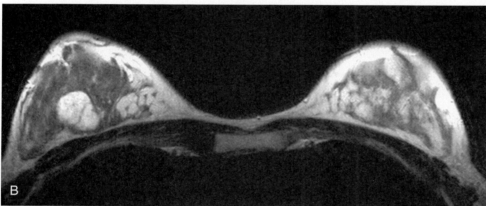

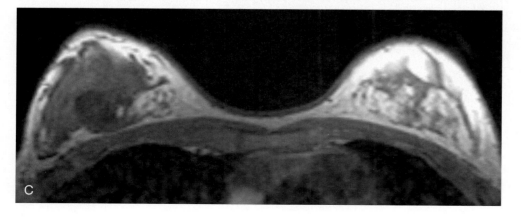

FIGURE 10–3. Myxoid fibroadenoma. Proton density (*A*) and T_2-weighted (*B*) images show a well-circumscribed hyperintense lesion of the right breast. *C,* On the T_1-weighted unenhanced image, the lesion shows low signal intensity. In dynamic imaging

FIGURE 10–3 *Continued.* (*D–H*, 1 minute to 5 minutes after contrast injection), a strong but delayed enhancement can be noted. The strong enhancement and the distinct borders of the lesion are best displayed in the subtracted image (*I*), and quantification of contrast uptake shows delayed enhancement (*J*). However, magnetic resonance imaging does not allow a confident distinction from a well-circumscribed malignancy.

Illustration continued on following page

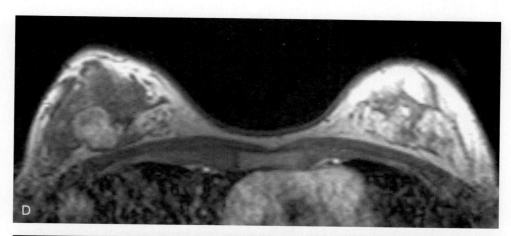

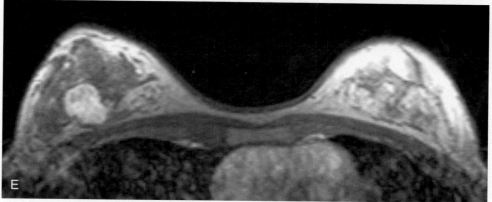

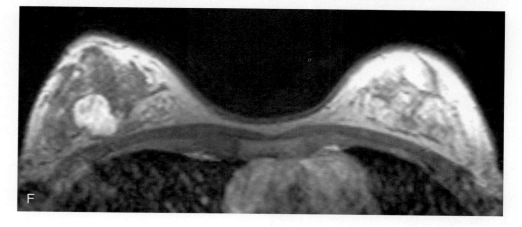

FIGURE 10–3 *Continued.*

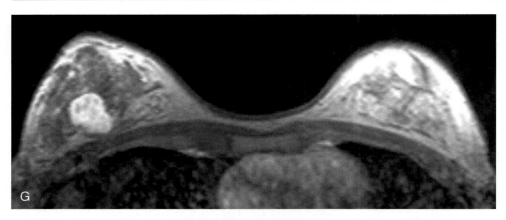

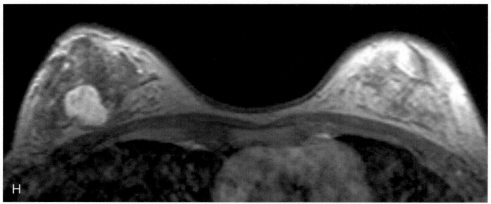

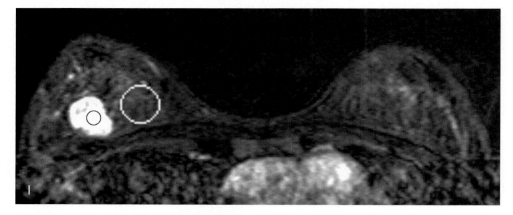

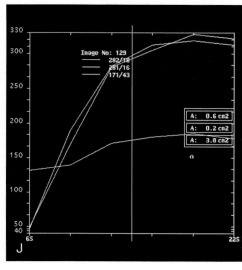

situ carcinomas may never become invasive, only invasive carcinomas have the risk of metastatic spread, which increases with tumor size and histologic grade. Noninvasive in situ carcinoma and invasive carcinoma are distinguished by the integrity of the basal membrane. Approximately 30% of invasive carcinomas show microcalcifications. Many invasive cancers tend to be irregular and show dull borders and thus can be detected by means of x-ray mammography. Identification of carcinomas without microcalcification is influenced by the appearance of surrounding fat or glandular tissue. Detection and diagnosis are impaired in dense breast tissue. The majority of in situ carcinomas in contrast are detected because of microcalcifications.

On unenhanced MRI, carcinomas have low signal intensity on T_1-weighted images and variable signal intensity on T_2-weighted images. Because benign tissue may have signal intensities similar to that of breast cancer, T_2-weighted images and unenhanced MRI do not allow a specific diagnosis. However, morphologic signs of malignancies, such as scarring, may sometimes be displayed very accurately in unenhanced images. CE MRI gives valuable additional information in the evaluation of breast cancer, because the majority of invasive carcinomas show stronger enhancement than normal glandular tissue or fat. Typical signs of malignant lesions are irregular circumscribed focal lesions that show generally a fast and strong enhancement (Fig. 10-4) Another observation in quantitative analysis that indicates malignancy is an early washout of contrast medium from the lesion. However, there is a significant overlap between benign and malignant lesions concerning contrast enhancement. Up to 10% of invasive carcinomas have delayed enhancement or are well circumscribed or diffuse in nature (differentiation from diffuse enhancing benign tissue as in parenchymal proliferation is impossible). In situ carcinomas also show enhancement in the majority of cases; however, only approximately 50% of in situ carcinomas show enhancement patterns in dynamic evaluation that is typical for malignancy. Thus, it is important to emphasize that MRI must always be interpreted in correlation with x-ray mammography.

In patients who have undergone surgery, MRI may be quite helpful for distinguishing between scarring and malignancy. However, it is important to realize that in the first 6 months postoperatively scar tissue may enhance significantly; thus, reliable results can be achieved only in studies performed after this period.

Breast Implants

The appearance of breast implants on MRI varies because of the many different types. Before imaging, one must know the age and type of implant and whether prior implants were ruptured with open or closed capsulotomy or capsulectomy (Fig. 10-5). X-ray mammography usually only allows detection of fully collapsed rupture if extracapsular silicone is present. Ultrasonography may be very sensitive in showing collapsed or even uncollapsed rupture. In the detection of small amounts

of soft tissue silicone, ultrasonography may be even more sensitive than MRI. However, silicone fluid that extends all the way to the skin or calcification in the fibrous capsule of an implant may block the ultrasound signal, rendering further evaluation impossible.

The imaging protocol in MRI of breast implants should consider implant type and date of placement. Typically, first T_2-weighted spin echo sequences should be performed. These allow assessment of the extent of the implant and determination of whether fluid collections are present either around the implant or in soft tissue. If, on these first T_2-weighted images, implant rupture is not clearly identified or ruled out, additional high-resolution sequences should be performed that include water-suppressed T_2-weighted images in both the axial and sagittal planes. The slice thickness of these sequences should not exceed 3 to 4 mm. If a rupture is detected and there is suspicion of free soft tissue silicone in the area of the axilla, the brachial plexus, or even retrosternally, additional sequences with the use of an array coil for imaging of the thorax should be performed to delineate these lesions.

In imaging of breast implants, contour abnormalities may be recognized that represent herniation of either an intact or ruptured implant or a variation of the shape of an intact fibrous capsule. These herniations should not be generally interpreted as a ruptured implant. Collapsed rupture of an implant is indicated by the so-called wavy line sign and C sign. The wavy line sign stands for internal continuous wavy lines in an implant representing an implant shell totally enveloped and surrounded by silicone gel in a single-lumen implant. The C sign is based on the observation that the back patch of an implant shows the shape of the letter C and is fully surrounded by silicone gel. In a fully collapsed implant, the implant shell has a closely layered appearance or may be fully fallen on itself (Fig. 10-6). Uncollapsed rupture may be more difficult to detect. The best sign in detection of uncollapsed rupture is the definitive presence of a small amount of intracapsular silicone gel within an implant fold or folds outside an implant. Silicone detected in soft tissues outside the fibrous capsule of an implant is a very reliable sign of a present or prior implant rupture. Silicone from breast implants found in the soft tissue outside the fibrous capsule of an implant will assume different appearances. If some kind of capsule or scar surrounds the silicone in the soft tissue, it shows a bright signal intensity similar to that of silicone-filled breast implant. However, if there is granuloma formation or infiltration of scar tissue into the silicone deposition, the signal intensity may vary and thus can make a rupture undetectable. Ultrasonography is more sensitive for detecting silicone deposition in lymph nodes (from an implant rupture). In summary, the main indications for MRI of breast implants include determination of rupture of a silicone gel-filled implant and, in the case of a ruptured implant, detection of soft tissue silicone, which should be further evaluated by MRI regarding amount and exact localization.

Text continued on page 258

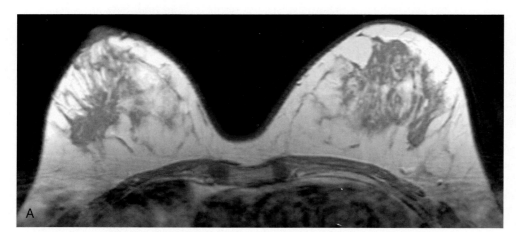

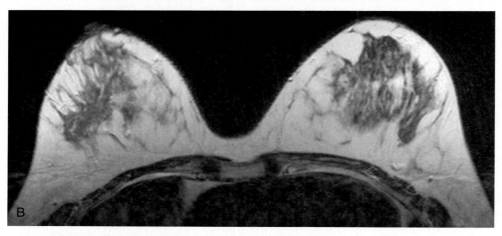

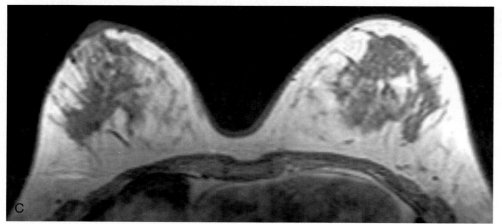

FIGURE 10–4. Invasive carcinoma. Proton density (*A*), T$_2$-weighted (*B*), and T$_1$-weighted (*C*) unenhanced images in a 43-year-old woman demonstrate an irregular, spiculated mass of the right breast that shows strong enhancement in the T$_1$-weighted image after contrast injection (*D*).

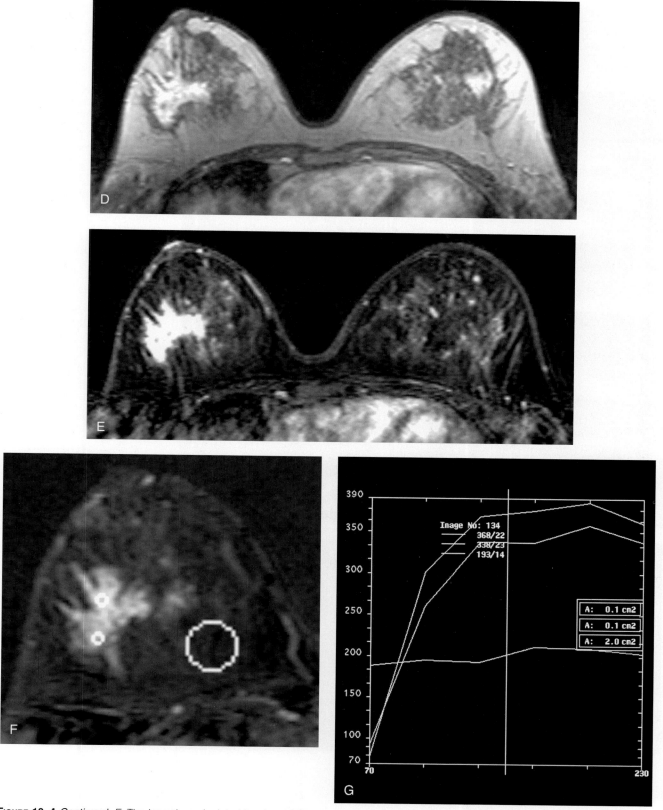

FIGURE 10–4 *Continued. E,* The irregular spiculated borders of the mass, typical for invasive carcinoma, are best demonstrated in the subtracted image. Quantification of contrast uptake (*F* and *G*) shows a strong increase of signal intensity in the first 2 minutes after CM administration with the beginning of washout by 5 minutes after injection.

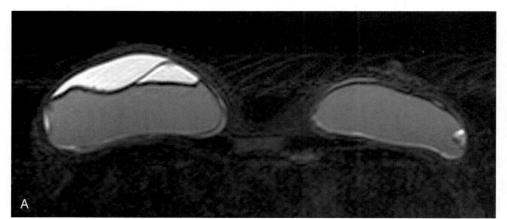

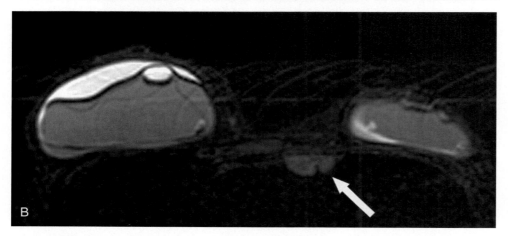

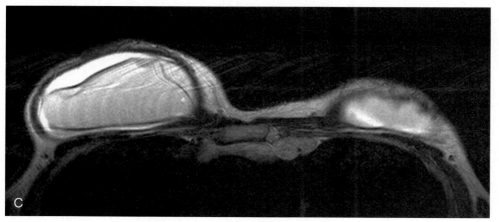

FIGURE 10–5. Free silicone after implant rupture and intracapsular water-like fluid. *A* and *B*, T$_2$-weighted fat-saturated images show an intracapsular water-like fluid collection surrounding an intact breast implant of the right breast. Additionally retrosternal soft tissue silicone can be demonstrated (*arrow*) as a result of prior implant rupture. *C*, T$_2$-weighted image without fat suppression shows the free silicone with high signal intensity. Thus, differentiation on this image from retrosternal fat is difficult.

FIGURE 10–6. Collapsed implant rupture. *A–C,* T$_2$-weighted fat-suppressed images cranial to caudal show a collapsed implant shell with extensive soft tissue silicone demonstrating a partial cystic appearance. The so-called wavy line sign is seen in the right breast implant.

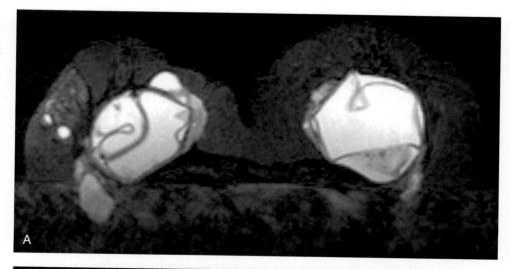

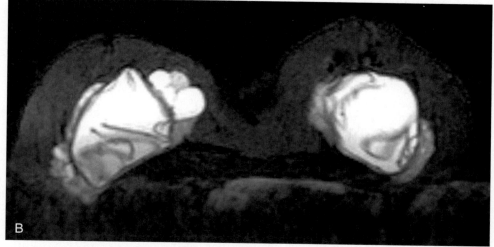

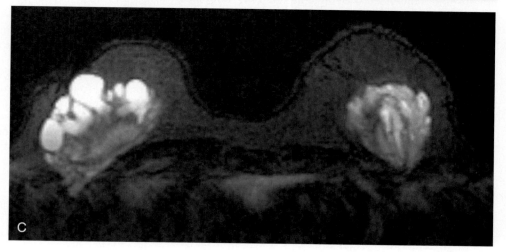

MEDIASTINUM, LUNG, AND CHEST WALL

MRI excels in the assessment of the mediastinum and hilum. The blood vessels and tracheobronchial tree are both visualized as regions of signal void highlighted by the surrounding fat. Masses in these regions have sufficiently different imaging characteristics to allow their distinction from normal structures and fat. Compared with computed tomography (CT), in which contrast is often needed to identify a mass and to avoid mistaking a blood vessel for a pathologic region, particularly in the pulmonary hilum, MRI provides excellent cross-sectional images of the mediastinum (without contrast), allowing assessment of mediastinal anatomy that is comparable to CT in quality and clarity. The main indications for MRI of the mediastinum and the thoracic inlet are imaging of vascular disorders, staging of non-small cell and small cell bronchiogenic carcinoma, evaluation of mediastinal masses, and staging as well as therapy monitoring in Hodgkin's and non-Hodgkin's lymphoma.

MRIs of the thorax are particularly susceptible to motion artifacts. Breathing motion and pulsation of the heart and great vessels can markedly degrade image quality; thus, short measurement times and artifact reduction techniques have to be used when performing MRI of the chest. If imaging of the thoracic inlet and the upper mediastinum above the level of the aortic arch is to be performed, electrocardiogram (ECG) gating and respiratory compensation are not needed, because artifacts in this area are not substantial and high image quality can be obtained with standard T_1-weighted and T_2-weighted sequences. If imaging below the aortic arch is performed, ECG or pulse oximetry gating is mandatory. If T_2-weighted fast spin echo sequences are used for imaging, additional prospective respiratory gating or breath-hold sequences with imaging of only one slice per breath-hold should be performed. New ultra-fast single-shot imaging techniques allow acquisition of high-quality images without breath-holding because acquisition time is typically less than 250 milliseconds. When T_1-weighted imaging of the chest below the aortic arch is performed, two different approaches can be used: (1) breath-hold T_1-weighted sequences with acquisition of one slice per breath-hold or (2) acquisition of T_1-weighted sequences using respiratory compensation techniques such as respiratory-ordered phase encoding (ROPE). The latter technique accomplishes a reduction in respiratory artifacts by reordering the phase-encoding lines of k space. Generally, if respiratory gating techniques are performed, the patient should be instructed to breathe softly and evenly to minimize chest wall movement.

The selection of coils depends on the area of interest. If the entire mediastinum is to be scanned, a phased-array body coil should be used to achieve sufficient resolution and an adequate signal-to-noise ratio. If tu-mors of the posterior mediastinum or paravertebral tumors such as neuroblastoma are to be imaged, spine surface coils can be used for evaluation.

Primary Mediastinal Masses

In the diagnosis of primary mediastinal tumors, the age of the patient and the localization of a mass are of special importance. Typical tumors that can be found in the anterior mediastinum are tumors of the thymus (Fig. 10-7), germ cell tumors, mediastinal lymphangioma, mediastinal goiter, and mediastinal parathyroid adenoma. In the middle mediastinum, mediastinal cysts and esophageal as well as tracheal pathologies are the most common lesions (Fig. 10-8), whereas in the posterior mediastinum typically neurogenic tumors arising from the peripheral nerves, sympathetic ganglia tumors, and thoracic meningoceles account for the majority of lesions. Malignant lymphomas, either Hodgkin's or non-Hodgkin's lymphoma, are encountered in all sections of the mediastinum (Fig. 10-9).

In the esophagus and the trachea, MRI is most useful in the preoperative staging of large tumors. Because of its multiplanar imaging capabilities and high tissue contrast, MRI is well suited to evaluate tumor extension and the relationship of the tumor to other surrounding structures.

Secondary Mediastinal Masses

MRI of the mediastinum is useful in detecting secondary mediastinal masses, particularly abnormal lymph nodes. Overall, the sensitivity of MRI in detecting lymph node enlargement is similar to that of CT, although in MRI the differentiation of small lymph nodes from vessels is much easier. However, because of its ability to acquire multiple planes, MRI has proven to be superior to CT in detecting lymph nodes at the hilum. MRI is also useful in detecting mediastinal invasion in the staging of lung cancer. Encasement or invasion of the vasculature (Fig. 10-10), esophagus, and trachea and involvement of the pericardium or myocardium are accurately detected with MRI. Because of the multiplanar imaging capabilities, better performance compared with CT has been reported. However, currently MRI is principally used as a complementary procedure for assessing the mediastinum and hilum and in those patients who have a contraindication to the use of iodinated contrast media or in whom the CT is equivocal, particularly for lesions in the hilum.

Imaging of the Thoracic Inlet

In imaging of peripheral cancers located in the lung apex, MRI, because of its multiplanar capacity, has an obvious advantage over transaxial and reformatted CT images. It is difficult to evaluate this area with CT because of artifacts caused by the surrounding bony

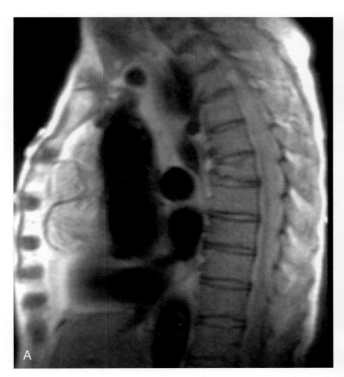

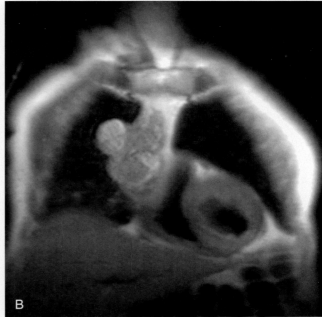

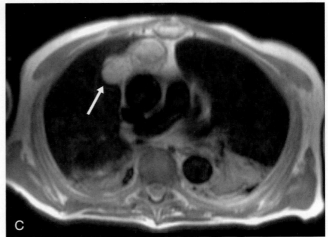

FIGURE 10–7. Malignant thymoma in a 42-year-old woman with myasthenia gravis. T₂-weighted images in sagittal (*A*), coronal (*B*), and axial (*C*) orientations show a lobulated inhomogeneous high-signal-intensity mass of the anterior mediastinum with partially indistinct borders. The mass is partially located within the anterior mediastinal fat and shows extension into the right para-aortic space (*arrow*).

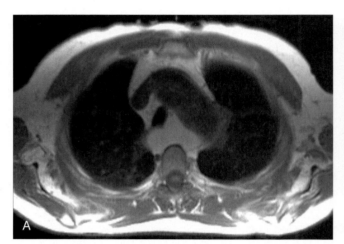

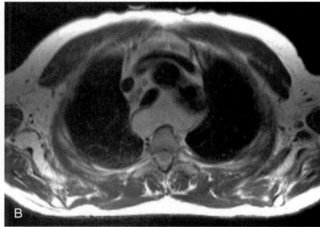

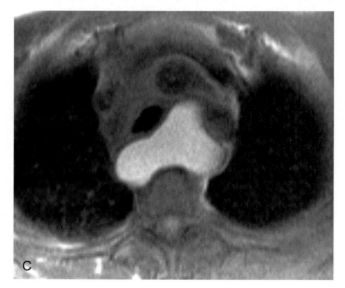

FIGURE 10–8. Bronchogenic cyst. T_1-(*A*) and T_2-weighted (*B*) axial images show a lobulated high-signal-intensity (SI) mass of the posterior mediastinum located dorsally to the trachea. In the T_1-weighted fat-saturated image (*C*), the high SI of the cyst is not suppressed, indicating high protein content of the fluid consistent with a bronchogenic cyst.

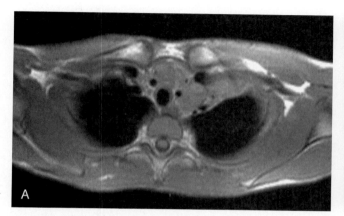

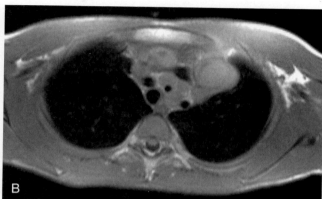

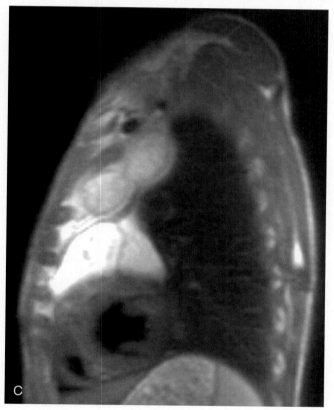

FIGURE 10–9. Hodgkin's disease. T$_2$-weighted images in axial (*A* and *B*) and sagittal (*C*) orientations show multiple soft tissue masses with different signal intensities in the mediastinum and the upper thoracic inlet. The size of a lymphoma can be determined very accurately by MRI because of the multiplanar imaging capabilities. Thus, reproducible measurements during therapy can be performed.

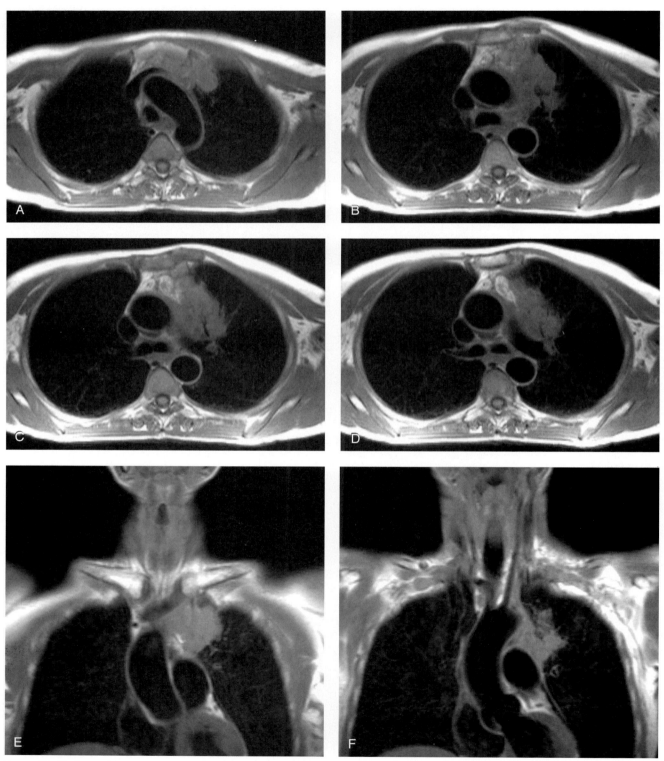

Figure 10–10. Bronchial carcinoma with mediastinal invasion. T_1-weighted axial images (*A–D*) cranial to caudal show a low-signal-intensity tumor invading the anterior mediastinum with encasement of the brachiocephalic vein. Additionally, tumor invasion between the ascending and descending aorta is depicted. *D,* Encasement of the left pulmonary artery is demonstrated with loss of the fat plane between the pulmonary artery and the tumor. *E* and *F,* Coronal T_1-weighted images confirm encasement of the pulmonary artery and show extension of the tumor along the left carotid artery.

structures. Unless an adequate bolus of contrast media is given, the effect of the mass on the blood vessels within the thoracic inlet may not be delineated by CT. The high incidence of chest wall involvement with extension to and involvement of the vascular structures, brachial plexus (Fig. 10-11), and spine is the main indication for imaging studies. Because localized chest wall invasion generally is not a contraindication for surgical resection, it is imperative to clearly display the relationship of the tumor to adjacent structures. Contraindications for surgical resection include involvement of the brachial plexus, invasion into the spinal canal, and gross vertebral body involvement as well as encasement of vascular structures. These are clearly displayed by MRI, although oblique sections are sometimes necessary for definitive diagnosis. Because the majority of these tumors undergo radiotherapy, MRI has an important value in radiation planning and follow-up during and after therapy. On T_1-weighted images, tumors tend to be isointense to the vasculature and the brachial plexus. However, fat planes are best demonstrated on T_1-weighted sequences, which is very important in order to determine plexus or vascular involvement.

Chest Wall

In imaging of tumors of the chest wall, especially when evaluating primary tumors, metastatic lesions, and direct extension of pulmonary tumors, MRI has proven to be more accurate than CT. However, rib destruction is usually best detected by chest x-ray film, and early destruction of vertebral bodies is most easily evaluated by CT. Because MRI, with its superior contrast resolution and multiplanar imaging capabilities, allows delineation of chest wall fat, muscle, and bones, it is the preferred method for evaluating chest wall extension of malignant tumors. Oblique scanning planes parallel or perpendicular to the ribs help to optimize evaluation of chest wall invasion. Differentiation between benign and malignant tumors on the basis of signal intensity characteristics on T_1-weighted and T_2-weighted images alone is impossible. Only with lipomas, the most common primary chest wall tumor, can tissue-specific characterization be made on MRI. The extension of lipomas, herniation between the intercostal muscles, and subpleural component (if present) are readily demonstrated on MRI. Malignant tumors of the chest wall are rather rare and in most cases originate from the pleura or osseous structures (as in Ewing's sarcoma). Identification of irregular lesion margins and infiltrative growth are hallmarks of malignancy on MRI.

Pulmonary Parenchyma

The lungs are seen as regions of low (black) signal intensity on MRI. An abnormality within the lung parenchyma causes increased signal intensity. In general, most pulmonary nodules can be seen using either CT or MRI. However, CT usually detects a larger number of small nodules than MRI, but small nodules adjacent to the blood vessels are better displayed on MRI.

Small lesions within the lung parenchyma are not as readily identified on MRI as on CT because of the form of acquisition. MRI times are longer, and patients breathe quietly throughout the acquisition of multiple images. Therefore, small lesions can suffer from partial volume averaging during an MRI study because they move in and out of the imaging plane. New ultra-fast imaging sequences allow imaging during breath-holding. In contrast, CT images are obtained during suspended respiration, which decreases the effect of partial volume averaging of small nodules. Additionally, CT examinations using both soft tissue and lung windows improve identification of small pulmonary nodules. In the imaging of tuberculosis or metastases of osteosarcoma, CT can identify even small areas of calcifications that cannot be seen on MRI.

Thoracic Aorta

Disease of the thoracic aorta is best evaluated by MRI. Because of its multiplanar imaging capabilities, studies can be optimally tailored to the different diseases that may need further evaluation. The basic examinations in imaging of the thoracic aorta consist of ECG-gated multislice acquisitions, ECG-gated breath-hold single-slice imaging, multiphase cine imaging, and velocity mapping dynamic imaging. First, transaxial scans should be performed from the thoracic inlet to the level of the diaphragm followed by a left anterior oblique study, which follows the axis of the aortic arch and descending aorta. In certain cases, it is also necessary to perform transaxial slices perpendicular to the aorta to achieve further information about diseases of the aortic wall. Furthermore, MRI using cine techniques allows reliable quantification of blood flow, ejection fraction, stroke volume, and quantification of regurgitation in aortic valve insufficiency.

Gd-enhanced 3D magnetic resonance angiography (CE MRA) is a newer technique that provides high-resolution 3D data sets very quickly and is well suited for depicting intrathoracic vessels. Because of the 3D nature of the data set, CE MRA provides volumetric data that can be processed for multiplanar reformations and maximum intensity projections. Vascular visualization using CE MRA relies on the T_1 shortening of blood by Gd-based contrast during the intravascular transit. It is important to note that this technique requires the combination of an intravenously administered Gd chelate-contrast bolus with the image acquisition. A major advantage of this technique compared with time of flight or phase contrast angiography is the less pronounced sensitivity to flow-related artifacts and thus the more reliable visualization of vascular structures. Another important issue is the acquisition of the whole data set in a single breath-hold, thus avoiding respiratory artifacts. The sequences used for CE MRA depend on the different MRI systems; however, generally the fastest possible 3D imaging sequence, typically a fast 3D gradient echo scan, should be used. Preferential arterial images can be achieved by selective timing of the contrast bolus arrival to the acquisition of the central k-space data.

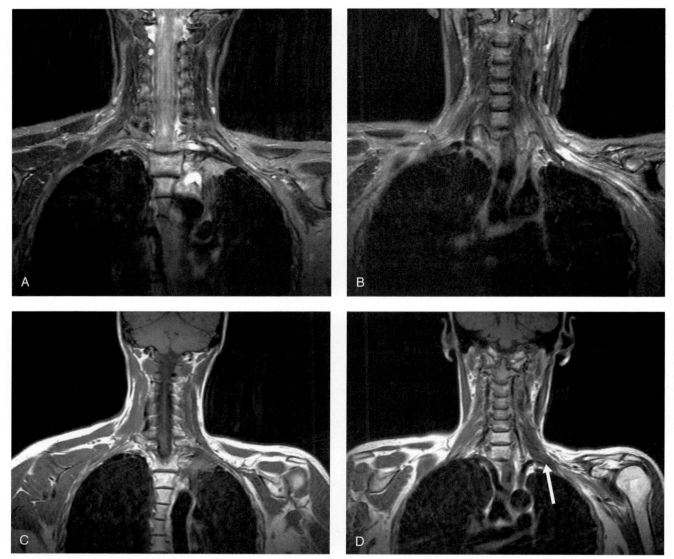

FIGURE 10–11. Pancoast tumor (superior pulmonary sulcus tumor) in a 52-year-old woman with progressive atrophy of the left upper extremity. *A* and *B,* Coronal short TI inversion recovery images demonstrate a small high-signal-intensity (SI) superior sulcus tumor along the lower brachial plexus. *C* and *D,* On coronal T$_1$-weighted images, the tumor has low SI. Decreased SI can be noted within the involved brachial plexus (*arrow*) on the left as compared with the contralateral, normal side.

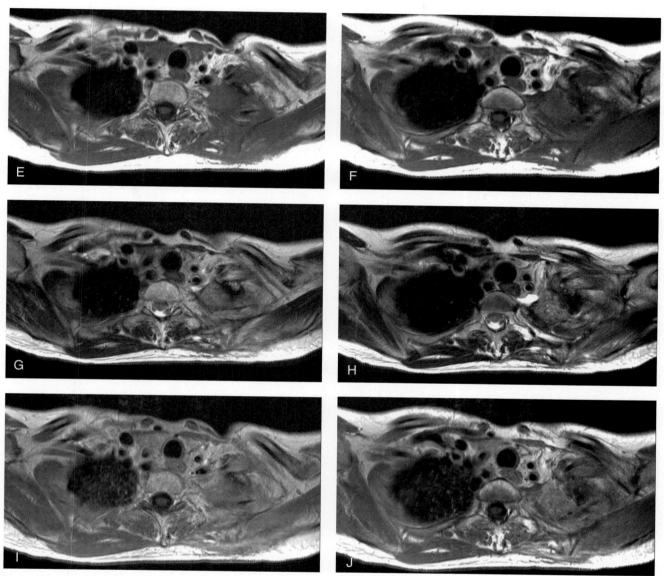

FIGURE 10–11 *Continued.* Axial T$_1$- (*E* and *F*) and T$_2$-weighted (*G* and *H*) images also demonstrate the direct contact between the tumor and the lower brachial plexus, with inhomogeneous enhancement of the tumor and parts of the brachial plexus on T$_1$-weighted contrast-enhanced images (*I* and *J*), indicating infiltration of the lower brachial plexus.

Aneurysms

In the evaluation of patients with an aortic aneurysm, in addition to measuring the true diameter of the vessel and the diameter of the patent lumen, it is extremely important to characterize the location, shape, and extent of the aneurysm and to determine its relationship to branch vessels and any effect the aneurysm may have on adjacent structures. Atherosclerosis is the leading cause of aneurysms involving the thoracic aorta. As a result of weakening of the media secondary to the atherosclerotic process, a progressive increase in the diameter of the aorta involving all layers of the vessel can be observed. Because tortuosity in combination with aortic aneurysm is a common observation, the lateral anterior oblique (LAO) view in most cases does not allow imaging of the entire aorta in one single slice. Different configurations of aortic aneurysms can be found, including fusiform, saccular, and cylindroid. The location of a thoracic aneurysm is an important determinant of the cause. For atherosclero-

sis it is rare that an aneurysm solely involves the ascending aorta. Rather, these aneurysms also involve the aortic arch and the descending aorta. If an aneurysm involves only the ascending aorta, the differential diagnosis should include cystic medial necrosis, other degenerative processes of the media, and aneurysmatic dilatation caused by aortic valve disease (Fig. 10-12).

In Marfan's syndrome, the loss of elastic fibers classically leads to a progressive increase in the diameter of the aorta with involvement of the aortic root, the tubular portion of the aorta, and the proximal ascending aorta. As a result of the marked dilatation of the aortic root, secondary aortic insufficiency, aortic dissection, and hemopericardium can be observed and should be recognized on MRI if present. Marfan's syndrome can also involve the pulmonary arteries and result in an isolated pulmonary artery aneurysm; however, not all patients with Marfan's syndrome will exhibit aortic root changes or other vascular involvement. Overall, MRI is an excellent noninvasive imaging modality for evaluating pa-

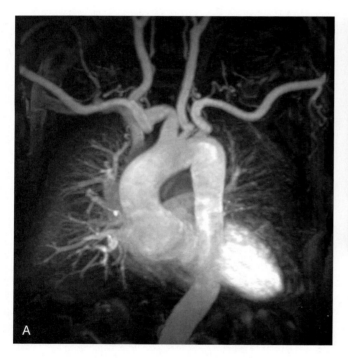

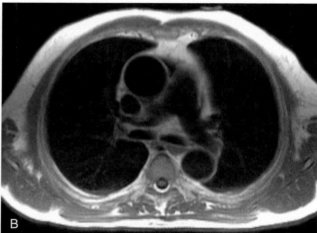

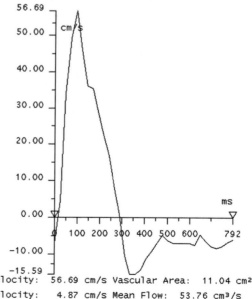

FIGURE 10–12. Aortic regurgitation. *A,* Contrast-enhanced magnetic resonance angiography shows an increased diameter of the ascending aorta and kinking of the supra-aortic vessels. *B,* The diameter of the aorta is clearly evaluated in an axial T$_1$-weighted image, and (*C*) flow evaluation of the aorta with a phase contrast acquisition shows the regurgitation volume as the area under the curve for the negative flow component.

Peak Velocity: 56.69 cm/s   Vascular Area: 11.04 cm²
Mean Velocity: 4.87 cm/s   Mean Flow: 53.76 cm³/s

C

tients with Marfan's syndrome. In aortic valve disease, including both aortic insufficiency (see Fig. 10-12) and aortic valve stenosis, MRI can be used to evaluate stroke volume, ejection fraction, left ventricular hypertrophy, and left ventricular enlargement and to assess quantitatively the velocity across the aortic valve. Because MRI can accurately determine the true diameter of an aneurysm caused by aortic valve disease, and further increases in the aortic diameter can be reliably measured in a noninvasive matter on follow-up, MRI is an excellent tool in monitoring of aortic aneurysms. In general, aneurysms larger than 6 cm in diameter have an increased incidence of aortic rupture and, therefore, require immediate surgery. Unlike x-ray angiography, MRI is also effective in depicting para-aortic processes, including compression of adjacent structures by an aneurysm, para-aortic hematomas, and thrombus formation within an aneurysm, and in detecting mural thrombus.

Aortic Dissection

More than 95% of aortic dissections start in the thoracic aorta, of which 60% to 70% involve the ascending aorta, and only approximately 25% start distal to the left subclavian artery in the region of the ligamentum arteriosum. Aortic dissections are classified by location, and two classifications exist. In DeBakey type I, the dissection begins within the ascending aorta and extends to the descending aorta; in type II, dissections are localized only in the ascending aorta; and in type III, dissections begin just distal to the subclavian artery. Stanford type A dissections involve the ascending aorta, where type B dissections do not. Because dissections of the ascending aorta may affect the aortic valve, coronary arteries, and branching vessels, they represent surgical emergencies and have a very high mortality in the first few hours after onset. Often patients with acute dissection of the ascending aorta are unstable; thus, MRI is not the imaging modality of choice. CT is used for diagnosis followed by immediate surgical intervention. The classic

clinical picture in an acute onset of aortic dissection is severe chest pain that radiates to the back, sometimes similar to the clinical picture of ischemic heart disease.

In hemodynamically stable patients, it has been suggested that MRI is the best imaging modality for the evaluation of aortic dissection. If on conventional spin echo images the intimal flap is not clearly displayed, cine MRI usually clarifies the issue. Likewise, differentiation between thrombus and slowly flowing blood in the false lumen can be made by the use of cine MRI techniques (Fig. 10-13). MRI is also highly effective in evaluating branch vessel involvement (Figs. 10-14 and 10-15) and retrograde extension of a dissection with depiction of involvement of the aortic root. Occasionally, it may be difficult to differentiate complete thrombosis of the false lumen of a dissection from an aortic aneurysm or mural thrombus (Fig. 10-16). Indirect signs that favor the diagnosis of a dissection include longitudinal thrombus extension (which is not typically identified in an aneurysm), a noncircular compressed patent lumen, and a change in the position of the thrombus as a result of the spiral configuration of the dissection membrane. MRI is extremely useful in the evaluation of patients after medical or surgical intervention and in the evaluation of periaortic hematomas, infections, and progressive dilatation of the false lumen. In patients who have undergone graft placement, MRI can be used to examine the graft and screen for anastomotic aneurysms.

Pulmonary Arteries

Since its introduction, there has been interest in the use of MRI for evaluating the pulmonary arteries for pulmonary embolism or thrombus. Standard MRI techniques are limited in their ability to evaluate the pulmonary arterial tree because they lack the ability to study the peripheral vasculature. In normal pulmonary arteries, signal void appears within the vessels on standard spin echo pulse sequences. MRI detects central thrombus as an intraluminal signal within the pulmonary

Text continued on page 272

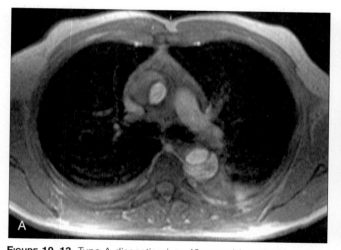 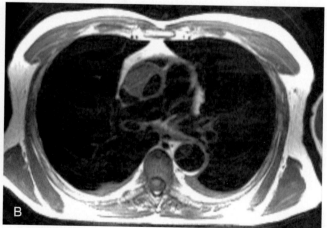

FIGURE 10–13. Type A dissection in a 46-year-old man with sudden onset of thoracic pain and no signs of myocardial infarction. *A,* Axial cine imaging shows a dissection membrane in the ascending and descending aorta. However, there is no high signal intensity within the false lumen in the ascending aorta, indicating thrombosis of the false lumen. This is also confirmed on T_1-weighted axial imaging (*B*), which demonstrates signal within the false lumen in the ascending aorta.

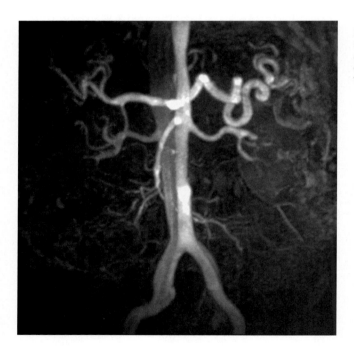

FIGURE 10–14. Abdominal aortic dissection. Contrast-enhanced magnetic resonance angiography clearly displays dissection of the abdominal aorta with retrograde filling of the false lumen by a re-entry at the level of the iliac arteries. Note that all abdominal vessels except the right renal artery arise from the true lumen.

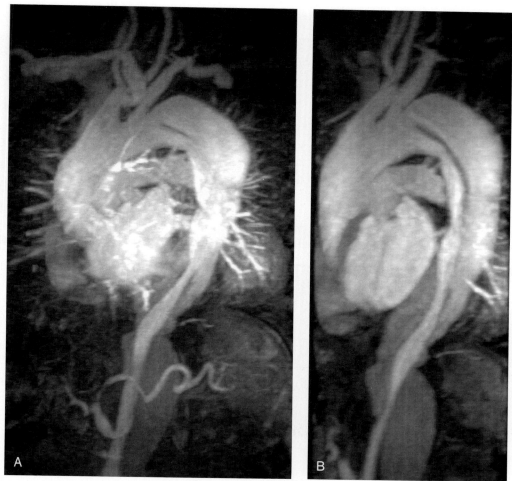

FIGURE 10–15. Chronic type B dissection in a 64-year-old man. Whole-volume MIP projection (*A*) and targeted subvolume MIP projection (*B*) of contrast-enhanced magnetic resonance angiography data set clearly display the aortic dissection beginning just distal to the left subclavian artery. However, the dissection membrane is better appreciated in the subvolume MIP.

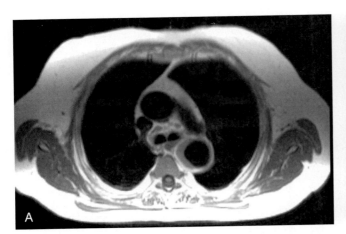

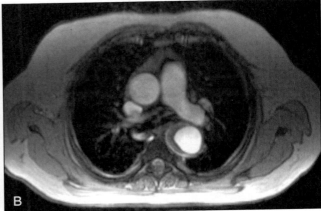

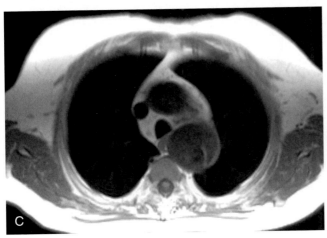

FIGURE 10–16. Intramural bleeding with subsequent type B aortic dissection in a 52-year-old man with sudden onset of thoracic pain. *A,* T_1-weighted axial imaging at initial presentation shows thickening of the aortic wall with intermediate to high signal intensity. *B,* Axial cine imaging at this time only shows the thickening of the wall but no intimal flap. One year later, the patient presented for routine follow-up without history of another pain episode.

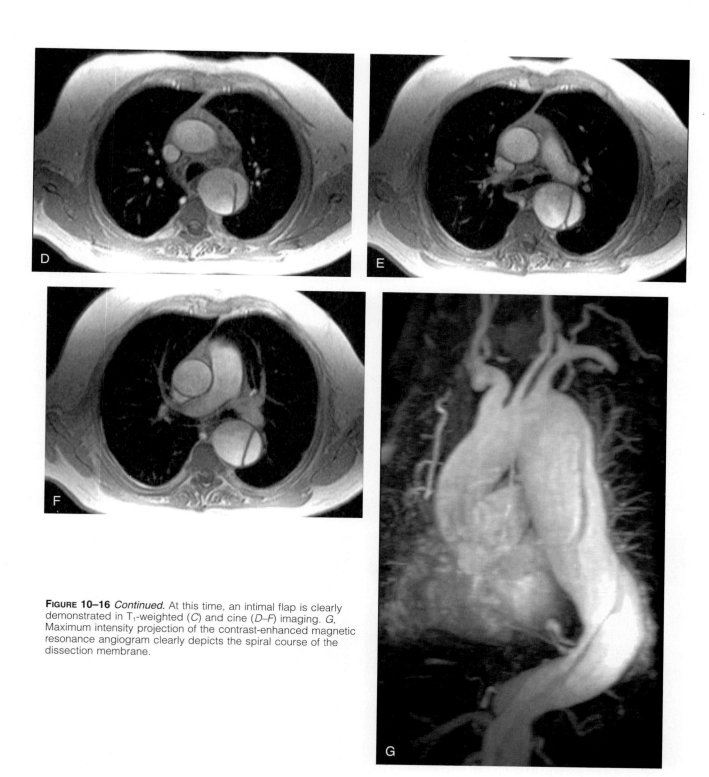

FIGURE 10–16 *Continued.* At this time, an intimal flap is clearly demonstrated in T$_1$-weighted (*C*) and cine (*D–F*) imaging. *G,* Maximum intensity projection of the contrast-enhanced magnetic resonance angiogram clearly depicts the spiral course of the dissection membrane.

arteries; however, using standard techniques, MRI is not the modality of choice for detecting pulmonary emboli. In a patient for whom there is an absolute contraindication to iodinated contrast and an equivocal ventilation-perfusion scan, MRI plays an important role by demonstrating emboli. If MRI with standard techniques is to be used for pulmonary artery evaluation, it is important to note that the technique is better suited for detecting central rather than peripheral emboli. The varying flow direction within the pulmonary arteries as well as potentially diminished flow may lead to incomplete washout and to erroneous simulation of thrombus as a result of missing signal void. More recently, Gd-enhanced MRA has been used for imaging patients with suspected pulmonary embolism. It is especially helpful for imaging patients with ambiguous pulmonary ventilation and perfusion scintigraphy and patients with contraindications to the use of iodinated contrast. Several studies report high sensitivity and specificity for CE MRA in detecting pulmonary embolism up to the subsegmental branches. Three-dimensional CE MRA is also particularly useful for identifying systemic pulmonary circulation connections (e.g., shunt lesions). Typically, CE MRA depicts these anomalous connections, because they generally fill with contrast (Fig. 10-17). The evaluation of the data set using multiplanar reformation and targeted maximum intensity projections gives very high sensitivity for detecting these lesions. In imaging of the pulmonary veins, CE MRA may be helpful in evaluating anomalous pulmonary venous return in patients with congenital heart disease.

HEART
Congenital Heart Disease

Since the late 1980s, MRI has developed into a clinically useful tool to study the heart, in particular for congenital malformations. The effectiveness of MRI in diagnosing congenital heart diseases (CHD) is widely recognized, but its appropriate role in imaging of CHD in relation with echocardiography and cardioangiography is still evolving. The anatomy of CHD either pre- or postoperatively can vary from simple to very complex. Many CHD types require intervention, either corrective or palliative, and with improvement of various surgical and intervention techniques survival rate has increased dramatically. This has resulted in a growing number of postoperative patients who generally require extensive follow-up. Because residual sequelae and complications determine the long-term outcome of corrected or palliated CHD, timely detection and quantification of morphologic and functional abnormalities require accurate and preferably noninvasive imaging methods.

Echocardiography is currently used as the initial noninvasive imaging study for almost all patients with known or suspected CHD. It is unlikely that MRI will replace echocardiography as the first diagnostic procedure because of the portability, universal availability, and low cost of echocardiography. It is superior to MRI in depicting cardiac valves, real-time cardiac motion, and small intracardiac shunts. However, MRI can demonstrate cardiovascular anatomy without the limitation of acoustic windows or ultrasound penetration of the body. Furthermore, MRI can provide tomographic images in any imaging plane and with a wide field of view. Clearly, in many cases, the diagnostic capabilities of MRI and echocardiography are complementary rather than competitive.

Angiocardiography has been the gold standard for evaluation of cardiac anatomy and function. Important information such as intracardiac pressures, pulmonary vascular resistance, and oxygen saturation can be obtained as with no other modality. However, catheterization has a known complication rate, requires the use of ionizing radiation and intravascular administration of

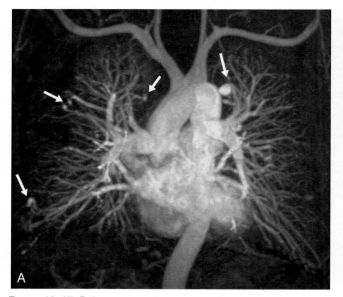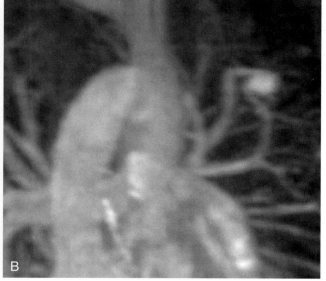

FIGURE 10–17. Pulmonary arteriovenous malformations (PAVMs) in a 43-year-old man with hereditary hemorrhagic telangiectasia (Osler's disease) in whom a brain abscess developed. *A,* Maximum intensity projection from the contrast-enhanced magnetic resonance angiogram of the pulmonary vasculature depicts multiple PAVMs (*arrows*) in both lungs with one larger malformation in the upper left lobe. *B,* Subvolume MIP clearly depicts the feeding artery as well as the draining vein.

iodinated contrast media, and thus is particularly undesirable for repeated applications in young patients.

Conventional echocardiography-gated spin echo sequences are still the basis for evaluation of cardiac anatomy. In most cases, T_1-weighted imaging should be performed. Adjunct T_2-weighted sequences are necessary only if inflammation or myocardial tissue abnormalities are suspected. Respiratory artifacts can be reduced using prospective imaging algorithms that improve image quality significantly and do not prolong imaging time. High-field-strength systems (1.5 T) have some clear advantages over lower strength systems, because improved spatial resolution and shorter imaging times are very important. This is especially true in imaging in children because occasionally very thin sections (3 mm) are needed to evaluate the anatomy effectively. In contrast to spin echo imaging, gradient echo imaging is a faster technique that allows evaluation of the same section with a high repetition rate at different times after the trigger signal, which enables reconstruction of a cine loop of this particular section. Turbulent flow, stenosis, regurgitation, and shunt flow in this type of imaging can be detected as a jet of signal void. Cine gradient echo MRI can also be used to assess left ventricular and right ventricular function in terms of volume and myocardial mass.

In a typical imaging protocol, first a scout image is obtained to determine the location of subsequent transverse sections. After coronal images are obtained, multislice transverse images are acquired from the top of the aorta to the diaphragm using spin echo sequences. Typically, in these initial studies, a slice thickness of 5 mm should be used. However, if small structures that need additional evaluation are detected, a specially targeted sequence with a smaller slice thickness (3 mm) should be used. These first transverse images are supplemented by sagittal and coronal images. Additionally, oblique images may be needed (e.g., to demonstrate the aortic arch or the descending aorta). Short-axis or four-chamber views of the heart may be acquired with cine MRI technique to quantify ventricular volume, ejection fraction, and shunts.

The main clinical indications for MRI in CHD are

1. Evaluation of thoracic aortic anomalies
2. Assessment of presence, central connections, and size of the pulmonary arteries in tetralogy of Fallot, pulmonary atresia, and right-sided obstructive anomalies
3. Evaluation of intracardiac and extracardiac morphology of complex ventricular anomalies
4. Examination of pulmonary venous connections and other pulmonary venous anomalies
5. Assessment of septal defects
6. Monitoring of patient status after various surgical procedures
7. Identification of systemic venous anomalies

In evaluation of the aorta, MRI has been found to be effective for definitive diagnosis of a number of different congenital anomalies.

MRI can demonstrate aortic arch anomalies such as, for example, double aortic arch and aberrant left subclavian artery (Fig. 10-18). The most frequently encountered congenital anomaly of the thoracic aorta is coarctation (Fig. 10-19). MRI is very effective for evaluating

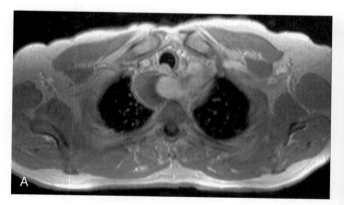

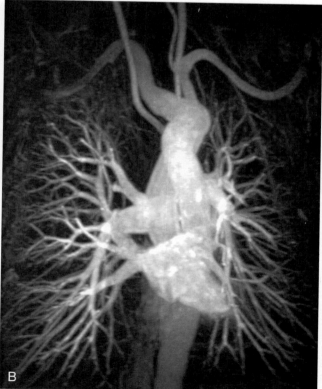

FIGURE 10–18. Abberant right subclavian artery with aneurysm formation in a 42-year-old woman with increasing dysphagia. *A,* The axial T_1-weighted contrast-enhanced image shows a vessel with aneurysm formation and mural thrombus passing from the left to the right behind the esophagus and trachea. *B,* MIP projection of the contrast-enhanced magnetic resonance angiogram demonstrates that the vessel is the last branch of the aortic arch and follows the route of the right subclavian artery. Note that the aneurysm formation would not be appreciated correctly on angiography alone.

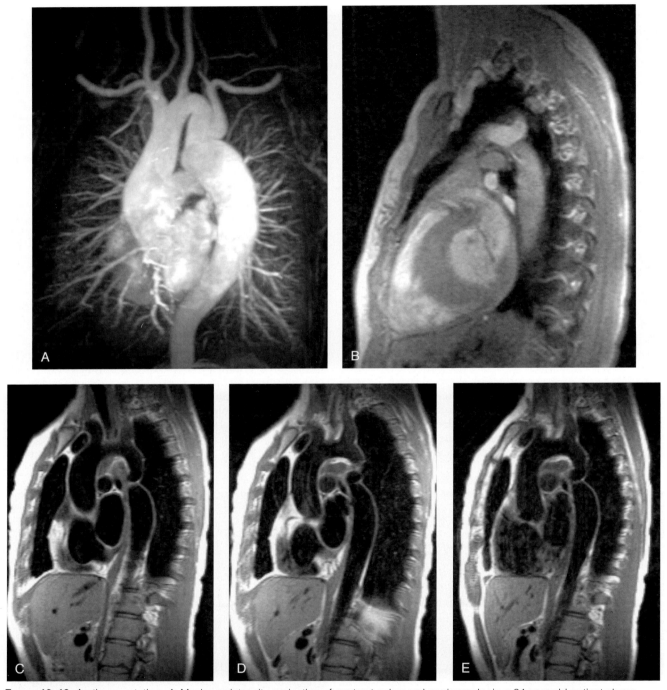

Figure 10–19. Aortic coarctation. *A,* Maximum intensity projection of contrast-enhanced angiography in a 34-year-old patient shows previously undiagnosed coarctation of the aorta with pre- and poststenotic dilatation of the aorta and aneurysmal widening of the left subclavian artery. *B,* In a 5-year-old boy, oblique cine imaging parallel to the aortic arch displays a poststenotic jet. *C–E,* A follow-up study in a 14-year-old girl after balloon angioplasty shows restenosis on oblique T_1-weighted images.

coarctation initially and after treatment. The transverse and the sagittal or LAO view should be used when this diagnosis is suspected. The stenosed aortic segment is often most clearly identified using the LAO equivalent plane because this plane is perpendicular to the coarctation. However, because of the tortuosity of the aorta in the prestenotic segment, occasionally the complete aortic coarctation cannot be displayed in one single slice.

MRI can clearly depict the luminal diameter of the coarctation site as well as poststenotic dilatation and dilated collaterals. Additionally, CE MRA can be performed with maximum intensity projection reconstructions to give a detailed overview of the anatomy for planned surgery. After treatment, MRI can be used to demonstrate the diameter at the site of repair, postoperative mediastinal hematoma, and false aneurysms developing at the site of patch angioplasty or caused by balloon angioplasty.

Pulmonary atresia is depicted on transverse MRI as a solid layer of muscle in the region of the right ventricular outflow tract at the base of the heart. Additional images oriented along the right ventricular outflow tract can be used to evaluate the atretic segment further. The solid layer of muscle found in pulmonary atresia represents the blind-ended infundibulum, and the length of the atresia may be shown to be extensive or focal at the valve level. The most useful information provided by MRI in patients with pulmonary atresia is the state of the main and central pulmonary arteries distal to the atresia.

In the evaluation of tetralogy of Fallot (Fig. 10-20), transverse scans depict the ventricular septal defect and the infundibular, annular, and pulmonary arterial stenosis. MRI provides information about the size of the main and central pulmonary vessels. The blood supply to the lung is assessed in both axial and coronal images. The aorta in tetralogy of Fallot is typically anteriorly displaced, overriding the ventricular septal defect. In complex anomalies such as transposition of the great arteries (Fig. 10-21) with coexistent septal defect or a double-outlet right ventricle, both the relationship of the great vessels and the anatomy of the outflow tracts can be readily displayed on MRI. This is of special interest for surgical planning. Because of the multiplanar imaging capabilities, MRI can reliably depict the complete anatomy.

The evaluation of pulmonary venous connections and other pulmonary venous anomalies has already been discussed. Regardless, it should be emphasized that MRI can provide important additional information even in combination with pulmonary catheter angiography to clearly depict the sometimes very complicated vascular anatomy. In the evaluation of systemic venous abnormalities, MRI is also a very effective, noninvasive method to depict the complete anatomy. Venous anomalies such as left superior vena cava and interruption of the inferior vena cava with azygos continuation are clearly demonstrated on MRI. Often these venous anomalies are found in combination with other CHDs; thus, their preoperative depiction has a great impact on the therapeutic approach. With regard to imaging of septal defects, MRI has the ability to quantify shunts by measuring left and right ventricular volume from cine MRI or by simultaneous measurement of flow in the ascending aorta and the main pulmonary artery using velocity-encoded cine MRI. The difference calculated between the right and left ventricular stroke volume is the net volume of the shunt for patients with atrial septal defect and patent

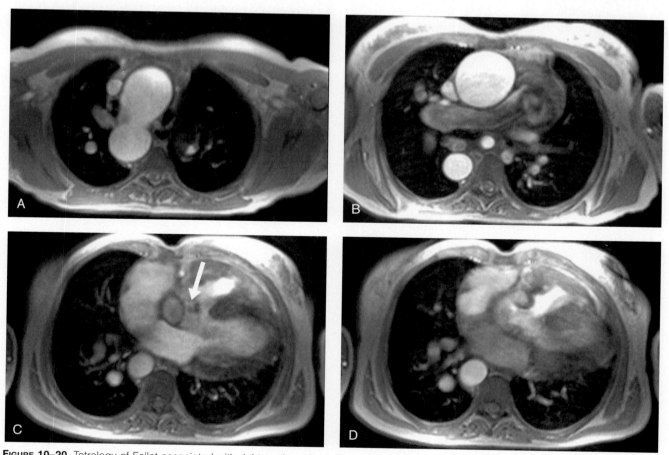

FIGURE 10–20. Tetralogy of Fallot associated with right aortic arch. *A–D,* Axial cine images cranial to caudal show a right-sided aortic arch with a right descending aorta and enlargement of central pulmonary vessels. Turbulence in the pulmonary truncus (*B*) can be noted as a result of obstruction of the right ventricular outflow tract. The aorta is deviated anteriorly and overrides the interventricular septal defect (*C, arrow*).

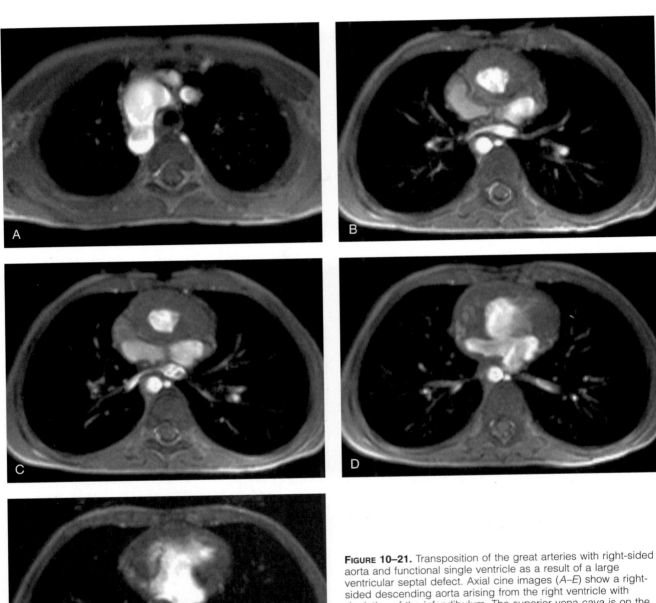

FIGURE 10–21. Transposition of the great arteries with right-sided aorta and functional single ventricle as a result of a large ventricular septal defect. Axial cine images (*A–E*) show a right-sided descending aorta arising from the right ventricle with depiction of the infundibulum. The superior vena cava is on the left. The pulmonary artery arises posterior to the aorta, and a single ventricle can be identified.

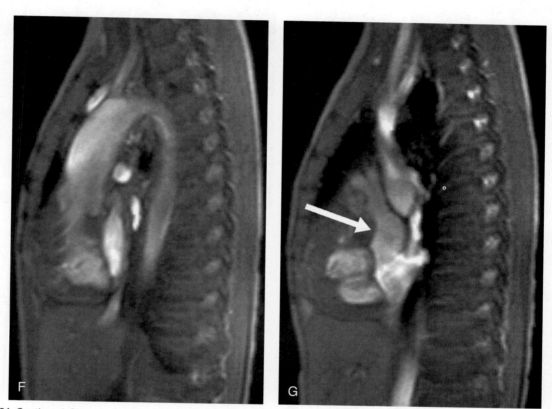

FIGURE 10–21 *Continued.* Sagittal cine images (*F* and *G*) again demonstrate the more ventral ascending aorta and the posterior pulmonary truncus (*G, arrow*).

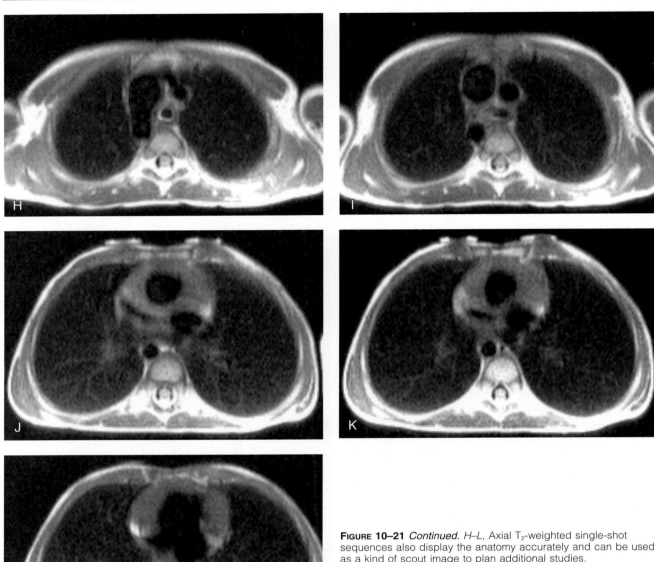

FIGURE 10–21 *Continued. H–L,* Axial T$_2$-weighted single-shot sequences also display the anatomy accurately and can be used as a kind of scout image to plan additional studies.

ductus arteriosus. The same holds true for patients with partial anomalous pulmonary venous connection.

In summary, MRI is an extremely powerful noninvasive tool for the anatomic depiction of CHD and evaluation of hemodynamics. However, the structural evaluation of cardiac valves is clearly one area in which echocardiography remains superior to MRI. Another drawback for MRI is the relatively long time of examination. A full examination of a patient with CHD may require 30 to 60 minutes; deep sedation is required for infants and small children. Thus, echocardiography currently is used as the initial noninvasive imaging study for almost all patients with known or suspected CHD. New and faster MRI techniques in the future may enable reliable and fast imaging of the heart in children. MRI may become a routine examination in patients with suspected CHD both for initial diagnosis and in follow-up after treatment (Fig. 10-22).

Acquired Heart Disease

The high contrast between the moving blood and the myocardium, the high spatial resolution, and the lack of ionizing radiation render MRI a superb technique for myocardial assessment. As a result of ongoing technical developments, MRI is evolving to be the noninvasive gold standard for cardiac structure and function assess-

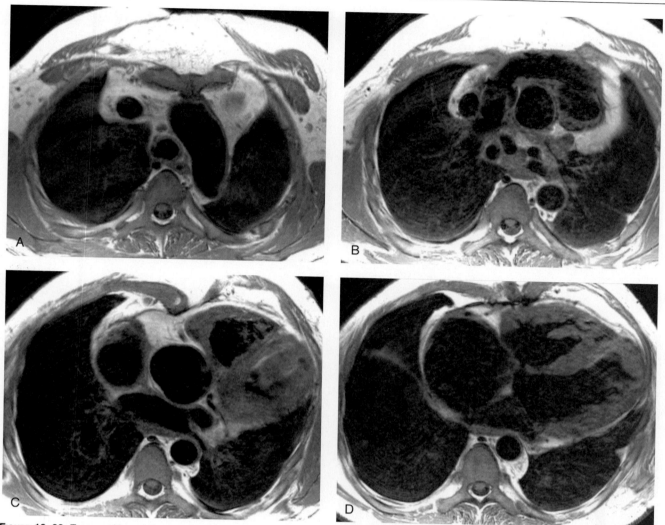

FIGURE 10–22. Transposition of the great arteries after an arterial switch procedure. *A–D,* T$_1$-weighted axial images cranial to caudal show a normal origin of the aorta. The pulmonary artery arises from the right ventricle. A retrosternal conduit between the pulmonary trunk and the right pulmonary artery had to be made during the arterial switch procedure to allow connection of the pulmonary vasculature.

ment. Because cardiac motion is a fundamental problem in MRI of the heart, MRI must be restricted to a constant portion of the cardiac cycle to avoid blurring of the images. Different techniques can be used for evaluating acquired heart disease. These include ECG-gated conventional spin echo images, which can be acquired in either a multislice mode without breath-hold or in a single-slice ECG-gated acquisition mode in breath-hold. These conventional spin echo images give a very good overview concerning the anatomy of the heart combined with high soft tissue contrast and can be used to display, for example, the replacement of muscle by adipose or fibrous tissue, hypertrophic cardiomyopathy, myocarditis (Fig. 10-23), and cardiac masses. Another technique that is generally used to evaluate acquired heart disease is cine gradient echo imaging. In cine imaging, a picture loop of various phases of the cardiac cycle in one single slice is displayed so regional and global wall thickening and functional parameters can be assessed. To evaluate blood flow, phase contrast (PC) methods are applied in

which the contrast between stationary and moving tissue is generated as a result of velocity-induced phase shifts of moving spins in a magnetic field gradient. Using this method, the induced phase shift is directly proportional to the velocity, so that PC methods allow quantitative measurement of the velocity of flow. Absolute flow can be calculated by multiplying the linear blood velocity by the cross-sectional area of the blood vessel. Typically, this approach is used to measure flow in the aorta, pulmonary arteries, or ventricular cavities in patients with CHD.

In imaging of acquired heart disease, it is generally preferable to use a phased-array surface coil because higher signal-to-noise ratios with minimum time to repetition and time to echo values can be achieved. In imaging of the coronary arteries, which is still under clinical evaluation, so-called navigator echoes that allow tracking of the diaphragmatic motion are used in combination with 3D image acquisition to depict the anatomy of the coronary arteries without breathing artifacts. To

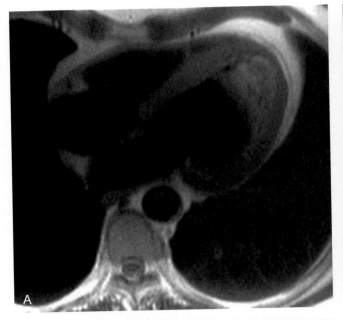

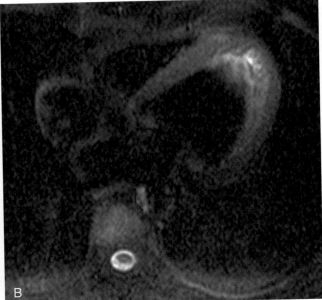

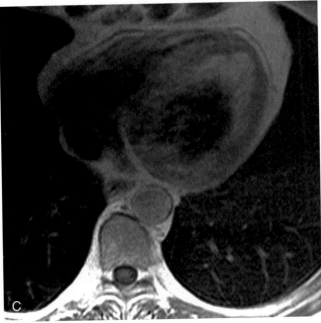

FIGURE 10–23. Myocarditis in a 45-year-old man with sudden onset of cardiac arrhythmia after a viral infection and exclusion of myocardial ischemia. T_2-weighted (*A*) and short TI inversion recovery (*B*) images show areas of high signal intensity within the myocardium of the left ventricular apex consistent with myocardial edema. *C,* In the T_1-weighted contrast-enhanced sequence, the affected myocardium shows increased contrast uptake. Myocardial biopsy showed acute myocarditis with necrosis of myocytes.

assess cardiac function further, cine gradient echo imaging with myocardial tagging can be applied. In myocardial tagging, using a saturation band pattern, either a grid or parallel tag lines, a labeled zone of myocardial tissue can be followed anatomically throughout the cardiac cycle. Thus, important insights into regional myocardial mechanics can be achieved by direct visualization of the movement of the myocardium.

The primary planes for cardiac imaging are the transverse, sagittal, and coronal planes. These planes are orthogonal to the thorax but oblique to the axis of the heart. Thus, to achieve similar orientations as used in echocardiography, it is necessary to perform oblique imaging. The oblique long-axis planes of the ventricle are either perpendicular or parallel to the plane of the ventricular septum, producing a horizontal or vertical long-axis plane orientation. Images perpendicular to the long-axis plane orientations of the heart are short-axis planes, which accurately display regional myocardial diameter. To achieve images in the long- and short-axis planes, preliminary imaging in other planes is required. First, an orthogonal imaging plane to the body is acquired. If the sagittal plane is used for these first images, the anterior angulation of the cardiac apex relative to the base is determined. A series of oblique images is then acquired parallel to this plane. From these images, the leftward angulation of the cardiac apex is determined and images parallel to the short axis of the heart can be prescribed perpendicular to a line that defines the left-ward angulation of the heart. From the basis of the short-axis images, horizontal and vertical long-axis images can then be acquired.

Normal Myocardium

The normal left ventricle has a wall thickness of 9 to 11 mm in end diastole. Focal areas of thinning of the myocardium are associated with remodeling after myocardial infarction, whereas a diffuse thickening or thinning may be associated with cardiomyopathy. In both long- and short-axis views, the papillary muscles are clearly visualized. If spin echo sequences are used, the signal of the normal myocardium in T_2-weighted images is similar to or slightly higher than the signal of the skeletal muscle. On T_1-weighted images, the signal is usually similar to that of skeletal muscle. Using spin echo imaging, the ventricular and atrial cavities typically have low signal intensity. The normal right ventricle normally shows an end-diastolic thickness of approximately 3 mm, and the trabeculation is much more obvious compared with the left ventricle. The walls of the atria are thin, and if no high-resolution imaging is performed sometimes the atrial septum may not be identified on spin echo images. Quantification of cardiac dimensions such as volume and wall thickening can be made on the basis of cine MRI techniques or of both end-diastolic and end-systolic spin echo images. Because of the ability of MRI to obtain images with good spatial resolution in any tomographic plane, MRI can be rated as the gold standard in evaluation of the left ventricle (Fig. 10-24). The same is true for the right ventricle, in which echocardiography is of limited value because of the difficulties visualizing endocardial borders as well as the complex geometry of the right ventricle. Another important issue in imaging of the heart in acquired heart disease is assessment of the atrial volume. Atrial function augments ventricular function because the atrium acts as a reservoir for delivery of blood to the ventricles. Assessment of the atrial dimensions is important in acquired valvular disease and systemic or pulmonary hypertension (see Fig. 10-24) and acts as an important indicator for diagnosis of these diseases.

Ischemic Heart Disease

Signal intensity changes that correlate with myocardial infarction can be visualized on both noncontrast T_1- and T_2-weighted images. However, there seems to be a better correlation of the high signal intensity in noncontrast T_2-weighted images with the size of the infarct compared with the decrease in signal intensity seen on T_1-weighted images of myocardial infarction. Nevertheless, although increased signal intensity in T_2-weighted images corresponds to myocardial infarction, it also may correspond to edema formation observed in patients with unstable angina or myocarditis without histologic signs of myocyte necrosis. Another important issue in T_2-weighted imaging of myocardial infarction is the fact that slow-flowing blood in the trabecular system near the myocardial infarction may lead to an increase in

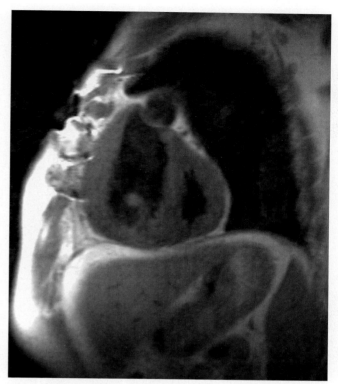

FIGURE 10–24. Right ventricular hypertrophy in a 36-year-old man with idiopathic pulmonary hypertension. The T_2-weighted short-axis view shows marked hypertrophy of the right ventricular myocardium. The myocardial thickness of the right ventricle exceeds that of the left ventricle.

signal intensity, which can make the evaluation of the adjacent endocardial region difficult. In these cases, inversion recovery (IR) sequences in which the signal both from the blood and fat are nulled and which currently, with state-of-the-art MRI machines, can be performed in breath-hold can show better results in quantification of the infarcted area on T_2-weighted noncontrast studies.

Using CE T_1-weighted MRI for the assessment of acute myocardial infarction, two basic approaches for imaging of affected areas can be performed. On the one hand, first-pass perfusion MRIs can be achieved; on the other hand, images acquired several minutes after contrast injection can be used to identify areas of increased contrast enhancement representing reperfused myocardial infarction.

If first-pass perfusion MRI is performed, multiple short-axis T_1-weighted slices with high temporal resolution are acquired during injection of typically a bolus of 0.1 mmol/kg of a Gd chelate. Using this approach, infarcted areas are demonstrated usually as a subendocardial, hypoenhancing zone that extends toward the epicardium.

In images acquired approximately 10 to 15 minutes after contrast injection, these areas become hyperintense in comparison with surrounding normal myocardium if areas of nonviable myocardium are present. This late enhancement represents reperfused infarcts and can be

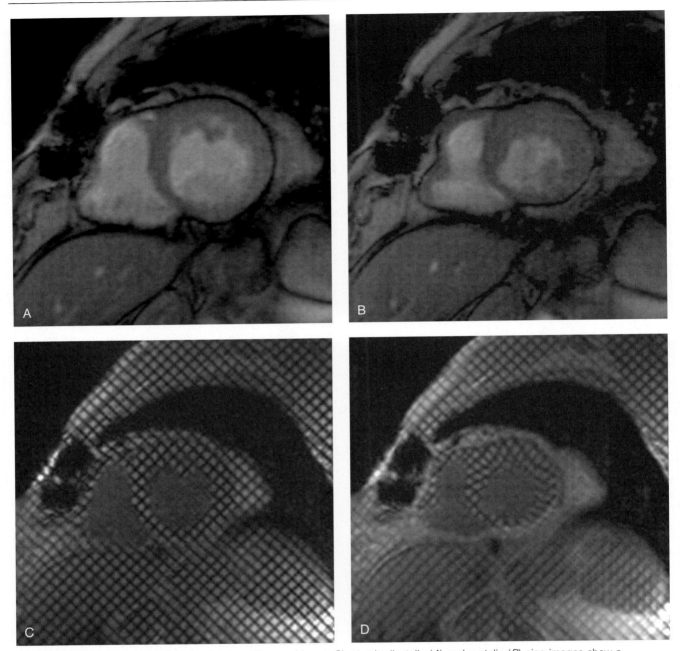

FIGURE 10–25. Chronic myocardial infarction in a 58-year-old man. Short-axis diastolic (*A*) and systolic (*B*) cine images show a decreased thickness of the inferior septum as a result of myocardial infarction. *C* and *D,* In myocardial tagging, decreased myocardial wall motion is visualized in the corresponding area.

used for detection and determination of the size of a myocardial infarction. If a comparison with cine MRI and, in particular, cardiac tagging is performed in the affected region (Fig. 10-25), these areas typically demonstrate decreased myocardial wall thickening and a lack of motion of the myocardial tagging lines.

Areas of chronic myocardial infarction are demonstrated as regions of focal wall thinning on MRI both on conventional T_1- and T_2-weighted spin echo sequences and on cine MRI. Typically, an abrupt transition in thickness from normal myocardium to scar in the area of transmural infarction is observed. In chronic infarction, MRI is also very useful in determining the infarct volume. Possible complications, including aneurysm formation and compensatory myocardial hypertrophy (Fig. 10-26), are evaluated with high accuracy.

Cardiomyopathy

Cardiomyopathy represents a diverse group of disorders, including dilated cardiomyopathy, hypertrophic cardio-

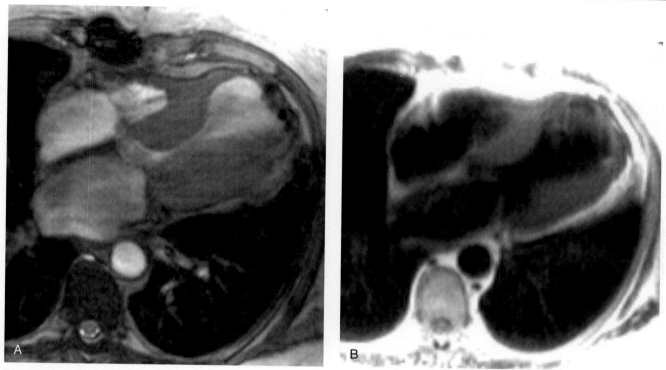

FIGURE 10–26. Hypertrophic obstructive cardiomyopathy following resection of a cardiac aneurysm after myocardial infarction. *A,* Cine imaging shows hypertrophy of the left ventricular myocardium specifically involving the septum at the left ventricular outflow tract and the posterior wall. The heart apex shows marked thinning and artifacts caused by surgical clips after resection of the cardiac aneurysm. *B,* The T$_2$-weighted image shows homogeneous signal of the myocardium, excluding tumor formation.

myopathy, and restrictive cardiomyopathy. Generally, cardiomyopathies are defined as muscular disorders of the heart. Spin echo imaging may be used to demonstrate the morphologic abnormalities in this group of diseases, and cine MRI may be used to demonstrate the concomitant functional abnormalities.

In dilated cardiomyopathy, MRI demonstrates dilatation of the left ventricle and, in many cases, the right ventricle. Pathologically, underlying myocardial fibrosis is present that accounts for the reduced contractility of the myocardium. Cine MRI and myocardial tagging may be used to show the reduced cross-fiber shortening compared with that of normal individuals. MRI may be used both for diagnosis as well as for monitoring of therapeutic intervention. Despite the thinned wall, there is typically an overall increased myocardial mass.

In hypertrophic cardiomyopathy, MRI has proved to be accurate in defining the extent, location, and severity of hypertrophy of the myocardium and in differentiating obstructive from nonobstructive forms. Because there is considerable variability in ventricular morphology in this group of patients, MRI is mainly used to document the presence of unusual forms. In some patients, hypertrophy exists only in the outflow tract septum, whereas in others the entire septum is hypertrophied. The best imaging planes for hypertrophic cardiomyopathy are short-axis and horizontal long-axis views, because the outflow tract can be assessed optimally in the horizontal axis and quantification is best made in the short axis. If MRI tagging is used to evaluate patients with hypertro-

phic cardiomyopathy, the circumferential and longitudinal myocardial shortening is typically depressed in hypertrophied segments compared with that in normal myocardium. Abnormalities in diastolic filling of the ventricle can be reproducibly displayed in cine MRI. There is also evidence that the same parameters involving the right ventricle are abnormal in hypertrophic cardiomyopathy as well.

Restrictive cardiomyopathy clinically may have a similar presentation to constrictive pericarditis (Fig. 10-27). Restrictive cardiomyopathy is characterized by enlarged atria with the coexistent finding of relatively normal-sized ventricles. The lack of increased pericardial thickness as typically seen in constrictive pericarditis hints at the diagnosis of a restrictive disease.

In dysrythmogenic right ventricular dysplasia, pathologically a replacement of muscle by adipose or fibrous tissue and enlargement of end-diastolic diameter are present. Typically, fat extends from the epicardial surface into the interstitium and displaces myocardial fibers. MRI has shown promising results in clarifying the diagnosis of right ventricular dysplasia. MRI can provide information as well about cardiac function, regional wall motion, and direct visualization of the anatomy of the right ventricular free wall. Typically, T$_1$-weighted images should be used to identify fatty infiltration because they give a high contrast between normal myocardium and adipose tissue. To differentiate right ventricular dysplasia, which has a high risk of sudden death, from right ventricular outflow tract tachycardia, which typically

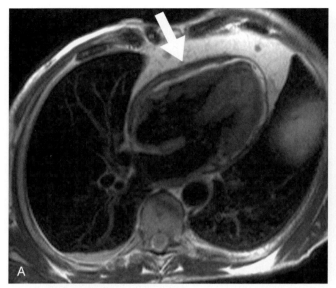
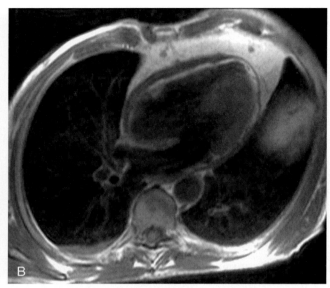

FIGURE 10–27. Constrictive pericarditis in a 45-year-old man with dyspnea and chest pain. T_2- (A) and T_1-weighted (B) images show a low-signal-intensity (SI) thickening of the pericardium mainly located anterior to the right ventricle (*arrow*). The low SI in both T_2- and T_1-weighted images indicates chronic constriction consistent with fibrotic tissue. Note the small tubular right ventricle.

shows a more benign course, MRI may be helpful in localizing dyskinesia to the right ventricular outflow tract in cine MRI.

Valvular Disease

Using ECG-gated spin echo imaging, MRI most commonly is used to assess the secondary changes that occur in combination with valvular disorders of the aortic, pulmonary, and mitral valves. Using cine MRI, the regurgitation jet in valve insufficiency as well the jet observed in stenosis of a valve can be visualized as a region of signal void (Fig. 10-28). Unfortunately, the size of this signal void does not correlate with the degree of

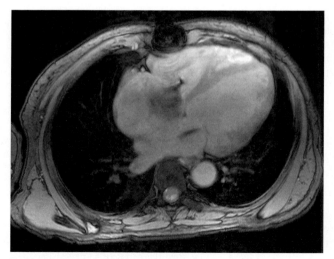

FIGURE 10–28. Combined tricuspid and mitral regurgitation. Systolic cine imaging in the four-chamber view shows a retrograde jet in the area of the tricuspid and the mitral valve with marked enlargement of the right atrium.

regurgitation or stenosis. However, cine MRI can be used for quantification of the volume of regurgitation in patients with only one affected valve (Figs. 10-12 and 10-29). The regurgitation volume can be assessed by the difference between right and left ventricular stroke volumes as calculated from serial MRIs covering the ventricles acquired in both diastole and systole. However, this is very time consuming; thus, velocity-encoded techniques are favored to measure regurgitant flow. Using this approach, images are obtained parallel to the annulus of the affected valve, and with PC techniques the total flow during the cardiac cycle can be calculated as the product of the valve area and the velocity. Thus, retrograde flow can be quantified. MRI is useful as well in detecting and quantifying acquired valvular disease and in differentiating among congenital anomalies such as subvalvular stenosis in pediatric patients. Combining measurement of the cross-sectional area of the aorta with the functional assessment of the aortic valve gives a complete overview of the disease and allows reproducible follow-up in cases with equivocal findings concerning indication for surgery.

Pericardium

In normal patients, the pericardium in T_1-weighted images is less than 2 mm thick. Overall, the pericardium is somewhat better visualized during systole and can be easily identified on T_1-weighted images anterior to the right ventricle (see Fig. 27). In contrast, posterolateral to the left ventricle the normal pericardial signal is often not seen against the low-signal-intensity lung parenchyma. Although echocardiography is the primary modality for identifying pericardial abnormalities, MRI has an established role in the evaluation of the pericardium. Typical indications include patients in whom clinical findings are inconsistent with echocardiographic diagno-

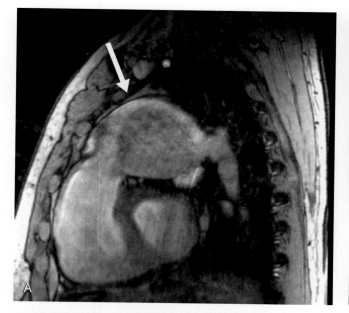

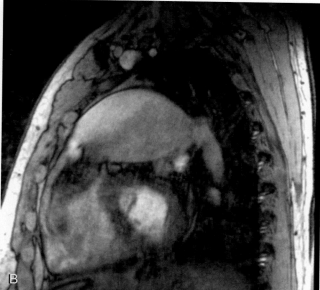

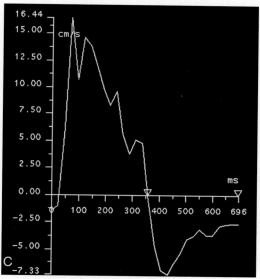

FIGURE 10–29. Pulmonary regurgitation in a 34-year-old, otherwise healthy man. A systolic ejection murmur was detected during routine check-up. *A,* Systolic cine imaging longitudinal to the right ventricular outflow tract shows turbulence across the pulmonary valve and marked dilatation (*arrow*) of the pulmonary truncus. *B,* In diastole a retrograde jet is noted across the pulmonary valve. *C,* Flow evaluation of the pulmonary flow with phase contrast acquisition shows the regurgitation volume as the area under the curve for the negative flow component.

sis, patients with inadequate echocardiographic evaluation, and patients in whom a more precise evaluation is necessary. However, for identification of calcific pericarditis, CT is the method of choice.

Pericardial Effusion

In contrast to what is seen with fluid collections elsewhere in the body, the signal intensity of a pericardial effusion on T_2-weighted images is frequently lower than that of simple fluid. Flow effects in the pericardium in patients with a large simple effusion may also lead to inhomogeneous signal intensity, with areas of both high and intermediate signal. These alterations of the signal are probably caused by a loss of phase coherence within the pericardial fluid from fluid motion. Pericardial perfusions may be serous, bloody, or lymphatic. Hemorrhagic effusion is characterized by high signal intensity on T_1-weighted spin echo images in contrast to the low signal intensity of nonhemorrhagic fluid. Typically, it is easier to identify nonhemorrhagic effusions on T_1-weighted images because pericardial fat has a high signal intensity; thus, serous or lymphatic effusions are distinguished by their low signal intensity compared with normal myocardium and pericardial fat. Effusions may be generalized or loculated, and associated pericardial inflammation may be separately recognized as a thickened pericardium with a higher signal intensity than pericardial effusion on T_1-weighted images.

In pericardial thickening, MRI detects a widened pericardial line of low signal intensity on T_1-weighted images. Calcifications may appear as focal areas of decreased signal with irregular borders. In constrictive pericarditis, a thickness of more than 4 mm indicates pericardial thickening. However, pericardial thickening can also be observed in the absence of constrictive pericarditis; thus, the diagnosis should always include a con-

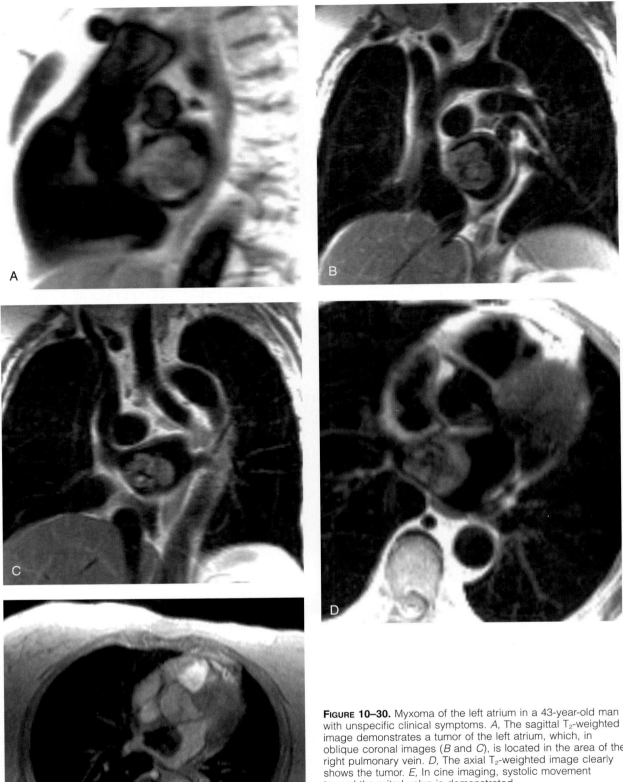

Figure 10–30. Myxoma of the left atrium in a 43-year-old man with unspecific clinical symptoms. *A,* The sagittal T$_2$-weighted image demonstrates a tumor of the left atrium, which, in oblique coronal images (*B* and *C*), is located in the area of the right pulmonary vein. *D,* The axial T$_2$-weighted image clearly shows the tumor. *E,* In cine imaging, systolic movement toward the mitral valve is demonstrated.

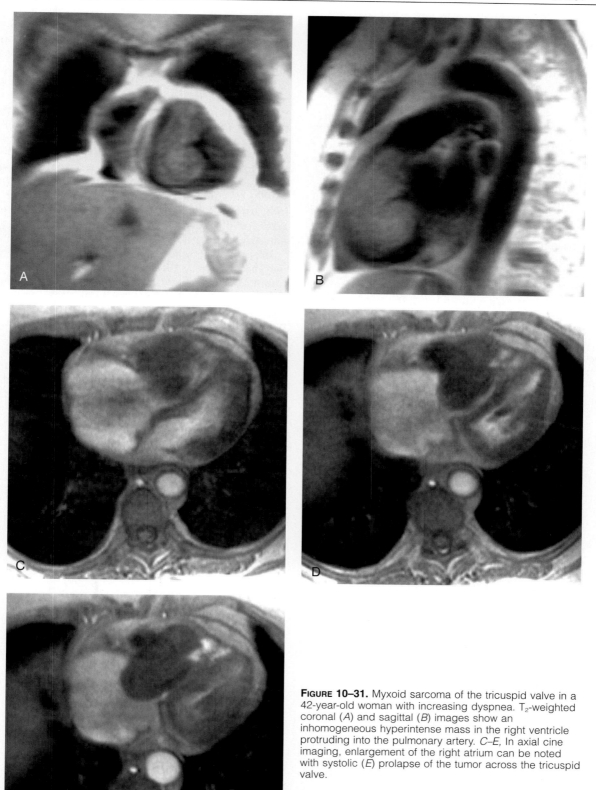

Figure 10–31. Myxoid sarcoma of the tricuspid valve in a 42-year-old woman with increasing dyspnea. T$_2$-weighted coronal (*A*) and sagittal (*B*) images show an inhomogeneous hyperintense mass in the right ventricle protruding into the pulmonary artery. *C–E,* In axial cine imaging, enlargement of the right atrium can be noted with systolic (*E*) prolapse of the tumor across the tricuspid valve.

sideration of clinical symptoms. The main issue in MRI for constrictive pericarditis is the differentiation from restrictive cardiomyopathy. In this clinical setting, pericardial thickening in combination with a small, tubular right ventricle and a dilated right atrium favors the diagnosis of constrictive pericarditis.

Cardiac Masses

ECG-gated spin echo sequences have proven effective in demonstrating the presence, location, and extent as well as in certain instances the nature of a cardiac mass. Primary cardiac tumors are rare. Approximately 80% are benign and can be effectively treated with surgical resection. Secondary malignant tumors involving the heart are somewhat more common, resulting from metastatic disease to the myocardium and pericardium or direct invasion of a tumor from adjacent lung or mediastinal structures.

The most frequent intracardiac mass is thrombus, which is usually located within the left atrium or left ventricle. The most frequent primary benign tumors are myxoma and lipoma; the former is usually located in the left atrium (Fig. 10-30) and the latter in the right. MRI can be used to distinguish these tumors from mural thrombus, which may occur in a similar location, by identifying a pedicle that attaches the tumor to the atrium in the case of a myxoma and by the homogeneous high signal intensity of the mass in the case of a lipoma. Definite tissue specific diagnosis of a cardiac tumor can only be made in cases of lipoma that typically show the same high signal intensity in T_1-weighted images as subcutaneous or pericardial fat. Occasionally, in the case of a myxoma, prolapse of the tumor across the mitral valve can be observed in diastole that can be identified on cine MRI. Other benign and malignant cardiac tumors include rhabdomyomas and rhabdomyosarcomas, angiosarcomas, myxoid sarcomas (Fig. 10-31), fibromas, and melanomas. Observations that favor the diagnosis of a malignant tumor include a wide base of attachment, which, in contrast to the pedicle in myxoma, is more indicative of a malignant infiltrative tumor, and the observation of a hemorrhagic pericardial effusion in combination with a cardiac mass.

In secondary tumors of the heart, cardiac involvement may be caused by direct spread of mediastinal or lung tumors or extension of tumors of the upper abdomen through the inferior vena cava into the right atrium (e.g., in cases of tumor thrombus with renal cell carcinoma). In imaging of metastases to the pericardium, myocardium, or the cardiac chambers, MRI has been proved effective in demonstrating these tumors. However, in most cases, myocardial metastases represent end-stage metastatic disease, and there is only limited effect on therapeutic management of the patient.

Abdomen

11

Günther Schneider

The use of magnetic resonance imaging (MRI) in the diagnosis of intra-abdominal diseases in the past has been limited because artifacts caused by respiratory, cardiac, and peristaltic motion significantly degraded the quality of images. As MRI technology has advanced, these limitations have been overcome.

Motion artifacts in T_1-weighted images can be controlled for spin echo sequences using a combination of respiratory gating, averaging, and presaturation pulses. However, with the introduction of breath-hold sequences, spin echo sequences in imaging of the abdomen are being replaced on up-to-date equipment. Multisection spoiled gradient echo sequences are primarily used for this purpose (e.g., fast low-angle shot [FLASH]), which allows T_1-weighted imaging of the entire upper abdomen in one single breath-hold of less than 20 seconds. Thus, dynamic imaging of the upper abdomen during contrast medium injection in the arterial and portal venous phase of liver perfusion is possible.

For T_2-weighted imaging, multishot fast spin echo (FSE) or so-called turbo spin echo (TSE) sequences are primarily used, which allow respiratory gated imaging of, for example, the liver in only a few minutes. Although, as reported in the literature, these sequences may show a slight loss of contrast between liver lesions and surrounding liver parenchyma, the higher image quality regarding motion artifacts more than compensates for this. Newer sequences allow T_2-weighted imaging of the upper abdomen in suspended respiration. Even non-breath-hold T_2-weighted studies using ultrafast single-shot sequences can be performed in patients who cannot follow breathing commands adequately.

For imaging of the bile ducts and the pancreatic duct in magnetic resonance cholangiopancreatography (MRCP), heavily T_2-weighted sequences should be applied because the fluid in the bile ducts and pancreatic duct is static and has a long T_2 time. Using this technique either in suspended respiration or with respiratory gating, two- and three-dimensional reconstructions of the biliary system can be acquired.

Chemical shift imaging of the abdomen is another technique that is of great interest. It allows detection of focal fatty infiltration in the liver (Fig. 11-1) as well as identification of benign adrenocortical masses in imaging of the adrenal glands. Currently used chemical shift techniques include opposed-phase imaging featuring signal cancellation in voxels that contain both triglyceride and water as well as frequency selective fat suppression techniques in which a narrow band excitation pulse is used to selectively saturate triglyceride protons without affecting water protons. Opposed-phase images are more sensitive in detecting small quantities of lipid (e.g., in focal fatty infiltration of the liver), whereas fat-suppressed images are better in identifying large quantities of lipid in a tissue (e.g., a lipoma).

LIVER

The detection and differential diagnosis of focal liver lesions in patients with suspected primary malignant liver tumors or metastases are important challenges that have major clinical consequences. Although the accurate differentiation between benign lesions such as liver hemangioma or focal nodular hyperplasia (FNH) and malignant liver lesions is of great importance, the ability to localize lesions precisely, to determine the exact number of lesions present, and to ascertain the involvement, if any, of vascular or biliary structures may have a major impact on therapeutic management. MRI can be regarded as the most accurate method for the detection, differential diagnosis, and staging of benign and malignant liver tumors.

Although unenhanced MRI, using morphologic characteristics on T_1- and T_2-weighted images to differentiate between benign and malignant liver lesions, has high accuracy rates, it is widely accepted that the use of contrast can improve the detection as well as the differential diagnosis of focal liver lesions.

Contrast for MRI of the liver has generally been classified in one of two ways: as a nonspecific agent that distributes exclusively to the extracellular fluid space and that is effective for dynamic phase imaging of the liver for lesion detection and characterization (e.g., gadolinium [Gd]-DTPA, Gd-DTPA-BMA or Gd-HP-DO3A); or as a liver-specific agent that is targeted specifically to liver cells (i.e., hepatocytes, e.g., Gd-BOPTA, Gd-EOB-DTPA, or mangafodipir trisodium [Mn-DPDP]) or Kupffer cells (e.g., superparamagnetic iron oxide (AMI-25), magnetite) and that is effective in a more delayed phase for liver lesion detection.

Although liver-specific agents like Mn-DPDP and ferumoxides (AMI-25) are approved for clinical use in the United States, their actual utilization is very low.

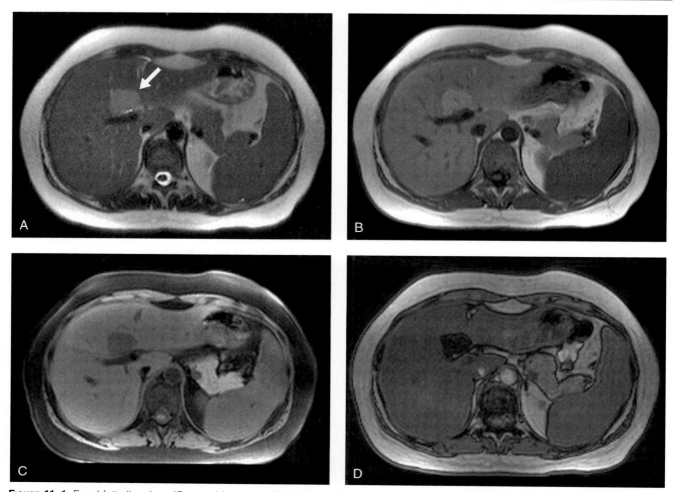

FIGURE 11–1. Focal fatty liver in a 47-year-old woman with a history of breast cancer who is undergoing chemotherapy. On T$_2$- (*A*) and T$_1$-weighted (*B*) images, there is a hyperintense, sharply demarcated liver lesion in the perihilar region (*arrow*). *C*, The signal of the lesion can be suppressed in fat-saturated T$_1$-weighted imaging; thus, hemorrhage can be excluded. *D*, On opposed-phase imaging, the signal of the lesion markedly decreases, indicating a focal fatty area.

Thus, the use of extracellular space agents for imaging of the liver is emphasized in this chapter.

The vascular anatomy of the liver is essential for the differential diagnosis of focal liver lesions and for liver surgery. Surgical anatomy divides the liver into nine segments, any of which can be resected individually or in combination with neighboring segments. If there is enough liver parenchyma left, no diminution of liver function should result. The falciform ligament divides the liver into the left and right lobes. The liver segments are differentiated by their vascular supply with the branches of the portal vein showing intrasegmental localization and the hepatic veins located intersegmentally.

Knowledge of the different perfusion phases of liver parenchyma and focal liver lesions is essential to understand the diagnosis and therapy of focal liver lesions. The liver parenchyma receives up to 80% of its blood supply from the portal vein; the remaining 20% is supplied by the common hepatic artery via the celiac trunk. In contrast to normal liver parenchyma, focal liver lesions are mainly fed by branches of the hepatic arteries.

Extracellular contrast in MRI is given intravenously and distributed initially within the intravascular com-

partment. In this use, application of the contrast by means of a power injector with a flow rate of at least 1 mL/sec is superior to a continuous infusion if dynamic imaging is to be performed.

The normal blood supply of the liver, characterized by perfusion via the hepatic artery and portal vein leads to a typical enhancement pattern after bolus contrast administration. With a delay of 25 to 30 seconds after starting contrast injection, hepatic arteries are contrasted, whereas venous and portal venous structures are still unenhanced and remain hypointense to surrounding liver tissue. The hypointense appearance of venous structures in the arterial phase scan should not be mistaken for focal liver lesions. In the arterial phase of liver perfusion, arterial hypervascularized liver lesions can easily be differentiated from hypointense, only slightly contrasted normal liver tissue. Hepatic areas with incidental regional hypervascularization, already known from computed tomography (CT) examination as areas of focal attenuation difference, must not be misinterpreted as hypervascularized focal lesions. Thus, a comparison with unenhanced and portal venous scans is always necessary. After initial arterial enhancement, a homogeneous filling of venous and portal venous structures can be observed in the portal venous phase, 50 to 55 seconds after the beginning of contrast injection, also accompanied by increasing contrast enhancement of surrounding normal liver tissue. This phase of liver perfusion enables good differentiation of liver segments based on the identification of left, middle, and right liver vein. Furthermore, hypovascularized focal lesions can be clearly depicted beause the entire liver now shows homogeneous contrast enhancement. Delayed-phase images 5 to 15 minutes after contrast administration show an enhancement of liver tissue in comparison with unenhanced images. At this time, the vessels may again appear hypointense or isointense in comparison with surrounding liver parenchyma. Liver lesions with a delayed, persistent enhancement can be detected and classified.

Classification of Focal Liver Lesions in MRI Based on Vascularization Patterns

Dynamic MRI examinations refer to a classification that describes perfusion patterns, and specifically the degree of tumor vascularization, without primary consideration of the origin of the tumor or tumor-like lesion.

Regarding perfusion patterns of focal liver lesions, three groups can be distinguished:

1. Hypervascular liver lesions
2. Hypovascular liver lesions
3. Lesions presenting delayed persistent enhancement

Figure 11-2 demonstrates the three different perfusion characteristics to which most focal liver lesions can be assigned. Figures 11-3 to 11-5 briefly summarize the lesion types that may be found in each of the three groups and give additional information for subdivisions.

All three groups in this classification include benign and malignant liver tumors as well as primary and secondary liver lesions. Additional differentiation is possible by comparing dynamic images with unenhanced T_1- and T_2-weighted scans and by analyzing internal lesion morphology based on contrast-enhanced images.

This radiologic classification does not consider the histopathologic differentiation of liver tumors because the degree of vascularization and not the histologic appearance is the basis for differentiation of focal liver lesions in dynamic MRI. Applying histopathologic criteria, focal liver lesions can be divided in different groups with regard to their differentiation and type (Fig. 11-6). Primary lesions can be subgrouped as mesenchymal, epithelial, or mixed as well as tumor-like lesions; secondary lesions mainly comprise metastatic and parasitic disease.

Some of the morphologic characteristics described in pathologic classifications may also be recognized in MRI of the liver (e.g., the central scar in focal nodular hyperplasia, regressive changes in hepatocellular carcinoma, and myxoid degeneration in a giant hemangioma). Nevertheless, the pathologic description in most cases does not reflect vascularization patterns that may be used for differential diagnosis in contrast-enhanced cross-sectional imaging (e.g., the centripetal filling of hemangioma or the arterial hypervascular rim in liver metastases of colorectal adenocarcinoma). Thus, classification of liver lesions in dynamic contrast-enhanced MRI uses morphologic criteria described for pathologic classifications as well as contrast kinetics, leading to the differentiation between arterial hypervascular and hypovascular lesions and lesions demonstrating delayed persistent enhancement without primary regard to origin or type of liver lesions. Figure 11-6 shows the clinically most

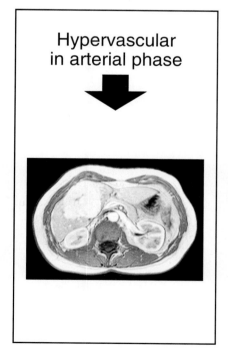

Hypervascular in arterial phase

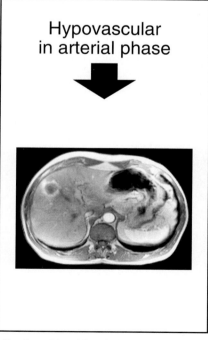

Hypovascular in arterial phase

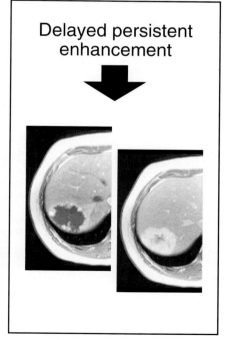

Delayed persistent enhancement

FIGURE 11–2. Classification of focal liver lesions in T_1-weighted dynamic imaging.

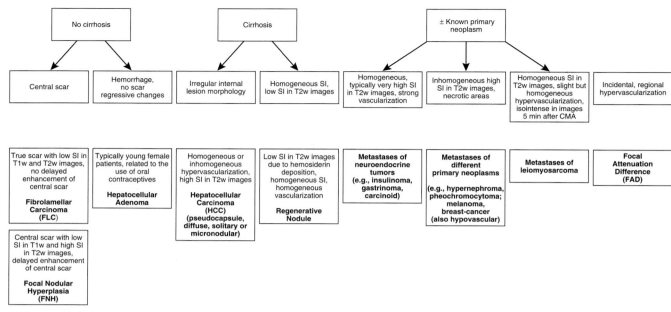

FIGURE 11–3. Liver lesions that are hypervascular in the arterial phase. (SI, signal intensity; CMA, contrast medium administration.)

Cystic appearance	Hypervascular rim in arterial phase	Hypovascular in arterial and portalvenous phase, isointense in images 5 min post CM injection	Hypervascular rim with persistent enhancement, no central CM uptake	History of abdominal trauma or surgery

Sharply demarcated, no irregular regional vascularization **Cyst solitary/multiple Caroli's disease polycystic kidney disease**	Washout sign 5–15 min after CM injection, T2w: Doughnut sign/ halo sign **Metastases of adenocarcinoma** **(pancreas, colon, stomach, and other primary tumors)**	Irregular areas of low SI in T1w images, increased SI or isointense in T2w images **Non-Hodgkin's lymphoma, Hodgkin's disease**	High SI in T2w images (almost cystic appearance), occasionally gas formation **Liver abscess**	Cystic appearance, tends to increase in size, dislocation of vessels, high SI in T2w images **Bilioma**

Low SI rim, internal septations, daughter cysts **Echinococcal disease**	Cystic appearance, irregular cyst wall with focal solid areas, internal septations **Cystic metastases** **(e.g., ovarian cancer or after chemotherapy)**			Irregular borders, inhomogeneous SI in T1w and T2w images, hyperintense rim due to extracellular methemoglobin, with time increase of central SI **Liver hematoma/ rupture**

FIGURE 11–4. Liver lesions that are hypovascular in the arterial phase. (CM, contrast medium; SI, signal intensity.)

Infiltration along portal tracts, segmental biliary obstruction	± Known primary neoplasm	Nodular peripheral enhancement in arterial phase, centripetal filling

Irregular, partially nodular enhancement in arterial phase, irregular filling	Homogeneous, sometimes early enhancement, irregular shape

Hypovascular with hypervascular peripheral enhancement in arterial phase **Intrahepatic cholangiocellular carcinoma (CCC)**	Hypo- or slightly hypervascular in arterial phase, low SI in T1w and high SI in T2w images, sometimes peripheral washout **Metastases of leiomyosarcoma and gastrointestinal stromal tumors (GIST)**	High SI in T2w images (light bulb appearance), in large lesions central areas may remain unenhanced after CM injection due to thrombosis/fibrosis, sharply demarcated **Hemangioma**

Centrifugal or irregular filling, irregular borders **Hemangiosarcoma, hemangio-endothelioma, hemangiopericytoma**	High SI in T2w images, iso- or hyperintense in delayed-phase images **Peliosis hepatis**

FIGURE 11–5. Liver lesions that show a delayed persistent enhancement. (SI, signal intensity; CM, contrast medium.)

	BENIGN LIVER TUMORS	MALIGNANT LIVER TUMORS
PRIMARY TUMORS		
Epithelial tumors		
Hepatocellular origin	Hepatocellular adenoma	Hepatocellular carcinoma Fibrolamellar carcinoma
Cholangiocellular	Bile duct adenoma Biliary papillomatosis	Cholangiocellular carcinoma Bile duct cystadenocarcinoma
Mesenchymal tumors		
Vascular tumors	Hemangioma Hemangioendothelioma (children) Angiomyolipoma	Angiosarcoma Hemangiosarcoma Malignant epithelioid hemangioendothelioma Embryonal sarcoma Rhabdomyosarcoma
Mixed type		Hepatoblastoma
SECONDARY TUMORS	Parasitic infections	Metastases
TUMOR-LIKE LESIONS	Cysts Focal nodular hyperplasia Regenerative nodules Mesenchymal hamartoma Peliosis hepatis Inflammatory pseudotumors	

FIGURE 11–6. Classification of focal liver lesions by histopathology.

293

relevant primary and secondary hepatic lesions as well as tumor-like lesions, which must be distinguished from true neoplasms.

In practice, the liver should be scanned before administration of an extracellular agent (unenhanced imaging) using both T_1- and T_2-weighted sequences and in the immediate postcontrast arterial (approximately 18–25 seconds after the start of contrast administration) and portalvenous phases (approximately 50–55 seconds after contrast administration) after bolus injection of the contrast using T_1-weighted gradient echo breath-hold sequences covering the entire liver in a single breath-hold. Additional T_1-weighted images should be acquired approximately 5 minutes after contrast injection.

Hypervascular Liver Lesions

Hypervascularized liver lesions are characterized by strong contrast enhancement in the arterial phase scan (25–30 seconds after the start of contrast application) as a result of the blood supply being mainly from the hepatic arteries. Hypervascularized liver lesions may be sharply demarcated or may show a more diffuse appearance. Often lesions presenting with early arterial enhancement are isointense and barely detectable in the portalvenous and delayed-phase scans. Arterial hypervascularization is rarely seen as a result of arteriovenous shunting, such as in high-flow arteriovenous malformations (AVMs). However, in general, benign or malignant neoplasms are the main cause of arterial blood supply of focal liver lesions with the exception of inflammatory changes.

The most common primary malignant tumor of the liver presenting with arterial hypervascularization is hepatocellular carcinoma (HCC). This malignant neoplasm is mostly associated with alcoholic cirrhosis, long-standing chronic hepatitis B or C, and other forms of chronic parenchymal damage (e.g., hemochromatosis). Three different types of HCC can be distinguished by means of morphologic appearance in macroscopic pathology or histology as well as by imaging studies: the expansile (encapsulated) form, a more infiltrative variant, and the multifocal or diffuse type. All types of HCC typically show hypervascularization in the arterial phase scan. Depending on necrosis or hemorrhage in HCC, hypervascularization may range from homogeneous to inhomogeneous. In expansile or encapsulated HCC (Fig. 11-7), a hyperintense pseudocapsule may be seen in the portalvenous phase scan consisting of compressed liver tissue, and lesions may appear single or multinodular. The infiltrative type (Fig. 11-8) shows irregular margins with partially hypervascular and hypovascular areas occasionally replacing most or all of one liver lobe. The diffuse type presents as several small tumors (<1 cm) at multiple sites in the liver, resulting in a more diffusely appearing hypervascularization in the arterial phase scan, isointense or slightly hypointense in portalvenous phase, and almost always associated with advanced signs of cirrhosis. On unenhanced images, depending on underlying parenchymal changes, HCC in patients with underlying cirrhosis typically appears hypointense on T_1-weighted images and hyperintense on T_2-weighted im-

ages. In patients with hemochromatosis, HCC appears hyperintense on T_1- and T_2-weighted images compared with the surrounding low-signal-intensity-liver tissue (resulting from excessive iron storage within the liver).

Fibrolamellar carcinoma (FLC) is a rare type of hepatocellular carcinoma and is found mainly in young patients without predisposing chronic liver disease. Early resection may result in long-term survival. FLC can resemble focal nodular hyperplasia (FNH). In the arterial phase, FLC shows marked enhancement with a central hypointense scar similar to the findings in FNH. In contrast to FNH, the central scar in FLC typically appears hypointense in T_2-weighted imaging, and central calcification may be noted on CT in 30% of the patients. The central scar in FLC represents lamellar fibrosis ("true scar"); thus, in contrast to FNH, no delayed enhancement of the central scar is observed on delayed-phase imaging.

Liver cell (hepatocellular) adenoma (HCA) is the most important benign primary liver tumor predominantly arising in young female patients (15–45 years). The association with oral contraceptive steroid usage is well established. Even so, HCA may occur, albeit rarely, spontaneously. Incidence and complication rates seem to correlate with duration and dosage of oral contraceptives. Rare cases of malignant transformation are described. Histologically, HCA consists of benign hepatocytes arranged in sheets without acinar architecture, portal tracts, or bile ducts. Large adenomas may cause abdominal discomfort; they often appear with areas of necrosis, hemorrhage, or fatty degeneration. Thus, inhomogeneous signal intensity may be noted in unenhanced T_1- and T_2-weighted and contrast-enhanced MRI. The risk of rupture into the peritoneal cavity is high in liver cell adenomas larger than 10 cm, and resection should be seriously considered for this reason alone. Typically, these lesions are hypervascular on the arterial phase scan. Depending on the size of the lesion internal, hypovascular areas resulting from hemorrhage or necrosis may be present. On unenhanced T_1- or T_2-weighted images, small HCAs without necrotic areas or hemorrhage may appear isointense to surrounding liver tissue (Fig. 11-9). Larger HCAs with hemorrhage or necrosis may appear hyper- or hypointense (Fig. 11-10).

Regarding pathologic classification, focal nodular hyperplasia (FNH) represents a tumor-like benign liver lesion presenting with arterial hypervascularization. It is most often incidentally found in young, otherwise healthy individuals. Relation to oral contraceptives is less evident than for HCA, but oral contraceptive steroid usage may promote growth. On macroscopic tissue pathology examination, FNH shows fibrous septa and a central stellate scar. On histologic exam, abnormally arranged normal hepatocytes with Kupffer cells and primitive bile ductules without communication with ducts are present. No portal tracts or central veins can be found. Typically, the central scar of the lesion is hyperintense on T_2-weighted scans and shows enhancement on delayed-phase images (Fig. 11-11), a relatively reliable sign for FNH in differential diagnosis from fibrolamellar carcinoma. In contrast to FLC, the "pseudoscar" in FNH consists of vessels, bile ducts, and

Text continued on page 300

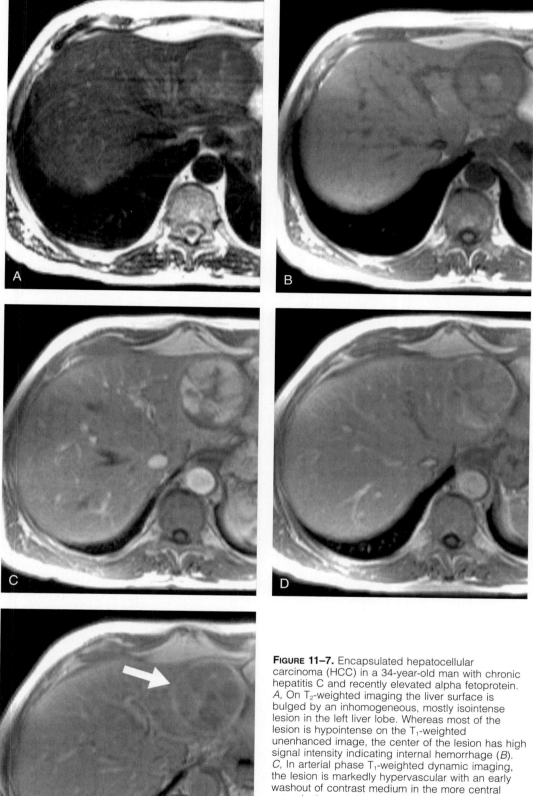

FIGURE 11–7. Encapsulated hepatocellular
carcinoma (HCC) in a 34-year-old man with chronic
hepatitis C and recently elevated alpha fetoprotein.
A, On T₂-weighted imaging the liver surface is
bulged by an inhomogeneous, mostly isointense
lesion in the left liver lobe. Whereas most of the
lesion is hypointense on the T₁-weighted
unenhanced image, the center of the lesion has high
signal intensity indicating internal hemorrhage (*B*).
C, In arterial phase T₁-weighted dynamic imaging,
the lesion is markedly hypervascular with an early
washout of contrast medium in the more central
areas in the portalvenous phase (*D*). There is a
persistent enhancing pseudocapsule (*arrow*)
surrounding the lesion in the equilibrium phase (*E*),
which is typically found in encapsulated HCC
caused by compressed surrounding liver
parenchyma.

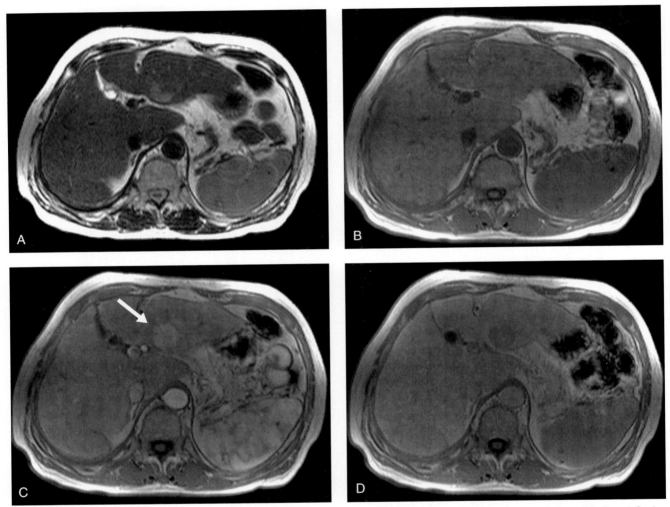

FIGURE 11–8. Liver cirrhosis and hepatocellular carcinoma (HCC) in a 63-year-old man with long-standing chronic hepatitis B and C. *A* and *B*, Unenhanced T$_2$- and T$_1$-weighted images show liver cirrhosis with a humpy liver surface and an irregular nodular appearance of the liver parenchyma as a result of multiple macroregenerative nodules. There is a hyperintense lesion in the left liver lobe on T$_2$-weighted imaging (*A*), which shows arterial enhancement in the arterial phase (*C, arrow*) and early contrast washout in the portalvenous phase (*D*), consistent with HCC.

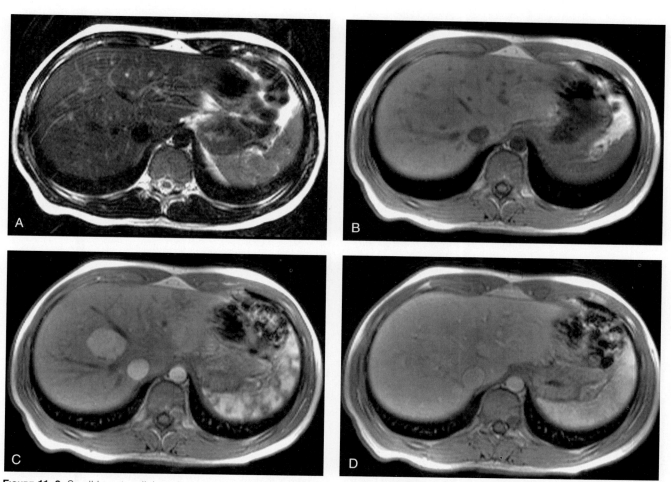

FIGURE 11–9. Small hepatocellular adenoma without degeneration in a 16-year-old boy with a history of Hodgkin's lymphoma in complete remission, recurrent right upper quadrant pain, and a focal liver lesion on sonography. T_2- (*A*) and T_1-weighted (*B*) images hardly detect the round focal lesion in segment 8. It is almost isointense to surrounding parenchyma on T_2-weighted imaging and slightly hypointense on T_1-weighted imaging. There are no signs of hemorrhage or regressive changes. *C,* In the arterial phase, there is strong hypervascularization, and the lesion is isointense in the portalvenous phase (*D*).

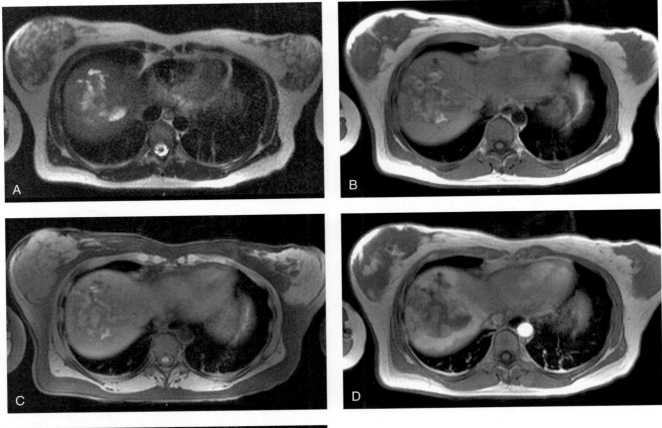

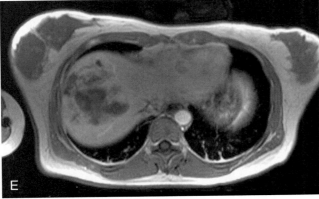

FIGURE 11–10. Hepatocellular adenoma with large internal hemorrhage in a 34-year-old woman with right upper quadrant pain. *A,* In T$_2$-weighted imaging an inhomogeneous signal intensity with areas of high signal, visible also in the T$_1$-weighted image (*B*), is demonstrated. *C,* The fat-suppressed image again demonstrates high-signal-intensity areas, indicating hemorrhage. The lesion shows inhomogeneous strong arterial enhancement (*D*) with a slightly persistent elevated signal in the portalvenous phase (*E*).

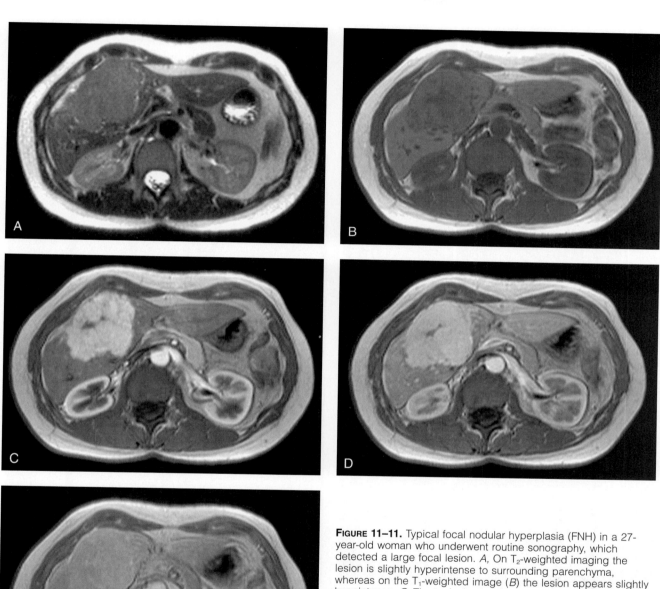

FIGURE 11–11. Typical focal nodular hyperplasia (FNH) in a 27-year-old woman who underwent routine sonography, which detected a large focal lesion. *A,* On T$_2$-weighted imaging the lesion is slightly hyperintense to surrounding parenchyma, whereas on the T$_1$-weighted image (*B*) the lesion appears slightly hypointense. *C,* The typical arterial hypervascularization with a hypointense central scar is clearly visible in the arterial phase T$_1$-weighted dynamic image. *D,* In the portalvenous phase the central scar is still clearly visible. However, the central stellate scar displays enhancement in the equilibrium phase (*E*) typical of FNH.

edematous liver tissue. On T₁-weighted arterial phase imaging, FNH shows strong enhancement and the central scar appears hypointense. In the portalvenous phase, FNH is almost isointense to surrounding liver tissue (Fig. 11-12). The central scar in most cases still appears hypointense but demonstrates contrast uptake on delayed-phase images. On unenhanced T₁-weighted images, the lesion is typically isointense or slightly hypointense. T₂-weighted images depict FNH as isointense or slightly hyperintense lesions. However, approximately 30% of FNHs are atypical (Fig. 11-13) and do not show a central scar.

Hypervascular liver metastases represent secondary malignant liver lesions. The following primary tumors typically show arterial hypervascular liver metastases: functional islet cell tumors such as gastrinoma and insulinoma, nonhyperfunctioning islet cell tumors, hypernephroma, neuroendocrine pancreatic tumor, carcinoid (Fig. 11-14), malignant pheochromocytoma, gastrointestinal stroma tumor (GIST), uveal melanoma, pancreaticoblastoma, breast cancer, and other rare primary neoplasms. Depending on the primary tumor, hypervascular liver metastases may show extremely high signal intensity in T₂-weighted images (e.g., insulinoma, gastrinoma) comparable to the signal intensity found in a hemangioma. Especially with small metastases, differen-

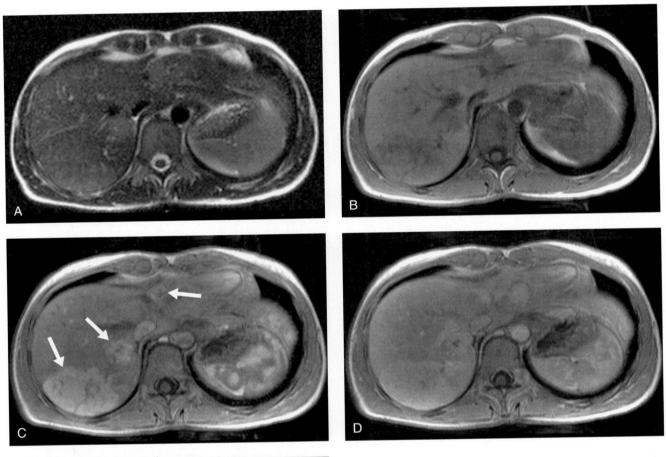

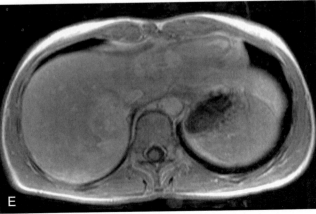

FIGURE 11–12. Multiple typical focal nodular hyperplasia (FNH) in a 32-year-old woman with nonspecific right upper quadrant pain. Typically, FNH displays almost isointensity to surrounding parenchyma on unenhanced images (*A* and *B*), reflecting the similarity of its stroma to normal hepatic parenchyma. *C,* The arterial phase image clearly depicts the strongly hypervascularized lesions (*arrows*), which in this case are scattered throughout the liver. The large lesion in segment 7 shows the typical central scar, which is still visible in the portalvenous phase (*D*), with enhancement in the equilibrium phase (*E*). This late enhancement reflects the histologic appearance of this central pseudoscar in FNH, which represents vessels and focal areas of cirrhosis. In fibrolamellar carcinoma as a main differential diagnosis, the central true scar would not show delayed enhancement, and calcifications of the central scar can be noted in approximately 30% of cases on CT.

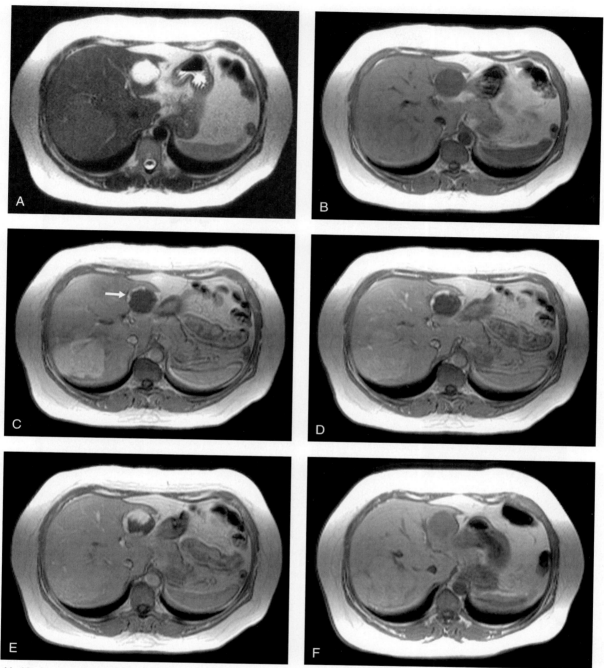

FIGURE 11–13. Atypical focal nodular hyperplasia (FNH) and liver hemangioma in a 52-year-old woman with newly diagnosed breast cancer. Magnetic resonance imaging of the liver was performed for staging. On T_2-weighted imaging (*A*), only the high-signal-intensity lesion of the left liver lobe is visible, which is hypointense on unenhanced T_1 (*B*) and shows peripheral nodular enhancement (*arrow*) in dynamic imaging (*C* and *D*). There is a clump-like fill-in of the lesion 5 minutes after contrast administration (*E*), consistent with a hemangioma. The lesion of the right liver lobe can only be visualized clearly on T_1-weighted contrast-enhanced images (*C* and *D*). There is a strong enhancement in the arterial phase with a slight pooling of contrast in the portalvenous phase. In the equilibrium phase, the lesion is again isointense to surrounding liver tissue. *F*, In images acquired 1 hour after injection of a hepatocyte-directed contrast (0.05 mmol/kg Gd-BOPTA), the lesion is hyperintense compared with surrounding liver tissue, indicating a liver lesion that contains functioning hepatocytes. There is no otherwise typical central stellate scar. Despite its atypical appearance, the diagnosis of an FNH can be made because of the contrast media uptake of the liver cell-specific contrast medium and the homogeneous hypervascularization of the lesion in a patient without underlying liver cirrhosis. An adenoma of this size would show regressive changes. Metastases would show a more inhomogeneous, increased signal intensity in unenhanced T_2-weighted images.

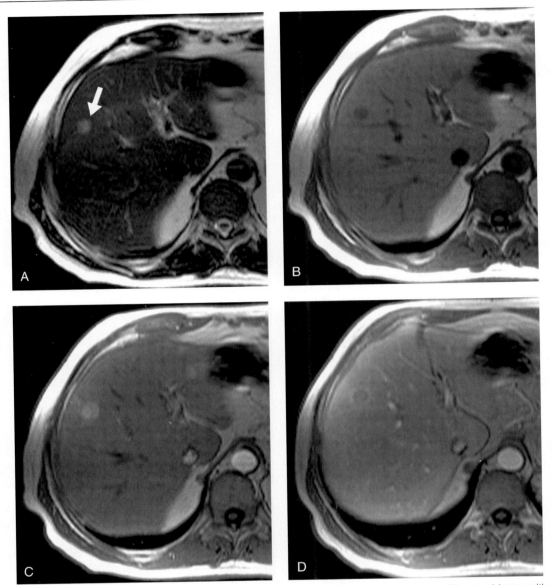

FIGURE 11–14. Hypervascular liver metastasis from carcinoid tumor found during a follow-up study in a 72-year-old man with previous resection of a small bowel carcinoid. *A,* On the T₂-weighted image, a hyperintense liver lesion (*arrow*) with homogeneous signal intensity is visible. The lesion is hypointense on T₁ and shows a strong homogeneous hypervascularization in arterial phase dynamic imaging (*C*). There is an early washout of contrast in the central area, indicating arteriovenous shunting, which is often present in malignant liver lesions (*D,* portalvenous phase image).

tial diagnosis versus a hemangioma may only be possible using arterial phase images because internal lesion morphology often cannot be determined on unenhanced scans as a result of the small size of the lesion. Inhomogeneous signal intensity in unenhanced images, early washout, indistinct interface with adjacent liver, and multiple lesions are indirect signs of hypervascular liver metastases. In contrast to benign liver lesions like HCA or FNH, most of the malignant hypervascularized liver lesions show high signal intensity on T₂-weighted images. Nevertheless, hypervascular liver metastases may also show well-defined margins, homogeneous internal morphology, and even low-signal capsules and may be misinterpreted as HCC or HCA.

Hypovascular Liver Lesions

Hypovascular liver lesions are characterized by reduced or missing perfusion of the lesion, resulting in a hypointense appearance of the lesion compared with surrounding liver tissue in all phases of the dynamic T₁-weighted liver examination. Lesions may show signs of peripheral hypervascularization or irregular segmental perfusion in the arterial phase as an indicator of malignant liver lesions (e.g., with metastases from colorectal carcinoma or cystic metastasis from ovarian cancer). Alternatively, no signs of irregular perfusion indicate benign liver tumors, as in simple hepatic cysts (Figs. 11-15 to 11-17) or post-traumatic lesions such as biloma. Benign primary, traumatic, parasitic, or inflammatory

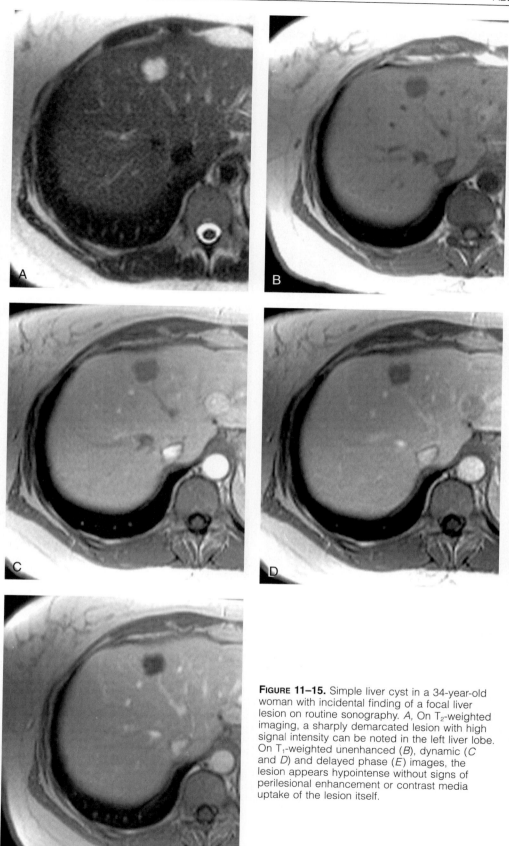

FIGURE 11–15. Simple liver cyst in a 34-year-old woman with incidental finding of a focal liver lesion on routine sonography. *A,* On T$_2$-weighted imaging, a sharply demarcated lesion with high signal intensity can be noted in the left liver lobe. On T$_1$-weighted unenhanced (*B*), dynamic (*C* and *D*) and delayed phase (*E*) images, the lesion appears hypointense without signs of perilesional enhancement or contrast media uptake of the lesion itself.

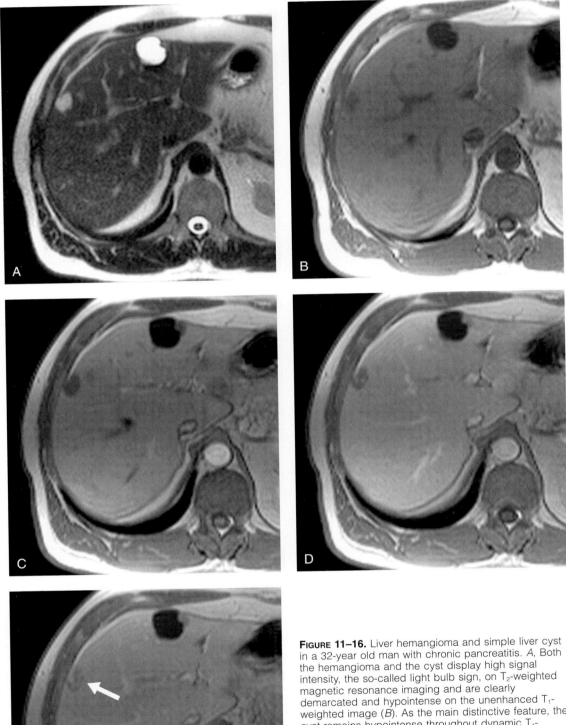

FIGURE 11–16. Liver hemangioma and simple liver cyst in a 32-year old man with chronic pancreatitis. *A,* Both the hemangioma and the cyst display high signal intensity, the so-called light bulb sign, on T$_2$-weighted magnetic resonance imaging and are clearly demarcated and hypointense on the unenhanced T$_1$-weighted image *(B)*. As the main distinctive feature, the cyst remains hypointense throughout dynamic T$_1$-weighted imaging, whereas the hemangioma displays typical peripheral nodular enhancement. In the arterial phase *(C)*, there is no enhancement. Nodular enhancement is initially noted in the hemangioma in the portalvenous phase *(D)*, with ongoing uptake of contrast media *(arrow)* in the equilibrium phase *(E)*. Enhancement of the lesion was more characteristic at a slightly lower slice position (not shown).

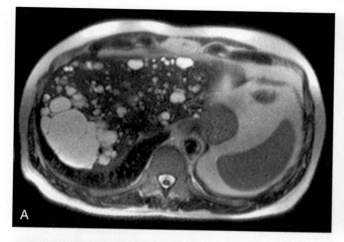

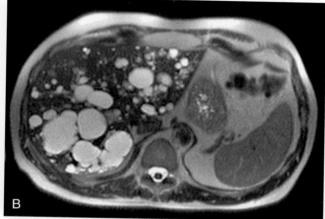

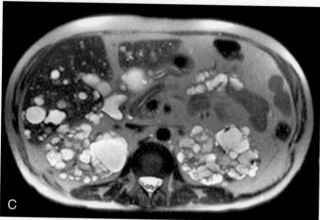

FIGURE 11–17. Multiple liver cysts in a 16-year-old girl with multicystic kidney disease. *A–C*, T₂-weighted images show diffusely spread liver cysts with confluent areas of high signal in liver segments 8/7. Note as well the almost complete cystic transformation of both kidneys.

hypovascular liver lesions include simple hepatic cysts, lipoma, biloma, liver abscess, echinococcal (Fig. 11-18) and amebic liver abscess, and others. Malignant lesions include primary liver tumors (e.g., juvenile hepatocellular carcinoma or bile duct cystadenocarcinoma) and metastases from most primary sites (e.g., colon, rectum, pancreas, lung), adenocarcinomas, small cell lung cancer, pharyngeal carcinoma, melanoma, cystadenocarcinoma of the pancreas and ovaries, liposarcoma, teratoma, breast cancer, cervical carcinoma, and secondary involvement of the liver in Hodgkin's lymphoma and NHL and others.

Important clues for distinguishing between simple hepatic cysts and cystic or necrotic metastasis include a hypervascularized rim, hypervascularized areas in the arterial phase together with irregular internal lesion morphology, enhancing mural nodules or septations, and a solid tissue rim surrounding central liquefaction necrosis (Figs. 11-19 and 11-20). Biphasic contrast-enhanced MRI may very sensitively show these areas of irregular vascularization as a result of tumor infiltration in arterial phase images, which is occasionally the only sign of malignant liver tumor in small lesions. Nevertheless, additional delayed-phase images should be performed to demonstrate peripheral washout as a very specific sign of malignancy in focal liver lesions, especially in metastases of adenocarcinoma. This sign may be explained by the difference in vascularity between the periphery and

the center of the lesion, which becomes rather ischemic or even degenerative and necrotic as the tumor outgrows its own blood supply. Histologic examinations have shown that the peripheral zone of metastases demonstrating washout phenomenon in images acquired approximately 5 minutes after contrast injection represents the growing tumor margin, whereas the center contains necrotic areas. Echinococcal disease (see Fig. 11-18) may show irregular hypervascularization as a result of inflammatory changes; however, in most cases no significant irregular blood supply is noticed in the arterial phase, and only cystic lesions with septations and daughter cyst are demonstrated. Hodgkin's lymphoma and NHL typically appear hypovascular in arterial and portalvenous phase scans. On delayed images lesions may appear isointense to surrounding liver tissue as a result of the diffuse periportal infiltration that results in a homogeneous late enhancement of the affected areas. Thus, this type of lesion can as well be classified as a tumor with a delayed persistent enhancement. In children, hepatoblastoma also has to be considered in the differential diagnosis of liver tumors because these primary liver lesions, found only in children and young adults, are also mainly hypovascular (Fig. 11-21).

On T₂-weighted imaging, hypovascular lesions may appear homogeneously hyperintense like hepatic cysts or may present irregular hyperintensity compared with surrounding liver tissue such as most solid metastases.

Text continued on page 310

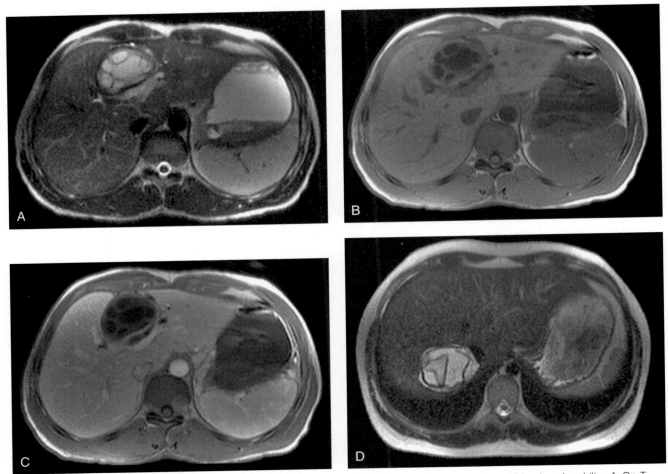

FIGURE 11–18. Echinococcal disease in a 36-year-old man with persistent right upper quadrant pain and blood eosinophilia. *A,* On T$_2$-weighted imaging there is a septated, mainly hyperintense mass with sharp demarcation to surrounding parenchyma. *B,* on T$_1$-weighted imaging, the mass is mainly hypointense with no enhancement after contrast administration (*C*). The perilesional liver parenchyma shows a slight increase in signal compared with surrounding normal liver because of compression of liver tissue. *D,* In another patient, a similar lesion is evident in the dorsal right liver lobe with typical septations.

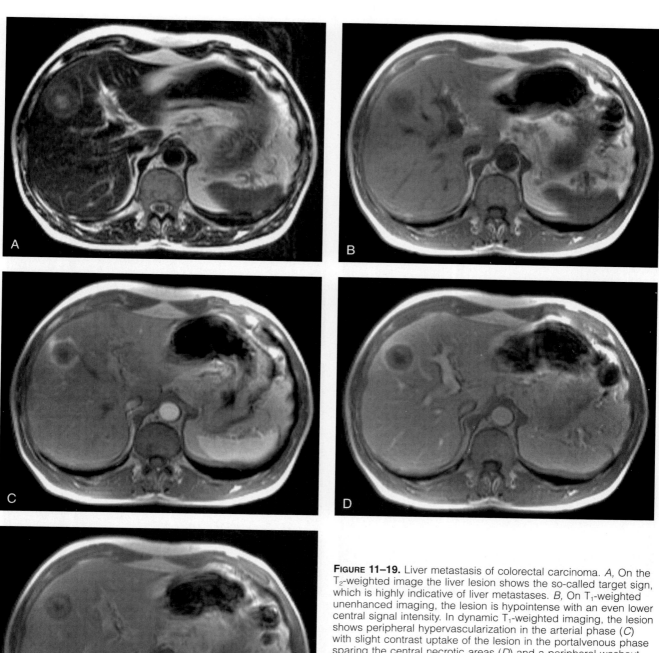

FIGURE 11–19. Liver metastasis of colorectal carcinoma. *A,* On the T$_2$-weighted image the liver lesion shows the so-called target sign, which is highly indicative of liver metastases. *B,* On T$_1$-weighted unenhanced imaging, the lesion is hypointense with an even lower central signal intensity. In dynamic T$_1$-weighted imaging, the lesion shows peripheral hypervascularization in the arterial phase (*C*) with slight contrast uptake of the lesion in the portalvenous phase sparing the central necrotic areas (*D*) and a peripheral washout sign in the equilibrium phase (*E*). This peripheral washout sign, which is characterized by a hypointense rim surrounding the lesion in images acquired approximately 5 to 10 minutes after contrast injection, is typically found in metastatic disease of the liver and so far has not been described in benign liver lesions. Unfortunately, it is not found in all liver metastases.

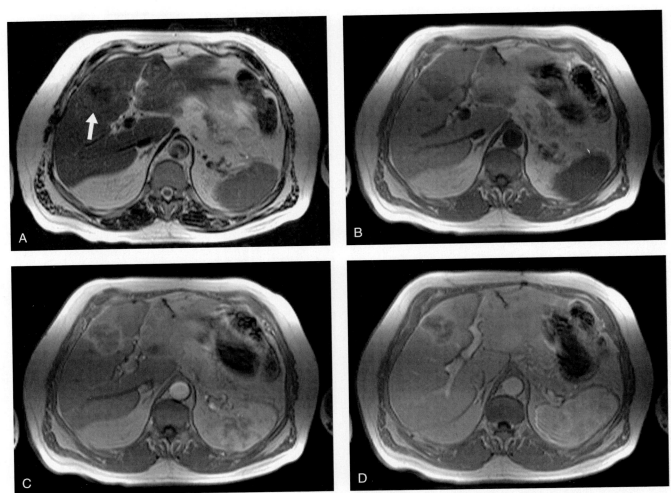

FIGURE 11–20. Liver metastasis from rectal adenocarcinoma with internal hemorrhage after chemotherapy in a 64-year-old man. *A,* T_2-weighted image shows a slightly hyperintense liver lesion (*arrow*) with a low signal intensity (SI) center. *B,* On the T_1-weighted image these central areas correspond with a slightly increased SI in the overall hypointense lesion. *C,* The periphery of the lesion has an irregular arterial contrast uptake, indicating an infiltrative growth. *D,* The central areas remain hypointense to surrounding parenchyma in the portalvenous phase. Note that the low SI of the central area in the T_2-weighted image is caused by hemorrhage during chemotherapy. Thus, the overall appearance of the lesion is rather atypical for a metastasis of an adenocarcinoma, and the clinical information about previous chemotherapy is essential for diagnosis.

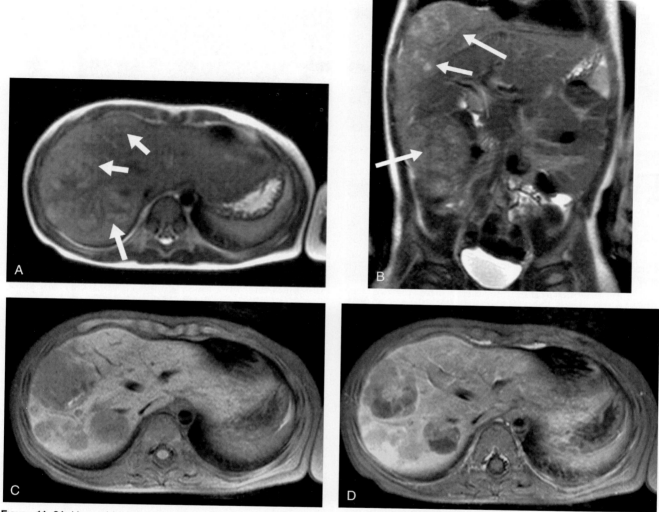

FIGURE 11–21. Hepatoblastoma in a 16-month-old boy with abdominal pain and increased abdominal circumference. *A and B,* T₂-weighted axial and coronal images show multiple inhomogeneously hyperintense liver lesions (*arrows*) with indistinct borders to surrounding liver parenchyma. *C,* The lesions are mainly hypointense on T₁-weighted fat-saturated magnetic resonance imaging, but small areas of hemorrhage with high signal intensity can be detected, indicating internal hemorrhage. *D,* After contrast administration, most of the lesions remain hypointense. In contrast to hepatocellular carcinoma, hepatoblastomas found in pediatric patients are mainly hypovascular, although sometimes small areas of hypervascularization may be noted.

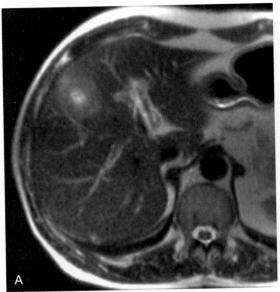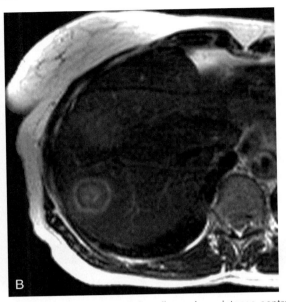

FIGURE 11–22. Typical signs in T$_2$-weighted imaging of liver metastases. *A,* The "doughnut sign" describes a hyperintense central area of a lesion caused by necrosis in fast-growing malignant lesions, mainly found in hypovascularized hepatic metastases such as those of colorectal adenocarcinoma. The central necrosis develops because the lesion outgrows its own blood supply and histologically corresponds to liquefactive necrosis. *B,* The so-called target sign or halo sign describes a high-signal-intensity (SI) rim surrounding central areas of signal decrease and signal increase. The high SI region in the periphery seems to correlate with viable tumor, whereas the low SI areas more centrally consist of coagulative necrosis, fibrosis, and mucin. The central hyperintense area again represents liquefactive necrosis.

In metastases with central liquefactive necrosis, central areas may have increased signal relative to the more solid components of the metastases. This feature has been termed the "doughnut sign" (Fig. 11-22) and is most commonly identified in metastatic lesions of adenocarcinoma. In some metastatic lesions, a bright halo surrounding a less intense nodule is present on T$_2$-weighted images, the "halo sign" (see Fig. 11-22), in which the peripheral halo represents viable tumor surrounding low-signal coagulative necrosis.

Lesions Presenting Delayed Persistent Enhancement

Focal liver lesions presenting delayed with persistent enhancement are characterized by a delayed uptake of contrast medium. Thus, lesions appear isointense or hyperintense on delayed-phase images, whereas most of the lesion is hypointense in the arterial or portalvenous phase. On scans 10 to 15 minutes after contrast administration, lesions may still demonstrate hyperintensity compared with surrounding liver tissue because of the beginning washout of contrast medium in normal liver and contrast pooling (delayed washout) in liver diseases.

The most common benign nonepithelial primary liver tumor is the hemangioma, a liver lesion typically presenting delayed persistent enhancement after contrast injection (see Figs. 11-13 and 11-16). In the arterial phase, as known from dynamic CT imaging, hemangiomas typically show a nodular peripheral enhancement (Fig. 11-23) with subsequent centripetal filling in the portalvenous and delayed-phase images. This classic appearance of hemangioma in dynamic imaging, together with the homogeneous high signal intensity in T$_2$-weighted images, is highly specific for the diagnosis of hemangioma. Large or so-called giant hemangioma may have scar tissue, thrombosis, myxoid changes, or larger fibrotic areas (Fig. 11-24). Thus, lesions may not show complete fill-in on delayed-phase images, and inhomogeneous internal morphology may be noted on T$_2$-weighted scans. Peliosis hepatis is defined by the presence of cystic blood-filled spaces. In contrast to extreme sinusoidal dilatation, microscopy of peliosis hepatis should show evidence of lysis of reticulin fibers supporting normal anatomy. Macroscopic peliosis hepatis is usually induced by anabolic, estrogenic, or adrenocortical steroids. It also has been reported with a variety of chronic diseases such as malnutrition, leukemia, vasculitis, AIDS, and others. Because of the presence of dilated blood-filled spaces, peliosis hepatis may mimic a hemangioma with high signal intensity in T$_2$-weighted images and delayed enhancement. In the cases documented so far in our department, the main differences on imaging from a hemangioma were inhomogeneous margins, no nodular peripheral enhancement on arterial phase images, and sometimes irregular early enhancement in the arterial phase in parts of the lesion. Hemangiosarcoma, a malignant nonepithelial primary liver tumor, is the most common sarcoma arising in the liver. As a result of large cavernous, blood-filled spaces and rarely seen solid cellular masses, angiosarcomas show delayed persistent enhancement after intravenous contrast injection and high signal intensity in T$_2$-weighted images, comparable to that for hemangioma. As an important difference to hemangioma, angiosarcomas show inhomogeneous enhancement in the arterial phase with early enhancement of central regions, sometimes resulting in rather centrifugal than centripetal filling as for hemangioma.

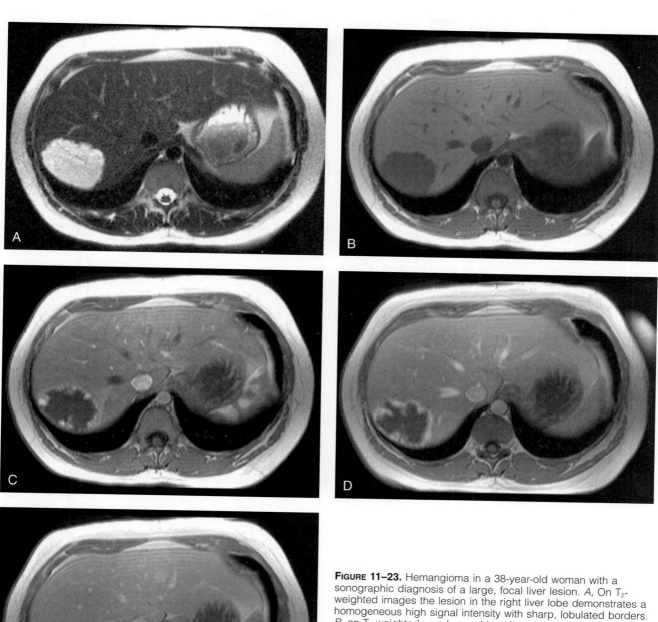

FIGURE 11–23. Hemangioma in a 38-year-old woman with a sonographic diagnosis of a large, focal liver lesion. *A,* On T$_2$-weighted images the lesion in the right liver lobe demonstrates a homogeneous high signal intensity with sharp, lobulated borders. *B,* on T$_1$-weighted unenhanced imaging, the lesion is hypointense with nodular peripheral enhancement in the arterial phase image (*C*). In the portalvenous phase (*D*) and the equilibrium phase (*E*), the lesion shows centripedal filling clearly indicating a hemangioma.

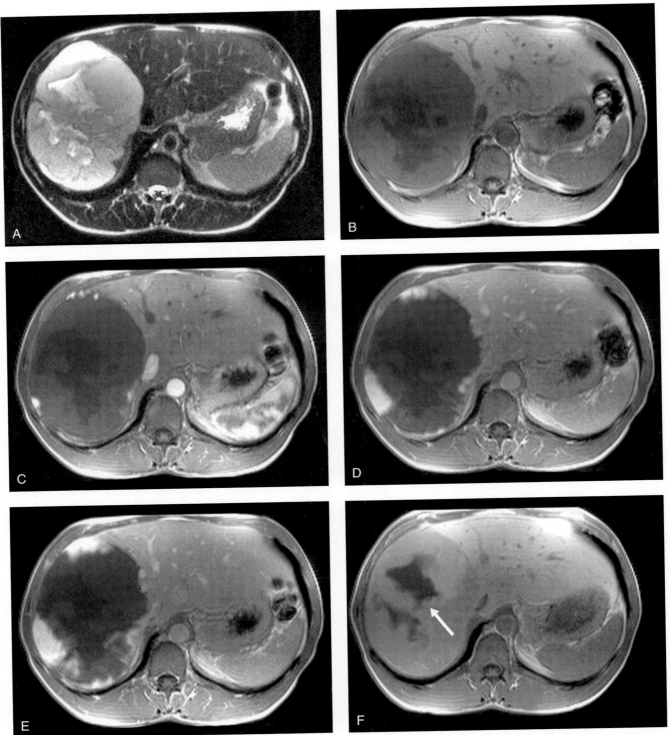

FIGURE 11–24. Giant hemangioma in a 34-year-old man with right upper quadrant pain. Because large hemangiomas often show areas of thrombosis or myxoid changes, the high SI of the lesion on T_2 (*A*) is inhomogeneous. *B*, on the T_1 weighted unenhanced image, the lesion shows an inhomogeneous hypointense signal. Nodular peripheral enhancement in the arterial phase (*C*), together with centripetal filling in the portalvenous (*D*) and the equilibrium phase (*E*) after injection of contrast medium, can be noted. In images acquired 15 minutes after contrast administration, (*F*) the central areas of the lesion still show no contrast media uptake because of thrombosis and myxoid changes (*arrow*). However, as a result of the postcontrast nodular peripheral enhancement that increases with time, the diagnosis of a giant hemangioma can be made.

Intrahepatic cholangiocellular carcinoma (CCC) represents a malignant epithelial primary liver tumor that typically appears hypointense in unenhanced arterial phase and portalvenous phase T_1-weighted images (Fig. 11-25). On T_2-weighted images, CCCs typically appear hyperintense. In cases without larger areas of necrosis or CCC with desmoplastic changes, delayed-phase images show a homogeneous uptake of contrast into the lesion.

Thus, CCC may appear hyperintense in comparison to surrounding liver tissue in delayed-phase T_1-weighted images. Comparable findings concerning contrast dynamics can be made in metastases of leiomyosarcoma (e.g., of the uterus). Lesions smaller than 5 cm usually appear homogeneously hypointense on unenhanced T_1-weighted images and homogeneously hyperintense on T_2-weighted images and show delayed enhancement as

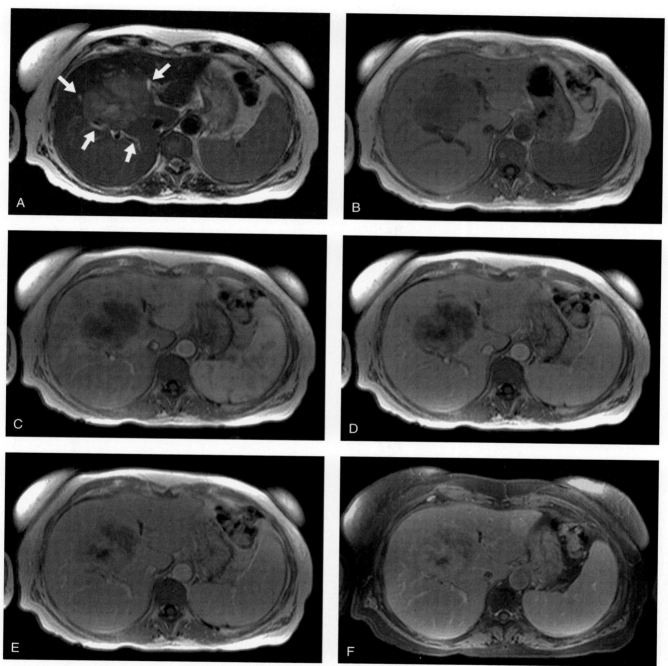

Figure 11–25. Intrahepatic cholangiocellular carcinoma in a 62-year-old woman with right upper quadrant pain and jaundice. *A,* The T_2-weighted image shows a large inhomogeneous hilar liver lesion with increased signal intensity and peripheral focal biliary dilatation (*arrows*). *B,* On T_1-weighted imaging the lesion demonstrates a hypointense signal, and irregular peripheral enhancement can be noted in arterial phase T_1-weighted imaging (*C*), indicating infiltrative growth of the lesion. *D,* In the portalvenous phase, initial contrast enhancement can be noted in the peripheral areas of the lesion, which increases with time. Thus, on the T_1-weighted image 5 minutes after contrast administration (*E*), the lesion shows almost complete contrast media uptake. *F,* This delayed enhancement is more obvious on the T_1-weighted fat-saturated image 15 minutes after contrast administration.

HYPOINTENSE	ISOINTENSE	SLIGHTLY HYPERINTENSE	HYPERINTENSE
Regenerative nodules (low SI caused by hemosiderin deposit)	FNH	Metastases of adenocarcinoma (e.g., colorectal), "halo sign," "doughnut"	Cysts
	Adenoma		Hemangioma
Calcification	Well-differentiated HCC	Undifferentiated HCC	Metastases of neuroendocrine tumors
AV malformations with high flow (flow void)		Focal fatty liver	Cystic metastases
Fibrosis	Metastases of neuroendocrine tumors after chemotherapy		Bilioma
Nonacute hemorrhage			AV malformations (low flow)
			Hemangiosarcoma

FIGURE 11–26. Classification of focal liver lesions in T_2-weighted imaging. (SI, signal intensity; AV, arteriovenous; FNH, focal nodular hyperplasia; HCC, hepatocellular carcinoma.)

a result of enlarged extracellular space after intravenous contrast injection, thus appearing slightly hyperintense or isointense in delayed-phase images.

In addition to the classification made in dynamic imaging of the liver, focal liver lesions can be classified in T_2-weighted imaging. Figure 11-26 gives a general overview of the signal intensity characteristics found in T_2-weighted imaging of liver lesions.

Regarding vascular diseases of the liver, mainly portal thrombosis and Budd-Chiari syndrome have to be considered. Spin echo images (because of flow void) as well as flow-sensitive gradient echo images are useful in depicting patency of the main portal vein and its major branches. On contrast-enhanced images, thrombus material may be displayed as hypointense material in the portal vein. Indirect signs of portal thrombosis are increased arterial vascularization of affected liver lobes (in thrombosis of a major branch of the portal vein) as well as a generally reduced enhancement of the liver in the arterial and portalvenous phases after contrast administration.

Budd-Chiari syndrome results from obstruction of the venous outflow from the liver, located in either the main hepatic veins or in small to intermediate-size veins, also known as veno-occlusive disease. In acute Budd-Chiari syndrome, perihepatic ascites, enlargement of the liver, and inhomogeneous and delayed enhancement of the liver may be found (Fig. 11-27). The inhomogeneous enhancement is caused by the decreased portalvenous perfusion of the liver caused by the increased vascular resistance. Peripheral liver tissue may show signs of severe hypovascularization. This may lead to atrophy of peripheral liver areas in chronic disease, whereas the more central parts may show collateral venous drainage. In the chronic stage of Budd-Chiari syndrome, hypertrophy of segment 1 can be found resulting from the separate venous drainage of this segment directly into the inferior caval vein. The same can be found for the lower liver segments 6 and 5, which often demonstrate accessory liver veins.

SPLEEN

In spite of its important role in immunology, the spleen has always been of less interest for clinicians and radiologists compared with other parenchymal abdominal organs. However, as we know from macro- and microscopic disease, the spleen is involved in a wide variety of neoplastic and infectious diseases, although this involvement often cannot be visualized by noninvasive imaging modalities and thus remains undetected. MRI, with its great potential in soft tissue contrast and the possible imaging of splenic perfusion, seems to be a reliable tool for evaluating diffuse and focal splenic disease.

The spleen develops during the fifth week of gestation as a mesenchymal proliferation of the dorsal mesogastrium. It is located intraperitoneally and follows the axis of the 10th rib in the left upper quadrant. Ligamentous fixation includes the gastrosplenic ligament with the arteria and vena gastrica brevis and arteria gastroepiploica sinistra and the phrenicosplenic ligament with the splenic artery and vein. Traumatic rupture of those fixating structures may lead to splenic torsion or the so-called wandering spleen. Accessory spleens most often develop in the omentum majus or gastrosplenic ligament (in 10% of individuals).

A physiologic spleen in adults is about 11 cm long, 7 cm wide, and 4 cm thick with a weight of approximately 150 g. It is surrounded by a fibrous capsule. Microscopically, it consists of the red and white pulp. The red pulp is mainly built of the splenic sinusoids, whereas the white pulp comprises the lymphoid elements. Typically, T lymphocytes are found in the periarteriolar T cell-rich lymphoid sheaths around central arteries. Primary and secondary B-cell follicles are located at the periphery of the T-cell zone. Hemodynamically, a fast compartment with early passage of the blood from the arteries to the sinus can be distinguished from a slow compartment, where the in-flowing blood remains for up to hours in the mantle zone before reaching the

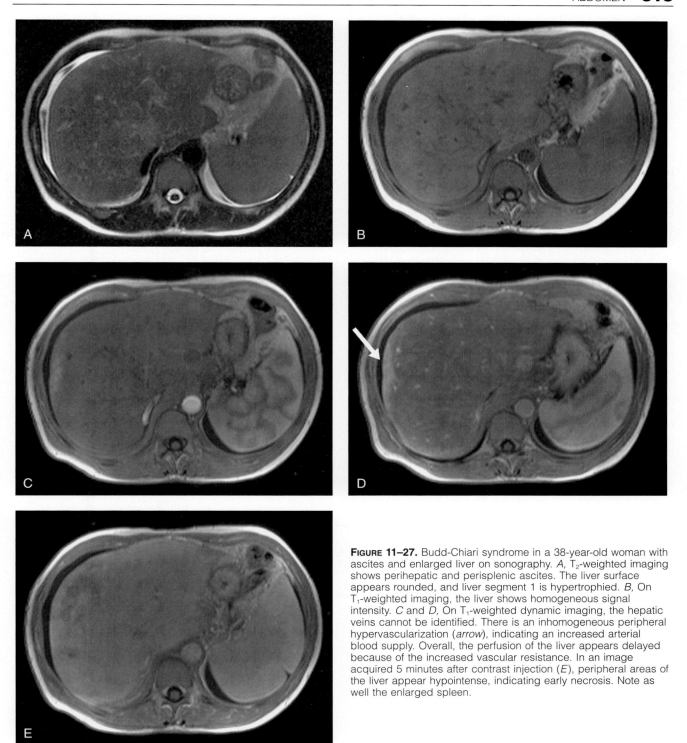

FIGURE 11–27. Budd-Chiari syndrome in a 38-year-old woman with ascites and enlarged liver on sonography. *A,* T₂-weighted imaging shows perihepatic and perisplenic ascites. The liver surface appears rounded, and liver segment 1 is hypertrophied. *B,* On T₁-weighted imaging, the liver shows homogeneous signal intensity. *C* and *D,* On T₁-weighted dynamic imaging, the hepatic veins cannot be identified. There is an inhomogeneous peripheral hypervascularization (*arrow*), indicating an increased arterial blood supply. Overall, the perfusion of the liver appears delayed because of the increased vascular resistance. In an image acquired 5 minutes after contrast injection (*E*), peripheral areas of the liver appear hypointense, indicating early necrosis. Note as well the enlarged spleen.

sinusoidal structures. The normal passage of blood is via the splenic artery to central arteries and arterioles to capillaries, which lead to the sinusoids, where the blood is drained by small veins to the splenic vein into the portalvenous circulation. There are no afferent lymphatic vessels to the spleen. Splenic function consists of maturation of reticulocytes, elimination of defective erythrocytes, and some pooling function for thrombo-

cytes. During the first 4 months of gestation, there is additional physiologic hematopoiesis.

Because sonographic evaluation of the spleen is quite unreliable, most splenic diseases are detected by CT and MRI, often incidentally. Once a focal lesion is found, further evaluation has to be made by means of imaging because fine-needle biopsy of the spleen in contrast to hepatic biopsy is rarely performed.

Evaluation of splenic disease in imaging relies considerably on the evaluation of splenic perfusion. The inhomogeneous contrast enhancement of the red and white pulp during the early arterial phase results in a high detection rate of even small focal lesions. They present as a gap in the normal perfusion pattern, either as a hypoperfused area or a homogeneously enhancing small lesion.

The use of unenhanced MRI in the detection of focal lesions is restricted because splenic and tumorous tissue in a large number of cases demonstrates similar signal intensities. Imaging of contrast dynamics offers an additional approach to detect splenic disease. Bolus administration of extracellular Gd-based contrast agents leads to an early irregular, arciform pattern of enhancement of the spleen within the first 25 to 30 seconds after contrast administration. A second perfusion phase is characterized by its homogeneous peak enhancement about 60 seconds after contrast injection. Imaging of focal lesions depends primarily on the contrast between a hypointense lesion and the arciform-enhancing splenic tissue. In the second phase of perfusion, the signal intensities become more alike as contrast slowly distributes in the extracellular compartment of the lesion. Thus, early imaging of the spleen after contrast administration is crucial for lesion detection. Figure 11-28 gives an overview for classification of splenic tumors, diagnosed on contrast-enhanced MRI. Intravenous administration of superparamagnetic iron oxide (SPIO) particles represents a second approach to increase the contrast between the normal parenchyma and focal lesions. Iron particles

are taken up only by reticuloendothelial cells and thus lead to a loss of signal intensity in normal splenic tissue, whereas focal lesions remain unaffected. In contrast to the use of the extracellular contrast agents, the time window is much longer because of the intracellular uptake of iron in the mononuclear phagocytic system.

The spleen may be affected by many different diseases. Often, as in infectious disease, the involvement remains clinically relatively silent, and in trauma it may even be life threatening. Splenic malformations include accessory and ectopic splenic tissue as well as agenesis of the spleen. Agenesis of the spleen is very rare, often seen in combination with cardiovascular malformations, known as Ivemark's syndrome. Most children die of overwhelming postsplenectomy infections (*Streptococcus pneumoniae*, malaria). In contrast, accessory spleens are seen in up to 10% of individuals. An ectopic spleen can be found intrathoracically (agenesis of the diaphragm) or in an umbilical herniation. In splenogonadal fusion, fibrous tissue connects the spleen and the gonads; heterotopic splenic tissue on the gonads can be found as well, but only left sided. In acute trauma of the upper quadrants, the spleen is the most affected parenchymal organ, often in combination with rib fractures. Trauma may result in subcapsular hematoma without discontinuity of the splenic capsule, or in more severe cases in a laceration, which may lead to intraperitoneal loss of blood. In up to 85% of splenic trauma, CT or MRI may demonstrate perisplenic blood clots, thus pointing to the diagnosis. Often there is a delay of weeks between acute trauma and onset of symptoms in splenic rupture. Post-

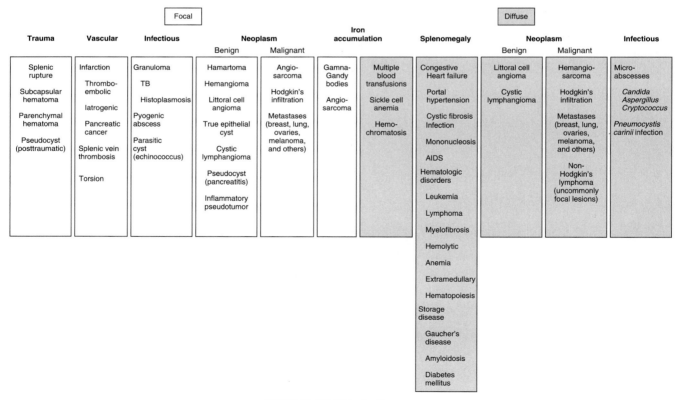

FIGURE 11–28. Splenic disease.

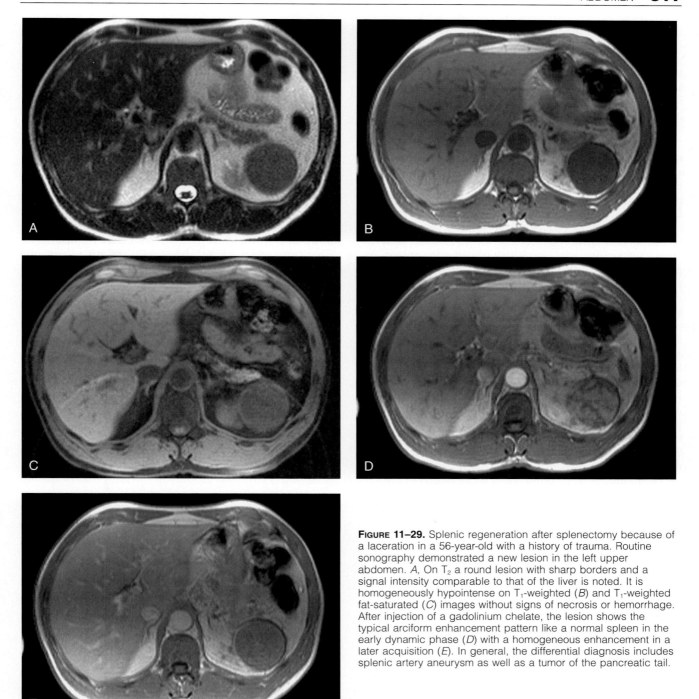

FIGURE 11–29. Splenic regeneration after splenectomy because of a laceration in a 56-year-old with a history of trauma. Routine sonography demonstrated a new lesion in the left upper abdomen. A, On T$_2$ a round lesion with sharp borders and a signal intensity comparable to that of the liver is noted. It is homogeneously hypointense on T$_1$-weighted (B) and T$_1$-weighted fat-saturated (C) images without signs of necrosis or hemorrhage. After injection of a gadolinium chelate, the lesion shows the typical arciform enhancement pattern like a normal spleen in the early dynamic phase (D) with a homogeneous enhancement in a later acquisition (E). In general, the differential diagnosis includes splenic artery aneurysm as well as a tumor of the pancreatic tail.

traumatic findings include splenic torsion with traumatically ruptured ligaments and splenosis (Fig. 11-29). Splenosis after laceration or rupture of the spleen represents splenic tissue that is seeded out intraperitoneally and may be incidentally found without causing any primary symptoms.

With regard to inflammation, the spleen reacts in all different bacterial infections, with the exception of peritonitis; thus, peritoneal mesothelium has a reticulo-histiocytic function. Often the changes are more diffuse

and do not allow an etiologic classification (splenitis). The spread of the infectious agents most often occurs hematogenously. An acute focal perisplenitis may arise in splenic infarctions. Specific infections such as tuberculosis, syphilis, or brucellosis and yersiniosis may lead to a more granulomatous infiltration resembling sarcoidosis. Abscess formation is most often associated with bacterial endocarditis, trauma, or hemoglobinopathies; it may be found in patients with hemorrhagic hereditary telangiectasia resulting from AVMs of the lung. In this context, patients are predisposed to brain abscess and other visceral abscess formations. Granulomas typically develop in patients with sarcoidosis or Wegener's granulomatosis. Granulomas may be as large as 5 mm and are typically seen throughout the spleen as miliary lesions that are hypointense on contrast-enhanced images and often also have low signal intensity on unenhanced T_2-weighted images.

Disorders of splenic or portal circulation may result in splenomegaly or splenic infarctions. Splenomegaly caused by hyperemia is found with elevated pressure of the venous circulation such as in cardiac insufficiency or portal hypertension. Thrombosis of the splenic vein also leads to a splenomegaly, which may be caused by torsion, compression, or thrombus formation in coagulation or lymphoproliferative disorders as well as in acute pancreatitis. Infarctions are typically anemic and caused by emboli (endocarditis, arteriosclerosis) or thrombus formation (CML, sickle cell anemia).

With regard to neoplasms, the spleen is most often secondarily involved in Hodgkin's lymphoma and NHL with an incidence of up to 60% to 100% in small lymphocytic NHL. In Hodgkin's disease (HD), up to one third of patients have splenic involvement at staging laparotomy. In patients with the lymphocyte-predominant type of HD, the incidence seems to be somewhat lower. Unfortunately, increased splenic size does not invariably stand for infiltration. The spleen may also have a normal size. Typically, in disease, randomly distributed fleshy nodules are found, which may be confluent, but isolated small (1 mm) foci or miliary small nodules may be present as well, which cannot be diagnosed by means of imaging. Because liver or bone marrow infiltration is rare without splenic involvement, this diagnostic test seems to be a more reliable prognostic factor than imaging.

In NHL as well, the spleen may have a normal size despite infiltration. Involvement may be depicted as miliary small nodules typically found in follicular lymphoma, large solitary nodules, or a diffuse infiltration of the splenic parenchyma without evidence of a focal lesion, which may be seen in diffuse large cell lymphoma. A sign on imaging indicating diffuse involvement of the spleen in HD and NHL is the missing inhomogeneous enhancement of the spleen in images 25 to 30 seconds after contrast administration. This rather homogeneous enhancement may also be found in cases of circulation disorders. Rare cases of primary splenic lymphoma are described in literature. This entity should be applied only to lymphoma involving the splenic parenchyma or the splenic lymph nodes without evidence of involvement of other sites. Its incidence is as low as 1% of all lymphoma, and most of them are NHL. In all cases of splenic involvement by lymphoid cells, mononucleosis is the main differential diagnosis, especially in young patients.

Splenic hemangioma is the most common benign splenic tumor. Comparable to hepatic hemangioma, the size may vary from 5 mm up to several centimeters (Fig. 11-30). On rare occasions, a so-called giant hemangioma (>10 cm) may be found. Symptoms may result from consumption coagulopathy, rupture, or thrombocyto-

penia, but most patients remain asymptomatic. Splenic hemangiomas usually have high signal intensity on T_2-weighted images comparable to the findings in liver hemangiomas. If no degeneration or thrombosis is present, they demonstrate a homogeneous delayed, persistent enhancement on images after injection of a Gd chelate. If other organs such as liver or skin are involved as well, diffuse angiomatosis has to be considered in the differential diagnosis.

Most hemangiomas are cavernous with large blood-filled spaces lined by endothelium and separated by fibrous septae or splenic pulp. Larger hemangiomas may show regressive changes such as infarction, thrombosis, or fibrosis. Hemangiomas have to be distinguished from splenic peliosis, which is typically of a more diffuse nature and is found in patients with wasting disease or under medication with anabolic steroids. Splenic lymphangioma is a rare disease and most often occurs in diffuse lymphangiomatosis with involvement of other organ systems. It is usually found in the capsular or trabecular areas of the spleen, where most of the lymphatics are located, and may present as a focal nodule as well as a multicentric lesion. On T_2-weighted images, lymphangioma appears similar to a hemangioma. However, there is no enhancement of the lesions after Gd injection, and typically multiple septations can be demonstrated.

Hemangioendothelioma and hemangiopericytoma are rarely found in the spleen. The diagnosis of hemangioendothelioma is typically made in cases of hemangioma with cellular atypia and mitoses, representing a borderline tumor between hemangioma and angiosarcoma. Angiosarcoma of the spleen is another rare primary splenic tumor, occurring most often in older patients presenting with abdominal pain or even rupture of the spleen. Symptoms like coagulopathy or thrombocytopenia may be found in larger tumors. Metastatic spread most often involves the liver, lung, and bone, and the prognosis is grave. On macroscopic exam, there are typically multiple ill-defined nodules with large areas of hemorrhage or necrosis. The classic differential diagnosis in imaging is hemangioma. The irregular borders and the infiltrative growth pattern of an angiosarcoma favor the diagnosis of a malignant vascular lesion. However, there may be an overlap in the imaging appearance with multiple hemangiomas and peliosis hepatis. Biopsy in suspected angiosarcoma of the spleen should be extensive because angiosarcoma may have spots of benign appearance that may be misinterpreted as hemangioma. Inflammatory pseudotumor of the spleen is a reactive lesion sometimes associated with prior bacterial infection. It typically presents as a solitary nodule with areas of hemorrhage or necrosis, thus mimicking infiltration by a lymphoid or even a solid tumor. Definitive diagnosis in most cases is possible only by histology.

Epithelial cysts of the spleen are typically solitary tumors with an epithelium lining. They are mostly asymptomatic lesions but may sometimes present as a mass lesion (Fig. 11-31) or may be complicated by rupture or bacterial superinfection. Uncomplicated cysts show homogeneous high signal intensity on T_2-weighted images, and there is no enhancement after injection of

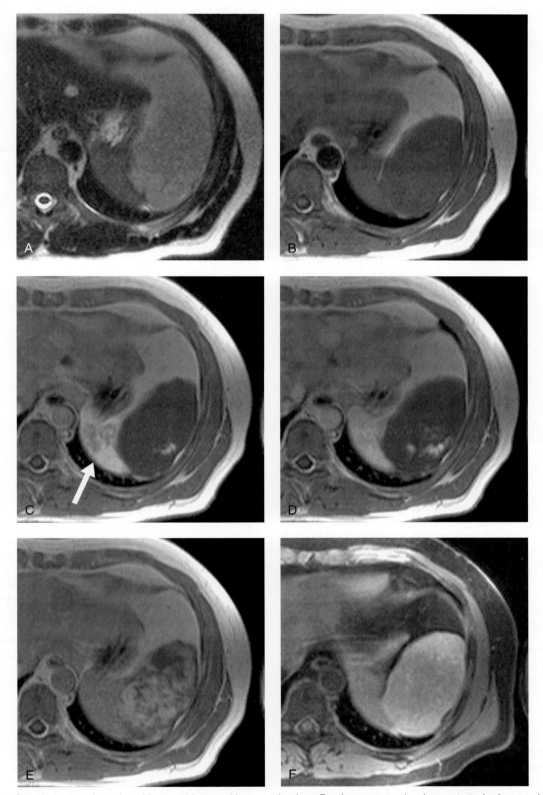

FIGURE 11–30. Splenic hemangioma in a 38-year-old man with a gastric ulcer. Routine sonography demonstrated a large splenic lesion. Comparable to hepatic hemangiomas, splenic hemangiomas have high signal intensity on T_2-weighted magnetic resonance images (*A*) and are hypointense or even isointense to normal splenic tissue on unenhanced T_1-weighted images (*B*). *C–E*, The lesion shows peripheral nodular enhancement on dynamic T_1-weighted images. *F*, Delayed persistent enhancement is visible 20 minutes after contrast administration. Note the typical stripelike appearance (*arrow*) of normal splenic parenchyma in the early dynamic image (*C*).

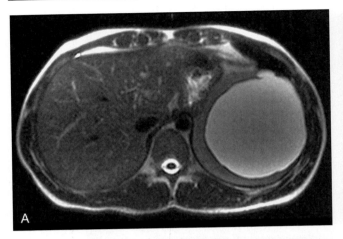

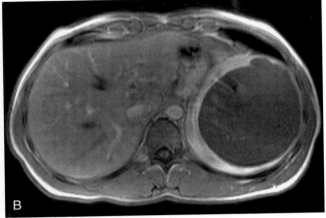

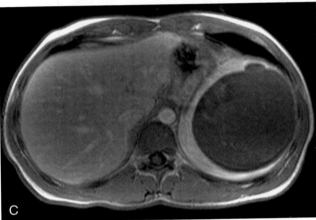

FIGURE 11–31. Splenic cyst in a 16-year-old girl. A large splenic lesion was found on routine sonography, and there was no history of trauma. *A,* T$_2$-weighted magnetic resonance imaging shows a large hyperintense cyst with sharp demarcation from the surrounding parenchyma. After injection of contrast, the early dynamic T$_1$-weighted image (*B*) shows typical inhomogeneous enhancement of remaining splenic tissue with homogeneous enhancement in a later dynamic image (*C*).

contrast. Parasitic cysts may, as with hepatic disease, arise in infection with echinococcus, presenting as uni- or multilocular disease with septated cystic lesions that may be ill defined from surrounding splenic tissue.

In contrast to true epithelial cysts, false cysts or pseudocysts arise after trauma, the result of liquefaction of a hematoma. They typically lack an endothelial lining, and the fibrous wall may show calcifications. Patient history is the most important information in diagnosis of posttraumatic pseudocysts because imaging findings may be similar to true epithelial cysts.

In cases of splenic metastases, the spleen may be involved by tumor growth in the vicinity (stomach, pancreas, kidney) or by hematogenous spread. There is great variability in the reported frequency of splenic metastases. Regardless, the most common primaries are malignant melanoma and breast and lung cancer. Involvement may be present as a solitary nodule (Fig. 11-32) as well as miliary lesions or diffuse replacement of splenic parenchyma. Frequency of splenic metastases seems to increase with greater long-term survival of cancer patients. On MRI usually solid, hypovascular (in comparison with splenic tissue) tumors are identified that may show central necrosis. On T$_2$-weighted images, a solid metastasis may be either hyper- or isointense; however, if central necrosis is present, a central high-signal-intensity area may be identified.

PANCREAS

The normal pancreas on conventional T$_1$-weighted spin echo images is of intermediate signal intensity similar to liver and hypointense compared with surrounding retroperitoneal fat. With fat suppression, the relative signal intensity of the pancreas on T$_1$-weighted images increases substantially so that normal pancreatic tissue is the brightest soft tissue structure in the upper abdomen and can be clearly demarcated from surrounding structures (Fig. 11-33). On T$_2$-weighted images, the pancreas is isointense or slightly hyperintense to the liver. The fat surrounding the pancreas is typically hyperintense compared with the pancreas on T$_2$-weighted non-fat-suppressed images. The pancreatic duct as well as the common bile duct in the pancreatic head show a T$_2$ value that is much longer than that of adjacent soft tissue and thus is displayed with high signal intensity on T$_2$-weighted images or may even be depicted exclusively as in MRCP. Concerning contrast dynamics, the pancreas enhances before the liver after bolus injection of extracellular distributed Gd chelates. As for the liver, it is important to image the pancreas in a dynamic fashion after contrast administration. This approach improves lesion detection and provides, on the basis of enhancement characteristics, information regarding differential diagnosis. Because of the central position of the pancreas

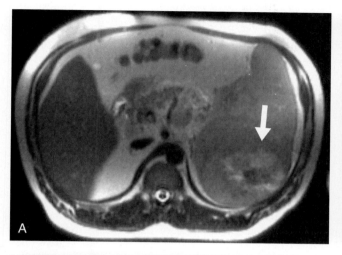

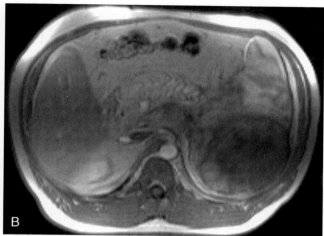

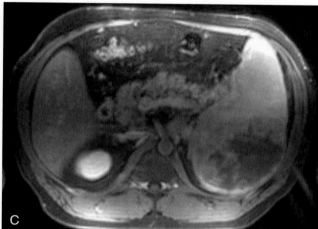

FIGURE 11–32. Splenic metastases in a 36-year-old woman with a clinical history of breast cancer and an enlarged spleen with a focal lesion on routine follow-up sonography of the upper abdomen. *A,* The T$_2$-weighted image shows an inhomogeneous, hyperintense splenic lesion (*arrow*). There are signs of central necrosis on T$_1$-weighted contrast enhanced (*B*) and T$_1$-weighted fat-suppressed contrast enhanced (*C*) images. On contrast-enhanced images after intravenous injection of a gadolinium chelate, the lesion is primarily hypovascular.

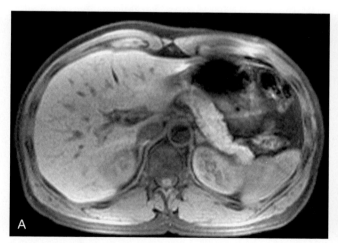

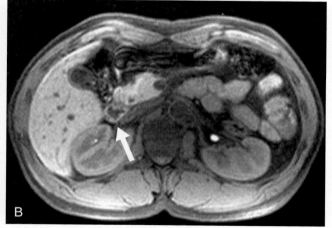

FIGURE 11–33. Normal pancreas on T$_1$-weighted fat-suppressed images. *A and B,* The pancreatic parenchyma is best visible on T$_1$-weighted fat-suppressed images because the retroperitoneal fat remains dark and the parenchyma can well be appreciated due to its homogeneous high signal intensity. Note the close relationship of the pancreatic tail to the kidney and splenic hilum and the clear distinction of the pancreatic head from the neighboring duodenum (*arrow*).

in the upper abdomen, special problems may arise for MRI. Artifacts from respiration, peristalsis, and vascular pulsation may obscure fine detail of the pancreatic parenchyma; thus, different strategies should be applied to improve the diagnostic quality of pancreatic MRI. These include signal averaging, presaturation, antiperistaltic medication, and in particular the use of fast breath-hold imaging techniques. Oral contrast material may be used in addition to achieve better differentiation of adjacent bowel loops.

With regard to their pathologic classification, pancreatic tumors can be categorized as tumors of the exocrine or endocrine pancreas, tumor-like lesions, and secondary tumors. Figure 11-34 gives an overview of the pathologic classification of pancreatic tumors. For the differential diagnosis of pancreatic lesions on MR imaging, a classification that reflects the imaging characteristics should be used. For this reason, pancreatic lesions may first be subdivided into solid, cystic, or complex masses and may then be subdivided into hyper- or hypovascular tumors as well as solitary or multiple lesions (Fig. 11-35).

The differential diagnosis of pancreatic adenocarcinoma is an important diagnostic challenge in imaging of pancreatic masses. Whereas adenocarcinomas of the head of the pancreas frequently come to attention at a

rather small size as a result of obstruction of the bile duct producing jaundice (Fig. 11-36), tumors of the pancreatic body and tail tend to grow insidiously, presenting with almost no or ill-defined late symptoms and a large tumor size at initial presentation (Fig. 11-37). Pancreatic carcinoma typically has decreased signal intensity on T_1-weighted images. However, on T_2-weighted images, pancreatic carcinoma may be isointense or only slightly higher in signal intensity than the normal pancreas. Only in large tumors with high-signal-intensity central necrosis does T_2-weighted imaging help in the diagnosis of pancreatic carcinoma. On T_1-weighted images with fat suppression, pancreatic carcinoma has substantially decreased signal intensity compared with the high signal intensity of normal pancreatic tissue. Thus, this imaging sequence is used principally for the diagnosis of small pancreatic carcinomas. One major problem in imaging of pancreatic carcinoma are those cases that present together with pancreatitis, because in these cases the signal intensity of pancreatic parenchyma on T_1-weighted images is lowered. Thus, the contrast between pancreatic carcinoma and inflammatory pancreatic tissue is decreased.

The classic sign of pancreatic carcinoma in the pancreatic head is the "double-duct" sign, with obstruction of the common bile duct as well as the pancreatic duct

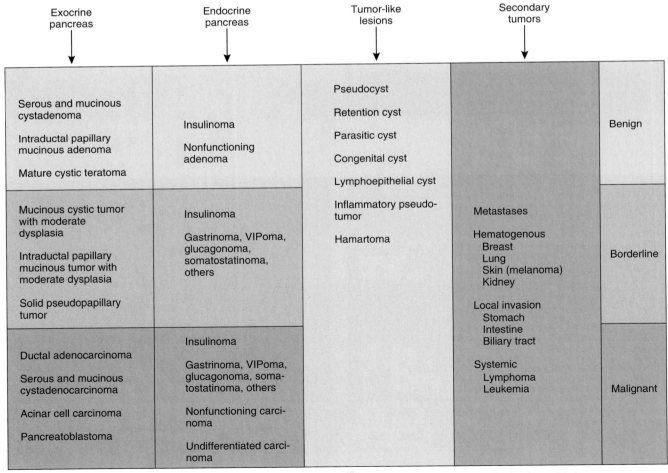

FIGURE 11–34. Pathologic classification of pancreatic tumors. (VIP, vasoactive intestinal polypeptide.)

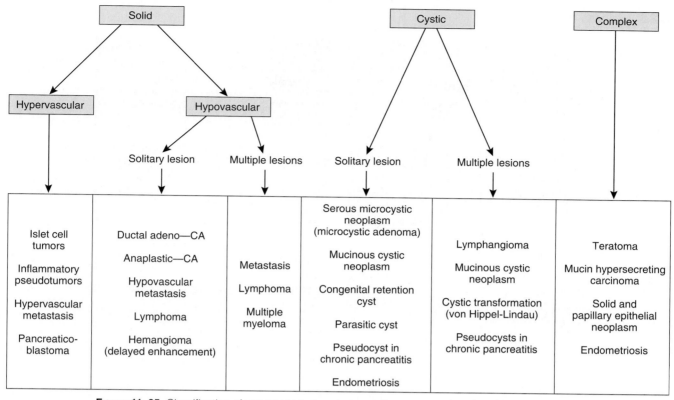

FIGURE 11–35. Classification of pancreatic lesions in magnetic resonance imaging. (CA, carcinoma.)

Solid

Hypervascular

Islet cell tumors

Inflammatory pseudotumors

Hypervascular metastasis

Pancreatico-blastoma

Hypovascular

Solitary lesion

Ductal adeno—CA

Anaplastic—CA

Hypovascular metastasis

Lymphoma

Hemangioma (delayed enhancement)

Multiple lesions

Metastasis

Lymphoma

Multiple myeloma

Cystic

Solitary lesion

Serous microcystic neoplasm (microcystic adenoma)

Mucinous cystic neoplasm

Congenital retention cyst

Parasitic cyst

Pseudocyst in chronic pancreatitis

Endometriosis

Multiple lesions

Lymphangioma

Mucinous cystic neoplasm

Cystic transformation (von Hippel-Lindau)

Pseudocysts in chronic pancreatitis

Complex

Teratoma

Mucin hypersecreting carcinoma

Solid and papillary epithelial neoplasm

Endometriosis

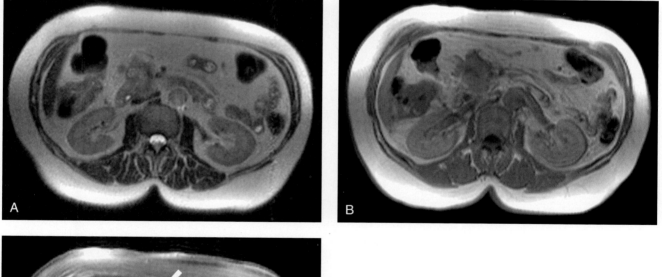

FIGURE 11–36. Pancreatic adenocarcinoma of the pancreatic head in a 70-year-old man with weight loss and abdominal pain. *A*, On T$_2$-weighted imaging, a small tumor of the pancreatic head with slightly elevated signal compared with normal pancreatic parenchyma can be identified. *B*, T$_1$-weighted imaging shows early infiltration of the peripancreatic fat; however, there seems to be an intact fat plane between the tumor and the superior mesenteric vessels. *C*, T$_1$-weighted fat-suppressed imaging again demonstrates the lower signal intensity of the carcinoma (*arrow*) compared with normal parenchyma.

323

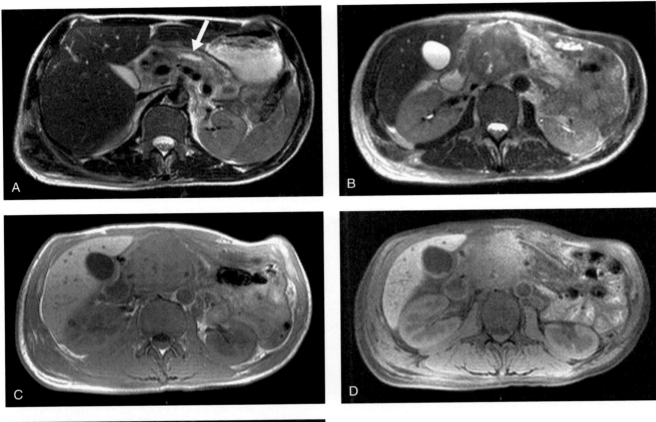

FIGURE 11–37. Pancreatic adenocarcinoma in a 73-year-old man with weight loss and increasing back pain of several weeks duration. *A* and *B*, Axial T$_2$-weighted images show significant atrophy of the pancreatic tail with dilatation of the pancreatic duct (*arrow*) as well as a large tumor of the pancreatic head with infiltration of the peripancreatic fat. The tumor is very inhomogeneous with central areas of high signal intensity. On T$_1$-weighted (*C*) and T$_1$-weighted fat-suppressed (*D*) images, encasement of the superior mesenteric vessels can be clearly visualized. The unsharp borders with infiltration of peripancreatic fat and retroperitoneal structures are best displayed on the T$_1$-weighted fat-suppressed image. *E,* On early-phase T$_1$-weighted dynamic imaging, after contrast administration the tumor is hypovascular and shows inhomogeneous enhancement of peripheral areas.

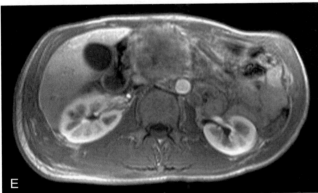

(Fig. 11-38). One should always look for an obstructed pancreatic duct as an indirect sign of pancreatic carcinoma. Typically, in a case of pancreatic carcinoma, the obstructed and dilated duct is surrounded by atrophic pancreatic tissue without signs of chronic pancreatitis such as pseudocyst formation or inflammatory changes in the surrounding peripancreatic fat. For contrast-enhanced MRI of the pancreas, bolus injection of Gd chelates with early dynamic imaging using breath-hold T$_1$-weighted sequences is the most reliable technique for detection of pancreatic carcinoma. Typically, pancreatic carcinoma is hypointense precontrast and also hypovascular (and thus remaining hypointense) during the first 1 to 2 minutes after contrast administration when normal pancreatic tissue maximally enhances. In images 2 to 5 minutes after contrast injection, leakage of contrast to the extracellular fluid compartment of the tumor reduces the contrast between pancreatic carcinoma and normal pancreatic tissue. Thus, pancreatic carcinoma may become isointense. In staging of pancreatic carcinoma, local as well as remote spread of tumor has to be considered concerning resectability of the tumor. Because of the special lymphatic drainage of the pancreas and the lack of a capsule surrounding the organ, pancreatic carcinoma can metastasize to almost any lymph node group of the upper abdomen. Metastases may occur in the liver or to the peritoneum; either finding makes the tumor unresectable. Another area of special interest concerning staging of pancreatic carcinoma is the involvement of vessels of the upper abdomen, specifically encasement of the superior mesenteric artery, superior mesenteric vein, or portal vein. Figure 11-39 gives an overview concerning resectability criteria for ductal adenocarcinoma of the pancreas on MRI.

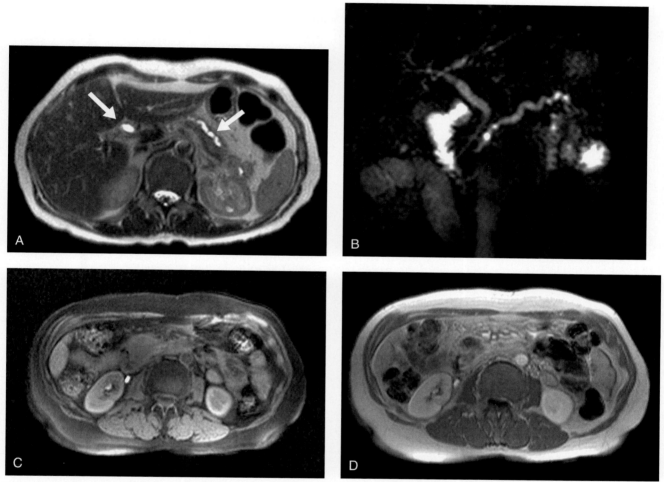

FIGURE 11–38. Pancreatic adenocarcinoma of the pancreatic head in a 74-year-old man with sudden onset of painless jaundice and weight loss. *A,* The axial T₂-weighted image shows dilatation of the choledochal as well as the main pancreatic duct (*arrows*), the so-called double-duct sign. The pancreatic tail shows parenchymal atrophy without signs of acute or chronic pancreatitis, which is rather common in pancreatic carcinoma. *B,* Magnetic resonance cholangiopancreatography confirms obstruction of the common bile duct and pancreatic duct. *C,* On the T₁-weighted fat-suppressed unenhanced image, a low-signal-intensity (SI) lesion in the pancreatic head can be identified with small areas of remaining high SI pancreatic tissue in the more medial aspect of the pancreatic head. *D,* The T₁-weighted contrast-enhanced image demonstrates a hypovascular area in the pancreatic head close to the papillar region consistent with pancreatic adenocarcinoma.

MRI RESECTABILITY CRITERIA

- No dilation of pancreatic duct or common bile duct

- No pancreatic atrophy

- Size < 2 cm

- Tumor completely surrounded by normal pancreatic tissue

MRI NONRESECTABILITY CRITERIA

- Ascites (peritoneal carcinomatosis)

- Liver metastasis

- Vascular involvement (encasement of SMA or celiac axis; occlusion of SMV or portal vein)

  If fat plane lost ⟶ Involvement cannot be excluded

  If tumor encases vessels ⟶ Definite involvement (pancreatitis usually spares perivascular fat)

- Local tumor extension (except duodenum)

FIGURE 11–39. Ductal adenocarcinoma resectability criteria. (MRI, magnetic resonance imaging; SMA, superior mesenteric artery; SMV, superior mesenteric vein.)

In imaging of islet cell tumors of the pancreas, distinction has to be made between tumors that produce hormonally active peptide (functioning islet cell tumors) and those tumors that do not produce peptides (nonfunctioning islet cell tumors). Because of the production of hormonally active peptides and the resulting clinical symptoms, functioning islet cell tumors typically are much smaller at presentation. In distinction, nonfunctioning tumors are often larger (Fig. 11-40) and clinical symptoms that lead to presentation include mass effect and metastases. Generally, islet cell tumors of the pancreas show high signal intensity on T_2-weighted and low signal intensity on T_1-weighted fat-suppressed images. After intravenous bolus injection of Gd chelates, they show very early enhancement. Thus, imaging of islet cell tumors in the early arterial phase is of great importance. Functioning endocrine pancreatic neoplasms have to be considered in patients with classic multiple endocrine neoplasia type I (MEN I). An increased incidence of functioning pancreatic neoplasms also has to be considered in von Hippel-Lindau disease, in which other find-

ings like pancreatic cysts may also be evident. Because of the potential malignancy and multicentricity of endocrine pancreatic neoplasms and the lack of pathologic findings that can clearly prove nonmalignant tumors, preoperative imaging is very important in the evaluation of patients with an assumed pancreatic endocrine neoplasm.

Insulinoma of the pancreas is the most frequent islet cell tumor; 90% of these tumors are benign, and in the majority of cases patients have solitary neoplasms. Gastrinomas, the most frequent islet cell tumor associated with MEN I, however, are multicentric in 20% to 40% of cases and malignant in up to 60%. Gastrinomas as well as insulinomas are hypointense on T_1-weighted fat-suppressed images and hyperintense on T_2-weighted sequences. However, gastrinoma may show larger cystic areas in contrast to insulinoma. Rare functioning islet cell tumors include glucagonoma, VIPoma, and somatostatinoma; each has a distinct clinical presentation. As a reminder, approximately one third of pancreatic tumors are classified as insulinoma, one third are other functioning islet cell tumors, and one third are nonfunctioning islet cell neoplasms.

True pancreatic cysts are rare and typically occur in combination with a systemic disease such as von Hippel-Lindau disease. Other congenital diseases that may be associated with true pancreatic cysts are cystic fibrosis and polycystic kidney disease. True pancreatic cysts have uniform high signal intensity on T_2-weighted images, have a thin wall, lack contrast enhancement, and are not associated with chronic pancreatitis.

The term pancreatic pseudocyst refers to a collection of fluid consisting of pancreatic juice without a true cyst lining. This means that the fluid is kept within a fibrous capsule. Pancreatic pseudocysts are typical complications of pancreatic inflammation or trauma. Normally, in acute pancreatitis they are rather ill defined and in most of the cases resolve spontaneously within 3 to 4 weeks. However, chronic pseudocysts (Fig. 11-41) may occur within the pancreatic parenchyma. True neoplasms of the pancreas that appear cystic include microcystic adenoma, which is also referred to as serous cystadenoma, as well as mucinous cystic neoplasms, which include a spectrum of neoplasms characterized by the production of mucus. In microcystic adenoma, typically multiple, lobulated cysts with thin walls and thin internal septations can be found (Fig. 11-42) that show almost no contrast enhancement after injection of Gd chelates. However, in rare cases, some solid areas within the cystic tumor may be found that can show marked enhancement after contrast injection. Very rare tumors that should be mentioned in the context of pancreatic tumors are solid and papillary epithelial neoplasm, anaplastic carcinoma, metastases, and pancreaticoblastoma, a malignant pancreatic tumor predominantly found in children.

FIGURE 11–40. Nonfunctioning islet cell tumor of the pancreatic head in a 34-year-old woman with abdominal discomfort. No excessive level of insulin, gastrin, vasoactive intestinal polypeptide, or somatostatin could be detected. *A,* The coronal T_2-weighted image shows the double-duct sign of dilated choledochal and pancreatic ducts, which is confirmed on magnetic resonance cholangiopancreatography (*B*). In the coronal T_2-weighted image, a round, well-demarcated tumor (*arrow*) of the pancreatic head at the area of the obstruction of choledochal and pancreatic ducts is visible. This is also confirmed on axial T_1-weighted imaging (*C*), which shows a round, homogeneously hypointense lesion of the pancreatic head with strong contrast enhancement on early contrast-enhanced T_1-weighted imaging (*D*). This is typically seen in islet cell tumors, whereas pancreatic adenocarcinoma is typically hypovascular. Homogeneous persistent contrast uptake is clearly visible on the T_1-weighted fat-suppressed contrast-enhanced image (*E*), indicating a tumor with increased extracellular space.

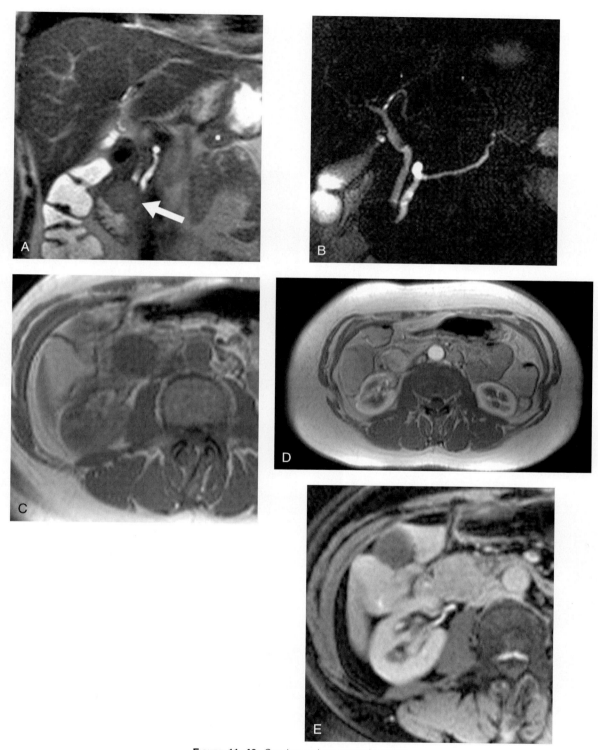

Figure 11–40. *See legend on opposite page*

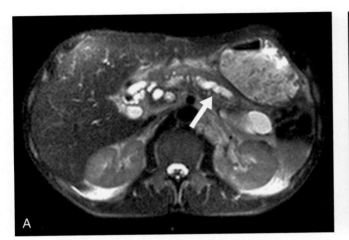

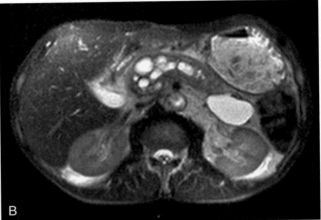

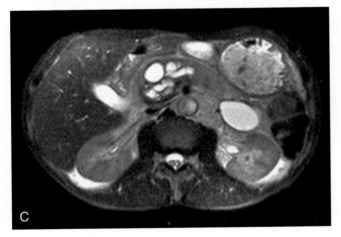

FIGURE 11–41. Pancreatic pseudocysts in a 42-year-old man with a history of chronic pancreatitis. *A–C,* T$_2$-weighted images show marked dilatation of the pancreatic duct (*arrow*) and formation of pseudocysts in both the pancreatic head and tail. There is little remaining pancreatic tissue; however, no solid tumor can be identified.

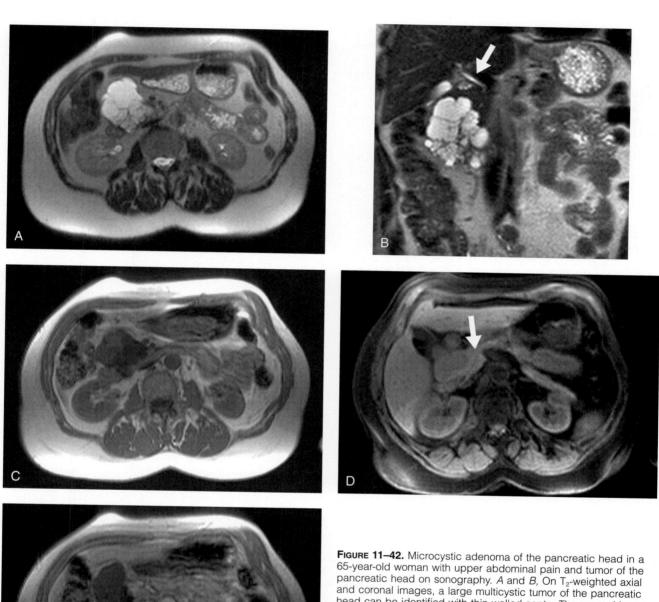

FIGURE 11–42. Microcystic adenoma of the pancreatic head in a 65-year-old woman with upper abdominal pain and tumor of the pancreatic head on sonography. *A* and *B,* On T$_2$-weighted axial and coronal images, a large multicystic tumor of the pancreatic head can be identified with thin-walled septa. The coronal image shows no dilatation of the common bile duct (*arrow*). T$_1$-weighted (*C*) and T$_1$-weighted fat-suppressed (*D*) images show low signal intensity (SI) of the cystic tumor with depiction of high SI normal pancreatic tissue in the more medial aspect of the pancreatic head (*arrow*). *E,* After contrast administration no significant enhancement is seen.

ADRENAL GLAND

In clinical practice, CT is the preferred method of adrenal lesion imaging because of its low cost, greater availability, and higher spatial resolution compared with MRI. This is especially the case for localization of small functioning adrenocortical tumors as in Cushing's and Conn's syndromes. However, MRI is recommended for characterization of incidental adrenal masses, pheochromocytoma, localization and preoperative evaluation of adrenal carcinoma, and imaging of patients with known hypersensitivity to iodinated contrast agents or poor renal function.

MRI of the adrenal glands is usually performed in both the axial and coronal planes with 5- to 8-mm sections. With large masses, coronal as well as sagittal views may be helpful for differentiation of adrenal from hepatic or renal lesions. Imaging protocols should include T_1- and T_2-weighted sequences before and after injection of Gd chelates. Chemical shift MRI using in- and opposed-phase breath-hold imaging and fat-suppressed sequences are important MRI techniques available for identifying lipid-containing adrenal adenomas.

Chemical shift imaging in this context takes advantage of the fact that protons in water and lipid precess at different frequencies within a magnetic field. Thus, by choosing a time to echo appropriate for the magnetic field strength, images can be obtained in which lipid and water are maximally in-phase or out of phase. Using this imaging technique, tissue that contains both water and fat, such as an adrenal adenoma that contain lipids, shows reduction of signal intensity on opposed-phase images when compared with the in-phase sequences. Alternatively, the other types of lesions in the differential diagnosis of an adrenal mass, including specifically metastases, pheochromocytoma, or adrenal carcinoma, do not contain sufficient lipid to demonstrate signal loss on opposed-phase images. However, 20% of adrenal adenomas only display a slight decrease in signal intensity on opposed-phase images, which does not allow a specific diagnosis of adrenal adenoma.

On conventional spin echo images, the adrenal glands have homogeneous low signal intensity compared with the surrounding perinephric fat. They are isointense or hypointense to liver on T_1- and T_2-weighted images. Applying fat suppression, the adrenal glands are hyperintense to both the liver and the adjacent fat. For imaging of the adrenal glands, both axial and coronal images should be acquired, and the slice thickness should not exceed 5 mm when a large mass is not present.

In imaging of adrenal masses in general, functional adrenal disorders have to be distinguished from adrenal masses with normal function. Functional adrenal disorders include disorders that arise from the adrenal cortex, such as primary hyperaldosteronism, Cushing's disease, and adrenocortical carcinoma, as well as adrenomedullary disorders, such as pheochromocytoma and neuroblastoma.

In primary hyperaldosteronism, typical laboratory findings are elevated plasma aldosterone levels and increased plasma renin activity. Clinical symptoms include hypertension, hypokalemia, fluid retention, weakness, and cardiac arrhythmia. Approximately 79% to 90% of patients with primary hyperaldosteronism have a benign aldosterone-producing adenoma, so-called Conn's syndrome, and can be treated by surgical resection. However, in 10% to 30%, diffuse adrenal hyperplasia accounts for primary hyperaldosteronism in which medical treatment is the preferred therapeutic option. Rarely, extensive aldosterone production can be found in adrenocortical carcinoma.

In primary hyperaldosteronism that is caused by diffuse adrenocortical hyperplasia, the adrenal glands may appear normal on imaging studies. Bilateral nodules may be found with a diameter of up to 2 to 3 cm. If this diffuse nodularity of the adrenal gland is missed because of one dominating large nodule, this nodule may be mistaken for an adrenal adenoma.

Endogenous causes of Cushing's syndrome include cortisol-producing adenoma (20%), adrenocortical carcinoma (10%), and adrenocortical hyperplasia resulting from increased corticotropin (ACTH) production (70%). In the majority of patients with increased ACTH production and Cushing's syndrome, adrenocortical hyperfunction is caused by a pituitary adenoma. In 10%, ectopic production of ACTH is found associated with neoplasms (e.g., bronchial carcinoid and tumors of the pancreas or thyroid). In general, cortisol-producing adenomas of the adrenal gland are easily demonstrated because they are usually larger than 2 cm in diameter. The majority of such adenomas are isointense to liver on T_2-weighted spin echo images. To confirm the diagnosis of a lipid-containing adenoma, opposed-phase images should be acquired to show the reduction of signal intensity in the opposed-phase image. In adrenal hyperplasia associated with Cushing's syndrome, up to 50% of patients have normal-appearing adrenal glands, whereas in the rest of patients there is diffuse unilateral or bilateral enlargement. Occasionally, the glands have a macronodular appearance.

Primary adrenocortical carcinoma is a rare malignancy that shows hormonal hyperfunction in up to 50% of patients. Depending on the hormone that is mainly produced, clinical findings include Cushing's syndrome, feminization or virilization, and rarely primary hyperaldosteronism. Typically, large masses are found that have an inhomogeneous enhancement after injection of Gd chelates as a result of central necrosis (Fig. 11-43). In 30% of cases, calcifications may be noted on CT. Primary adrenocortical carcinoma typically is hypointense compared with the liver on T_1-weighted images and has high signal intensity on T_2-weighted images. In opposed-phase images, some small areas of the tumor may show signal reduction. However, the majority of the lesion does not show a signal intensity decrease in opposed-phase images. The homogeneous reduction of signal characteristic of adrenal adenomas is not observed.

Pheochromocytomas are neuroendocrine tumors that arise within the adrenal medulla or from paraganglionic tissue. In approximately 85% to 90% of cases, a paraganglioma arises in the adrenal gland; this is called a pheochromocytoma. These tumors are usually hormonally

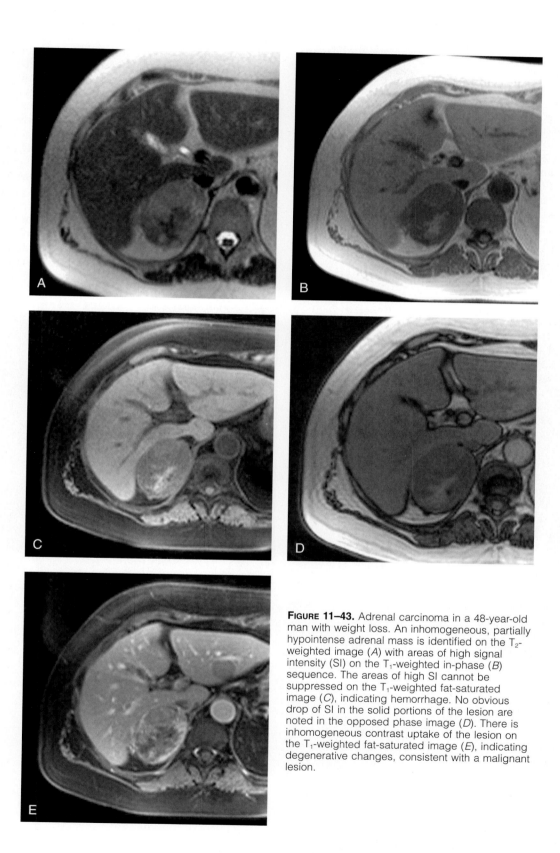

FIGURE 11–43. Adrenal carcinoma in a 48-year-old man with weight loss. An inhomogeneous, partially hypointense adrenal mass is identified on the T$_2$-weighted image (*A*) with areas of high signal intensity (SI) on the T$_1$-weighted in-phase (*B*) sequence. The areas of high SI cannot be suppressed on the T$_1$-weighted fat-saturated image (*C*), indicating hemorrhage. No obvious drop of SI in the solid portions of the lesion are noted in the opposed phase image (*D*). There is inhomogeneous contrast uptake of the lesion on the T$_1$-weighted fat-saturated image (*E*), indicating degenerative changes, consistent with a malignant lesion.

active, producing both norepinephrine and epinephrine. Thus, symptoms such as sustained or paroxysmal hypertension, headache, sweating, and attacks of anxiety may be found resulting from transient elevation of catecholamine levels. Typical syndromes that are associated with pheochromocytoma are MEN IIa and MEN IIb, neurofibromatosis, and von Hippel-Lindau disease. Laboratory findings consistent with a pheochromocytoma include elevated levels of catecholamines and metabolites, including norepinephrine, vanillylmandelic acid, and metanephrine. In such cases (when a pheochromocytoma is assumed to be present), MRI is performed for screening of the adrenal glands. Adrenal pheochromocytomas are usually larger than 3 cm and typically have very high signal intensity on T_2-weighted images (Fig. 11-44). Sometimes, however, this high signal intensity may be reduced because of calcification or hemorrhage. In opposed-phase images, they do not show signal intensity loss compared with the in-phase image.

Adrenomedullary hyperfunction in children in most cases is caused by neuroblastoma. Pheochromocytomas are very rare in childhood. Neuroblastoma represents the most common extracranial malignant tumor in children. Most neuroblastomas arise from the adrenal gland, but they can develop from virtually any tissue of neural crest cell origin. Neuroblastomas are usually poorly defined tumors in which calcifications can be found (in contrast with a nephroblastoma, which is the principal differential diagnosis in childhood). Neuroblastomas show very early and extensive encasement of the vessels of the upper abdomen and are rather large at presentation (Fig. 11-45). Different stages of maturation exist, including ganglioneuroblastoma and benign ganglioneuroma, which, in contrast to neuroblastoma, do not show the early encasement of vessels of the upper abdomen (Fig. 11-46) and show a more expansile growth pattern and distinct borders. Because hemorrhagic neuroblastoma in neonates may present as traumatic adrenal

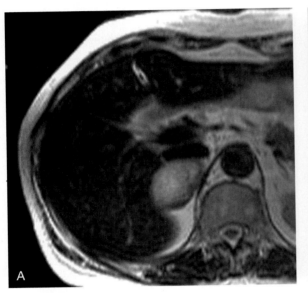

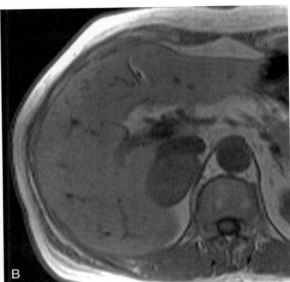

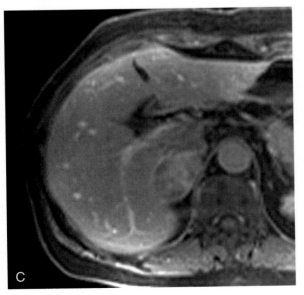

FIGURE 11–44. Pheochromocytoma in a 38-year-old woman with flushing and episodes of extremely elevated blood pressure. *A,* A large high-signal-intensity (SI) mass of the right adrenal can be identified on the T_2-weighted image. *B,* The lesion shows lower SI than normal liver tissue on T_1. *C,* Inhomogeneous but almost complete enhancement of the lesion, indicating a solid tumor rather than a cystic lesion, can be noted on the T_1-weighted fat-suppressed contrast-enhanced image.

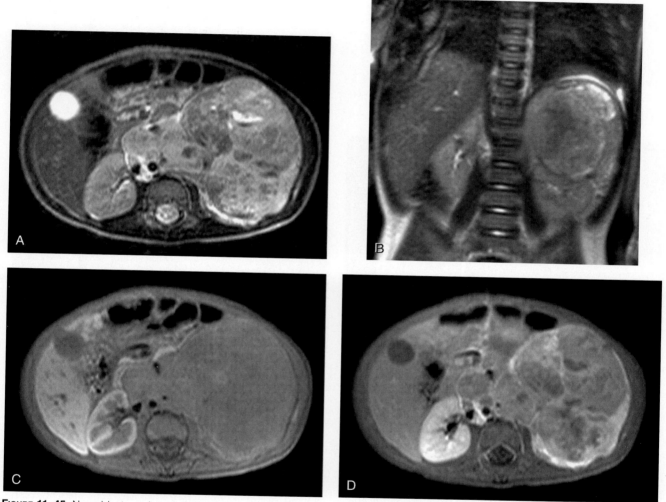

FIGURE 11–45. Neuroblastoma in a 4-year-old boy with abdominal pain and a palpable abdominal mass. *A* and *B*, T_2-weighted images show a large inhomogeneous mass of the left upper abdomen that displaces the kidney. The T_2-weighted images also show areas of necrosis within the tumor. Comparison of pre- (*C*) and post-contrast (*D*) fat-suppressed T_1-weighted images reveals peripheral enhancement with large parts of the lesion remaining hypointense. Typical for neuroblastoma is the extensive encasement of abdominal vessels which in this case reaches the contralateral renal hilum.

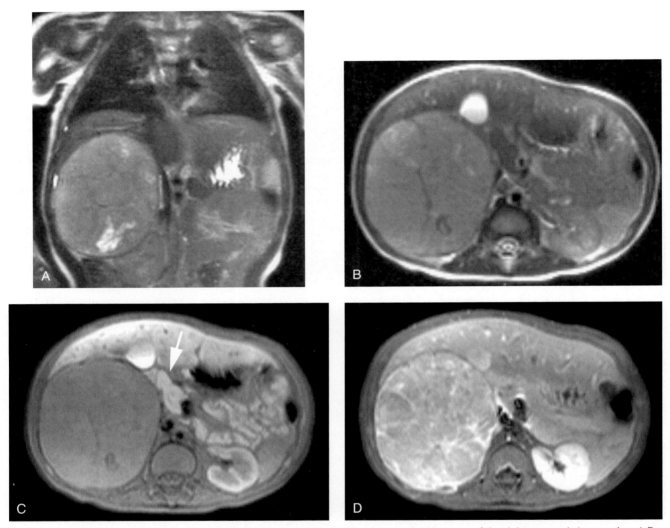

FIGURE 11–46. Ganglioneuroblastoma. This 5-year-old boy presented with a large palpable mass of the right upper abdomen. *A* and *B*, T_2-weighted images show a large, well-defined mass displacing the right kidney. The coronal image (*A*) demonstrates the adrenal origin of the lesion. *C*, There is no sign of encasement of vessels of the upper abdomen in the T_1-weighted fat-suppressed unenhanced image as typically found in neuroblastoma. The pancreatic head (*arrow*) is displaced to the left. *D*, The lesion shows inhomogeneous enhancement on the T_1-weighted fat-suppressed contrast-enhanced image, which is more indicative of ganglioneuroblastoma rather than ganglioneuroma.

hemorrhage, urinary catecholamine screening should be performed to ensure the diagnosis.

In contrast to hyperfunctioning masses of the adrenal glands, nonhyperfunctioning adenomas or so-called incidentalomas are common. In most cases, these lesions are detected in imaging studies of the upper abdomen performed for other reasons. In spin echo imaging, nonhyperfunctioning adrenal adenomas have a signal intensity similar to the liver on T_1- and T_2-weighted sequences, whereas adrenal carcinoma and metastases are typically hyperintense on T_2-weighted images. The signal intensity can be variable, however, because of hemorrhage, necrosis, or calcification. The most promising method to characterize adrenal adenomas is chemical shift imaging, in which up to 80% of adenomas show an obvious signal intensity reduction (Fig. 11-47) in opposed-phase images as compared with in-phase images.

Metastases to the adrenal glands are rather common. Overall, the adrenals are the fourth most common involved organ in metastatic disease. Typical primary tumors are lung cancer, breast cancer, and thyroid and colon cancer as well as malignant melanoma. In MRI adrenal metastases are seen as rounded or oval masses that are hyperintense to the liver on T_2-weighted images (Fig. 11-48). Chemical shift imaging is also very sensitive for the detection of adrenal metastases. However, this technique does not allow differentiation from benign nonhyperfunctioning adenomas because both types of lesions fail to show signal reduction on opposed-phase images.

A rare benign neoplasm of the adrenal gland that contains both fat and myeloid elements is adrenal myelolipoma. In MRI of adrenal myelolipoma, it is important to look for lipomatous tumor or a solid tumor that contains foci of fat that can readily be identified in

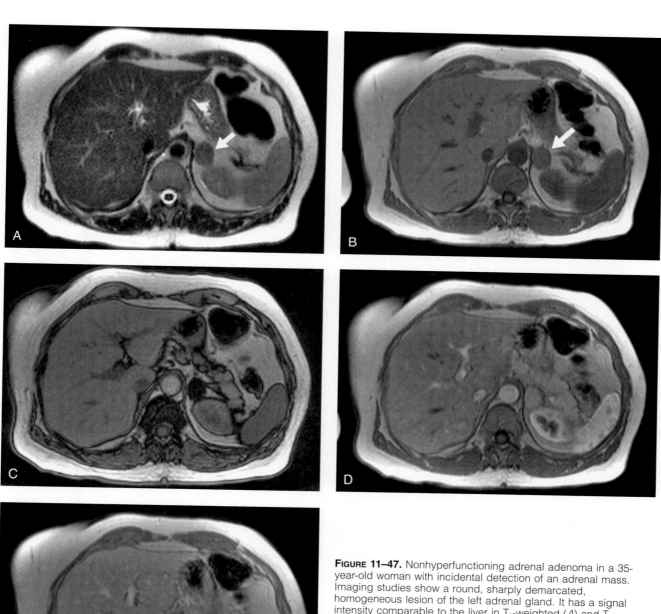

FIGURE 11–47. Nonhyperfunctioning adrenal adenoma in a 35-year-old woman with incidental detection of an adrenal mass. Imaging studies show a round, sharply demarcated, homogeneous lesion of the left adrenal gland. It has a signal intensity comparable to the liver in T$_2$-weighted (*A*) and T$_1$-weighted in-phase (*B*) images (*arrows*). *C*, The signal of the lesion decreases significantly in opposed-phase imaging. The early (*D*) and delayed (*E*) enhancement after injection of an extracellular gadolinium chelate is homogeneous comparable to normal adrenal tissue.

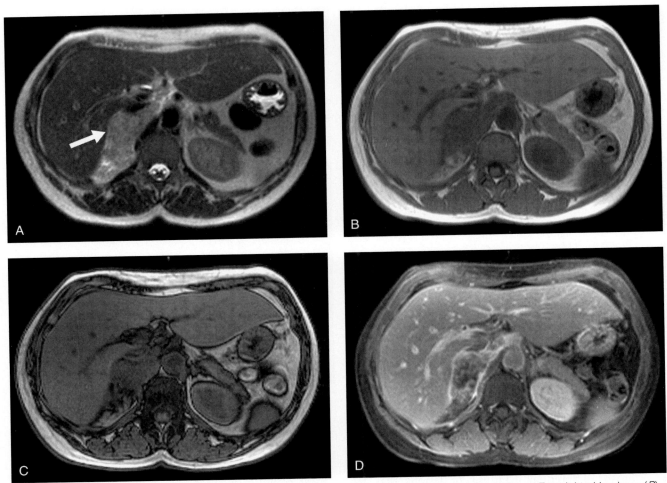

FIGURE 11–48. Adrenal metastases in a 72-year-old man with bronchial adenocarcinoma. T$_2$-weighted (*A*) and T$_1$-weighted in-phase (*B*) images show a large, poorly marginated, inhomogeneous mass of the right adrenal gland (*arrow*). Some high-signal-intensity (SI) areas can be identified in the periphery of the lesion that represent adjacent retroperitoneal fat rather than a fat-containing lesion. *C*, No obvious decrease in SI is noted in the opposed-phase image. *D*, After contrast administration the T$_1$-weighted fat-suppressed image demonstrates inhomogeneous enhancement of the lesion with irregular margins.

fat-suppressed images (Fig. 11-49). If only small foci of fat mainly in the periphery of an adrenal lesion are found in a patient with known malignancy, the differential diagnosis includes metastases, and biopsy must be performed to prove the diagnosis.

Another rare entity of the adrenal glands are cysts; most are endothelial. Pseudocysts may also be found, which develop after hemorrhage of the adrenal gland. The imaging appearance of adrenal cysts on MRI depends on the content of the cyst; however, most adrenal cysts are hypointense on T_1-weighted images and have a very high signal intensity on T_2-weighted sequences. If hemorrhage is present, an increase of signal intensity in T_1-weighted images and a decrease in T_2-weighted images can be seen.

KIDNEY

Because of its wide distribution and low cost, ultrasonography is generally the method of choice for screening renal masses. Nevertheless, both MRI and CT are superior to ultrasonography for morphologic assessment. In distinction to ultrasound, MRI and CT permit simultaneous assessment of macroscopic changes and evaluation of functional derangements. In the 1980s, CT was the method of choice for characterization of suspected malignant renal lesions primarily detected using ultrasonography. At that time, MRI of the kidneys did not play an important role. In the interim, studies have shown MRI to be helpful in the detection and staging of renal cancer. With the development of new pulse sequences, including fast spin echo sequences with motion compensation and gradient echo sequences as well as the use of dynamic imaging, the role of and indication for MRI in the work-up of renal lesions have changed. Dynamic and delayed postcontrast images are considered to be the most helpful for lesion identification and characterization (i.e., determination of the lesion extent). In comparison with CT, MRI has been shown to be statistically superior for correct characterization of benign renal lesions regarding infiltrative versus expansive masses, whereas there is only a slight difference between these two methods concerning detection and differential diagnosis of renal masses. MRI is also considered to be superior for differential diagnosis of lesions that are equivocal on CT, especially in the differentiation between complicated cysts and cystic or hypovascular renal cell carcinoma (RCC). MRI is considered superior to CT in the evaluation of perirenal and vascular involvement, as well as the involvement of perinephric fat and adjacent organs. For evaluation of the renal vein and the inferior vena cava (regarding tumor thrombus formation), MRI again has advantages over CT.

Thus, today MRI is the imaging technique of choice for preoperative and postoperative tumor staging. Indeed, small solid masses, less than 1 cm in diameter, may be visible using MRI but not be visible with ultrasonography or CT.

Renal cell carcinomas are the most frequent malignant neoplasms of the kidney. Histologically, these tumors belong to the parenchymal malignant tumors. Moreover, there are many other malignant and benign tumors that can affect the kidney. With an incidence of 2% to 3% of all neoplasms, solid tumors of the kidney are rather rare. Most of the lesions that arise in the kidney are benign mesenchymal cysts and almost all are asymptomatic, whereas approximately 90% of solid renal lesions are classified as malignant.

From a histopathologic perspective, renal tumors may be divided into four groups:

1. Parenchymal tumors
2. Mesenchymal tumors
3. Tumors of the renal pelvis
4. Secondary tumors

Parenchymal tumors include both benign and malignant tumors. Adenomas, nephroblastomatosis, and multiloculated or uniloculated cystic kidney diseases are examples of benign renal masses. Renal cysts may be divided into genetic cystic diseases, obstructive cystic disease, acquired cystic disease, and cysts associated with systemic diseases. Within these entities, the age at presentation, renal function impairment, localization, and appearance of the cysts vary considerably. Autosomal-recessive polycystic kidney disease (ARPKD), also called type I cystic kidney disease according to Potter, is the most common heritable cystic disease in infancy and childhood, appearing unilateral and bilateral as well as uniloculated or multiloculated. Its incidence is 1 in 20,000 births, and it accounts for about 5% of all end-stage renal disease in the United States. In ARPKD the liver often is affected by congenital hepatic fibrosis, which may be helpful in the differential diagnosis.

Acquired cystic disease is most often caused by uremia. Etiologically, it has to be differentiated from obstructive cystic diseases, including multicystic dysplasia and cystic dysplasia. In rare cases, renal cysts are diagnosed in systemic diseases such as tuberous sclerosis and von Hippel-Lindau disease.

In addition to strictly benign and malignant parenchymal masses, there are also borderline types such as oncocytoma. Oncocytomas in general are benign masses but should be considered to be borderline because they have potential for malignant transformation.

Both RCC as well as nephroblastoma (Wilms' tumor) represent malignant parenchymal tumors. RCC is the most common malignant tumor of the human kidney, and it is important to note that this group of tumors is very heterogeneous concerning histopathology. Approximately 6% to 7% of RCCs are impossible to classify by histology, and special molecular genetic studies are required for proper characterization.

Angiomyolipoma, hemangioma, lipoma, reninoma, and capsuloma are examples of benign mesenchymal tumors affecting one or both kidneys, whereas renal sarcoma is a quite common malignant mesenchymal tumor.

Tumors of the renal pelvis are another group of entities that may affect the human kidney. Transitional cell carcinoma is the most frequent malignant genitourinary tumor in adults and the second most common tumor of the kidney. This mesenchymal tumor develops from transitional epithelium and generally affects the human

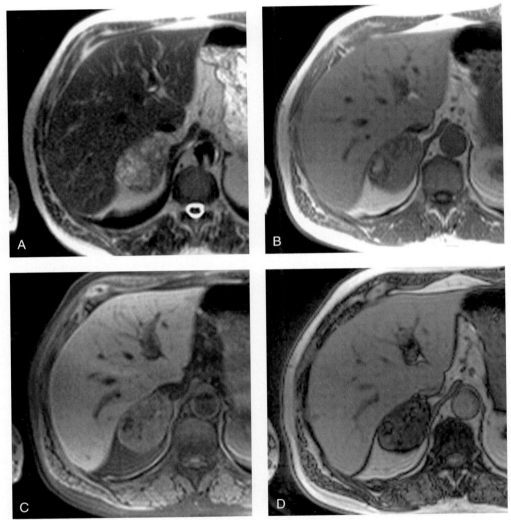

FIGURE 11–49. Adrenal myelolipoma in a 47-year-old man with adrenal enlargement. There is a large solid lesion of the right adrenal gland, which has areas of fat on T_2- (A) and T_1-weighted (B) images. The fat signal can be suppressed on the T_1-weighted fat-saturated (C) and opposed-phase images (D).

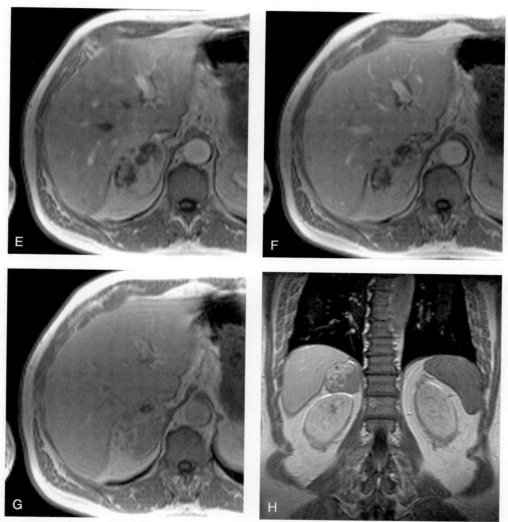

FIGURE 11–49 *Continued. E–G,* Large areas of the tumor show homogeneous enhancement on dynamic imaging; some small regions of internal hemorrhage or degenerative changes remain hypointense. *H,* The T$_1$-weighted contrast-enhanced coronal image clearly demonstrates the adrenal origin of the lesion. The presence of fat and solid tissue within an adrenal lesion makes the diagnosis of myelolipoma most likely.

bladder. However, transitional cell carcinoma also occurs in the renal pelvis. Because there may be secondary involvement of the kidney in transitional cell carcinoma of the bladder or ureter, these tumors are considered as secondary (as opposed to primary) kidney tumors.

Secondary renal lesions may be benign (e.g., in case of parasitic infection such as echinococcal disease or a granulomatous tumor). Secondary malignant neoplasms include lymphomas, leukemia, and metastases. Renal involvement in patients with known lymphoma ranges from 30% to 60%.

Finally, tumors exist that cannot definitely be distributed to a specific group such as the malignant rhabdoid tumors (typically found in children and carrying a bad prognosis). These tumors have in common a distinct so-called rhabdoid cytologic feature and are further characterized by variable histologic and immunohistochemical patterns.

Figure 11-50 summarizes the pathologic classification of renal masses. The problems concerning specific pathologic characterization of renal masses reflect the difficulties in radiographic examination and characterization.

The basic MRI approach for imaging of the kidneys includes T_1-weighted spin echo sequences acquired in the transverse plane analogous to CT scanning. Additionally, T_2-weighted sequences should be performed. For lesions located at the upper or lower pole of the kidney, images in the coronal plane may give important additional information.

Postcontrast scans should be acquired in a dynamic fashion (after intravenous bolus injection of a Gd chelate) during the various phases of contrast enhancement. It should be noted that some lesions are only clearly visible in the early arterial phase, whereas others are better depicted in images acquired approximately 1 to 2 minutes after contrast injection. In cases of suspected disease involving the vasculature, additional gradient echo images or contrast-enhanced magnetic resonance angiography (MRA) can be performed for further evaluation. To evaluate perirenal or pararenal extension of tumors, fat-suppressed T_1-weighted images after contrast injection are useful because they provide much better contrast between fat and solid contrast-enhancing lesions.

In the normal kidney, there is good differentiation (precontrast) between the cortex and the medulla on T_1-weighted images; the cortex shows a higher signal intensity. Fat in the renal sinus has high signal intensity both on T_1- and T_2-weighted images; the vessels of the hilum are seen as flow voids. On T_2-weighted images, the boundary between the cortex and medulla is less clearly seen. However, on unenhanced images cysts are best detected with T_2-weighted sequences. In dynamic imaging of the kidney after bolus injection of a Gd chelate, an increase of signal intensity in the renal cortex can be observed 5 to 10 seconds after the start of contrast injection. An increase of signal intensity in the medulla starts at approximately 20 to 30 seconds. In images between 2 and 3 minutes postinjection, a homogeneous increase of signal intensity in the kidney can be observed.

Classification of Renal Masses in MRI

On MRI, renal masses are classified with regard to their general imaging appearance (i.e., solid or cystic masses) and growth patterns (i.e., expansile vs. an infiltrative growth) (Fig. 11-51). In addition to imaging findings, the patient's age, sex, and medical history should always be considered in the differential diagnosis. The prevalence of malignant tumors in childhood differs markedly from those of adults; thus, tumors of the kidney in childhood are discussed separately.

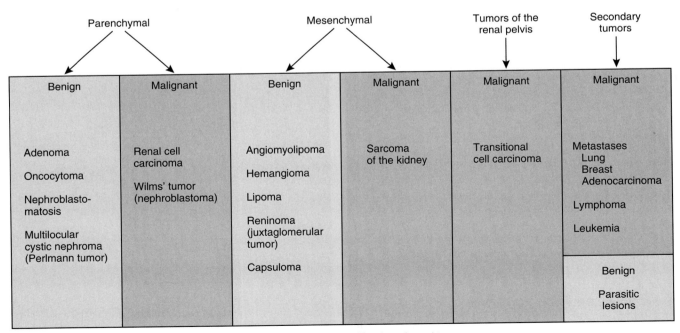

FIGURE 11–50. Pathologic classification of renal tumors.

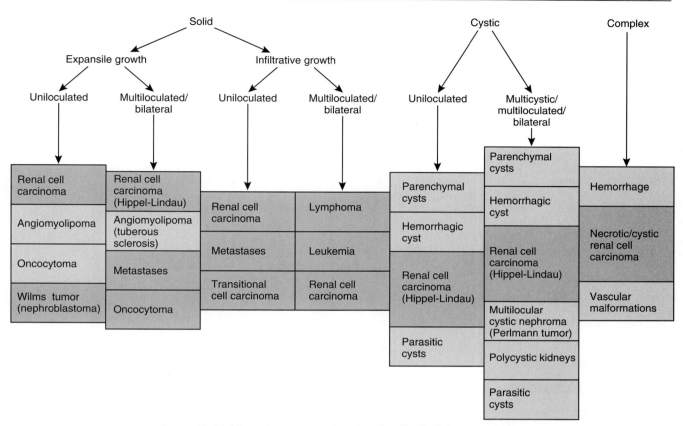

FIGURE 11–51. Magnetic resonance imaging classification of renal masses.

Simple cysts of the kidney are the most frequent renal masses in adults; most cases are detected incidentally. With simple cysts, MRI has a minor role in evaluation because these lesions can be clearly characterized by ultrasonography or CT. However, in those lesions that cannot be categorized confidentially on CT or ultrasonography, MRI provides important additional information. Simple cysts in MRI have low signal intensity on T_1-weighted images and homogeneous high signal intensity on T_2-weighted scans. After contrast injection, no increase in signal intensity is observed. Fat-suppressed T_1-weighted images after contrast have a very high sensitivity for detection of small cysts.

Complicated cysts account for approximately 5% of renal masses. Complicated cysts are characterized by irregular borders, septations, and internal hemorrhage, or they may contain a high concentration of protein or calcium in suspension as well as wall calcification. The main differential diagnosis in complicated cysts is necrotic neoplasm or cystic RCC. These lesions can be indistinguishable from complicated, non-neoplastic cysts. Although the signal intensity of complicated cysts in T_1-weighted images is variable and determined by the fluid composition, the high signal intensity in T_2-weighted images in most cases is maintained. However, some cysts with hemoglobin degradation products may show decreased signal intensity both on T_1- and T_2-weighted sequences. Sometimes layering can be demonstrated. On T_1-weighted images, complicated cysts often present as hyperintense masses, and susceptibility artifacts with the application of fat suppression further increase the signal intensity of the cyst fluid. In polycystic kidney disease (Fig. 11-52), multiple cysts of variable signal intensity can be depicted representing cysts with hemorrhage and infection. However, a clear differentiation between infected and hemorrhagic or even malignant cysts cannot be made accurately on MRI, CT or ultrasonography.

A benign neoplastic lesion that also presents as a cystic tumor is multilocular cystic nephroma. This tumor is composed of multiple noncommunicating cysts with a fibrous stroma and a fibrous capsule. Typically, no solid areas can be detected. However, differential diagnosis versus cystic RCC (Fig. 11-53) in the majority of cases is not possible by means of imaging findings.

The most frequent renal mass of mesenchymal origin is angiomyolipoma. Pathologically, angiomyolipoma is a hamartomatous tumor composed of vessels, smooth muscle fibers, and lipocytes in different proportions. Angiomyolipoma may present spontaneously or as bilateral or multilocular tumors in combination with tuberous sclerosis. The MRI appearance of angiomyolipoma depends on the histologic composition of the tumor. The signal intensity may be dominated by fat, leading to a high signal intensity on both T_1- and T_2-weighted images. The fat content can be proven by applying fat suppression (Fig. 11-54). In those tumors in which smooth muscle predominates differentiation from malignant tumors (e.g., RCC) may not be possible by means of imaging studies.

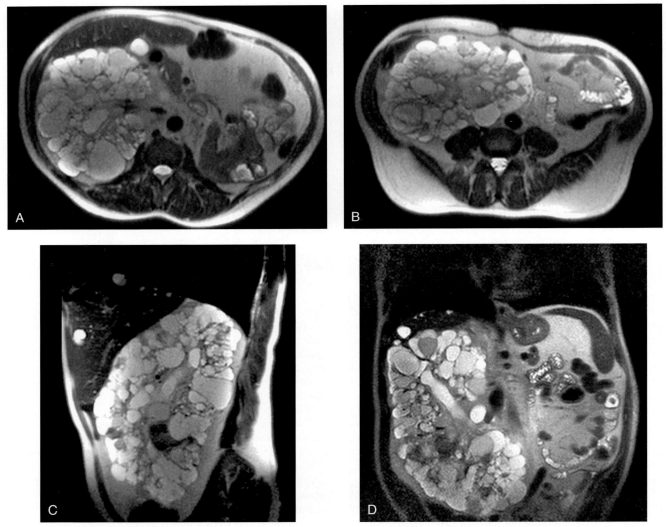

FIGURE 11–52. Adult polycystic kidney disease in a 45-year-old man with a history of nephrectomy of the left kidney as a result of renal cell carcinoma. *A–D,* T$_2$-weighted axial, sagittal, and coronal images show a diffuse cystic transformation of the right kidney, which displaces the liver and reaches down into the pelvis. The cysts have different signal intensities indicating simple and complicated renal cysts with hemorrhage of different age. Note the multiple hepatic cysts.

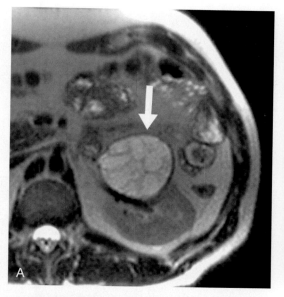

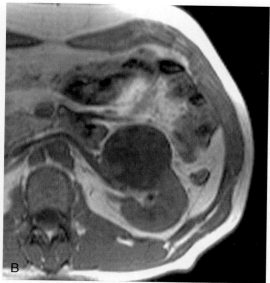

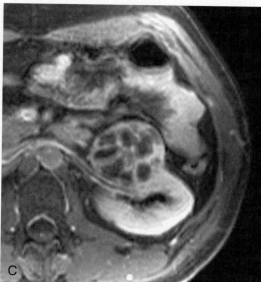

FIGURE 11–53. Cystic renal cell carcinoma in a 38-year-old man with hematuria. Sonography demonstrated a renal tumor. *A,* T$_2$-weighted imaging shows a mainly cystic tumor of the left kidney (*arrow*) with internal septations. *B,* On the T$_1$-weighted image the tumor displays low signal intensity. Fatty components and hemorrhage can thus be excluded. However, the septations show strong contrast uptake on the T$_1$-weighted fat-suppressed contrast-enhanced image (*C*), and solid areas are visible. Differential diagnosis includes benign multilocular cystic nephroma; however, solid areas favor the final histologic diagnosis of a cystic renal cell carcinoma.

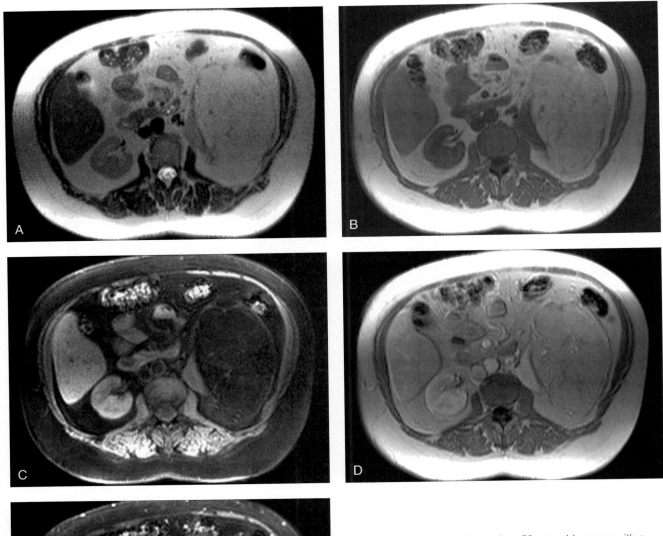

Figure 11–54. Angiomyolipoma in a 58-year-old woman with a renal tumor on routine sonography. *A,* The lower pole of the left kidney is mainly replaced by a hyperintense tumor (on T$_2$) with thin, hypointense septations. *B,* The signal remains almost isointense to perirenal fat on T1. *C,* On the fat-suppressed T$_1$-weighted image, the tumor displays low signal intensity and is sharply demarcated from the adjacent renal parenchyma by a thin capsule. *D,* After contrast administration, the majority of the tumor does not seem to show any contrast uptake on the T$_1$-weighted contrast-enhanced image. However, the T$_1$-weighted fat-suppressed contrast-enhanced image clearly demonstrates contrast enhancement of septations and small solid areas (*E*).

Another benign tumor that can be diagnosed by means of MRI is lipoma of the kidney, although this tumor is rather rare. Other benign neoplasms that show no typical characteristics on MRI are hemangioma, lymphangioma, and juxtaglomerular tumors. In these tumors, biopsy has to be performed for definitive diagnosis.

As mentioned previously, oncocytoma historically was considered a benign tumor. However, since reports about malignant foci in oncocytomas, this tumor is now classified as a low-grade or borderline renal neoplasm. Typically, these tumors are well circumscribed and may show a central star-shaped scar composed of fibrous tissue. If a central scar exists, it is often depicted with low signal intensity on T_2-weighted images. The tumor itself on T_1- and T_2-weighted images has a signal intensity similar to the renal parenchyma and often can only be identified because of mass effect. Differentiation between oncocytoma and RCC is difficult because central necrosis or hemorrhage may occur, and there are no reliable imaging findings that can clearly differentiate between these two entities. However, if oncocytoma is favored in the differential diagnosis, resection of the tumor should be performed by means of nephron-sparing surgery.

The most important malignant tumor of the kidney is RCC. About 50% of RCCs have cystic areas as a result of internal hemorrhage, necrosis, or even primary cystic growth (see Fig. 11-53). Improvements in imaging studies significantly increased the early detection of asymptomatic RCC; however, no specific morphologic finding exists that specifically allows the diagnosis of RCC. The signal intensity characteristics of RCCs are variable (Figs. 11-55 to 11-57). They may have areas of high and low signal intensity both on T_1- and T_2-weighted images. There are even reports about macroscopic foci of fat within RCC. Thus, the finding of fat in a solid renal tumor does not exclude RCC. Detection of RCC is improved with dynamic imaging after bolus injection of Gd chelates. However, there are no specific features on enhanced scans that reliably allow diagnosis or exclusion of RCC. In general, RCC has to be considered in all solid masses and even in cystic lesions showing small solid areas (Fig. 11-58).

An important role of imaging studies in RCC is the staging of tumor spread to establish prognosis and treatment planning. Hematogenous spread of RCC commonly involves lung, mediastinum, liver, brain, bones, and adrenal glands and even the contralateral kidney. Infiltration of renal veins and the inferior vena cava as well as tumor thrombus formation are common findings. Lymphatic spread involves the para-aortic lymph nodes. In imaging of para-aortic lymph nodes, it is important to note that the size of the lymph nodes does not necessarily correlate with metastatic spread of RCC. Reports exist of lymph nodes with a diameter of greater than 2 cm that histologically proved to be inflammatory changes.

For evaluation of tumor thrombus formation in the inferior vena cava, coronal imaging using gradient echo sequences as well as contrast-enhanced MRA have proven to be very useful. Another important issue in RCC with invasion of the renal vein is imaging of the right atrium to allow proper planning of surgery.

The second most common malignancy of the kidney in adulthood is transitional cell carcinoma. More than 40% of transitional cell carcinomas arise in the renal pelvis and have associated urothelial neoplasm in the ipsilateral ureter or bladder. Typically, these tumors show an infiltrative growth pattern that is clearly depicted by MRI. In patients with hydronephrosis caused by tumor growth, the tumor is typically depicted as a solid mass in the urine-filled renal pelvis.

Primary lymphoma of the kidney is very rare because of the lack of lymphoid tissue within the kidney. In most cases, the involvement of the kidney is secondary (metastatic). In MRI focal renal lymphoma is depicted as any other solid mass of the kidney. However, the lack of necrosis and the rather homogeneous signal intensity of the tumor on unenhanced and contrast-enhanced images favor the diagnosis of lymphoma. On unenhanced images, lymphoma typically has the same signal intensity as surrounding renal parenchyma. On contrast-enhanced studies in the early phase up to 1 to 2 minutes after contrast injection, lymphoma appears as a hypovascular mass with subsequent delayed homogeneous enhancement.

If multifocal renal tumors are detected, renal metastases have to be considered in the differential diagnosis. Metastases are the most common multifocal renal neoplasms and arise from primary tumors from the lung, colon, melanoma, breast, and others. Existence of a known extrarenal malignancy suggests the diagnosis. Imaging studies are not able to differentiate metastases from primary malignant tumors of the kidney (e.g., RCC).

Renal Masses in Childhood

The most common malignant neoplasm of the kidney in childhood is nephroblastoma, also called Wilms' tumor. These tumors are generally detected because of their huge mass at clinical presentation. T_2-weighted images typically demonstrate a large, inhomogeneous hyperintense tumor that often is septated (Fig. 11-59). The main differential diagnosis is neuroblastoma, which, in contrast to nephroblastoma, is often combined with lymph node enlargement and early encasement of abdominal vessels. Metastases from lymphoma and leukemia may also affect the kidneys of children. This differential diagnosis is especially important because these two tumors account for about half of the cancer cases of children in the United States.

Nephroblastomatosis is a very rare tumor that generally does not appear in adults. Pathologically, these tumors represent nephrogenic blastema that usually regresses by the age of 4 months. If this regression does not occur, so-called nephroblastomatosis with the potential to develop into Wilms' tumor may persist. T_1-weighted images show hypointense, partially irregular lesions often located in both kidneys. On T_2-weighted images, the tumors demonstrate high signal intensity comparable with the intensity of the renal parenchyma (Fig. 11-60). Most of these tumors have a distinct

Text continued on page 351

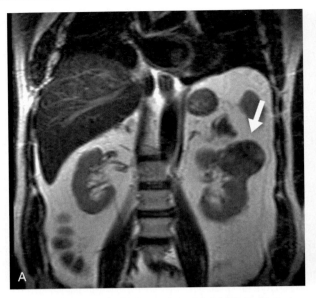

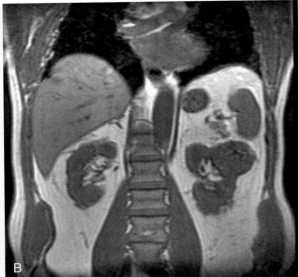

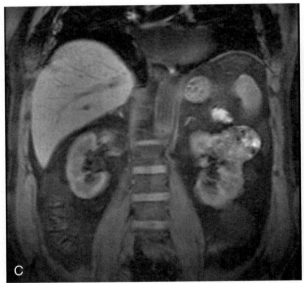

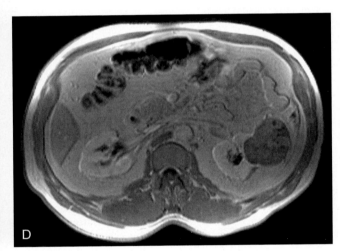

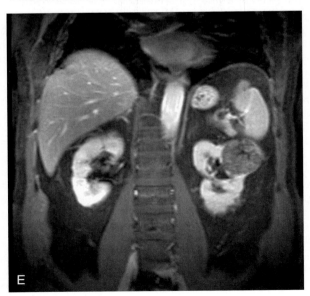

Figure 11–55. Renal cell carcinoma in a 68-year-old man with recurrent episodes of hematuria. *A,* The coronal T_2-weighted image shows a round tumor of the upper pole of the left kidney (*arrow*), which shows an inhomogeneous but almost isointense signal to the renal cortex. On T_1-weighted (*B*) and T_1-weighted fat-suppressed (*C*) images, the tumor again is isointense to the kidney with small streaks of low signal radiating to the center of the lesion. After contrast administration, there is an inhomogeneous contrast enhancement of the tumor demonstrated on T_1-weighted contrast-enhanced (*D*) and T_1-weighted fat-suppressed contrast-enhanced (*E*) images, clearly indicating a solid renal tumor.

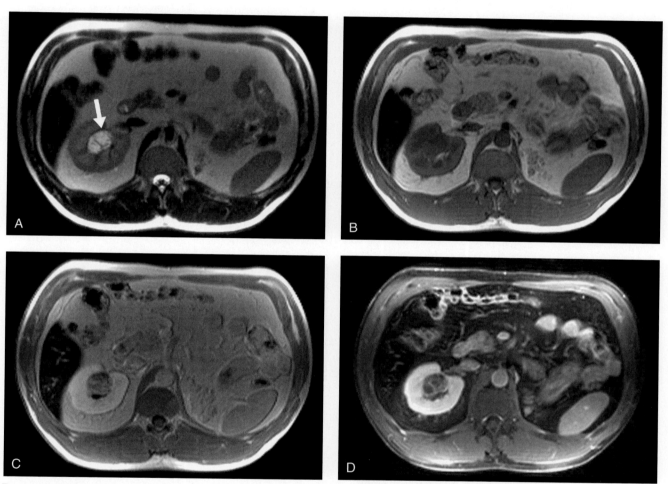

FIGURE 11–56. Renal cell carcinoma in a 64-year-old woman with hematuria. She had a history of nephrectomy after left-sided renal cell carcinoma. *A,* On the T$_2$-weighted axial image, a large hyperintense tumor (*arrow*) is demonstrated in the renal pelvis of the right kidney. The tumor is isointense to the renal parenchyma on the T$_1$-weighted image (*B*) and shows inhomogeneous enhancement with internal septations on T$_1$-weighted contrast-enhanced (*C*) and T$_1$-weighted fat-suppressed contrast-enhanced (*D*) images. Note the marked low signal intensity of the liver on T$_1$-weighted images resulting from iron overload after multiple blood transfusions.

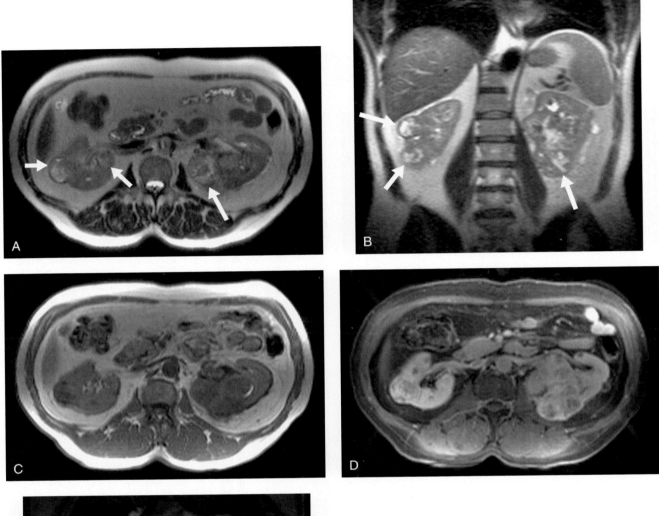

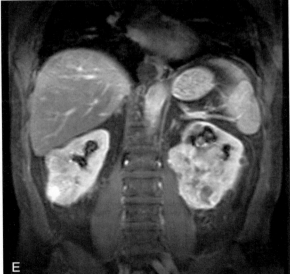

FIGURE 11–57. Bilateral renal cell carcinoma in a 59-year-old man with macrohematuria. *A* and *B*, On T_2-weighted images there are inhomogeneous, partially hyperintense renal tumors (*arrows*) in both kidneys. The large left-sided tumor invades the perirenal fat and the renal pelvis as shown on the T_1-weighted unenhanced image (*C*). The tumors enhance strongly after contrast injection and display large areas of necrosis as well as ill-defined borders (*D* and *E*: T_1-weighted fat-suppressed axial and coronal contrast-enhanced images).

FIGURE 11–58. Multiple cysts and renal cell carcinoma in a 45-year-old man with von Hippel-Lindau disease. *A,* The T₂-weighted image shows multiple cystic lesions of both kidneys; one lesion at the lower pole of the left kidney demonstrates internal septations. *B,* On the T₁-weighted unenhanced image the lesions are hypointense. *C,* The T₁-weighted fat-suppressed contrast-enhanced image demonstrates no contrast enhancement in the majority of lesions, consistent with simple cysts. However, there is inhomogeneous enhancement with demonstration of solid areas in the lesion at the lower pole of the left kidney (*arrow*), indicating a solid tumor that proved to be a renal cell carcinoma on surgery.

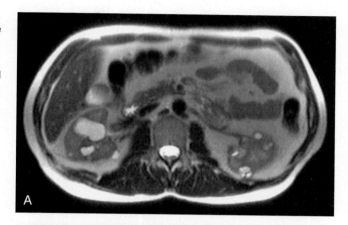

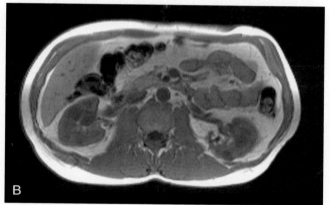

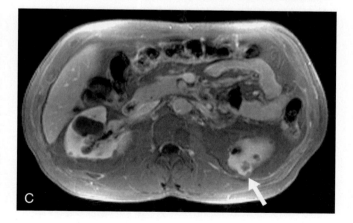

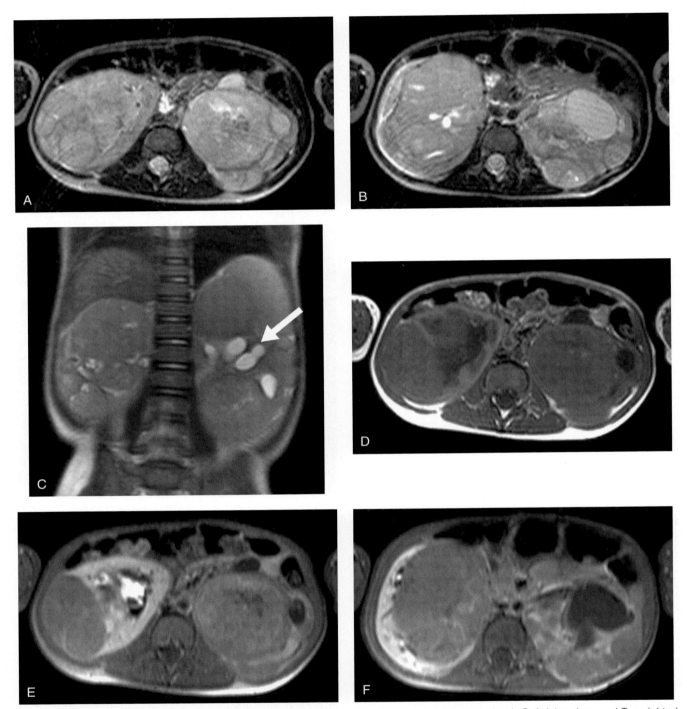

FIGURE 11–59. Bilateral nephroblastoma in a 2-year-old girl with abdominal discomfort and hematuria. *A–C,* Axial and coronal T$_2$-weighted images show large bilateral renal tumors with obstruction of the renal pelvis and hydronephrosis of the left kidney (*arrow*). The tumors have inhomogeneous signal intensity with a partially cystic appearance. Encasement of vessels of the upper abdomen is not present, in distinction from a neuroblastoma. *D,* On the T$_1$-weighted unenhanced image, the tumors are isointense to the renal medulla. *E* and *F,* The tumors are hypointense on T$_1$-weighted fat-suppressed contrast-enhanced images, and remaining renal parenchyma can be clearly identified by the strong contrast enhancement.

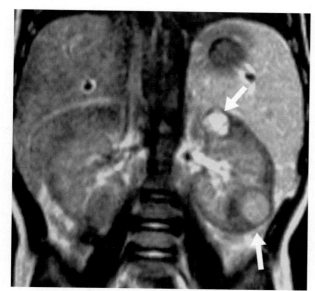

FIGURE 11–60. Nephroblastomatosis in a 2-year-old girl. Several renal masses were demonstrated on routine sonography. The T₂-weighted coronal image shows two high-signal-intensity tumors (*arrows*) of the left kidney with distinct borders. The tumors are confined to the kidney and have a round to oval shape.

oval shape of nephroblastomatosis in contrast to the round appearance in nephroblastoma. Because of its morphologic characteristics, mature teratoma of the kidney is quite easy to classify. These tumors generally consist of solid and cystic parts. High signal intensity on T_2- and T_1-weighted images is typical for the fat contents of these tumors, which can be proven by fat suppression. Mature tumors show no infiltrative growth. The multicystic appearance of the tumor together with the finding of fat leads to the correct diagnosis. As with adults, it is important to emphasize that diffuse enlargement of both kidneys is highly suspicious for lymphoma (Fig. 11-61). Because of patchy diffuse hypo-intense infiltration of the kidney on T_2- and T_1-weighted images, it is often not possible to visualize the physiologic border between renal cortex and medulla. Contrast administration generally shows decreased contrast uptake of the tumor. Nevertheless, in the equilibrium phase, homogeneous enhancement may be seen.

In summary, MRI is the imaging modality of choice for the diagnosis of kidney tumors. Lesion morphology, both in regard to tissue consistency and lesion growth pattern, is clearly seen. Unfortunately, the macroscopic appearance of lesions does not correlate well with their pathologic classification. That is why correlation between MRI findings and pathologic classification is difficult and requires much experience. It is important also to recognize that some tumors may have many different morphologic appearances. It bears repeating that RCC accounts for almost 90% of all malignant kidney tumors

border, and only a few are characterized by a slightly invasive growth. Because of its expansile character, nephroblastomatosis is often combined with a grossly dilated renal pelvis. The key to diagnosis is the more

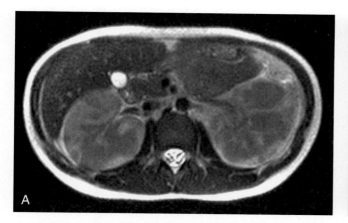

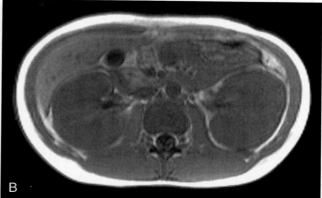

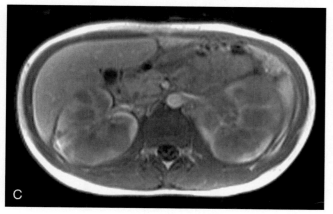

FIGURE 11–61. Diffuse leukemic infiltration of the kidney in a 6-year old boy with newly diagnosed acute lymphatic leukemia. T₂-weighted (*A*) and T₁-weighted (*B*) images show generalized enlargement of both kidneys with loss of the corticomedullary junction. *C,* After contrast injection, early T₁-weighted dynamic imaging depicts the leukemic infiltration as focal areas of hypointensity, whereas the residual parenchyma shows strong enhancement.

in adults and presents as a chameleon that may mimic many other benign and malignant conditions. It may appear uniloculated or unilateral/bilateral and multiloculated. It may have solid or cystic components or a combination. In regard to growth patterns, RCC can be infiltrative or expansile. Furthermore, areas of fatty degeneration may be found. Because of the high prevalence of RCC and its mimicking character, this diagnosis should always be considered in the differential diagnosis of kidney tumors.

Imaging in Renal Transplantation

In renal transplantation, the differentiation of acute tubular necrosis from rejection is critical. Basic knowledge of the appearance of a normal kidney is necessary to appreciate the changes in failing transplants. Healthy transplants should have the same signal characteristics as normal kidneys. On T_1-weighted images, the renal cortex should be of intermediate signal intensity, differentiating it from the triangle-shaped areas of lower intensity representing the medullary pyramids. In most normal kidneys, the corticomedullary junction is visible. The loss of corticomedullary differentiation on T_1-weighted images is the most consistent finding in acute or chronic renal transplant rejection, but the loss of corticomedullary differentiation is not specific for rejection. Relative or complete loss of corticomedullary differentiation may occur in hydronephrosis, glomerulonephritis, nonspecific renal failure, renal artery stenosis, pyelonephritis, and infiltrative tumor. Various degrees of loss of corticomedullary differentiation can also be seen in acute tubular necrosis. Cyclosporine toxicity has not been definitely associated with this finding. Perinephric fluid collections, such as postoperative urinomas, seromas, and lymphoceles, are typically depicted with a low intensity on T_1-weighted sequences and intermediate or high signal intensity on T_2-weighted images. This appearance is similar to other simple fluids. A perinephric abscess is typically heterogeneous and higher in intensity than other fluid collections on T_2-weighted images. Another common finding is gas formation within the abscess and secondary changes in the adjacent kidney, which are best demonstrated on Gd-enhanced images. Hematoma characteristics on MRI vary with age. Chronic hematomas have low signal intensity on T_1-weighted sequences and low to intermediate signal intensity on T_2-weighted images, sometimes similar to seromas, urinomas, and lymphoceles. Acute hematomas can be homogeneous in appearance and of intermediate to high signal intensity on T_1-weighted sequences and lower signal intensity on T_2-weighted images. In subacute hematomas, different components may be visible, with a central, low-intensity area surrounded by a high signal intensity rim on T_1-weighted images. Thus, in the early postoperative period, in most cases, MRI is able to differentiate hematomas from other fluid collections. Imaging after contrast administration allows evaluation of the perfusion of renal transplants and implementation of contrast-enhanced MRA makes possible the evaluation of transplant arteries.

Pelvis

12

Günther Schneider

Pelvic anatomy is ideal for magnetic resonance imaging (MRI) assessment because image quality is usually not degraded by respiration. On T_1-weighted images, the pelvic organs are highlighted by surrounding extraperitoneal fat. On T_2-weighted images, in particular, the internal architecture of the organs (e.g., the uterus) is depicted as the consequence of the superb tissue contrast provided by MRI. For imaging of the pelvis successful MRI examination requires careful preparation of the patient. However, imaging in general is not as difficult as in the upper abdomen.

Although respiratory motion and bowel motion are minimal when imaging the pelvis, they will degrade image quality if precautions are not taken. To minimize bowel motion, the patient should fast or have clear liquids at least 4 to 6 hours before MRI examination of the pelvis. In addition, intramuscular administration of 1 mg glucagon should be performed immediately before imaging to decrease bowel motion if no medical contraindication is present. Ideally, the bladder should be only moderately distended and the patient should not drink water immediately before the study.

Opacification of the small bowel and the colon is not routinely performed for MRI of the pelvis. Sometimes the bowel may account for errors in interpreting images of the pelvis by mistaking an unopacified bowel loop for a mass, lymph node, or abscess. Thus, in certain circumstances, when ovarian or bowel abnormality is suspected, oral contrast should be given. In Europe, a formulation of gadolinium (Gd)-DTPA for oral administration is approved and used in routine clinical practice. No such approval or specific formulation for oral use exists in the United States. Administration of this oral formulation results in high signal intensity of the bowel lumen. Typically, the patient should drink the Gd-DTPA solution approximately 1 to 2 hours before the examination.

Imaging sequences should include both T_1- and T_2-weighted multiplanar spin echo images, which are essential for imaging of the pelvis. On T_1-weighted images, there is good contrast between pelvic fat and the normal pelvic organs, so infiltration of fat planes and adjacent organs by certain diseases such as cervical carcinoma can be readily identified. T_2-weighted images are essential for evaluating internal organ morphology (e.g., the zonal anatomy of the uterus). T_2-weighted images should be acquired in at least two imaging planes with either con-

ventional or fast spin echo sequences. Chemical shift imaging with fat- or water-suppression techniques is useful to differentiate between lipid- and blood-containing lesions that have high signal intensity on T_1-weighted images and that are isointense to fat on T_2-weighted images. This is of importance in, for example, identifying mature teratomas, which typically contain fat, and detecting endometriosis. In endometriosis, the high signal intensity on T_1-weighted images caused by subacute hemorrhage cannot be suppressed on T_1-weighted fast spin images. To achieve high resolution in imaging of the pelvis, a dedicated phased-array coil should be used, which makes it possible to detect even small tumors and subtle invasion by malignancies (e.g., in bladder cancer).

Intravenous contrast administration, employing a Gd chelate, is useful in imaging the pelvis in some clinical situations. Contrast-enhanced images have been demonstrated to be useful in the evaluation of the internal architecture of pelvic masses, particular in differentiation between clot and debris from solid components (e.g., in endometrial or cervical carcinoma).

In our standard protocol, we perform imaging of the pelvis with 5- to 6-mm-thick sections and a gap of 1.5 mm. First, a sagittal T_2-weighted sequence is acquired followed by axial T_1- and T_2-weighted sequences. If a high-signal-intensity lesion is detected on T_1-weighted images, additional fat-suppression or water-suppression sequences, or a combination, are performed covering the detected lesion. Images in the coronal plane are complementary in the evaluation of the uterus and the vagina. They should be used as an adjunct in assessment of uterine morphology, the parametrium, and the levator ani muscle, and they offer the opportunity to identify lymphadenopathy. In special cases (e.g., a leiomyoma of the uterus), off-axis images should also be obtained. In evaluation of the uterus, these are typically images perpendicular to the long axis of the uterine cavity to allow accurate evaluation of intramural versus submucosal localization of a leiomyoma in a planned surgical resection. The same is true for evaluation of the depth of infiltration in endometrial carcinoma.

BLADDER

Most bladder tumors are malignant. Approximately 90% of bladder carcinomas are of transitional cell types; adenocarcinomas make up less than 5% of malignant neoplasms and squamous cell carcinomas less than 10%. Bladder carcinomas may have a papillary, infiltrative, or mixed pattern of growth.

Bladder carcinoma is the fourth most common cancer in men and accounts for 5% and 3% of all cancer deaths in men and women, respectively. Both prognosis and treatment depend on the stage of the tumor. Clinical staging of bladder carcinoma includes cystoscopy and biopsy with supplementary evaluation under anesthesia and intravenous urography.

Although cross-sectional imaging techniques play an important role in the evaluation of other major viscera of the genitourinary systems, they have been less critical in the assessment of the urinary bladder. MRI examinations in patients with bladder carcinoma are indicated only after clinical, conventional radiographic, and endoscopic studies that have yielded provisional diagnoses. MRI is mainly used to provide multiplanar delineation of complex anatomy and to document the extent of luminal, mural, and perivesical disease. MRI is appropriate for the anatomic staging of previously detected and diagnosed bladder neoplasm, for planning of radiation therapy, and for evaluating therapeutic response.

The normal urinary bladder is clearly delineated on MR images. On T_1-weighted images, the bladder is seen as a low-signal-intensity, variably ovoid structure. Its margins are well defined because of the contrast between low-signal-intensity urine and muscular bladder wall, and adjacent high-signal-intensity perivesical fat is marked. On T_2-weighted images, the intravesical urine shows a very high signal intensity, whereas the bladder wall shows a rather low signal intensity. The thickness of the bladder wall varies with the degree of bladder distension. When the bladder is fully distended, the wall should not exceed 5 mm in thickness. The signal intensity of the perivesical fat should be relatively homogeneous on both T_1- and T_2-weighted sequences. The lateral margins of the urinary bladder are best defined in transverse and coronal plane images; the bladder dome and the bladder neck are optimally delineated in sagittal and coronal plane images. T_2-weighted images are typically used to evaluate the integrity of the bladder wall. In this context, it is important to realize that visualization of the bladder wall is often affected by chemical shift artifacts in the direction of the frequency-encoding gradient. This artifact can cause one margin of the bladder to appear thinned and obscured, whereas the opposite margin will appear thickened. For example, if the frequency-encoding direction in a particular image is from the patient's left to right, the chemical shift misregistration is seen as a low-intensity band on the left side of the bladder and a symmetric, high-intensity band on the right side, which leads to the just-mentioned observation.

Bladder Carcinoma

On T_2-weighted images, transitional cell carcinoma tends to have intermediate to high signal intensity that is typically greater than the normal detrusor muscle (Fig. 12-1). On precontrast T_1-weighted images, the bladder wall and tumor have similar low to intermediate signal intensity and cannot be adequately differentiated. On T_2-weighted images, the preservation of the low-signal-intensity bladder wall at the center of the tumor suggests that the tumor is stage I or less. In certain cases, Gd enhancement can improve the accuracy of staging of bladder cancer. Applying fat-suppressed T_1-weighted sequences postcontrast is, for example, beneficial in detecting perivesical fat invasion. Perivesical tumor extension is less conspicuous on T_2-weighted images unless fat saturation is used. Tumor extension into the pelvic side wall musculature is most readily demonstrated on T_2-weighted images in which medium- to high-signal-intensity tumor will alter the normal low signal intensity of striated muscle. Lymph node enlargements are most easily detected on T_1-weighted images; lymph nodes larger than 10 mm are considered pathologic. These size criteria actually are used alone to determine the presence or absence of lymph node disease. In general, MRI is capable of distinguishing superficial from deeply invasive lesions. However, MRI cannot reliably document microscopic invasion of superficial bladder cancer. If segmental cystectomy is planned to provide control of pelvic disease while maintaining continence, contraindications such as extravesical tumor growth, invasion of the bladder neck, and invasion of the ureter can be depicted on MRI. Multiplanar MR images allow a better anatomic evaluation compared with computed tomography (CT), particularly when tumors involve the bladder dome, base, or bladder neck. In other locations, MRI is approximately equal to staging by conventional CT.

Other bladder diseases that can be evaluated by MRI include bladder diverticula, urachal anomalies that include cysts, diverticula, sinuses, and persistent patency as well as inflammatory disease of the urinary bladder.

Mesenchymal neoplasms of the urinary bladder are sarcomas that arise from the bladder wall, which have to be considered in particular with masses detected in children (Fig. 12-2). In general, sarcomas arising from the urinary bladder are indistinguishable from transitional cell carcinoma. However, these tumors are more often bulky and extensive at diagnosis.

In summary, MRI is considered as an adjuvant method of evaluating bladder disease and frequently is used to evaluate the extent of diseases previously detected and diagnosed by endoscopic methods or conventional radiographic studies. The major strength of MRI in evaluating the complex anatomic relationships of the pelvic viscera lies in its multiplanar capability and its high soft tissue contrast resolution.

FEMALE PELVIS

Primary gynecologic examination and evaluation of pelvic complaints are traditionally based on clinical symptoms, inspection, palpation, biopsy, and clinical as well as laboratory parameters. Ultrasonography still is the primary imaging modality for the evaluation of the female pelvis, representing the most important routine screening method in obstetric and gynecologic disorders. However, sonography is not suitable for one of the largest potential clinical applications: the staging of gynecologic tumors. In recent years, MRI has added a

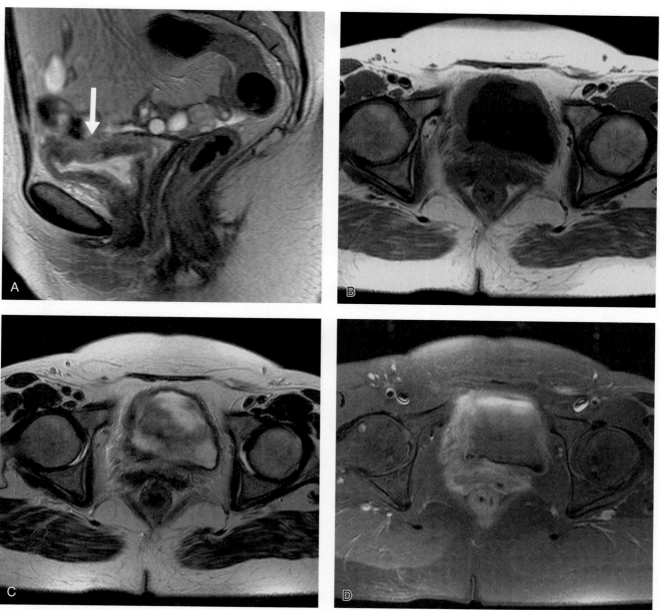

Figure 12–1. Bladder carcinoma in a 74-year-old woman with dysuria and hematuria. *A,* On the T$_2$-weighted sagittal image thickening of the posterior bladder wall by an intermediate signal-intensity mass is demonstrated. The normal low signal intensity of the detrusor muscle in this area (*arrow*) is not preserved, indicating muscle invasion. On axial T$_1$- (*B*) and T$_2$-weighted (*C*) images, bladder wall thickening of the right lateral aspect without infiltration of the tumor into the surrounding pelvic fat is seen. *D,* After contrast administration, strong enhancement of this area on the T$_1$-weighted fat-suppressed image is visible. However, as a result of contrast in the bladder, diagnostic information is reduced.

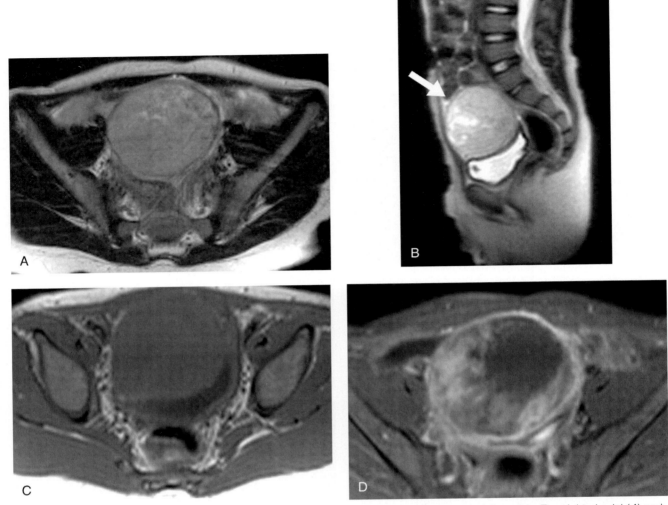

FIGURE 12–2. Rhabdomyosarcoma of the bladder wall in a 4-year-old boy with a palpable tumor of the pelvis. T_2-weighted axial (*A*) and sagittal (*B*) images show a large inhomogeneous hyperintense mass located cranially to the bladder (*arrow*). *C,* On axial T_1-weighted imaging the mass cannot be separated from the bladder wall. There is strong contrast uptake of the more peripheral areas on the T_1-weighted fat-suppressed contrast-enhanced image (*D*), with a large area of central necrosis.

new dimension to the evaluation of pelvic disorders, including the diagnosis, staging, preoperative planning, and follow-up of almost all gynecologic entities.

Multiple studies have shown the high accuracy of MRI for imaging of gynecologic abnormalities, thus becoming the imaging procedure of choice if available, complementing or even replacing sonography and CT. In particular, when sonography can only inadequately characterize pelvic abnormalities or if exact pretherapeutic staging is necessary, MRI has been shown to have high accuracy and diagnostic reliability. MRI is routinely used for staging of endometrial and cervical cancer and for follow-up examinations of both entities during and after therapy. MRI is also used to evaluate the origin and extension of adnexal masses if ultrasonography does not provide sufficient diagnostic information. MRI is also used in examinations of children and pregnant patients and for the detection and classification of congenital malformations. The advantages of multiplanar imaging are especially evident in demarcation and differentiation of gynecologic disorders relative to other

pelvic benign and malignant diseases (e.g., vesical and colorectal tumors).

Uterus

The normal uterus on a T_1-weighted image is seen as a homogeneous, medium-signal-intensity structure, with relatively indistinct uterine zonal anatomy. On the T_2-weighted image, the anatomic uterine division into corpus, isthmus, and cervix is readily delineated. On T_2-weighted sequences, the components of the corpus, myometrium, and endometrium are imaged with different signal intensities separated by the junctional zone, a low-signal-intensity line between them. The junctional zone is thought to represent vascular structures, mainly veins located within the inner third of the myometrium as well as compressed myometrium. The low-intensity line is seen on in vivo imaging of the normal menstruating uterus but is not seen or is indistinct on in vitro imaging as well as in histologic studies.

The uterine appearance on MRI varies with hormonal

stimuli. Reproductive-age females have reproducible changes in uterine appearance during their menstrual cycles. The endometrial width changes during the menstrual cycle and is seen at its largest dimension during the midsecretory phase. The volume and signal intensity of the myometrium also varies. During the secretory phase, the myometrium signal intensity is greatest, as seen on T$_2$-weighted scans. During the secretory phase, the total uterine volume changes to the greatest extent. Females of reproductive age taking oral contraceptives have a different uterine appearance. The separation between the myometrium and endometrium becomes indistinct, and endometrial atrophy is observed with inconsistent demonstration of the junctional zone.

MRIs of a premenarchal or postmenarchal uterus differ from the appearance of a reproductive-age uterus. The former uteri are small, and there is absent or atrophic cyclic endometrium. The length of the corpus uteri equals that of the cervix. The uterus of postmenopausal women on exogenous estrogens or with an estro-gen-producing ovarian malignancy appears similar to the uterus of reproductive-age women.

Congenital Anomalies of the Uterus

With an incidence of 0.1% to 0.5%, clinically significant congenital uterine abnormalities are unusual. The two major categories of congenital abnormalities are atresia or aplasia of the uterus and vagina and anomalies in development of the müllerian ducts.

Before the introduction of MRI, laparoscopy and hysteroscopy were often necessary for diagnostic evaluation because assessment with physical examination and imaging studies, including sonography, was often inconclusive. MRI has been shown to be an accurate, noninvasive method for the evaluation of congenital anomalies of the uterus and vagina.

Müllerian duct anomalies result from nondevelopment or partial or complete nonfusion of the müllerian ducts (Fig. 12-3). They are found in up to 15% of

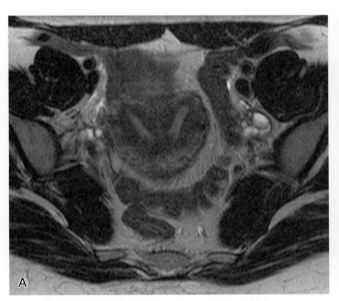

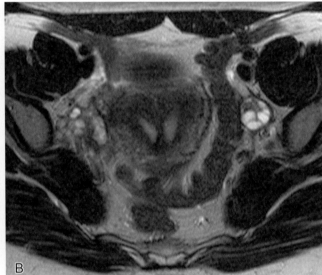

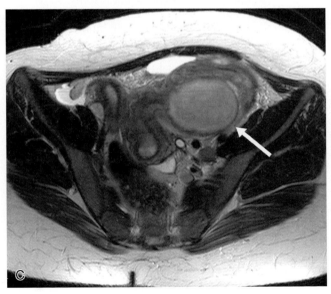

FIGURE 12–3. Uterus bicornis and uterus didelphys. *A* and *B*, Axial T$_2$-weighted images in uterus bicornis demonstrate a partially doubled uterine fundus, whereas in a uterus didelphys there are two separate uterine fundi, which lie apart from each other in different directions (*C*). Note as well the focus of endometriosis in the left ovary (*arrow*).

women. They are clinically associated with an increased incidence of impaired fertility and menstrual disorders. Müllerian duct anomalies may be associated with renal anomalies such as ipsilateral renal agenesis or ectopia. One of the most widely accepted morphologic classifications of müllerian duct anomalies was proposed by Buttram and Gibbons in 1979 and was modified by the American Society for Reproductive Medicine. The anomalies are classified by the number and configuration of the uterine elements (Fig. 12-4).

Uterine segmental agenesis or hypoplasia (class I) results from nondevelopment or partial development of the müllerian ducts. It may include varying degrees of uterine body, cervical, vaginal, and tubal hypoplasia. In the case of functioning endometrium, hematocolpos or endometriosis may be the cause of clinical symptoms. Unicornuate uterus (class II) results from hypoplasia or agenesis of one of the paired müllerian ducts. Uterus didelphys (class III) results from lack of fusion of the müllerian ducts, with the development of two normal-sized uteri and cervices and sometimes an upper vaginal septum. Bicornuate uterus (class IV) results from partial failure of müllerian duct fusion, in which the resulting septum is composed of myometrium. The patients may present with repeated spontaneous abortions, premature rupture of the membranes, and malpresentations. Septate uterus (class V) results from failure of resorption of the fibrous septum between the components of the müllerian ducts and has the highest rate of associated reproductive dysfunction.

Uterine Tumors

Leiomyoma is the most common solid uterine neoplasm, occurring in 20% to 40% of all females of reproductive age (Fig. 12-5). These tumors are benign and are composed predominantly of smooth muscle with varying amounts of fibrous connective tissue. They are usually well circumscribed and surrounded by a pseudocapsule. Myomas may be solitary (Fig. 12-6) or multiple (Fig. 12-7) and may occur in submucosal (Fig. 12-8), intramural, and subserosal locations of the myometrium. Although most myomas involve the body or fundus of the uterus, some occur in the cervix or even the broad ligament. The clinical presentation of uterine leiomyomas varies depending on the size, number, and location of lesions. Most patients have few or no symptoms, and the myoma is detected incidentally on physical examination as an enlargement of the uterus or on imaging examination. Patients with symptoms typically present with hypermenorrhea or other forms of dysfunctional uterine bleeding. Other symptoms include pelvic pain, infertility, recurrent spontaneous abortions, preterm labor, and in utero growth retardation. If large enough, a leiomyoma can produce symptoms as a result of compression of the adjacent organs, such as the urinary bladder, rectum, or distal ureters. Because these tumors are estrogen dependent, they may grow rapidly during pregnancy and usually regress after menopause. During menopause they may be calcified. Sudden growth of a leiomyoma in postmenopausal women not on exogenous estrogens indicates malignant transformation into a leiomyosarcoma.

There is a variable MRI appearance of leiomyoma within the uterus that depends on the presence or absence of hyaline, mucinous, myxomatous (Fig. 12-9), cystic, and fatty degeneration and on calcification. MRI can provide accurate assessment of the number, size, and precise location of leiomyomas, particularly in patients with planned surgical excision.

The optimal imaging technique for the diagnosis of intramural and submucosal leiomyomas is a T_2-weighted sequence in which nondegenerative leiomyomas are displayed with a low signal intensity (see Fig. 12-8). On T_1-weighted images, leiomyomas have intermediate signal intensity; thus, they are often indistinguishable from surrounding myometrium. However, it is important to obtain both T_1- and T_2-weighted sequences for tissue characterization of a myoma or other abnormality within the uterus. Chemical shift imaging may be useful to evaluate fatty degeneration or hemorrhage within large leiomyoma.

Adenomyosis is another benign entity within the uterus, defined as the presence of heterotopic endometrium located within the myometrium. Adenomyosis is most likely the result of direct invasion of the basal endometrium into the myometrium and may be microscopic, focal, or diffuse. These foci are surrounded by smooth muscle proliferation. Adenomyosis is found in up to 20% of hysterectomy specimens. Most symptomatic women present in the fourth or fifth decades of life, and the incidence is increased in multiparous women. Clinical presentation is similar to that of leiomyomas: hypermenorrhea, dysmenorrhea, pelvic pain, and infertility. The clinical distinction between adenomyosis and leiomyoma can be difficult because both may demonstrate increased size of the uterus on physical examination. This can be even more complicated by the occasional coexistence of adenomyosis and leiomyomas. Leiomyomas can be treated by selective myomectomy, whereas symptomatic adenomyosis often requires hysterectomy for definitive therapy. Medical treatment, including hormonal therapy with gonadotropin-releasing hormone (GnRH) analogues, is evolving for both conditions.

On T_2-weighted images, diffuse adenomyosis is seen as a wide low-signal-intensity band with an uneven distribution that surrounds the normal high-signal-intensity endometrium, producing a diffuse thickening of the junctional zone (Fig. 12-10). In the case of focal adenomyosis, an ill-defined, poorly marginated mass can be observed within the myometrium with low signal intensity on T_2-weighted images. In most cases, the mass is contiguous with the junctional zone, and, in contrast to the usually rounded shape of leiomyoma, focal adenomyosis shows a more oval shape. On T_1-weighted images, focal adenomyosis blends with the surrounding myometrium.

The hallmark of adenomyosis is the ill-defined border of the lesion because, in contrast to leiomyoma, which presents with a pseudocapsule of compressed myometrium, adenomyosis typically shows a more infiltrative-appearing growth pattern. Small foci of adenomyosis may simulate a leiomyoma because the pseudocapsule and the well-defined borders of leiomyoma may not be

Text continued on page 363

Uterus				Vagina	
Didelphian uterus	**Bicornuate uterus**	**Septated uterus**	**Uterine aplasia**	**Hematocolpos**	**Gartner's duct cyst**
(two uterine horns, two uterine bodies, two uterine cervices, two vaginas)	(two uterine horns, single uterine body and cervix)	(uterine horns not duplicated, duplicated uterine cavity)	(absence of uterus, associated with vaginal atresia and stenosis)	(accumulation of fluid within the vagina due to imperforated hymen or vaginal membrane)	(wolffian duct remnant; single or multiple cysts along the lateral or anterolateral wall of the vagina)

FIGURE 12–4. Congenital abnormalities of the female genitourinary tract. Uterine malformations are often associated with renal abnormalities (particularly renal agenesis) and vice versa (see Gartner's duct cyst).

Solid uterine masses	"Complex" uterine masses	Cystic uterine masses	Vaginal masses
Benign	**Benign**	**Benign**	**Benign**
Adenomyosis	Missed abortion	Hydrohematometra	Hematocolpos
Endometrial hyperplasia	Endometritis (pyometra)	Nabothian cysts	Gartner's duct cyst
Leiomyoma	Hydatidiform mole	Pyometra	Bartholin's cyst
Endometrial polyps		Intrauterine pregnancy	Rare: vaginal neurofibromas
			Extravaginal masses
			such as cervical fibroid
Malignant	**Malignant**		**Malignant**
Cervical carcinoma	Choriocarcinoma		Carcinoma of the vagina
Endometrial carcinoma	Hydatidiform mole		Extravaginal masses
Leiomyosarcoma			such as cervical cancer

FIGURE 12–5. Magnetic resonance imaging classification of uterine and vaginal masses.

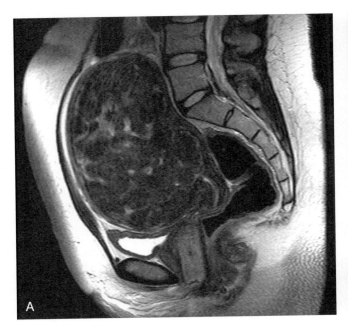

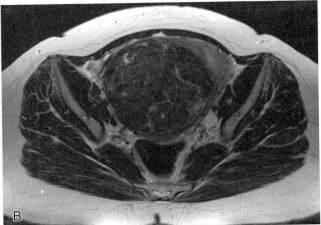

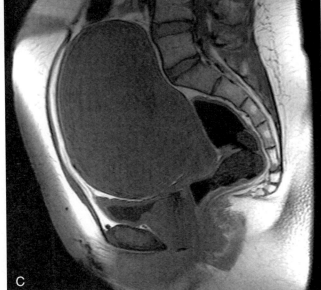

FIGURE 12–6. Large leiomyoma of the uterus with partial cystic degeneration in a 37-year-old nulliparous women. A large pelvic mass was detected ultrasonographically. On T$_2$-weighted sagittal (*A*) and axial (*B*) images, a large, mainly hypointense mass with small cystic areas is demonstrated consistent with a large leiomyoma with cystic degeneration. *C*, However, on the T$_1$-weighted unenhanced image, the tumor is almost isointense to normal uterine parenchyma, and internal morphology is not evaluable.

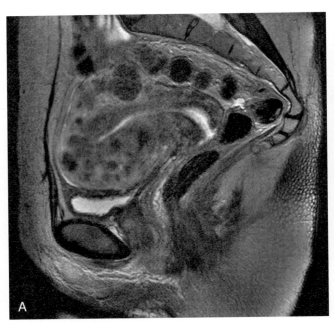

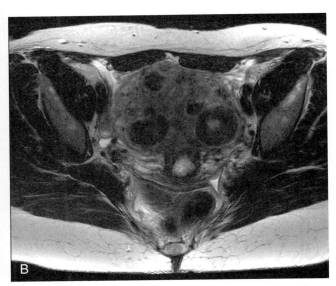

FIGURE 12–7. Uterus myomatosus in a 40-year-old woman. *A*, Sagittal T$_2$-weighted imaging shows a significantly enlarged uterus with multiple myometrial leiomyomas. Some of the larger tumors have central areas of high signal consistent with cystic degeneration, which is better visible on T$_2$-weighted axial imaging (*B*).

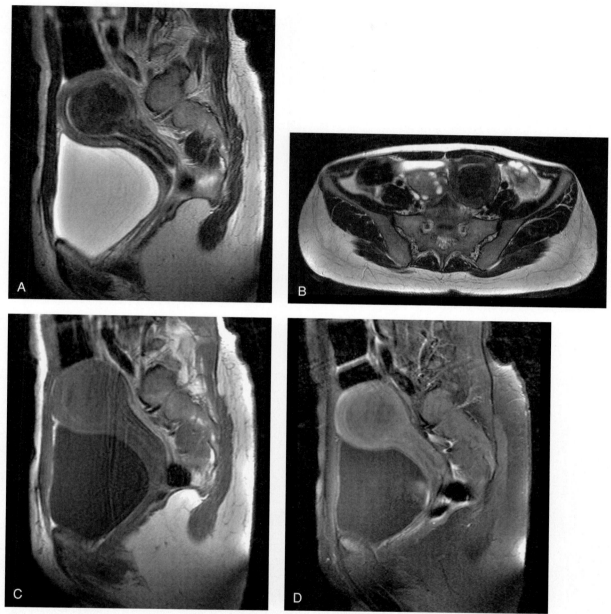

Figure 12–8. Submucosal leiomyoma in a 34-year-old woman with recurrent habitual abortions. *A,* A sagittal T$_2$-weighted image shows a large low-signal-intensity (SI) mass protruding into the cavum uteri with depiction of high SI endometrium just at the surface of the tumor. *B,* This submucosal localization is also confirmed on axial T$_2$-weighted imaging. Note as well the right-sided ovarian cysts. *C,* The lesion has a slightly lower SI on T$_1$-weighted imaging compared with surrounding myometrium and is hypointense on the T$_1$-weighted fat-saturated image after contrast administration (*D*).

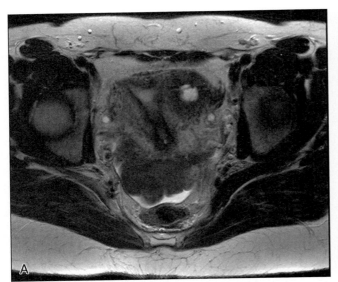
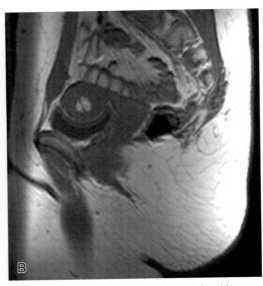

Figure 12–9. Leiomyoma with hyaline and myxomatous degeneration in a 42-year-old woman. *A,* On an axial T₂-weighted image, a left-sided mass arising from the myometrium of the uterine fundus is demonstrated. The lesion shows central high signal intensity (SI) surrounded by a low SI stroma. *B,* On T₁-weighted unenhanced sagittal imaging, the central areas of the tumor also display high SI consistent with tissue that shows a high protein content.

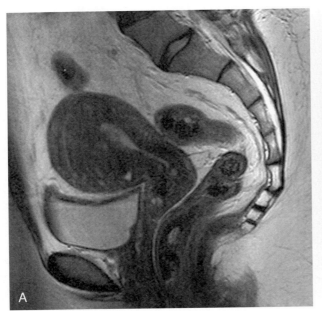
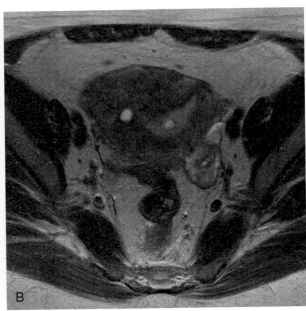

Figure 12–10. Adenomyosis in a 38-year-old woman with menorrhagia. *A,* The T₂-weighted sagittal image shows a diffuse, irregular thickening of the junctional zone. *B,* ill-defined borders are also displayed in the axial image. Note some small hyperintense cystic areas within the low-signal-intensity lesion.

so obvious in small lesions. Sometimes small areas of high signal intensity on T_2- and T_1-weighted images may be observed in adenomyosis that correspond to small foci of hemorrhage. If these small foci are only observed on T_2-weighted images, they are thought to represent endometrial tissue.

Endometrial carcinoma is the most common invasive carcinoma of the female genital tract, usually occurring in postmenopausal women. The development of endometrial carcinoma is promoted by unopposed estrogen stimulation. Histologically, 80% are endometrioid adenocarcinomas. Other histologic types include papillary serous, mucinous, and clear cell adenocarcinomas. Sarcomas and carcinosarcomas (malignant mixed müllerian tumors) also occur but are rare. Endometrial carcinoma tends to grow within the endometrial cavity as either a localized polypoid or exophytic mass or as a diffuse tumor involving the entire endometrial surface. Invasion through the myometrium or into the endocervical canal or cervical stroma may occur. Metastases to the adnexa or vagina are common. Lymphatic invasion produces spread to the pelvic, periaortic, and aortocaval lymph nodes. Positive peritoneal cytologic results are far more common than gross peritoneal spread. Distant metastases occur most often in the peritoneum, lung, liver, and supraclavicular lymph nodes. Sometimes there is coexisting ovarian carcinoma.

Most patients present in the early stages of the disease with postmenopausal bleeding. Prognosis of endometrial carcinoma and the choice of therapy are mainly influenced by the clinical stage of the tumor, depth of the myometrial invasion, histologic grade of the tumor, and presence of lymph node metastases at diagnosis. Patients with deep myometrial invasion (>50% of myometrial thickness) are at high risk for lymph node metastasis. In these patients, more extensive para-aortic lymph node sampling should be planned for during surgery.

On MRI, endometrial carcinoma is seen as an abnormality within the central endometrial cavity. On T_2-weighted MRI images, the signal intensity of small endometrial cancers is similar to that of normal endometrium (Fig. 12-11). Indirect signs that can be observed in the presence of endometrial cancer include increased thickening or lobulation of the endometrial cavity. The postmenopausal uterus usually shows a central canal of high signal intensity approximately 3 to 5 mm wide on T_2-weighted images. With endometrial carcinoma, the central high-signal-intensity endometrium is routinely wider (Fig. 12-12). Another important finding is disruption of the junctional zone between the myometrium and endometrium, which can be an important indicator of myometrial invasion (Fig. 12-13). In patients with endometrial carcinoma, visualization of the junctional zone indicates that the tumor is still confined to the endometrium. However, nonvisualization of the junctional zone does not necessarily indicate invasion, because occasionally the junctional zone is absent in normal postmenopausal women.

There is a variable appearance of endometrial carcinoma on MRI. There may be increased size of the high-signal-intensity endometrial cavity without evidence of medium-intensity masses within the cavity on T_2-weighted sequences. Often larger tumors are displayed as a heterogeneous high-signal-intensity mass on T_2-weighted images with overall lower signal intensity compared with normal endometrium. In other patients, there may be high signal intensity or medium signal intensity on a T_1-weighted sequence, but on the T_2-weighted sequence the tumor may blend with the surrounding high-signal-intensity endometrium. However, similar changes may be observed in submucosal degenerating leiomyoma, adenomatous hyperplasia, or endometrial polyps, so histologic diagnosis remains essential. The use of Gd chelates on contrast-enhanced T_1-weighted images may be beneficial to differentiate tumor from necrosis or fluid (e.g., hematometra or pyometra), which leads to an overall improvement in staging accuracy.

Malignant mesenchymal tumors of the uterus account for less than 5% of malignancies. The three most common histologic types are malignant mixed müllerian tumor, leiomyosarcoma, and endometrial stromal sarcoma. Malignant müllerian mixed sarcoma is believed to be derived from pluripotential müllerian tissue and exhibits differentiation toward endometrial (adenocarcinoma) and mesodermal (sarcomatous) cells. Malignant müllerian mixed sarcomas of the uterus arise similar to endometrial carcinoma, typically in postmenopausal women, and are frequently associated with a history of irradiation. Lymphatic and myometrial invasion occur in more than 80%. On MRI the tumor is typically seen as a large polypoid mass arising from the endometrial cavity.

Leiomyosarcomas arise from the myometrium and usually occur in perimenopausal women between 40 and 60 years old. Rapid enlargement of a leiomyoma or the uterus, especially in postmenopausal women, should raise concern. On MRI a heterogeneous myometrial mass with indistinct borders may be observed. Differential diagnosis mainly includes degenerative leiomyoma.

Cervix

The normal cervix is best delineated on T_2-weighted sequences and has at least two separate zones. The central zone is imaged with high signal intensity and presumably represents the cervical epithelium and mucus. The central canal is surrounded by a discrete region of low signal intensity, presumably representing the fibrous cervical stroma. Occasionally, a third narrow band of medium signal intensity is seen peripheral to the low-signal-intensity band and is very similar to the intensity of the myometrium of the uterus. The parametrium is seen as low or medium intensity, flanking the cervix on T_1-weighted images, and is separate from the low-intensity cervical stroma on both T_1- and T_2-weighted sequences. On T_2-weighted sequences, there is a relative increase in signal intensity of the parametrium, often blending with surrounding fat.

Benign cervical masses occasionally seen on MRI include the common small nabothian cysts. Rare lesions involving the cervix include leiomyomas, endometriomas, cervical mucoceles, Gartner's duct cysts, cervical pregnancy, and cervical stenosis, which may present as masses and have a variable appearance on MRI de-

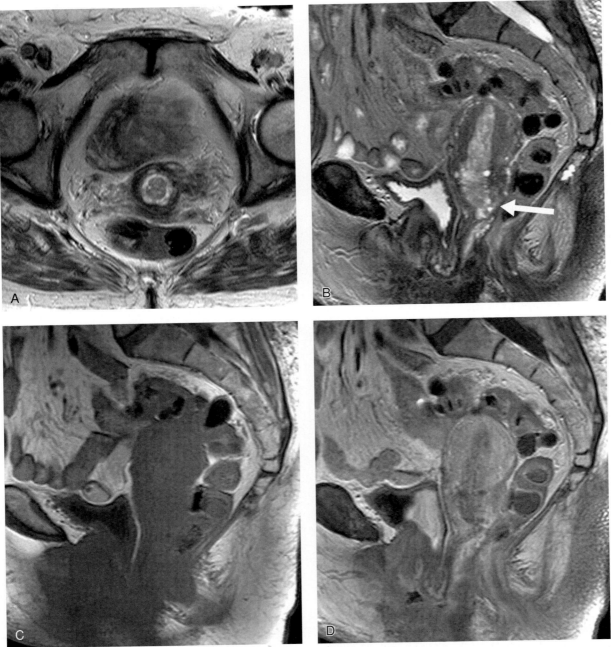

FIGURE 12–11. Endometrial carcinoma (stage IIB) in a 68-year-old woman with recurrent vaginal bleeding. *A* and *B,* On T$_2$-weighted axial and sagittal images, a significant increase in the thickness of the endometrium can be demonstrated, which cannot be visualized on the T$_1$-weighted unenhanced image (*C*). The tumor invades the cervix, prolapsing into the upper vagina (*arrow*). After contrast administration, the tumor is depicted as an area of lower signal intensity compared with the myometrium (*D*), and no fluid retention within the uterine fundus is visible.

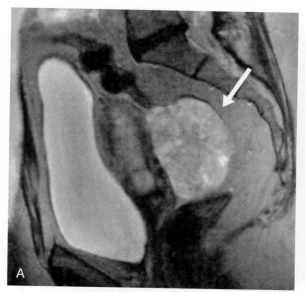
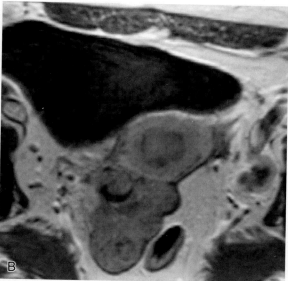

FIGURE 12–12. Endometrioid carcinoma of the ovary associated with endometrial carcinoma in a 72-year-old woman. *A,* The sagittal T$_2$-weighted image shows thickening of the endometrium consistent with stage IIA endometrial cancer with infiltration of the cervix. A large mass with inhomogeneous high signal is also noted dorsal to the uterus (*arrow*) originating from the ovary. *B,* On T$_1$-weighted contrast-enhanced imaging, the solid mass dorsal to the uterus has inhomogeneous contrast uptake, whereas the endometrial carcinoma is hypointense compared with the myometrium, with an infiltration depth less than 50% of the myometrial thickness.

pending on the relative composition (e.g., cystic, solid, or hemorrhagic components).

Cervical carcinoma is the third most common gynecologic malignancy and the most common malignancy in women younger than 50 years. It is second to ovarian

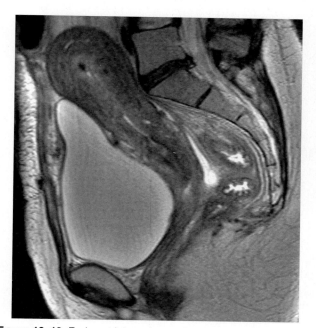

FIGURE 12–13. Endometrial carcinoma (stage IB) in a 45-year-old woman. The patient's histologically proven endometrial cancer was staged before surgery. A sagittal T$_2$-weighted image shows a more discrete thickening of the endometrial layer with slightly increased uterine fluid accumulation. An infiltration of the myometrium of less than 50% of the myometrial thickness is visible. The junctional zone is not depicted because of infiltration of the myometrium by the tumor.

carcinoma in mortality. Invasive cervical cancer is thought to develop over time from a noninvasive precursor lesion to a cervical intraepithelial neoplasia. Seventy-five to 85% of cervical carcinomas histologically are squamous-epithelial carcinoma; the remainder are adenocarcinoma (10%-15%) or adenosquamous carcinomas (2%-5%). Cervical carcinoma commonly arises at the squamocolumnar junction, which marks the junction between the endo- and ectocervix. Patients usually present with vaginal bleeding or discharge; however, this clinical presentation often already represents advanced disease. Cervical carcinoma spreads by invading through the cervical stroma and into the upper vagina, parametria, or myometrium. Extension into the lymphatic channels of the parametria produces nodal spread along the obturator, iliac, and para-aortic nodal chains. Direct invasion of adjacent structures, including the bladder (Fig. 12-14), ureters, sigmoid colon, and pelvic side wall, may be present. Prognosis and initial choice of therapy depend on the size and stage of tumor at presentation, its histologic grade, depth of stromal invasion, adjacent tissue extension, and presence of lymph node metastases.

Because of increased soft tissue contrast, MRI surpassed CT in the evaluation of cervical carcinomas and has been shown to be an excellent modality for staging cervical cancer. T$_2$-weighted sequences demonstrate the neoplasm as an abnormal area of high signal intensity, distinct from the normal lower-signal-intensity cervical stroma (see Fig. 12-14). MRI may be used for assessing tumor volume and extent within the cervical stroma, into the parametrium, and into the vagina. On T$_1$-weighted images, the tumor within the cervical stroma may not be differentiated from the stroma, but tumor extension into the parametrium may be better appreciated because of the tumor's slightly higher signal intensity than the parametrium. On T$_2$-weighted sequences,

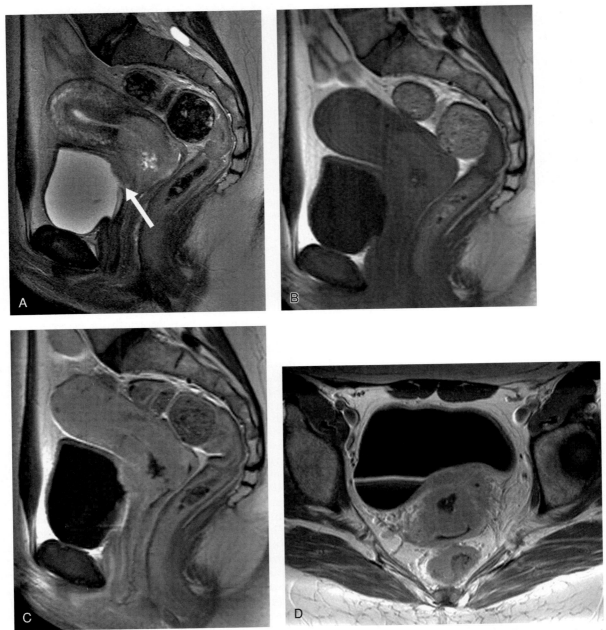

FIGURE 12–14. Cervical carcinoma with infiltration of the bladder wall in a 41-year-old woman. The cervical carcinoma was staged before surgery. *A,* A sagittal T₂-weighted image shows an inhomogeneous hyperintense tumor of the cervix, which infiltrates the upper third of the vagina. The low signal intensity of the bladder wall is interrupted at the area of the tumor (*arrow*). *B,* On a sagittal T₁-weighted image, no fat plane between the bladder and cervix is visible. *C* and *D,* After contrast administration, the tumor has irregular enhancement, and solid enhancing areas protruding into the bladder can be demonstrated.

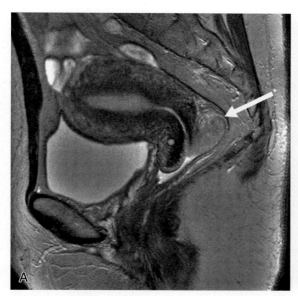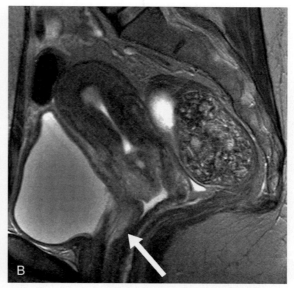

FIGURE 12–15. Cervical carcinoma. *A*, In this patient, the sagittal T$_2$-weighted image shows a localized cervical cancer in the posterior labium of the cervix (*arrow*) with early infiltration of the posterior fornix. *B*, In another patient, the T$_2$-weighted sagittal image shows infiltration of the upper third of the vagina (*arrow*) along the ventral wall.

however, the parametrium often increases in signal intensity to the same extent as that of tumor. Extension into the lower uterine isthmus or the vagina is optimally seen on both sagittal and coronal imaging planes (Fig. 12-15); the transverse images are used to complement the findings from the other two planes. For assessing primary cervical tumor, sagittal and transverse planes of imaging are optimal; for parametrial extension, an additional oblique transverse plane angled perpendicular to the long axis of the cervix may be helpful.

Vagina

T$_1$-weighted sequences delineate the vagina from surrounding structures equally as well as T$_2$-weighted sequences. However, in most cases, T$_2$-weighted sequences are essential and the optimal imaging plane is transverse. On T$_2$-weighted sequences, the high-signal-intensity center represents the vaginal epithelium and mucosa, and the lower signal intensity surrounding the high-signal-intensity center represents the vaginal wall.

The most common benign masses of the vagina, often found incidentally on MRI, are Bartholin's cysts. They are caused by retained secretions within the vulvovaginal glands and are typically located in the posterolateral aspect of the lower third of the vagina. In most cases they are asymptomatic. Depending on its fluid content, the cyst is usually of medium or high signal intensity on T$_1$-weighted images and high signal intensity on T$_2$-weighted sequences.

Primary malignant neoplasms of the vagina are rare, accounting for less than 2% of gynecologic cancers. They usually are squamous cell carcinomas (90%) or adenocarcinomas, and patients present with bleeding, discharge, or pain and fistula formation. Primary tumors in most cases cannot be differentiated from metastatic lesions on MRI, nor can inflammatory disease be separated from a neoplasm.

On T$_1$-weighted sequences, primary vaginal neoplasms are imaged with medium signal intensity like the normal vagina, and their presence can be appreciated only when they are large enough to alter the vaginal contour (Fig. 12-16). On T$_2$-weighted scans, a medium- to high-signal-intensity mass can be appreciated and its location and extent accurately assessed. The main role of MRI in evaluating malignant tumors of the vagina is not in making the primary diagnosis but rather in staging vaginal tumors and evaluating the extent of the tumor in adjacent tissue.

Ovary

Normal Anatomy

Currently, sonography is the method of choice for evaluating ovarian masses. MRI serves as a problem-solving technique after the sonographic study of adnexal abnormalities. Most ovarian masses are benign cysts, such as physiologic follicular cysts, corpus luteum cysts, serous cystadenomas, mucinous cystadenomas, and dermoids.

The normal ovaries are seen as low- or medium-signal-intensity structures on T$_1$-weighted sequences. Occasionally, the ovaries may blend with surrounding bowel loops. On T$_2$-weighted sequences, the signal intensity of the ovaries increases and has components of signal intensity equal to or greater than those of fat, depending on the field strength of the magnet used. The transverse and coronal imaging planes are ideal for evaluating the ovaries, and normal ovaries are demonstrated on MRI in up to 96%.

Ovarian Tumors

Figure 12-17 gives a brief overview about adnexal masses in MRI. Figure 12-18 summarizes differential diagnosis of nongynecologic masses in the female pelvis.

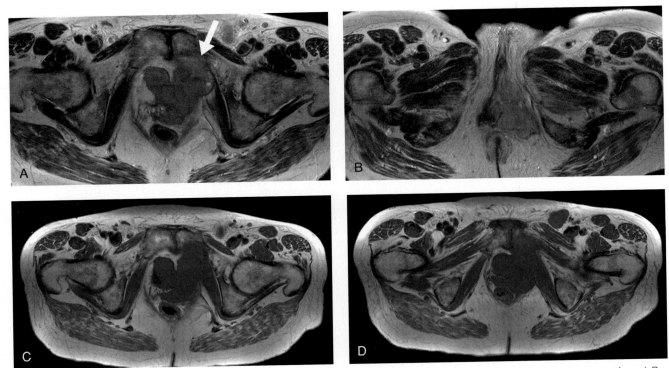

FIGURE 12–16. Vaginal carcinoma in a 72-year-old woman. Magnetic resonance imaging was performed for staging purpose. *A,* and *B,* T$_2$-weighted axial images show an ill-defined, infiltrating hyperintense mass arising from the vagina that infiltrates the pelvic side wall (*arrow*) as well as parts of the levator muscle. *C* and *D,* On T$_1$-weighted unenhanced images, no fat planes between the tumor and the pelvic side wall and muscular structures can be visualized, indicating infiltrative growth.

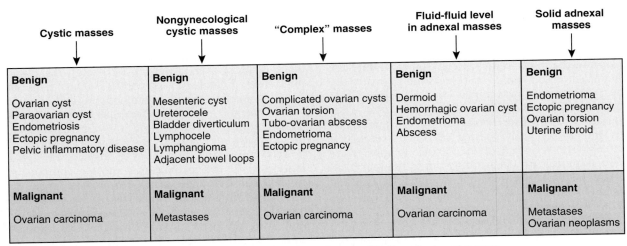

Cystic masses	Nongynecological cystic masses	"Complex" masses	Fluid-fluid level in adnexal masses	Solid adnexal masses
Benign Ovarian cyst Paraovarian cyst Endometriosis Ectopic pregnancy Pelvic inflammatory disease	**Benign** Mesenteric cyst Ureterocele Bladder diverticulum Lymphocele Lymphangioma Adjacent bowel loops	**Benign** Complicated ovarian cysts Ovarian torsion Tubo-ovarian abscess Endometrioma Ectopic pregnancy	**Benign** Dermoid Hemorrhagic ovarian cyst Endometrioma Abscess	**Benign** Endometrioma Ectopic pregnancy Ovarian torsion Uterine fibroid
Malignant Ovarian carcinoma	**Malignant** Metastases	**Malignant** Ovarian carcinoma	**Malignant** Ovarian carcinoma	**Malignant** Metastases Ovarian neoplasms

FIGURE 12–17. Magnetic resonance imaging classification of adnexal masses.

Metastasis of different primary tumors, peritoneal carcinosis	Pelvic kidney	Rectal, bladder, and other tumors of pelvic organs	Soft tissue tumors (sarcoma, fibroma, fibrosarcoma, and others)	Endometriosis	Neural tumors (neurofibroma, neurofibrosarcoma, ganglioneuroma, schwannoma, and other nerve sheath tumors)	Abscess formation

FIGURE 12–18. Nongynecologic masses of the female pelvis.

Cystic Benign Ovarian Lesions

Benign macroscopic cysts of the ovary include follicular cysts, corpus luteum cysts, theca lutein cysts, and simple cysts. Follicular and corpus luteum cysts are usually solitary and may contain hemorrhage. Both resolve without treatment. Theca lutein cysts result from high levels of human chorionic gonadotropin (hCG) or an increased sensitivity of theca cells to hCG. They typically are bilateral and multiple and, in the case of high levels of hCG, resolve when the cause of hyperstimulation is removed.

Simple ovarian cysts are thin walled with a smooth lining, contain serous fluid, and may reach 10 cm in diameter. Most adnexal cysts are asymptomatic. Occasionally, however, they may cause pelvic pain, pressure, or discomfort. Cysts may bleed, undergo torsion, or rupture, causing hemoperitoneum. On MRI, simple ovarian cysts are well-circumscribed homogeneous masses with a smooth interface (Fig. 12-19). If peripherally located, the cyst has a smooth and almost imperceptible wall. On T_1-weighted sequences, they are of low signal intensity, often similar to that of urine or slightly greater than urine. On a T_2-weighted sequence, the cyst has high signal intensity, in most cases higher than that of fat.

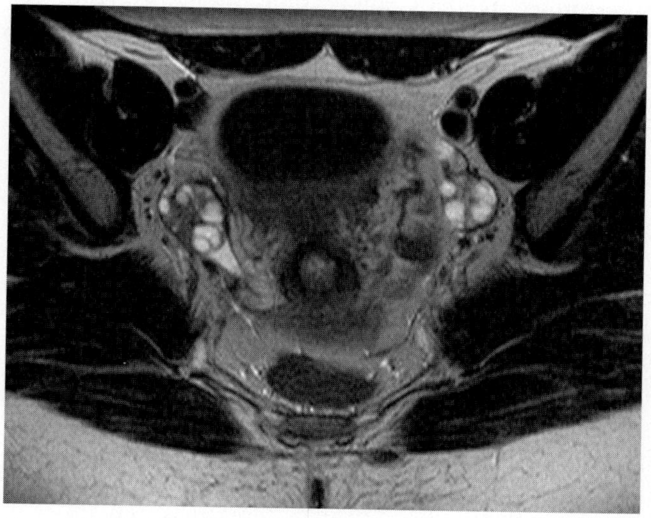

Ovarian hemorrhagic cysts are also well-circumscribed homogeneous structures with smooth walls of various thickness. The wall is seen as a low-signal-intensity line surrounding the ovarian lesion and corresponds to ovarian tissue or a pseudocapsule. Hemorrhagic cysts have high signal intensity on both T_1- and T_2-weighted sequences as a result of blood degradation products.

Polycystic ovarian disease results from a poorly understood derangement of reproductive endocrine function. It is characterized by the clinical triad of secondary menstrual abnormality (oligomenorrhea or amenorrhea), hirsutism, and obesity. Follicle-stimulating hormone (FSH) is produced by the pituitary gland and stimulates ovarian follicles, but there is no midcycle surge of luteinizing hormone (LH), and ovulation and menstruation do not occur. The ovaries in these patients are generally enlarged and contain numerous immature follicles around the periphery of the ovary. The unruptured follicles are typically 5 to 15 mm in diameter and may vary in size. The characteristic MRI appearance of polycystic ovarian disease consists of multiple small peripheral cysts adjacent to abundant low-signal-intensity central stroma.

Cystadenomas are benign neoplasms arising from the surface epithelium of the ovary. They may occur at any age, but most are found in women 20 to 44 years old. Serous cystadenomas constitute about 22% of benign ovarian neoplasms and are often between 5 and 10 cm in size. They are usually smooth, unilocular or multilocular cysts filled with serous fluid. Occasionally, papillary projections may be obvious. The signal intensity of the cyst fluid in MRI varies with the cyst contents. In the presence of mucin or hemorrhage, cysts may demonstrate increased signal intensity on T_1- and T_2-weighted images, and layering and fluid-fluid levels may be noted.

Mucinous cystadenoma accounts for about 15% to 20% of benign ovarian tumors. They are also smooth, but more frequently they present as multilocular cysts ranging in size, with a tendency to be larger than serous cystadenomas. The majority measure 15 to 30 cm in diameter at diagnosis. If rupture occurs, the tumor cells may implant on the peritoneum and result in pseudomyxoma peritonei. This is more commonly associated with malignant or borderline tumors. The MRI appearance of mucinous cystadenoma may be identical to that

FIGURE 12–19. Normal ovaries with follicular cysts in a 32-year-old woman. An axial T2-weighted image shows bilateral high-signal-intensity (SI) cysts of the ovaries. Solid areas within the cysts cannot be delineated. The ovarian stroma displays low SI.

of serous cystadenoma. The presence of thick septa and the more multilocular appearance may be used as differentiating features.

Solid Benign Ovarian Lesions

Ovarian fibromas account for about 5% of ovarian tumors. They are part of the sex cord–stromal tumors that include granulosa-theca tumors, Sertoli-Leydig tumors, lipid cell tumors, and gynandroblastomas. About 80% of these tumors produce hormones, although fibromas do not. Fibromas usually arise in postmenopausal women and are mostly asymptomatic until they cause pelvic pressure or produce torsion. Ascites is seen in 40% to 50% of patients with fibromas larger than 5 cm in diameter. Meigs' syndrome represents the rare triad of fibroma, ascites, and pleural effusion.

On MRI fibromas are usually well-defined solid tumors that demonstrate low signal intensity on both T_1- and T_2-weighted images. Because of hyalinization and myxomatous changes, irregular areas of high signal intensity on T_2-weighted images may occasionally be noted.

Pelvic Inflammatory Disease

Pelvic inflammatory disease is an ascending infection of the uterus, fallopian tubes, and broad ligaments. Pelvic inflammatory disease may be either acute or chronic, and tubo-ovarian abscess is a potential complication. Patients present with a history of abdominal pain and tenderness. In the case of a tubo-ovarian abscess, MRI will demonstrate an adnexal mass that is ill defined and inhomogeneous and that usually contains fluid because of abscess formation. Increased vascularity within the pelvis associated with the inflammatory response may be noted. After administration of Gd chelates, the abscess wall and surrounding inflammatory tissue typically enhance on T_1-weighted images, whereas the central abscess cavity remains of low signal intensity.

Endometriosis

Endometriosis is a condition of unknown pathogenesis in which endometrial glands and stroma are found in an ectopic site outside the uterine cavity and musculature. This condition occurs usually in premenopausal women; the postmenopausal population comprises only 2% to 4% of cases. It is found in up to 15% of women undergoing laparoscopy and affects as many as 30% to 40% of infertile women. The most common sites of involvement for implants of heterotopic endometrial tissue are, in decreasing order of frequency, the ovary, the uterine ligaments, the cul-de-sac, and the pelvic peritoneal surfaces.

Endometriomas are internal hemorrhages within an area of endometriosis resulting in endometrial cysts. As mentioned, they most commonly involve the ovary and are bilateral in one third of cases. They may partially or completely replace the normal ovarian tissue. The cyst wall usually contains endometrial glands and stroma and is often surrounded by a dense fibrous capsule with adhesions to adjacent structures. The cysts most often contain chocolate-colored material but may also contain subacute hemorrhage with clot and watery fluid. The two most common clinical presentations are pelvic pain and infertility. Less common manifestations include pleurisy, cyclic hemoptysis, and headaches.

Endometriosis has many different appearances on MRI. The most common is similar to that of a hemorrhagic ovarian cyst (Fig. 12-20). Lesions are often heterogeneous and composed of a variety of tissues, including a hemorrhagic fluid component, hemorrhagic solid components, and fibrotic tissue. Whereas MRI has been shown to be helpful in detecting implants in the vaginal fornix, rectovaginal ligaments, urinary bladder, and presacral region, including the cul-de-sac, mesenteric endometrial implants are, in most cases, not readily demonstrable. Although the MRI appearance is variable, several findings suggestive of endometrioma have been reported, including a distinct low-signal-intensity zone on both T_1- and T_2-weighted images surrounding a cyst containing hemorrhage and prominent low-signal-intensity shading in a cyst on T_2-weighted images (Fig. 12-21).

Teratoma

Three types of teratomas exist: mature benign teratomas, immature malignant teratomas, and monodermal or highly specialized teratomas, which include struma ovarii and carcinoid. The majority of teratomas consist of the cystic and mature forms, which are also referred to as dermoid cysts. They comprise approximately 90% of teratomas and 10% to 25% of all ovarian neoplasms. Teratomas most commonly occur during the reproductive years, although they may be seen at any age from infancy to senescence. Characteristically, dermoid cysts (Fig. 12-22) are unilocular cysts that contain ectodermal, mesodermal, and endodermal structures and often a solid protuberance, the so-called Rokitansky or dermoid plug. The plug often contains fat, hair, bone, or even well-formed teeth. Complications of cystic teratomas include torsion, rupture, infection, or even malignant transformation (in 2%). On MRI the key to diagnosis of a dermoid cyst is the identification of fat within an adnexal mass. Chemical shift imaging, applying T_1-weighted fat-suppressed images, is the most definitive way to differentiate fat within a dermoid cyst from hemorrhagic adnexal lesions, which may also show high signal intensity on T_1-weighted images. Other patterns that may be observed include fluid-fluid levels, floating debris, and mural nodules with areas of signal void representing bone or teeth formation within a mature teratoma. MRI is less sensitive than CT in detecting these calcifications.

In contrast to the much more common mature cystic teratoma, immature malignant teratomas are composed of immature or embryonal tissue derived from the three germ cell layers. These tumors are rather rare and comprise less than 1% of ovarian teratomas. They occur most commonly in the first two decades of life. At presentation, they are usually large and bulky and tend to form adhesions to surrounding structures or invade locally (Fig. 12-23). Typically, they grow rapidly, and fat

Text continued on page 375

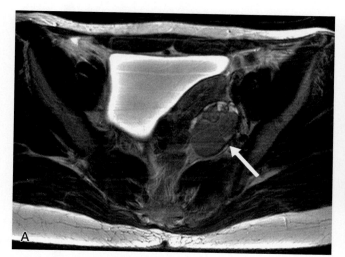

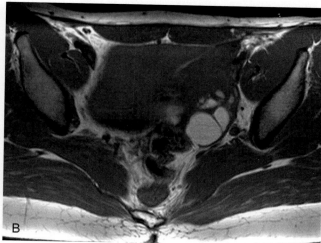

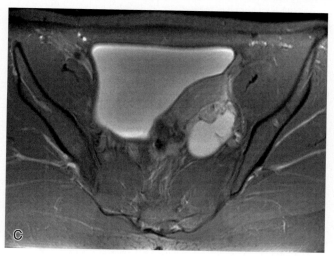

FIGURE 12–20. Endometriosis of the ovary in a 33-year-old woman. *A,* On T2-weighted axial imaging, a septated, partially hypointense mass can be seen in the left ovary (*arrow*); however, the typical shading of blood degradation products is not visible. *B,* The corresponding T1-weighted image shows high signal intensity (SI) of these areas, indicating hemorrhage. *C,* The T1-weighted fat saturated image after contrast administration does not show suppression of the high SI hemorrhagic areas as it does for fat.

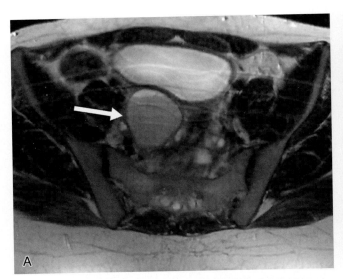

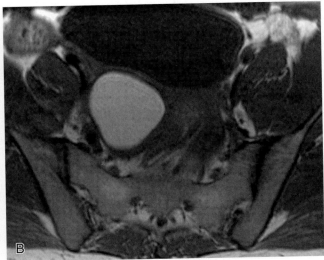

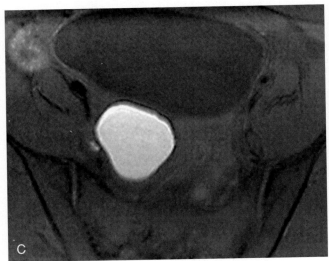

FIGURE 12–21. Endometriosis of the ovary in a 29-year-old woman. A tumor of the right ovary was found on routine sonography. *A,* On the T2-weighted axial image, a round lesion of the right ovary (*arrow*) with inhomogeneous signal intensity is demonstrated, displaying a shading of the signal from the more anterior to the more posterior parts. On T1- (*B*) and fat saturated T1-weighted (*C*) images, the lesion has a high signal consistent with hemorrhage.

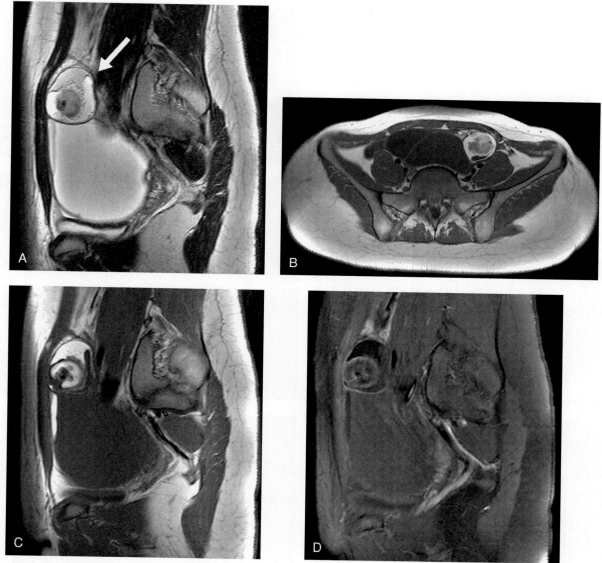

FIGURE 12–22. Dermoid cyst (cystic mature teratoma) of the ovary in a 16-year-old girl with sudden increase of abdominal girth and discomfort of the lower abdomen. *A,* On sagittal T2-weighted imaging, a huge septated lesion with large areas of high signal intensity (SI) is demonstrated. The cranial part of the lesion shows a more solid component. Some small areas of low signal represent Rokitansky's protuberance (*arrow*). T1-weighted axial (*B*) and sagittal (*C*) imaging show partial high SI areas within the lesion consistent with fat; the more caudal parts consist mainly of simple fluid. *D,* After contrast administration (T1-weighted fat suppressed contrast enhanced), the cranial, more solid component shows some contrast uptake, whereas the signal from fat is clearly suppressed. Again, small areas of low SI can be noted in this solid area, which represented teeth formation.

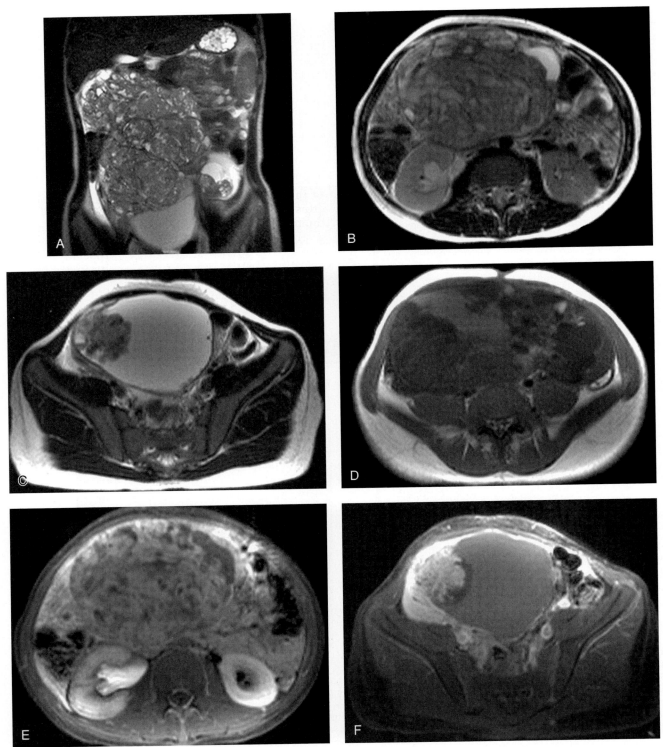

FIGURE 12–23. Malignant, immature teratoma of the ovary in a 9-year-old girl. The patient presented with a large palpable pelvic mass causing protrusion of the abdomen. A large inhomogeneous partially cystic mass can be seen on coronal (*A*) and axial (*B* and *C*) T2-weighted images. *D,* On T1-weighted unenhanced imaging, the lesion again shows an inhomogeneous signal intensity with areas of hemorrhage and fluid within cysts that show a high protein content. *E* and *F,* The main part of the lesion is solid and has inhomogeneous contrast uptake on T1-weighted fat saturated images. In the caudally located part, a papillary solid vegetation of the wall protrudes into a cystic area. Both kidneys show dilatation of the renal pelvis as a result of a compression of both ureters by the large tumor.

may occasionally be seen in parts of the lesion. Immature teratomas usually have an inhomogeneous appearance on T_2-weighted images with solid, cystic, and fatty areas. Solid parts of the lesions typically show enhancement on T_1-weighted images after injection of Gd chelates.

Malignant Ovarian Lesions

Ovarian cancer is the leading cause of death resulting from genital cancer in the United States. Malignant ovarian tumors are principally classified according to the ovarian component from which they arise: (1) surface epithelial tumors; (2) germ cell tumors; and (3) sex cord and stromal tumors.

Approximately 85% of ovarian malignancies originate from the epithelium of the ovary. Because there is no true capsule of the ovary and because the ovary is covered only by the visceral peritoneum, ovarian cancer often is already metastatic by the time it is discovered. Clinical symptoms are nonspecific. Ovarian carcinoma has a strong tendency for extension outside the ovary. Routes of spread include direct invasion of adjacent structures such as the uterus, sigmoid colon, urinary bladder, and small bowel. Peritoneal seeding to the small bowel, pelvis, and omentum also occurs frequently. Lymphatic dissemination is primarily to pelvic and paraaortic lymph nodes. Hematogenous spread occurs only very late to the liver, lung, or pleura. The prognosis of ovarian cancer depends on the presence of residual tumor after surgery, histologic type of the tumor, FIGO stage at initial diagnosis, and tumor grade.

The role of MRI in the evaluation of patients with suspected adnexal neoplasms lies in lesion detection, characterization, staging, and follow-up. On MRI the manifestation of ovarian carcinoma is variable and depends on the tumor type. Lesions are usually large (>4–5 cm) and may be solid, cystic, or mixed. Solid masses usually demonstrate a low to intermediate signal intensity on T_1-weighted images and high signal intensity on T_2-weighted images (Fig. 12-24). However, these findings may vary depending on the amount of hemorrhage or necrosis within the tumor. In cystic ovarian neoplasms, as with solid lesions, the MRI appearance varies and depends on the cyst contents. In cystic ovarian carcinomas that contain proteinaceous or hemorrhagic material, high signal intensity on both T_1- and T_2-weighted sequences may be seen. Cystic neoplasms may demonstrate thick walls or septations and contain solid vegetations or regions of nodularity (Fig. 12-25). Both findings are best demonstrated on either T_2-weighted or Gd chelate-enhanced T_1-weighted images. Extent of disease within the pelvis may also be determined using MRI, demonstrating involvement of the uterus, bladder, and rectosigmoid. Outside the pelvis, MRI may detect ascites, peritoneal implants, presence of omental cake, and mesenteric disease. MRI characteristics of a malignant lesion include size larger than 4 cm, solid or predominantly solid lesions, wall thickness greater than 3 mm, vegetations or solid nodules, and necrosis. Other findings that are found in malignant lesions include pelvic side wall or organ involvement, ascites, adenopathy, and omental disease.

In summary, the primary role of MRI for ovarian imaging is to act as a problem-solving modality after sonography and CT have been performed. MRI is more accurate than ultrasonography for tissue characterization in differentiating simple fluid from that of more complex fluids. MRI may supplement the ultrasonographic examination by defining the nature of an adnexal mass and its extent and determining the presence of blood or fat components. However, MRI still may not provide a specific diagnosis in certain cases of an adnexal mass.

MALE PELVIS

MRI is emerging as a valuable imaging tool in evaluation of the male pelvis. It has several advantages over other cross-sectional imaging modalities. MRI provides direct multiplanar images and superb soft tissue contrast. Currently, the most common indication for MRI in the evaluation of the prostate gland is preoperative staging of patients with biopsy-proven prostatic carcinoma. However, it is generally accepted that MRI is currently not suitable as a primary imaging modality for detection of prostate carcinoma. In imaging of the seminal vesicles, MRI is useful in evaluating a number of abnormalities, including suspected congenital anomalies, male infertility, primary or secondary neoplastic involvement, infection, and hemorrhage.

Prostate

The mature prostate is composed of both glandular and nonglandular tissue. Historically, the prostate was divided anatomically into different lobes. However, during the past 30 years, the concept of zonal anatomy has gradually replaced this previously described lobar anatomy.

The zonal anatomy of the prostate divides the gland into three major zones: peripheral, central, and transitional. A small amount of glandular tissue is also present in the periurethral glands. The zonal differentiation is clinically significant because most prostate carcinomas arise in the peripheral zone, whereas benign prostatic hyperplasia usually originates in the transitional zone. The urethra and the anterior fibromuscular stroma represent nonglandular tissue within the prostate. MRI of the prostate has evolved with the development in MRI coils and MRI pulse sequences. The use of phased-array coils and endorectal surface coils greatly improves the signal-to-noise ratio. The combination of both types of coils allows homogeneous signal within a large field of view and very high anatomic resolution. This has led to an overall improved accuracy in image interpretation of the prostate gland. In general, imaging of the prostate gland is performed using T_1- and T_2-weighted sequences. For high-resolution images, fast spin echo imaging has replaced conventional spin echo sequences. Imaging of the prostate gland is customarily performed in all three orthogonal planes; the relationships between the prostate and adjacent structures are best demonstrated on transaxial and sagittal images. The normal prostate gland demonstrates a homogeneous intermediate signal intensity on T_1-weighted images. On

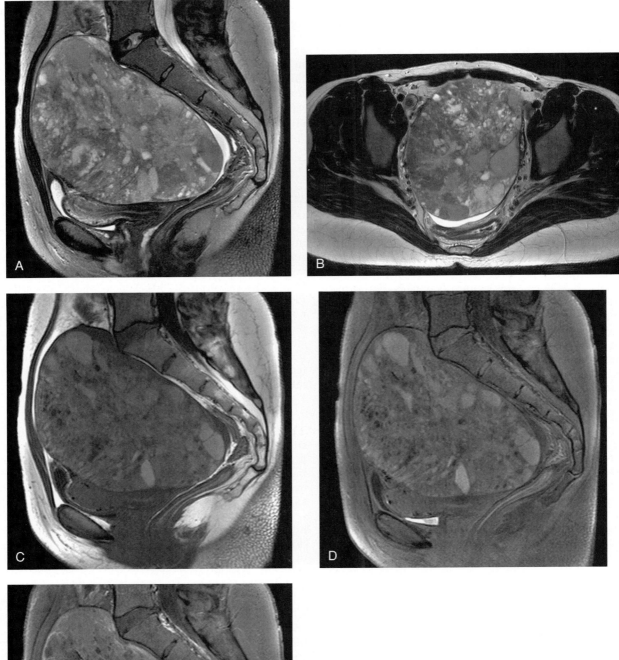

FIGURE 12–24. Ovarian carcinoma in a 32-year-old woman with a large, mainly solid pelvic mass on ultrasonography. *A* and *B,* Sagittal and axial T2-weighted images demonstrate a large inhomogeneous tumor displacing the uterus and bladder. The ovaries cannot be identified. On T1- (*C*) and fat suppressed T1-weighted (*D*) images, again inhomogeneous SI within the lesion can be noted with areas of hemorrhage. *E,* after contrast administration, the fat suppressed T1-weighted image demonstrates slight enhancement of the solid parts of the tumor.

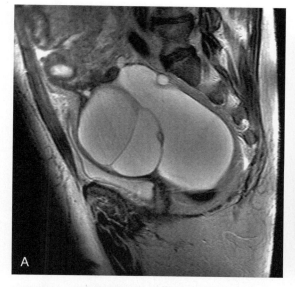

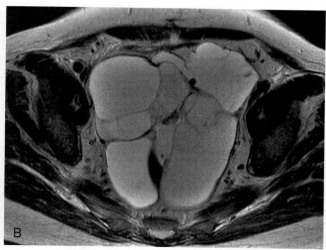

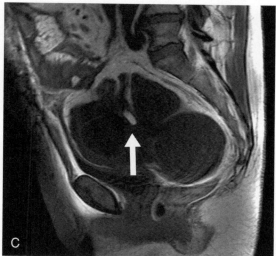

FIGURE 12–25. Ovarian carcinoma in a 52-year-old woman who presented with an enlarging mass of the pelvis. T2-weighted imaging in the sagittal (*A*) and axial (*B*) planes demonstrates a large septated mass. The cystic areas have a slightly different signal intensity. The septations are partially thickened, and some solid components can be identified. *C*, T1-weighted imaging demonstrates hemorrhage (*arrow*) in the central part of the lesion.

T_2-weighted sequences, the peripheral zone is of high signal intensity, equal to or greater than that of adjacent periprostatic fat, whereas the central zone has low signal intensity. The prostatic capsule is composed of fibrous and muscular elements and can be visualized as a low-signal-intensity line on T_2-weighted images closely surrounding the peripheral zone of the gland.

Benign prostatic hyperplasia is one of the most common abnormalities affecting the prostate gland. Benign prostatic hyperplasia develops predominantly within the transitional zone. As it enlarges, it causes compression of the surrounding central zone as well as the urethra, resulting in varying degrees of bladder outlet obstruction. The appearance of benign prostatic hyperplasia on MRI depends on whether stromal or glandular hyperplasia occurs. Glandular benign prostatic hyperplasia is characterized by nodular areas of heterogeneous increased signal intensity on T_2-weighted images (Fig. 12-26), whereas stromal benign prostatic hyperplasia is of more intermediate signal intensity.

In cases of acute prostatitis, usually no imaging studies are needed because the diagnosis is made clinically. In MRI of acute prostatitis, most commonly diffuse enlargement of the gland can be noted. If a prostatic abscess develops, the abscess is seen as an area of increased signal intensity on T_2-weighted images.

Congenital anomalies of the prostate gland are frequently found in the context of other anomalies of the genitourinary system. Congenital cysts of the prostate gland are either midline or lateral in location. Midline congenital cysts include prostatic utricle cysts and müllerian duct cysts. Both result from abnormal regression of the müllerian system. However, whereas utricle cysts are generally associated with other anomalies like hypospadias, ambiguous genitalia, or undescended testis, müllerian duct cysts are not associated with other genital anomalies and thus are usually diagnosed in adulthood as a result of clinical symptoms. Lateral congenital prostatic cysts are rare acquired cystic lesions of the prostate that include retention cysts and ejaculatory duct cysts. Typically, these cysts have low signal intensity on T_1-weighted images and a high signal intensity on T_2-weighted sequences. If the cysts contain hemorrhage or proteinaceous fluid, the signal intensity on T_1-weighted

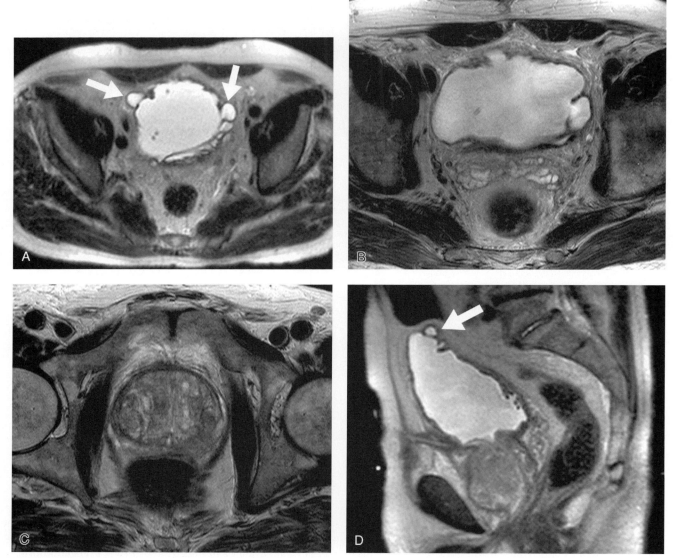

FIGURE 12–26. Benign prostatic hyperplasia in a 74-year-old man with bladder outlet obstruction. *A–D,* Axial and sagittal T2-weighted images show the bladder to be elevated, and a suprapubic catheter can be identified in the T2-weighted sagittal image. The bladder wall shows irregularities but no solid thickening, and bladder diverticula (*arrows*) are present. The prostate is quite symmetrically enlarged with nodular high signal intensity (SI) enlargement of the inner gland.

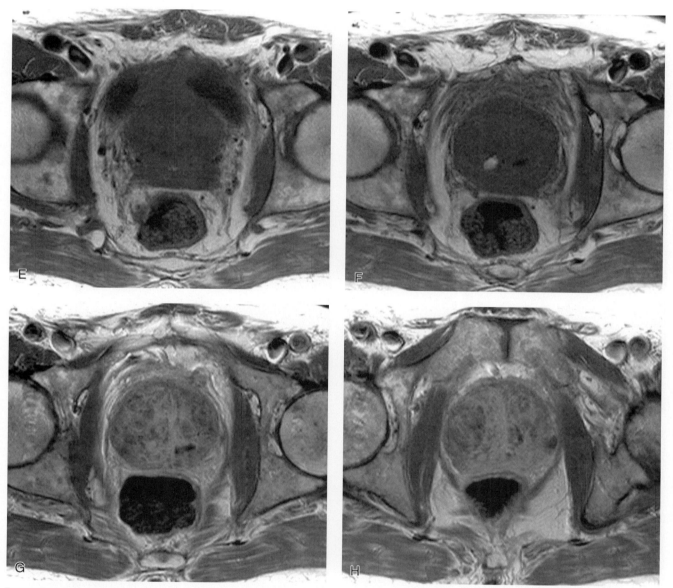

FIGURE 12–26 *Continued. E* and *F,* On T1-weighted images, there is a small area with accumulation of protein-rich fluid that shows a high SI. Otherwise, the prostate shows well-defined borders. *G* and *H,* After contrast administration, T1-weighted images show an inhomogeneous enhancement of the prostate with hypointense cystic areas.

images may also be higher than surrounding prostate tissue.

Prostatic carcinoma is the second leading cause of cancer-related death in men. Accurate preoperative staging of disease is imperative because the mode of therapy depends on the clinical stage of the condition. It is of special interest to differentiate disease confined to the prostate gland from disease that has extended beyond the prostate because treatment may vary depending on capsular extension (Fig. 12-27). Patients with cancer confined to the prostate gland alone may be candidates for radical prostatectomy. This procedure is potentially curative. Patients with disease extension beyond the confines of the prostate are generally not surgical candidates and may be offered an alternative therapeutic approach. Tumor invasion into the seminal vesicles can be detected on MRI by analysis of the size, configuration, and signal intensity of each vesicle.

Whereas on T_1-weighted images prostatic carcinoma may be hypointense or hyperintense relative to adjacent prostatic tissue, this tumor is generally detected on T_2-weighted sequences as a low-signal-intensity lesion within the high-signal-intensity peripheral zone. Tumors arising outside the peripheral zone are usually not detectable on MRI because the inhomogeneous signal pattern of the transitional zone prevents differentiation of prostatic tumor from benign prostatic hyperplasia. Similarly, a normal-appearing prostate gland does not exclude the presence of a carcinoma. Hemorrhage within the prostate gland that occurs because of a previous biopsy may lead to impaired tumor detection on MRI.

Seminal Vesicles

The seminal vesicles are seen posterior and superior to the prostate on sagittal images and posterior on trans-

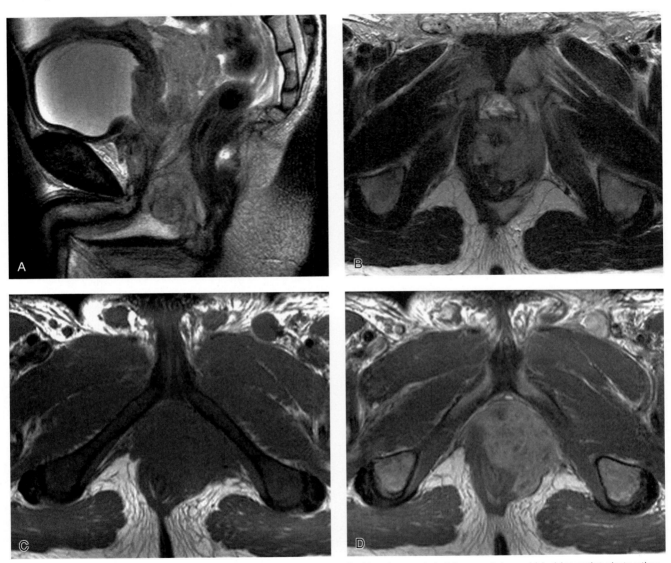

FIGURE 12–27. Prostate carcinoma in a 38-year-old man who presented with enlargement of the prostate and bladder outlet obstruction. *A* and *B*, T_2-weighted imaging demonstrates a large tumor with a nodular appearance and homogeneous high signal intensity (SI). The tumor arises from the prostate and infiltrates the bladder and the levator muscle. *C*, A T_1-weighted axial image clearly shows the infiltration of the periprostatic fat. *D*, After contrast administration, enhancement of the tumor is seen. Note the inguinal lymphadenopathy and the infiltration of the bone marrow in this very aggressive case of prostatic carcinoma.

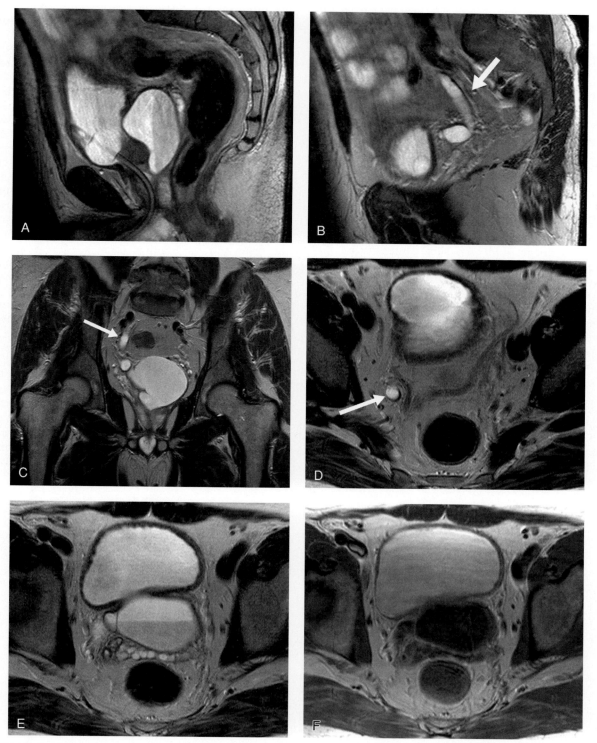

FIGURE 12–28. Seminal vesicle cyst associated with ipsilateral renal agenesis in a 34-year-old man with nonspecific clinical symptoms of the lower urinary tract. *A–C,* Sagittal and coronal T2-weighted images demonstrate a large cystic lesion located dorsally to the bladder with clearly visible shading of the signal from ventral to dorsal. Additionally, a tubular, fluid-filled structure (*arrow*) is displayed that follows the route of the normal ureter and enters the cystic lesion. On sonography, agenesis of the right kidney was noted. The tubular fluid-filled structure represents a rudimentary ectopic ureter that enters the seminal vesicle cyst. *D* and *E,* On axial T2-weighted imaging, the cyst can be seen in the seminal vesicles, and the dilated ectopic ureter is displayed in the pelvic side wall. *F,* After contrast administration, there is only discrete contrast uptake in the wall. No solid component can be found. (Courtesy of Dr. M. Uder, Hamburg.)

verse images, with low signal intensity in relation to the fat on T_1-weighted sequences. On a T_2-weighted sequence, there is a relative increase in signal intensity because of the fluid within the seminal vesicles, and the wall is seen as low intensity. Often the signal intensity is greater than that of the surrounding retroperitoneal fat.

Seminal vesicle cysts are the most common congenital anomalies of the seminal vesicles. They are most frequently unilateral and can either be unilocular or multilocular. Whereas small cysts are mainly found incidentally, large cysts can often be symptomatic. In MRI the signal intensity of a seminal vesicle cyst depends on the fluid composition. Because blood or high proteinaceous content may be present, frequently cysts have high signal intensity on both T_1- and T_2-weighted sequences (Fig. 12-28) or high signal intensity on T_1-weighted images and low signal intensity on T_2-weighted images. Otherwise, seminal vesical cysts have low signal intensity on T_1-weighted images and high signal intensity on T_2-weighted sequences. In rare cases, seminal vesicle cysts may be found in association with ipsilateral renal agenesis or dysplasia (see Fig. 12-28). The corresponding congenital abnormality in female patients is the didelphian uterus with Gartner's duct cyst and renal agenesis. Embryologically, these congenital anomalies represent developmental anomalies of the wolffian and müllerian ducts, respectively.

Testis and Scrotum

Ultrasonography is the imaging modality of choice because of its superb capabilities for displaying the scrotal anatomy and characterization of intratesticular and paratesticular lesions. However, MRI of testicular lesions may demonstrate in great detail the anatomy of the scrotum and inguinal region and is sensitive in demonstrating testicular abnormalities, especially on T_2-weighted images. MRI currently complements sonographic studies and is used when further evaluation is necessary.

The normal testis on MRI is a sharply defined oval structure of homogeneous intermediate signal intensity on a T_1-weighted image and higher signal intensity on a T_2-weighted image. A low-intensity 1-mm-thick layer demonstrated around the testis represents the tunica albuginea and the tunica vaginalis. The mediastinum testis, which arises from the tunica, is seen as a region of lower signal intensity than the testis on a T_2-weighted sequence and measures approximately 1 to 3 cm in length. Both T_1- and T_2-weighted sequences are necessary for evaluating the testis and intrascrotal contents. The coronal plane allows visualization of the testis, epididymis, and spermatic cord. This plane allows comparison of the right and left hemiscrotum. The bare area of the testis and the inguinal canal are best seen in the sagittal plane. The transverse plane allows comparison of the right and left structures and complements the coronal plane.

Testicular cysts are seen as smooth, round lesions on MR images. On T_1-weighted scans, these cysts have low signal intensity compared with the surrounding testicular tissue. On T_2-weighted scans, the cysts are of high signal intensity, similar to that of testicular tissue, and nearly isointense with the normal testicular parenchyma.

Testicular tumors are seen as areas of inhomogeneous signal intensity equal to or lower than the intensity of the normal testis on T_1-weighted sequences and markedly lower on T_2-weighted sequences. The margination and extent of the tumor, as well as the effect on the normal testicular size and shape, can be clearly demonstrated on MRI.

Musculoskeletal System

13

Mark H. Awh, Michael E. Stadnick, and Val M. Runge

Magnetic resonance imaging (MRI) is an extremely effective modality for evaluating the musculoskeletal system. In the early 1980s, it was initially thought that MRI would have limited application in the musculoskeletal system because of its relative inability to detect calcification. It was soon recognized that, despite the lack of visualization of calcium or cortical bone, MRI had much better soft tissue contrast than other imaging modalities. Because the musculoskeletal system is comparatively easy to immobilize, motion artifacts are relatively inconsequential. However, MRI had limited use in the musculoskeletal system until the advent of dedicated surface coils, which allowed adequate signal-to-noise ratio (SNR) and improved spatial resolution. The noninvasiveness, lack of ionizing radiation, and multiplanar imaging capabilities are desirable features of MRI.

In the two decades since its introduction, the indications for MRI in evaluating the musculoskeletal system have increased markedly. MRI is the primary imaging modality for evaluating internal derangements of the knee, hip, and shoulder, lesions of the wrist, hand, ankle, and foot, meniscal abnormalities in the temporomandibular joint (TMJ), and avascular necrosis, and it is superior for depicting the extent of soft tissue masses and bone marrow abnormalities.

This chapter reviews the current knowledge about MRI of the musculoskeletal system, with an emphasis on pathologic conditions and technical parameters for imaging the major joints, including the knee, hip, TMJ, shoulder, wrist, and ankle. The MRI appearances of soft tissue lesions, bone tumors, marrow diseases, and infections are also examined.

MRI OF THE KNEE

MRI has several advantages compared with other modalities in evaluating the internal architecture of the knee. MRI is noninvasive and painless and provides excellent soft tissue contrast. The first MRI of the knee was reported in 1985, but initial results were compromised by poor SNR and resolution. The implementation of local coils for extremity imaging and higher-field-strength magnets (1.0-1.5 T) helped to overcome these limitations. MRI plays a dominant role in the evaluation of knee abnormalities.

Technique

A complete examination of the knee must include evaluation of the menisci, ligaments, articular cartilage, and bone marrow. A suggested approach for scanning the knee includes sagittal and coronal thin-section (3 mm) T_1- and T_2-weighted images. Fast spin echo technique is usually used for T_2-weighted exams and should be implemented with fat suppression. Sagittal images with the knee externally rotated 10 to 15 degrees (or angled to achieve this result) allow optimal depiction of the anterior cruciate ligament (ACL). The knee should be imaged in the neutral position for coronal scans. All scans must be obtained using an extremity coil. Good spatial resolution requires a small (15 cm) field of view (FOV), which best demonstrates the menisci and ligaments. From the T_1-weighted scans, a second set of images is often filmed to improve visualization of the menisci, using a narrow window to give high contrast and large magnification.

Some sites also acquire a three-dimensional (3D) gradient echo scan. Articular cartilage can be highlighted using this approach. The scan also provides very thin contiguous sections. If the patellofemoral joint space needs to be imaged, axial scans should be acquired. Unfortunately, patient throughput must be considered, and the incorporation of all of the prior pulse sequences requires excessive scan time. The 3D acquisition and axial scans should be reserved for situations in which the cartilage and patellofemoral joint, respectively, are of specific clinical concern.

Meniscus

The assessment of the meniscus is usually the primary clinical concern in MRI of the knee. The meniscus consists of type I collagen, which contains few excitable protons and should remain dark (low signal intensity) on all pulse sequences (Fig. 13-1). Meniscal tears and degeneration are manifested as increased signal intensity on T_1- and T_2-weighted sequences within the substance of the meniscus primarily because of the influx of fluid.

The posterior horn of the medial meniscus is the most common site of injury. Isolated tears of the anterior horn of the meniscus are uncommon. One early MRI study reported a sensitivity of 95%, specificity of 91%, and accuracy of 93% for MRI detection of meniscal

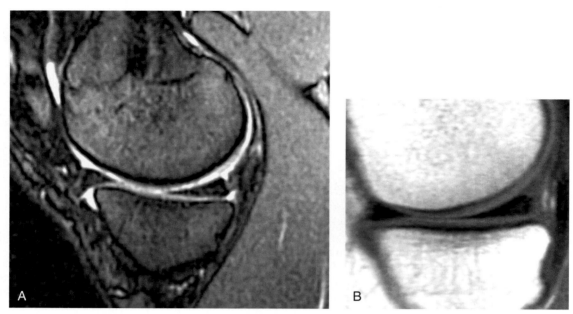

FIGURE 13–1. Normal meniscus (knee). The normal medial meniscus demonstrates homogeneous low signal intensity on T_2^*- (*A*) and T_1-weighted (*B*) sagittal images.

tears. This compared favorably with arthroscopy, which had an accuracy of 87% to 95%. The free edge of the meniscus is the most difficult area for MRI to evaluate, and 44% of the diagnostic errors occurred in this portion of the meniscus. The posterior horn of the lateral meniscus is a difficult spot for the arthroscopist to see and, therefore, is the most common site of diagnostic error in arthroscopy. Because the false-negative rate for MRI of the knee was reported to be almost zero, a normal MRI of the knee should obviate a surgical procedure.

Meniscal abnormalities on MRI have been classified by a grading system that has diagnostic and therapeutic implications. The grading system is as follows:

Normal: no intrameniscal signal

Grade 1: single round or punctate high-signal focus within the meniscal substance (Fig. 13-2)

Grade 2: linear high-signal focus within the meniscal substance that does not abut the articular surface (Fig. 13-3)

Grade 3: full- or partial-thickness tears of the meniscus communicating with an articular surface (Fig. 13-4)

Grade 4: meniscal fragmentation or peripheral rim tears (i.e., meniscal capsular separation)

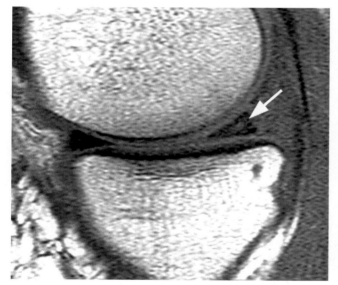

FIGURE 13–2. Grade 1 meniscal degeneration. Globular increased signal intensity (*arrow*) is noted within the posterior horn of the medial meniscus on this T_1-weighted sagittal image.

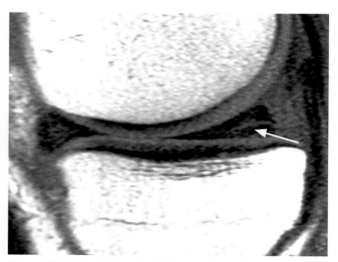

FIGURE 13–3. Grade 2 meniscal degeneration. A linear signal abnormality (*arrow*) without extension to the articular surface is apparent on this T_1-weighted sagittal image of the medial meniscus.

FIGURE 13–4. Complex meniscal tear. A proton density-weighted sagittal image demonstrates a complex tear of the posterior horn of the medial meniscus. This stellate tear communicates with both the femoral and the tibial articular surfaces (*arrows*).

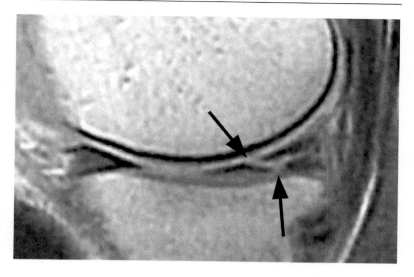

An early study correlated the bright intrameniscal signal (grades 1 and 2) with meniscal degeneration, which is manifested as a yellow discoloration in arthroscopic and macroscopic inspection. This degeneration, called mucoid or myxoid degeneration, is believed to occur in as many as 60% of patients and increases with age. Initially, collagen bundles enlarge because increased glycan accumulation separates fibrils and induces microcyst formation. Later histologic changes consist of further degeneration of meniscal matrix and collagenization, fragmenting the collagen bundles. The final stage leads to horizontal or oblique meniscal tears along the direction of the collagen fibers. Stoller and colleagues reported that the increased signal represents a continuum from mucinous degeneration to tear, in which absorbed synovial fluid appears as high signal intensity. In children, bright intrameniscal signal can be due to perforating vessels. Perforating vessels reach the center of the meniscus in children but not in adults.

Meniscal tears should be diagnosed only if the high intrameniscal signal intensity reaches an articular surface, as in grades 3 and 4. High signal intensity confined to the meniscus, as in grades 1 and 2, usually represents degenerative changes. Abnormalities confined to the meniscus that do not reach an articular surface also may not be seen at arthroscopy. The clinical significance of intrameniscal signal is uncertain, and it is likely that MRI is more sensitive than arthroscopy. The decision to perform meniscectomy currently is based exclusively on the presence of a surface tear.

Meniscal tears can be categorized by their configuration. A bucket-handle tear (Fig. 13-5) usually occurs as a result of an acute injury, most often involving the medial meniscus, beginning posteriorly and extending anteriorly. These tears are often seen as vertical high-signal intensities on coronal images. Fragmentation (grade 4) can produce the appearance of a small meniscus. The posterior horn of the medial meniscus is nor-

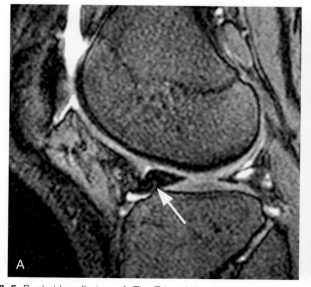

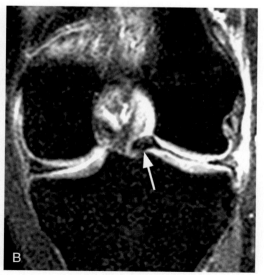

FIGURE 13–5. Bucket-handle tear. *A,* The T$_2$*-weighted sagittal image reveals excess meniscal tissue (*arrow*) displaced anteriorly adjacent to the anterior horn of the lateral meniscus; the posterior horn has a foreshortened appearance. *B,* The coronal fat-suppressed T$_2$-weighted image demonstrates the displaced bucket-handle fragment (*arrow*) along the lateral aspect of the intercondylar notch.

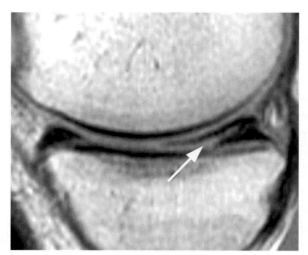

FIGURE 13–6. Horizontal tear. A horizontal-oblique tear (*arrow*) of the posterior horn of the medial meniscus is clearly visualized on this proton density-weighted sagittal image.

mally 30% larger than the anterior horn. Horizontal tears (Fig. 13-6) are the most common symptomatic abnormality of the menisci and are usually produced by the late stages of degenerative changes. Vertical tears (Fig. 13-7) are usually traumatic in origin as opposed to the degenerative origin of horizontal tears. The parrot-beak tear is a small tear located at the free edge of the body of the lateral meniscus. This is seen as blunting of the free edge of the meniscus, which normally is sharply defined. The discoid meniscus (Fig. 13-8) is an anatomic variant in which the body of the meniscus is seen on several (>3) images and often completely covers the tibial plateau.

Overreading of meniscal tears must be avoided so that unnecessary surgical procedures are minimized. Pitfalls in the diagnosis of meniscal tears can be caused by normal low-signal-intensity structures abutting the meniscus. These structures include the lateral inferior genicular artery, the transverse ligament, and the popliteus tendon. Pitfalls also arise from volume-averaging artifacts.

The lateral inferior genicular artery arises from the popliteal artery at the level of the tibiofemoral joint and courses laterally to the anterior aspect of the knee, where it lies in a fat pad between the meniscus and the lateral collateral ligament. When it lies adjacent to the anterior horn of the lateral meniscus, the space between it and the meniscus may simulate a tear. Usually the artery can be traced on adjacent sagittal images, which helps differentiate it from a tear. Coronal images often show the artery as a separate structure from the meniscus.

The transverse ligament, meniscofemoral ligament, popliteus tendon, and the meniscus are composed of type 1 collagen, and, therefore, render no signal on T_1- and T_2-weighted sequences. The transverse ligament (Fig. 13-9) arises from the anterior aspect of the medial meniscus and attaches to the anterior aspect of the lateral meniscus. A space between it and the anterior aspect of the medial meniscus can appear like a tear. The coronal view will help differentiate this from a true tear. The meniscofemoral ligament consists of two ligaments that extend from the posterior lateral meniscus to the lateral medial meniscus (Fig. 13-10). The anterior band is also called Humphry's ligament and passes anterior to the posterior cruciate ligament (PCL). The posterior band is called Wrisberg's ligament and passes posterior to the PCL. The ligament of Wrisberg is seen as it passes just posterior to the PCL in about one third of cases and should not be confused with a partial tear of the PCL. The popliteus tendon separates the lateral

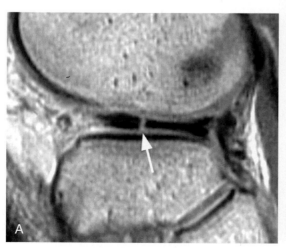

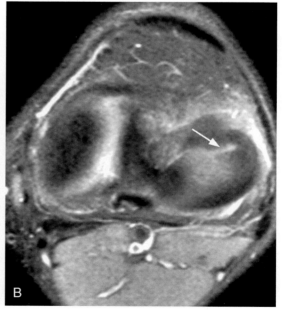

FIGURE 13–7. Vertical tear. *A*, A radial type tear (*arrow*) is readily apparent within the anterior junction of the lateral meniscus on a sagittal proton density-weighted image. *B*, The corresponding axial fat-suppressed proton density-weighted image confirms the free edge tear (*arrow*).

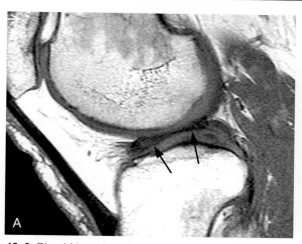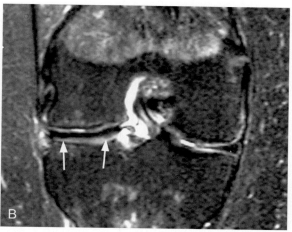

FIGURE 13–8. Discoid lateral meniscus. A discoid-type lateral meniscus (*arrows*) is noted on T₁-weighted sagittal (*A*) and fat-suppressed T₂-weighted coronal (*B*) images.

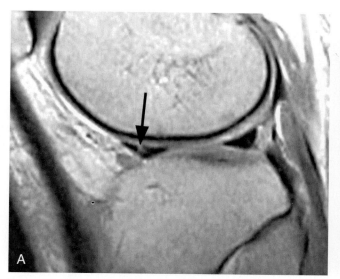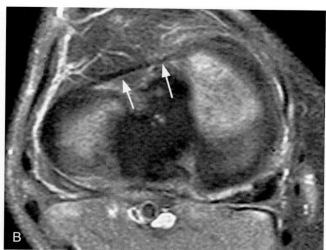

FIGURE 13–9. Transverse ligament. *A*, A linear signal abnormality (*arrow*) formed at the junction of the transverse meniscal ligament and the anterior horn of the lateral meniscus creates a meniscal pseudotear on this proton density-weighted sagittal image. *B*, A fat-suppressed proton density axial image demonstrates the typical course of the transverse meniscal ligament (*arrow*) connecting the anterior horns of the medial and lateral menisci.

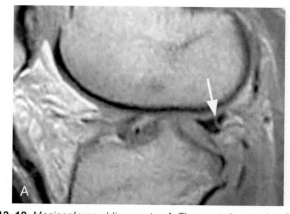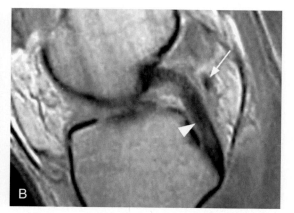

FIGURE 13–10. Meniscofemoral ligaments. *A*, The posterior meniscofemoral ligament of Wrisberg (*arrow*) may create a pseudotear at its junction with the posterior horn of the lateral meniscus, as seen on the proton density-weighted sagittal image. *B*, A more medial sagittal view demonstrates the normal course of the ligament of Wrisberg (*arrow*) along the posterior aspect of the posterior cruciate ligament (*arrowhead*).

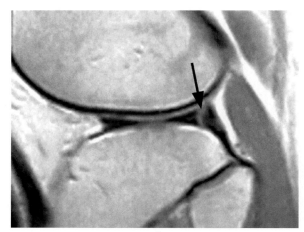

FIGURE 13–11. Popliteus tendon. Intermediate signal intensity formed at the interface (*arrow*) of the posterior horn of the lateral meniscus with the popliteus tendon results in a typical pseudotear pattern on this proton density-weighted sagittal image.

meniscus from the joint capsule and the lateral collateral ligament. A space between the posterior lateral meniscus and the popliteus tendon (Fig. 13-11) can mimic a meniscal tear on sagittal images. Coronal views can better delineate the true anatomy.

Volume averaging can also simulate meniscal disease. Sagittal images through the periphery of the meniscus may demonstrate an artifactual linear high signal intensity in the meniscus because of averaging of fat at the concavity of the periphery of the meniscus. This pitfall can be avoided by correlating with coronal images or by using thinner slices.

Bucket-handle tears can be missed on sagittal images because the tear is oriented in the plane of section. This tear is identified on the coronal images as a vertical high-signal-intensity line.

The postoperative meniscus presents a difficult challenge for MRI. Comparison with the normal, opposite meniscus and correlation with clinical history are helpful for arriving at the correct diagnosis. After a partial meniscectomy, the residual meniscal tissue appears smaller than the opposite, normal meniscus. After a complete meniscectomy, no residual meniscus is demonstrated. An early study noted that the MRI characteristics for meniscal tears in the virgin meniscus do not hold well in the postoperative meniscus. In particular, a linear area of increased signal intensity in the meniscus extending to the articular surface suggests retear, but caution must be used; this finding was false-positive in 5 of 17 cases (Figs. 13-12 and 13-13). Another common finding is diffuse increased signal intensity in the meniscal remnant, which should be considered to be a stable finding, not indicating a retear.

Ligaments and Tendons

Injuries of the ligaments are common in acute knee trauma. Clinical examination plays a crucial role in evaluating ligamentous injuries, but it can be inaccurate. MRI examination of the knee can accurately evaluate the ligaments, including the ACL, PCL, and the medial and lateral collateral ligaments.

The cruciate ligaments provide stability to the knee. The ACL prevents hyperextension of the knee and acts as a rotational guide for the femoral condyles. The PCL acts as a check against extreme hyperextension and maintains stability of the knee when the joint is flexed. Clinically, a tear of the ACL or PCL is diagnosed by an abnormal anterior or posterior drawer sign, respectively. The sensitivity of MRI for an ACL tear is in the range of 95%, with specificity near 100%. This compares favorably with a clinical sensitivity by anterior drawer sign of less than 80%. Numerous studies show the accuracy for diagnosing ACL tears by MRI to be again in the 95% range compared with an accuracy by arthroscopy of 60% to 95%.

The ACL originates at the posterior inner surface of the lateral femoral condyle and attaches to the tibia anterior and lateral to the anterior tibial spine. The PCL extends from the lateral surface of the medial femoral condyle to a depression behind the interarticular

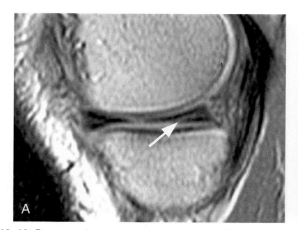
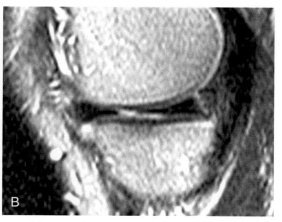

FIGURE 13–12. Postoperative meniscal pseudotear. *A,* The proton density-weighted sagittal image reveals a linear signal abnormality (*arrow*) extending to the tibial surface of this postoperative medial meniscus. *B,* The abnormality, however, does not persist on the heavily T$_2$-weighted sagittal view. This appearance is compatible with postoperative granulation tissue rather than a recurrent meniscal tear.

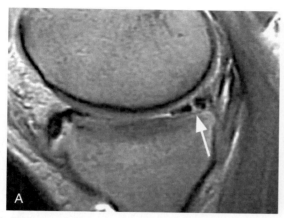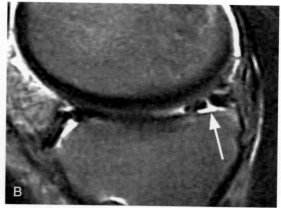

FIGURE 13–13. Postoperative meniscal retear. Proton density (*A*) and heavily T$_2$-weighted sagittal (*B*) images in this postoperative patient reveal a vertical signal abnormality (*arrows*) within the posterior horn of the medial meniscus. The persistence of the abnormality on the T$_2$-weighted image is compatible with a recurrent meniscal tear.

upper surface of the tibia. The cruciate ligaments are best demonstrated on sagittal images, and the ACL is seen best with the knee externally rotated 15 degrees (or equivalently the imaging plane angled to achieve the same result). The collateral ligaments extend from the femur to the tibia, lateral and medial to the joint, and are optimally visualized on neutrally positioned coronal images. Normally, the ligaments are smooth, continuous, low-signal-intensity fibers on T$_1$- and T$_2$-weighted images.

Tears of the ACL typically occur in the middle portion of the ligament, although they can occur at the proximal and distal attachments (Fig. 13-14). Tears usually are caused by external rotational injuries, occurring in abduction and 90-degree flexion. There are often associated tears of the collateral ligaments or meniscus. The diagnosis of an ACL tear is made on MRI by identifying disruption of the ligament along its normal course. Acute angulation of the proximal portion of the PCL (a "squared" PCL) is another reliable sign for a tear of the ACL. The tear in the ACL causes anterior subluxation of the tibia, which pulls the PCL with it, creating a buckle in the proximal portion of the PCL.

A finding suggesting a partial tear of the ligament is a focus of increased signal intensity within the substance of the ligament, often seen best on T$_2$-weighted images (Fig. 13-15). T$_2$-weighted images create an arthrographic effect, normally showing the straight smooth synovial reflection along the anterior margin of the ACL. Irregularity or waviness of this reflection suggests a partial tear of the ACL.

Tears of the PCL are diagnosed by disruption along the course of the ligament (Fig. 13-16) or by areas of increased signal intensity within the substance of the ligament. Most PCL tears involve the midsubstance of the ligament.

Tears in the collateral ligaments manifest as disruptions of the ligament or as abnormal high signal intensity in the adjacent soft tissues that often displaces the ligament, indicating bleeding or edema. The superficial portion of the medial collateral ligament (MCL) arises from the medial femoral condyle and inserts 5 cm below the joint line posterior to the pes anserinus. The superficial

fibers are separated from the deep fibers by a bursa; enlargement of the bursa from inflammation should not be confused with a tear in the MCL. The deep fibers of the MCL are firmly attached to the joint capsule and medial meniscus and attach to the femur and tibia closer to the joint. The lateral support structures consist of three parts. The lateral collateral ligament runs from the lateral femoral condyle to the fibular head (Fig. 13-17). The iliotibial band is thinner and lies more anterior. The third structure is the fibular collateral ligament, which passes from the lateral epicondyle of the femur to the head of the fibula. The MCL is more commonly injured than the lateral components. Incomplete tears of the collateral ligaments result in increased signal intensity within the (normally dark) ligaments and adjacent soft tissues on T$_2$-weighted scans. The course of the ligament, however, will be unchanged. Complete tears are identified by increased signal intensity on T$_2$-weighted scans at the site of the tear together with lack of continuity of the ligament (and typically retraction). A common classification scheme for MCL tears is based on their severity, which spans the spectrum from ligament sprain (grade I; Fig. 13-18) to partial tear (grade II; Fig. 13-19) to complete rupture (grade III; Fig. 13-20).

Care should be exercised when reviewing knee films to examine the quadriceps and patellar tendons closely for possible injury. If such an examination is not purposely placed in one's routine search pattern, injuries to these two structures can be overlooked. Injuries to the quadriceps and patellar tendons are most easily recognized on sagittal T$_2$-weighted images of the knee. Chronic stress on the patellar tendon leads to degenerative tendinitis, which is recognized by the presence of abnormal increased signal intensity within the tendon on proton density-weighted images. This weakens the tendon and may eventually lead to the tendon becoming stretched or ruptured (Fig. 13-21). Chronic degenerative changes usually precede rupture. Tears of the quadriceps tendon are occasionally seen at its insertion on the superior pole of the patella (Fig. 13-22). In a complete tear, the quadriceps tendon may retract superiorly. Chronic stress where the patellar tendon inserts on the tibial tubercle can lead to an inflammatory reaction (Osgood-

Text continued on page 394

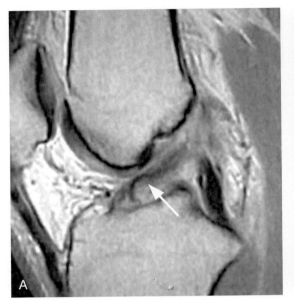

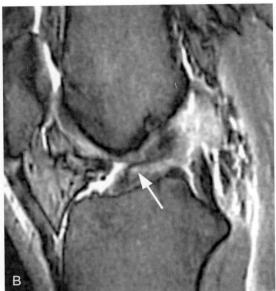

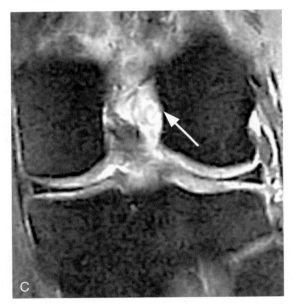

FIGURE 13–14. Complete anterior cruciate ligament (ACL) tear. Abnormal laxity is seen along the course of the ACL (*arrow*) on (*A*) proton density- and (*B*) T$_2$*-weighted sagittal images in this case of complete ACL disruption. *C*, Edema is apparent at the femoral attachment (*arrow*) on the corresponding fat-suppressed T$_2$-weighted coronal image.

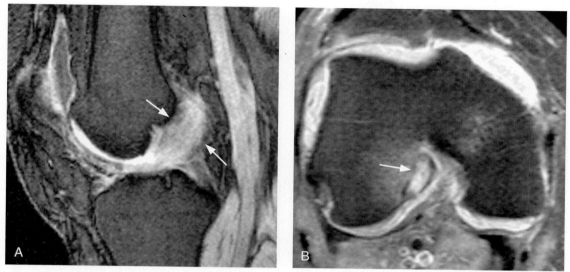

FIGURE 13–15. Partial anterior cruciate ligament (ACL) tear. T$_2$*-weighted sagittal (*A*) and fat-suppressed proton density-weighted axial (*B*) images demonstrate an edematous and thickened ACL (*arrows*), which maintains fairly normal orientation in this case.

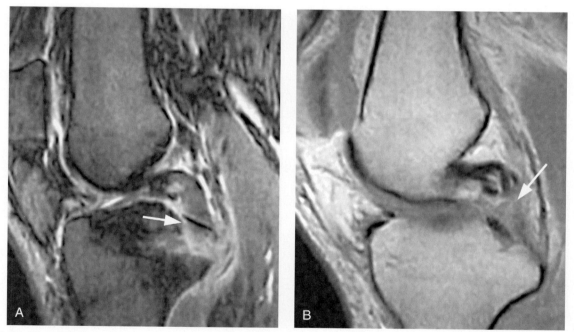

FIGURE 13–16. Posterior cruciate ligament (PCL) tear. Two cases of a complete PCL tear at the tibial insertion are shown. *A*, The T$_2$*-weighted sagittal image reveals an avulsion fracture at the tibial insertion (*arrow*). *B*, A proton density-weighted sagittal image demonstrates an edematous and retracted distal PCL (*arrow*).

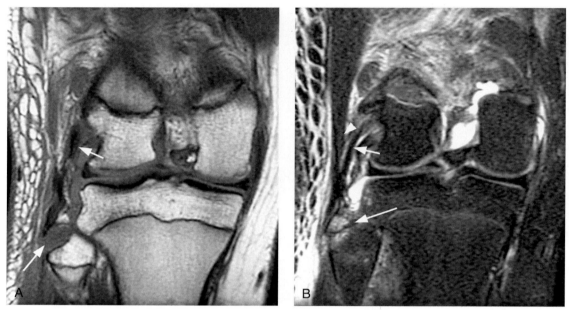

FIGURE 13–17. Lateral collateral ligament tear. T$_1$- (*A*) and fat-suppressed T$_2$-weighted (*B*) images reveal an avulsion fracture of the fibular head (*long arrow*) in this case of a lateral collateral ligament complex injury affecting the conjoined insertion of the fibular collateral ligament (*short arrow*) and the biceps femoris tendon (*arrowhead*).

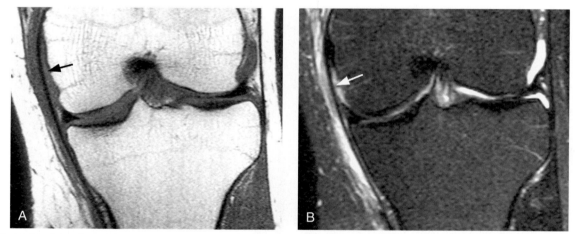

FIGURE 13–18. Medial collateral ligament tear grade I. Edema is present superficial to the fibers of the medial collateral ligament (*arrow*) on T$_1$- (*A*) and fat-suppressed T$_2$-weighted (*B*) images.

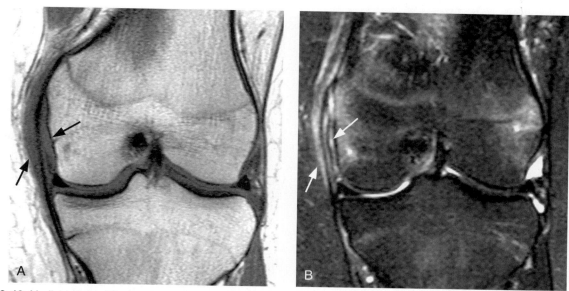

FIGURE 13–19. Medial collateral ligament tear grade II. Edema and soft tissue thickening (*arrows*) are present superficial and deep to the medial collateral ligament complex on T₁- (*A*) and fat-suppressed T₂-weighted (*B*) images.

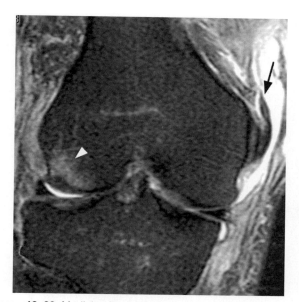

FIGURE 13–20. Medial collateral ligament tear grade III. A fat-suppressed T₂-weighted coronal image demonstrates complete medial collateral ligament disruption (*arrow*). A lateral condylar bone bruise (*arrowhead*) compatible with valgus injury is also apparent.

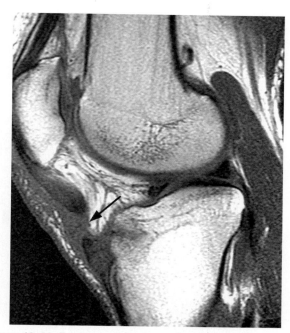

FIGURE 13–21. Patellar tendon rupture. Complete disruption of the patellar tendon (*arrow*) is apparent on a T₁-weighted sagittal image.

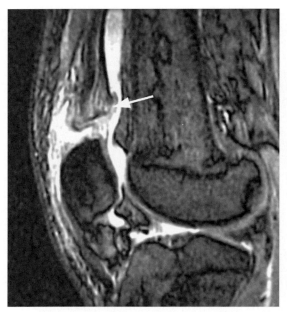

FIGURE 13–22. Quadriceps tendon rupture. A T₂*-weighted sagittal image reveals a complete tear of the quadriceps tendon (*arrow*) at its distal insertion.

Schlatter disease), which is best seen on T_2-weighted images. Two other similar lesions include cortical desmoid (seen at the insertion of the gastrocnemius muscle on the distal femur) and Pellegrini-Stieda disease (post-traumatic soft tissue calcification at the femoral origin of the MCL).

Patellar dislocation can occur as a result of a direct blow or exaggerated contraction of the quadriceps. A high patella (patella alta), low height to the lateral femoral condyle, and a shallow patellofemoral groove are several of the many predisposing abnormalities. Most dislocations are lateral (Fig. 13-23); accompanying osteochondral fractures of the medial patella and lateral femoral condyle are common.

Cartilage

Before the advent of MRI, noninvasive techniques capable of imaging the articular cartilage did not exist. Despite all the attention paid to meniscal and ligament damage, injury to hyaline cartilage potentially causes the most serious long-term effects. Damage to the cartilage can predispose patients to premature degenerative arthritis. Injured hyaline cartilage has a limited ability to repair itself because of a poor vascular supply. A noninvasive modality that can assess cartilaginous defects and follow treatment, such as MRI, is extremely useful. On spin echo technique, hyaline cartilage appears as a gray area overlying the dark subchondral bone. Gradient echo techniques, with the parameters chosen to depict cartilage as high signal intensity (adjacent to the low-signal-intensity cortical bone), are often used to highlight hyaline cartilage and disease thereof.

Injuries of the cartilage appear as irregularities or low-signal-intensity defects. One grading system for cartilage injuries is as follows:

Grade 0: normal cartilage
Grade 1: surface and texture changes but no cartilage substance loss
Grade 2: partial-thickness cartilage loss but no exposed bone
Grade 3: exposed bone

The majority of cartilage defects occur along the femoral condylar surface. A search for cartilaginous injuries is essential for a complete evaluation of the knee.

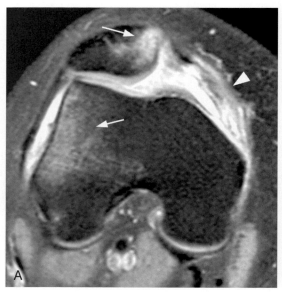

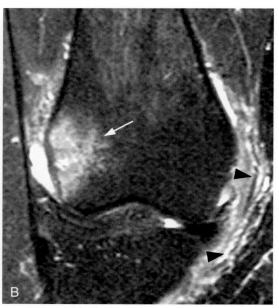

FIGURE 13–23. Lateral patellar dislocation. Characteristic bone bruises (*arrows*) are noted within the medial patella and the anterolateral aspect of the lateral femoral condyle on fat-suppressed proton density-weighted axial (*A*) and fat-suppressed T₂-weighted coronal (*B*) images. The medial retinaculum (*arrowhead*) is thickened and edematous, compatible with partial tearing.

Bone Marrow

Many unsuspected abnormalities have been identified within the bone marrow by MRI while scanning the knee. A common finding is an area of decreased signal intensity on T_1-weighted images and a corresponding area of increased signal intensity on T_2-weighted scans in the subchondral bone marrow. These areas represent osteonecrosis or microfractures with associated edema or hemorrhage. Correlative radiographs usually do not show an abnormality. Follow-up MRI scans have shown reversibility in some of these lesions. Another bony abnormality described is medullary infarction, which often presents as a discrete low-signal-intensity ring or an area of decreased signal intensity surrounding a high-signal-intensity core on T_1-weighted images.

Spontaneous osteonecrosis is usually seen in the middle-aged and elderly patient population (Fig. 13-24). Symptoms may include pain, swelling, and restricted motion. The typical location for lesions is along the weight-bearing surface of the medial femoral condyle. Possible causes include trauma and vascular insults. Degenerative joint disease and intra-articular osteocartilaginous bodies are the long-term result.

Osteochondritis dissecans is usually seen in the adolescent patient population. Symptoms are variable and may be lacking. The typical location is the non-weight-bearing surface of the medial femoral condyle. The cause is thought to be trauma. Development of intra-articular osteocartilaginous bodies is a common sequela. Osteochondritis dissecans (Fig. 13-25) manifests on MRI as a fragment of bone with low or moderate signal intensity on T_1-weighted images and various degrees of increased signal intensity on T_2-weighted images. Separation of the bone fragment, a fluid interface between the fragment and parent bone, or disruption of the articular cartilage represents loosening, which re-

quires surgical treatment. In the early years of knee MRI, spatial resolution was poor and the technique not very effective in locating small calcified intra-articular loose bodies. Computed tomography (CT) or standard radiography was, at that time, much more sensitive. As imaging technique, spatial resolution, and SNR improved, MRI became substantially better at detecting loose bodies (Fig. 13-26). Cartilaginous loose bodies (which are clearly seen by state-of-the-art MRI; Fig. 13-27) may indeed be quite difficult to detect using x-ray-based techniques, unless intra-articular contrast is administered.

Joint Fluid

Cystic lesions around the knee are common. By far, the most prevalent of these lesions is the popliteal (Baker's) cyst. This manifests as a round focus of intermediate signal intensity on T_1-weighted images and increased signal intensity on T_2-weighted images. These cysts are usually located posterior to the knee joint in the region of the gastrocnemius-semimembranosus bursa (Fig. 13-28).

Less common cystic lesions include meniscal and ganglion cysts. These cysts occur in locations atypical for simple popliteal cysts. A meniscal cyst (Fig. 13-29) is composed of synovial fluid, forced out through an underlying meniscal tear, which accumulates at the meniscocapsular margin on the medial or lateral surface of the knee joint. Meniscal cysts are always associated with underlying horizontal meniscal tears. Ganglion cysts may occur in atypical locations, attached to tendon sheaths, within muscle bundles, or adjacent to the tibiofibular joint. Ganglion cysts are not associated with meniscal tears. They may or may not have a connection with the joint space. On MRI, meniscal and ganglion cysts have intermediate signal intensity on T_1-weighted scans and high signal intensity on T_2-weighted scans.

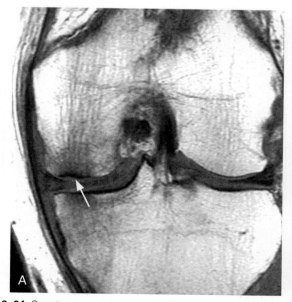
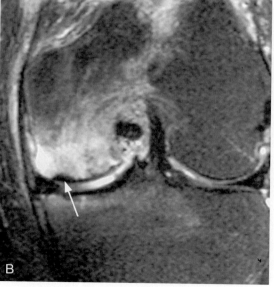

FIGURE 13–24. Spontaneous osteonecrosis. Prominent marrow edema is present within the medial femoral condyle on T_1- (*A*) and fat-suppressed T_2-weighted (*B*) coronal images. Collapsed subchondral bone results in hypointensity (*arrows*) above the articular surface on both imaging sequences.

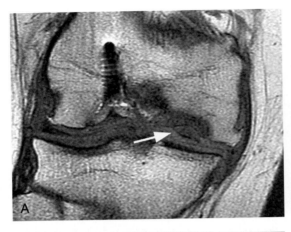

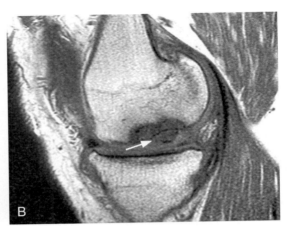

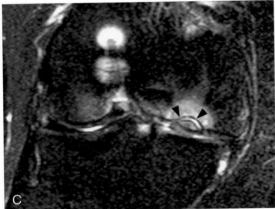

FIGURE 13–25. Osteochondritis dissecans. An osteochondral fragment (*arrows*) from osteochondritis dissecans is readily apparent on T_1-weighted coronal (*A*), T_1-weighted sagittal (*B*), and fat-suppressed T_2-weighted coronal (*C*) images of the knee. The rim of hyperintense fluid (*arrowheads*) on the T_2-weighted coronal image is considered an indicator of lesion instability.

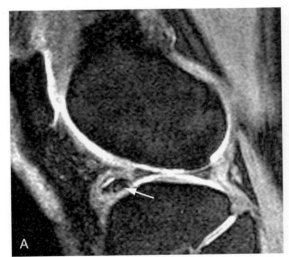

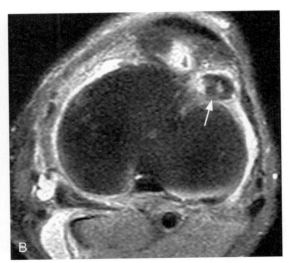

FIGURE 13–26. An ossified loose body (*arrows*) is apparent along the anterolateral aspect of the joint on T_2*-weighted sagittal (*A*) and fat-suppressed proton density-weighted (*B*) axial images.

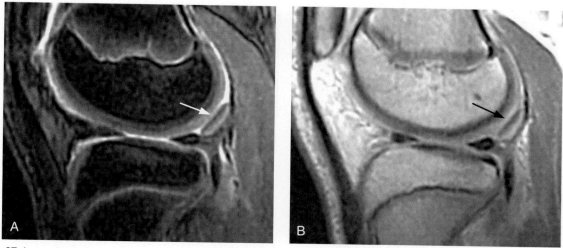

FIGURE 13–27. Loose body (cartilaginous). T_2*- (A) and proton density-weighted sagittal (B) images demonstrate a cartilaginous loose body (*arrows*) along the posterior aspect of the lateral femoral condyle.

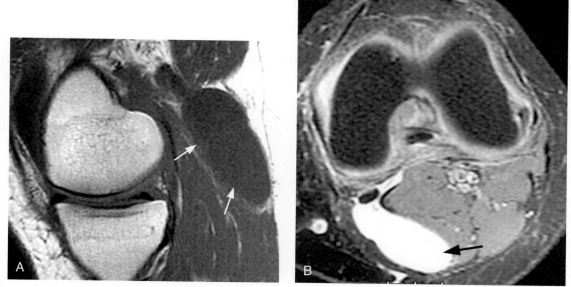

FIGURE 13–28. A popliteal (Baker's) cyst (*arrows*) in its typical location posterior to the medial head of the gastrocnemius muscle is apparent on T_1-weighted sagittal (A) and fat-suppressed proton density-weighted axial (B) images.

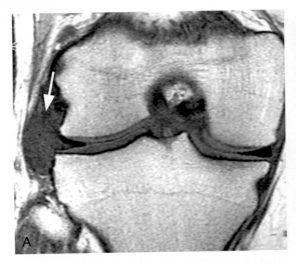

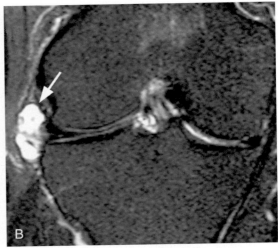

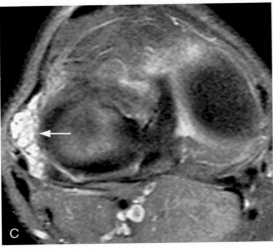

FIGURE 13–29. Meniscal cyst. *A,* A T₁-weighted coronal image reveals a horizontal cleavage tear of the lateral meniscus that decompresses into a parameniscal cyst (*arrow*) at the lateral joint line. The cyst (*arrow*) has a lobulated and hyperintense appearance on the corresponding fat-suppressed T₂-weighted coronal (*B*) and proton density-weighted axial (*C*) images.

Effusions can accompany knee injuries or be an isolated finding. Like other fluid, effusions have intermediate signal intensity on T₁-weighted scans and increased signal intensity on T₂-weighted scans. An exception is a bloody effusion (which can occur in hemophilia or after trauma). These have high signal intensity on T₁-weighted images.

Chondromalacia Patella

Chondromalacia patella is a common cause of patellofemoral pain, primarily affecting adolescents and young adults. Most often, the cause is repeated minor trauma or an acute traumatic event leading to damage of the posterior patellar hyaline articular cartilage. MRI is effective in diagnosing chondromalacia patella; findings correlate well with arthroscopy.

The normal patellar hyaline cartilage conforms to the posterior aspect of the patella, completely covers the posterior cortical bone, and has a smooth surface. Various degrees of abnormality can be seen on MRI in chondromalacia patella. Early findings include focal regions of swelling, with areas of low signal intensity on T₁-weighted and T₂-weighted images in the patellar cartilage. Later, irregularity of the articular cartilage surface and focal sites of thinning can be seen. In the final stage, absence of the cartilage exposes the subchondral bone. Occasionally, high-signal-intensity synovial fluid can be identified passing through the cartilage defect toward the bone surface on T₂-weighted images. To evaluate the patellar cartilage properly, axial and sagittal images must be obtained.

Pigmented Villonodular Synovitis

Pigmented villonodular synovitis (PVNS) is an uncommon disorder of unknown cause. The two best accepted theories for PVNS are that it represents either a chronic inflammatory response to an unknown, nontraumatic irritant or a benign neoplasm of synovial or fibrohistiocytic origin. Pathologically, PVNS consists of villous or nodular hyperplasia of the synovium, with hemosiderin and lipid deposition. PVNS occurs most commonly in the third to sixth decades of life, with an equal sexual prevalence. Presenting symptoms are progressive pain, swelling, and decreased range of motion of the involved joint. PVNS is usually a monoarticular process, occurring in the knee 80% of the time. Other joints may be involved, particularly the hip, elbow, ankle, and shoulder.

The radiographic findings in PVNS include soft tissue swelling (which often has increased density as a result of hemosiderin deposition in the synovium), subchondral cysts, cortical pressure erosions, and late joint-space narrowing. Other conditions that may be confused radiographically with PVNS are uncalcified synovial chondromatosis, tuberculous arthritis, hemophilic arthropathy, and synovial hemangiomas.

For diagnosing PVNS, classic MRI signal characteristics have been described. On T_1-weighted images, the nodules of PVNS have intermediate signal intensity, similar to or slightly higher than muscle. On T_2-weighted scans, PVNS has increased signal intensity, representing fluid and congested synovium. Most important, on T_2-weighted images there are interspersed areas of low signal intensity as a result of hemosiderin deposition (Fig. 13-30). Combining the clinical history, plain films, and MRI findings usually allows a specific diagnosis of PVNS to be made.

MRI OF THE HIP

The primary indication for MRI of the hip is the detection of early avascular necrosis (AVN). The femoral head is the most common site of AVN in the body. Early diagnosis of AVN of the hip allows appropriate treatment, with the goal of arresting or reversing the disease process before collapse of the femoral head. MRI is an ideal modality for diagnosing AVN because bone marrow changes can be detected very early in the disease process. Many studies have confirmed that MRI is the most sensitive imaging modality for detecting early AVN and is superior to radiography, radionuclide bone scans, and CT.

Technique

Images of the hip are obtained with the patient supine in the MRI scanner, using the body coil as both trans-

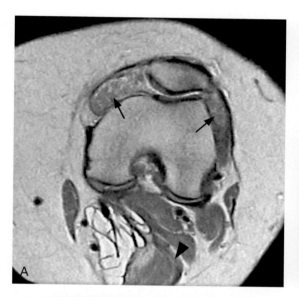
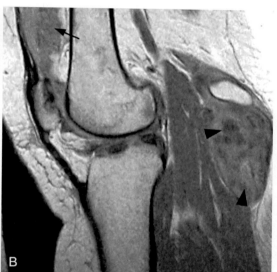
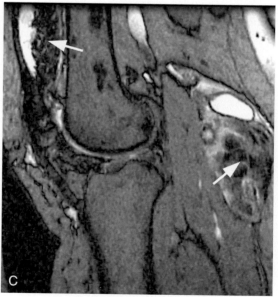

FIGURE 13–30. Pigmented villonodular synovitis. Proton density-weighted (*A*) axial and (*B*) sagittal images reveal bulky regions of intermediate signal intensity within the suprapatellar bursa (*arrows*) and within a large popliteal cyst (*arrowheads*). *C,* Central areas of low signal intensity compatible with hemosiderin deposition become more readily apparent on the T_2^*-weighted sagittal image (*short arrows*).

mitter and receiver or with a more specialized coil. Images are usually acquired in the coronal plane. Routinely, both hips are scanned simultaneously, which permits comparison of the two sides. However, if only one hip is to be scanned, images with superior SNR and resolution can be obtained using a surface coil. T_1-weighted spin echo, T_2-weighted fast spin echo, and fast short TI inversion recovery (STIR) scans are commonly acquired. Differentiation between fatty and hematopoietic bone marrow is best achieved by using a short time to repetition (TR) (400 ms) with T_1-weighted technique. Scans should be obtained with a 3- to 4-mm slice thickness, a matrix of 256×256 to 512×512, and one to two acquisitions.

Osteonecrosis

The cause of AVN can be traumatic or nontraumatic. Traumatic AVN occurs after fractures of the femoral neck, dislocation of the femoral head, or compression fractures of the femoral head, with resultant disruption of the blood supply to the femoral head. Nontraumatic AVN occurs with many conditions, including Gaucher's disease, sickle cell disease, postirradiation necrosis, caisson disease, gout, iron overload, and steroid or alcohol use, or it may be idiopathic. Idiopathic AVN in children is referred to as Legg-Calvé-Perthes disease. The pathogenesis of nontraumatic AVN is unknown, but numerous hypotheses have been proposed, including increased intraosseous pressure that impedes the local blood supply, intraosseous microemboli, and hyperlipidemia. The clinical presentation is usually hip pain, which may radiate to the groin, thigh, or knee. Patients often have increased pain with hip motion. Left untreated, the natural progression of AVN will be focal bone necrosis and repair, followed by subchondral fractures and collapse of the femoral head and severe degenerative arthritis of the hip, usually occurring in 3 to 5 years.

The stage of the disease process at diagnosis determines the treatment. If AVN is diagnosed before collapse or fracture of the femoral head, treatment consists of stress reduction (i.e., crutches, and bedrest), core decompression with or without autologous bone grafts, or an osteotomy. These treatments have arrested or reversed the disease process in some patients, preventing collapse of the femoral head and degenerative arthritis. Core decompression performed before bony fracture can decrease the intramedullary pressure and improve venous drainage and revascularization, with resultant healing. However, treatment of early AVN is still controversial. Once fracture or collapse have occurred, the process is beyond cure, and hemiarthroplasty or total hip arthroplasty are the only treatment options.

The various MRI appearances of AVN are determined by underlying pathologic events. In early AVN, there is cellular ischemia, with death of osteocytes and marrow cells, leading to bone necrosis and accumulation of necrotic debris in the intratrabecular spaces. Repair begins with the ingrowth of capillaries and undifferentiated mesenchymal cells into the necrotic marrow. The necrotic marrow is replaced by proliferating marrow. This marrow differentiates into osteoblasts, which lay down new bone over the dead trabeculae, producing a sclerotic margin. At the same time, osteoclasts are produced to remodel compact bone. During this time, there is a delicate balance between new bone formation and bone resorption. If mechanical forces, such as weight bearing, are excessive, they can overwhelm an area of weak bone and lead to subchondral fractures and subsequent bone collapse.

Before MRI, the radiographic diagnosis of AVN relied on plain film changes and radionuclide bone scans. Radiographic changes are classified as follows:

Stage 0: normal radiographic and radionuclide findings
Stage 1: normal radiographic findings
Stage 2: lucent or sclerotic changes in the femoral head
Stage 3: subchondral lucency and fracture, crescent sign
Stage 4: subchondral collapse with flattening of the femoral head
Stage 5: hip joint narrowing

The diagnosis of AVN is made on bone scans by identifying an area of decreased activity indicating absent or diminished blood supply. Later an area of increased uptake, a hot area, indicates repair and revascularization. MRI is much more sensitive to early changes of AVN than plain radiographs or bone scans. Specificity is also very high, reported in several studies to be 100%. Another method for diagnosing AVN is bone marrow pressure measurement, an invasive procedure, which has been shown to be more sensitive than MRI but with a low specificity (near 50%). Therefore, MRI is the procedure of choice for diagnosing early AVN and is particularly useful in detecting early changes in high-risk patients.

The normal femoral head has high signal intensity in the fatty bone marrow on T_1-weighted images, surrounded by a thin rim of low signal intensity representing cortical bone. The most common presentation of AVN is a focal area of decreased signal intensity in the medullary cavity on T_1- and T_2-weighted images, usually in the superolateral femoral head. Another common presentation on MRI is that of a rim of decreased signal intensity on T_1- and T_2-weighted images, with an inner zone of varying signal intensity. The dark peripheral rim is believed to represent the reactive interface between dead and viable bone, where inflammatory and fibroblastic tissue replace marrow fat, and in part may represent an area of sclerosis resulting from thickened trabecular bone.

Mitchell and colleagues correlated the MRI signal characteristics of the central lesion with the radiographic stage of disease and histopathologic findings. They devised four MRI classes of AVN. Class A had a "fatlike" MRI appearance, bright on T_1-weighted scans and intermediate signal intensity on T_2-weighted scans. This presumably corresponds to early AVN before revascularization of the central lesion. Class B had a "bloodlike" signal, bright signal intensity on T_1- and T_2-weighted images, and was the least common appearance. Class C is "water like" with low signal intensity on T_1-weighted scans and high signal intensity on T_2-weighted scans (Fig. 13-31). This occurred at early and late stages, presumably indicating inflammation or hyperemia, with

FIGURE 13–31. Bilateral avascular necrosis (AVN) is present on T_1-weighted spin echo (*A*) and (*B*) short TI inversion recovery coronal images of the hip. On the right, magnetic resonance imaging stage C AVN, demonstrating predominantly fluid signal intensity characteristics, is present. Stage A AVN, demonstrating signal characteristics of fat, is noted within the left femoral head.

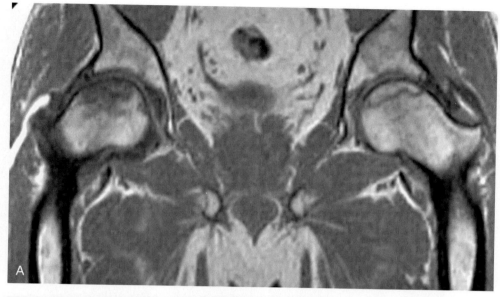

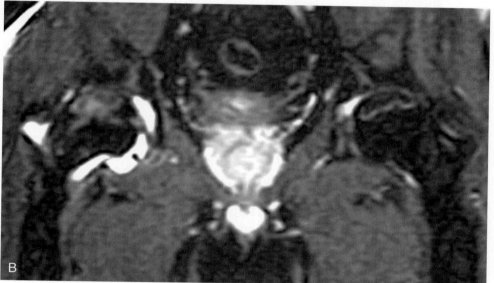

decreased lipid content of the femoral head. Class D is "fibrous like," with low signal intensity on both T_1- and T_2-weighted scans, representing advanced AVN, which is complicated by secondary fracture, with predominant fibrosis and sclerosis.

Their classification system correlated well with disease progression and radiographic staging. Early disease before fracture and collapse most often has class A MRI signal characteristics (Fig. 13-32). After fracture or collapse, most cases have class D MRI findings, with decreased signal intensity in the central lesion on T_1-weighted images. Classes B and C were not as strongly correlated with radiographic stage. Unfortunately, many cases of AVN do not fall cleanly into one of these four classes.

With very early AVN, conventional MRI sequences can be normal. Contrast enhancement with a gadolinium chelate (combined with fat suppression) can be used in this situation to detect early ischemic changes. Normal

marrow enhances rapidly as opposed to ischemic marrow, which shows no enhancement. With time (7 days or more), an enhancing zone can be identified around the ischemic zone.

Additional findings in late AVN include deformity of the femoral head after fracture or collapse. End-stage AVN will show joint space narrowing and osteophyte formation as a result of severe degenerative arthritis. After core decompression, a linear area of decreased signal intensity is seen in the femoral head at the site of the core. Because AVN is commonly bilateral, the contralateral hip must be carefully evaluated for early AVN if advanced changes are obvious in the other hip. We have had no difficulties scanning patients with unilateral arthroplasty other than local distortion of the magnetic field adjacent to the prosthesis.

Excessive joint fluid and early fatty conversion of bone marrow are common secondary findings in AVN. It has been shown that 95% of healthy patients younger than

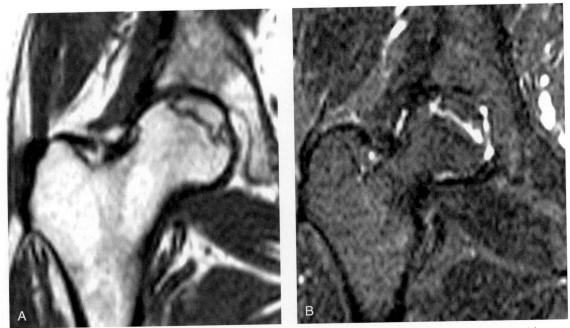

FIGURE 13–32. Magnetic resonance stage A avascular necrosis of the right femoral head is clearly seen on T_1- (*A*) and fat-suppressed T_2-weighted (*B*) images of the right hip. The large amount of the articular surface involved by the necrotic region suggests a poor prognosis for conservative therapy in this patient.

50 years have hematopoietic marrow in the intertrochanteric region of the femur compared with only 33% of patients with AVN. It is postulated that decreased marrow vascularity can hasten the conversion of hematopoietic to fatty marrow and that premature conversion to fatty marrow predisposes to AVN. Mitchell and colleagues reported that 84% of normal patients have a small amount of hip joint fluid. However, 58% of patients with AVN and only 5% of normal patients have enough fluid to surround the femoral neck or distend the joint capsule.

Transient Osteoporosis

Transient osteoporosis is a rare disease of unknown cause, most common in young or middle-aged men. The disease presents with pain (on weight bearing with a limp) and bone marrow edema. The onset is acute as opposed to AVN, which is gradual. Osteopenia is seen on radiographs 4 to 6 weeks after onset. MRI demonstrates increased signal intensity on T_2-weighted scans and decreased signal intensity on T_1-weighted scans in the femoral head and neck (Fig. 13-33). Effusions are common. Clinically, the disease resolves by 2 to 6 months; treatment is conservative (non-weight bearing).

Trauma

In recent years, MRI has replaced radionuclide scans as a method of excluding subtle hip and pelvic fractures, especially in the elderly. Insufficiency fractures are common in the pelvis, particularly in elderly osteoporotic women. Bone marrow edema is evident early after an insufficiency fracture and is seen with increased signal intensity on T_2-weighted scans and decreased signal intensity on T_1-weighted scans (Fig. 13-34). The fracture itself is low signal intensity and thus best seen on T_2-weighted or STIR sequences. Subtle fractures, including femoral neck fractures, stress fractures, and fractures not suspected (on the basis of plain radiographs; Fig. 13-35), are well defined by MRI early in the disease process. Stress fractures are also seen earlier on MRI compared with radionuclide scans; MRI is more specific as well for this diagnosis. Both T_1- and T_2- (or STIR) weighted images are required to define the fracture line (with associated edema), which may be subtle (Fig. 13-36). Resolution of stress fractures, based on MRI features, is seen by 6 to 12 months.

MRI is also the modality of choice for imaging of soft tissue injuries, whether these involve muscle, tendon, ligament, or neurovascular bundle. Injuries to thigh muscles and their pelvic attachments are common in both athletes and nonathletes. The hamstring muscles are most frequently injured (Fig. 13-37). Significant muscle injuries in the pelvic region (Fig. 13-38) are not uncommon in patients with suspected hip fractures with or without an actual associated fracture.

Another common cause of hip pain is trochanteric bursitis (Fig. 13-39). Clinical exam is often sufficient for diagnosis. MRI can be useful to confirm the diagnosis and to exclude other causes. T_2-weighted scans are typically acquired in both the axial and coronal planes and clearly define the bursae involved. An additional important bursa, which can also cause clinical symptoms and hip pain when inflamed, is the iliopsoas bursa (Fig. 13-40). This lies beneath the iliopsoas muscle as it crosses the anterior surface of the hip joint. Inflamed bursae should not be mistaken for neoplastic disease.

Pediatric Disorders

Legg-Calvé-Perthes disease is an ischemic disease of the femoral head seen most commonly in boys between the

Text continued on page 410

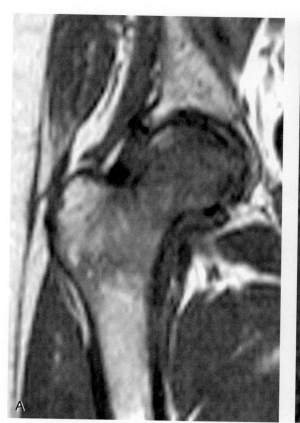

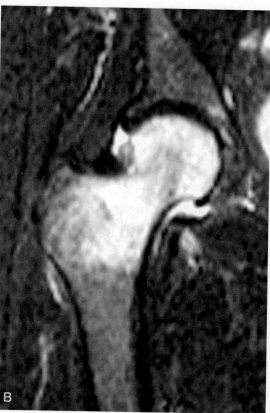

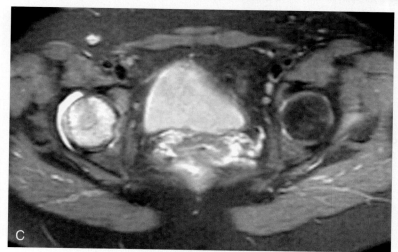

FIGURE 13–33. Transient osteoporosis of the hip. The hallmark of transient osteoporosis on magnetic resonance imaging is the presence of marrow edema. In this case of transient osteoporosis, there is extensive edema within the right femoral head and neck seen on the T_1-weighted coronal image (*A*) as abnormal low signal intensity and on fat-suppressed T_2-weighted coronal (*B*) and fat-suppressed proton density-weighted axial (*C*) images as abnormal high signal intensity.

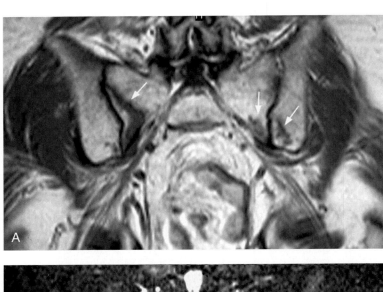

FIGURE 13–34. Sacral and iliac insufficiency fractures. Linear signal abnormalities (*arrows*) on the T_1-weighted coronal image (*A*) with corresponding areas of striking marrow edema (*arrows*) on fat-suppressed T_2-weighted coronal (*B*) and axial (*C*) images are present in this elderly female with insufficiency fractures involving the sacrum and left iliac wing.

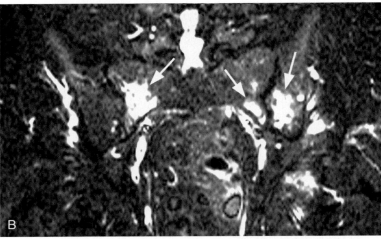

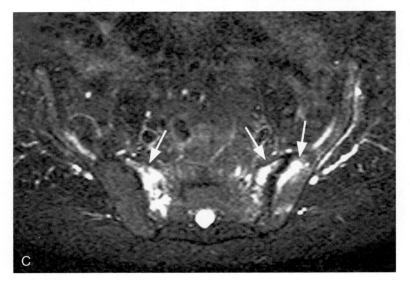

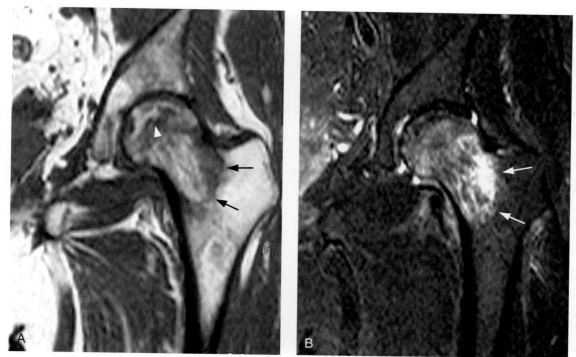

FIGURE 13–35. Occult femoral neck fracture. Plain films were normal in this case of an occult intertrochanteric fracture of the left femoral neck. *A*, T$_1$-weighted coronal image reveals the linear fracture (*arrows*), whereas the fat-suppressed T$_2$ weighted (*B*) image demonstrates intense marrow edema (*arrows*). Incidental avascular necrosis of the femoral head (*arrowhead*) is also apparent.

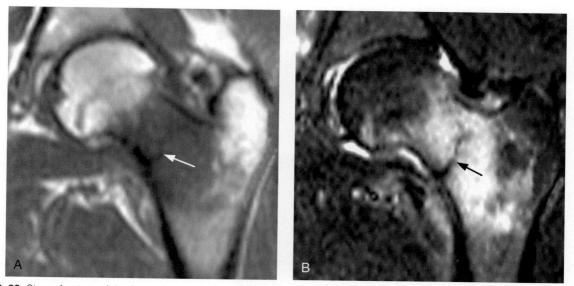

FIGURE 13–36. Stress fracture of the femoral neck. A stress fracture of the left femoral neck results in a linear signal abnormality (*arrow*) perpendicular to the medial cortex on T$_1$-weighted (*A*) and fat-suppressed T$_2$-weighted coronal (*B*) images of the left hip. Prominent surrounding marrow edema is also present.

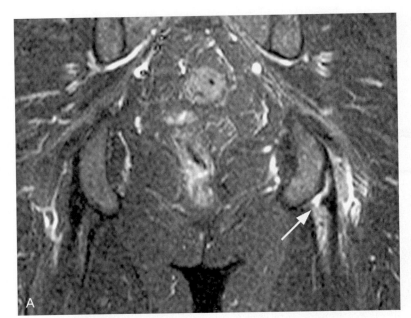

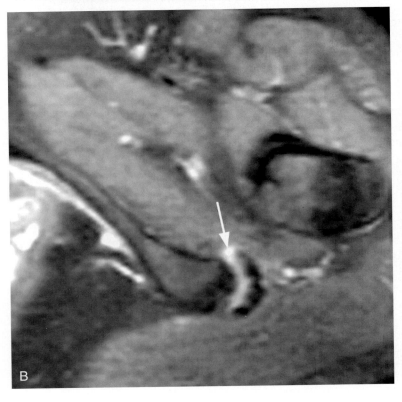

Figure 13–37. An avulsion of the hamstring tendon from the ischial tuberosity (*arrow*) is identified on fat-suppressed T$_2$-weighted coronal (*A*) and fat-suppressed proton-density axial (*B*) images of the pelvis.

FIGURE 13–38. Muscle strain of the hip. Striking edema from a strain of the gluteus minimus muscle (*arrows*) is apparent on fat-suppressed T$_2$-weighted coronal (*A*) and proton density-weighted axial (*B*) images.

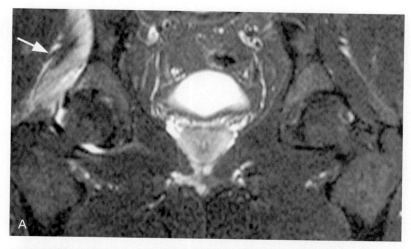

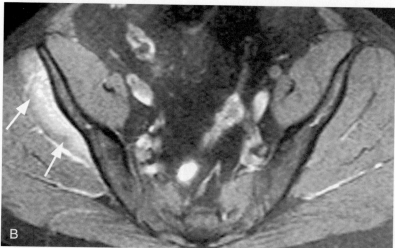

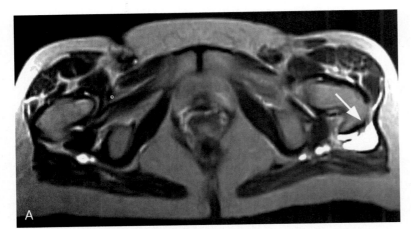

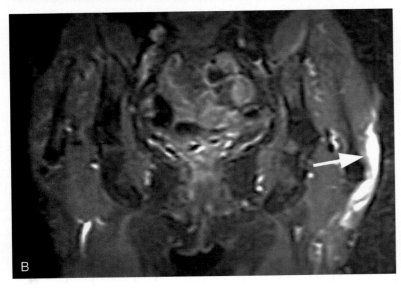

FIGURE 13–39. Trochanteric bursitis. A hyperintense fluid collection (*arrow*) is seen adjacent to the left greater trochanter on T$_2$-weighted axial (*A*) and short TI inversion recovery coronal (*B*) images of the hip.

FIGURE 13–40. Severe, chronic iliopsoas bursitis. Lobulated fluid (*arrows*) distends the iliopsoas bursa on T_1-weighted axial (*A*) and fat-suppressed T_2-weighted coronal (*B*) views.

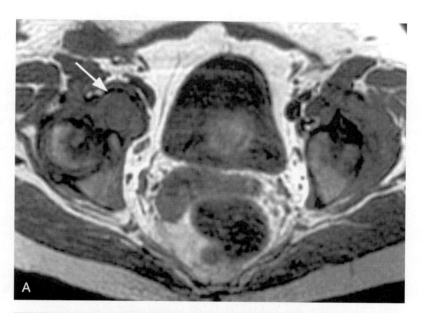

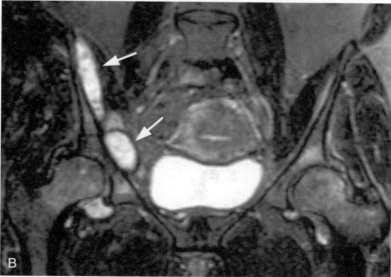

ages of 5 and 8 years. The disease is usually unilateral. Without intervention, the femoral head remodels with variable deformity leading long term to degenerative hip disease. Radionuclide scans and MRI are more sensitive for early disease detection than plain radiographs. MRI is superior to radionuclide scans because of better depiction of osseous and articular anatomy. The femoral head has been divided into central and peripheral zones for classification purposes; more severe disease involves the peripheral zones.

The most common hip disorder in adolescent patients is slipped capital femoral epiphysis (Fig. 13-41). The disease is a frequent cause of early osteoarthritis. The disease is bilateral in about a third of patients. Clinical presentation is with pain and a limp. The disease is staged as preslip, acute, or chronic. During the preslip stage, there is mild widening of the physis, but a slip is not apparent. The slip, once it occurs, is classified as mild, moderate, or severe depending on the degree of displacement. Plain film diagnosis is clearly established. MRI is reserved for evaluation in the preslip phase when radiographic findings are subtle, to exclude bilateral involvement, and to evaluate complications.

SHOULDER MRI

The painful shoulder is a common clinical problem with numerous potential causes such as subacromial bursitis, adhesive capsulitis, arthritis, and the various stages of the impingement syndrome, including complete or partial rotator cuff tears and tendinitis. The clinical examination is limited in differentiating these entities. Plain radiographs are helpful for diagnosing calcific tendinitis and arthritis, but they are poor for evaluating the rotator cuff. Arthrography, ultrasonography, and CT arthrography have been used to evaluate the rotator cuff with relative success. However, arthrography and CT arthrography are invasive procedures and are poor at diagnosing partial rotator cuff tears. Ultrasonography is exceedingly operator dependent and can be limited by bone interference. MRI is well suited for the evaluation of the shoulder because it has excellent soft tissue contrast, multiplanar capability, no bone artifacts and no ionizing radiation and is noninvasive.

Technique

MRI of the shoulder, first reported in 1986, has gained widespread acceptance as a primary imaging modality for the shoulder. The use of a dedicated surface or extremity coil is essential to obtain adequate SNR and spatial resolution. Oblique nonorthogonal imaging planes are also required to optimally visualize the rotator cuff.

Initially, axial thin sections using gradient echo technique to highlight the labrum are obtained from the level of the acromion to the inferior aspect of the glenoid. The axial images are then used to position the subsequent oblique scan planes. Two oblique planes are acquired: one parallel to the surface of the glenoid cavity (parasagittal) and another perpendicular to the surface of the glenoid cavity, oriented along the axis of the supraspinatus muscle (paracoronal). Usually, T_1- and T_2-weighted scans are acquired in both planes. However, the T_1-weighted scan is less important and may be obtained in only one plane. The use of fast spin echo technique for acquisition of the T_2-weighted scans is standard; however, this technique is best used with fat saturation. Another option in terms of general approach is performing double echo T_2-weighted scans in both oblique planes, eliminating the T_1-weighted scans. Slice thickness should be 4 mm or less, with the scan matrix 256×256 or greater. The patient should be supine, with the arm at the side in a neutral position and thumb up.

Anatomy

The rotator cuff is composed of four muscles. The supraspinatus, infraspinatus, and the teres minor muscles arise from the scapula, and their tendons insert on the greater tuberosity of the humerus. The subscapularis tendon inserts on the lesser tuberosity. Because only 33% of the humeral head is in contact with the surface of the glenoid, joint stability relies heavily on the integrity of the muscles, tendons, ligaments, and joint cartilage.

The articular surface of the glenoid cavity and the humeral head are lined by hyaline cartilage, which has intermediate signal intensity on T_1- and T_2-weighted images. The glenoid labrum and articular surface of the acromioclavicular (AC) joint are composed of fibrocartilage, which has low signal intensity on all conventional spin echo pulse sequences. The rotator cuff tendons normally have low signal intensity and can be difficult to separate from the adjacent cortical bone of the humeral head.

Axial scans optimally show the relationship between the humeral head and the glenoid cavity. The tendon of the long head of the biceps, the bicipital groove (which contains this tendon), the glenoid labrum, and the axillary neurovascular bundles are easily seen on the axial images. The oblique plane parallel to the glenoid cavity (i.e., parasagittal) demonstrates the glenoid, coracoid process, and the muscles and tendons of the rotator cuff in cross-section.

The oblique plane perpendicular to the glenoid cavity (i.e., paracoronal) best demonstrates the rotator cuff muscles and tendons. The acromioclavicular (AC) joint, coracoid process, and subacromial and subdeltoid bursae are also seen. Normally, the subacromial and subdeltoid bursae are potential spaces, and only their fat pads are visualized. These appear as thin straight bands of high signal intensity, located between the rotator cuff tendons and the AC joint and deltoid muscle. The paracoronal plane is optimal for visualizing rotator cuff tears and for other manifestations of the impingement syndrome. The parasagittal plane is an excellent second plane for detecting rotator cuff tears.

Impingement Syndrome and Rotator Cuff Abnormalities

MRI is well suited for evaluating the shoulder impingement syndrome. In this condition, pain occurs during

FIGURE 13–41. Slipped capital femoral epiphysis. The left proximal femoral physis (*arrow*) is abnormally widened and demonstrates abnormal alignment on T₁-weighted spin echo (*A*) and short TI inversion recovery (*B*) coronal images. Marrow edema and a reactive joint effusion are apparent on the STIR exam.

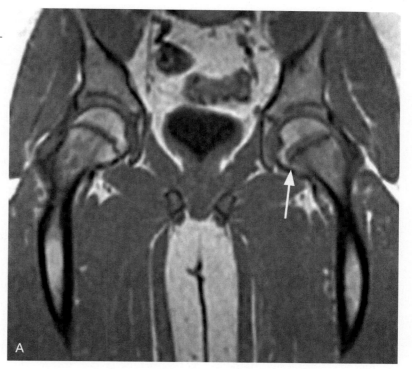

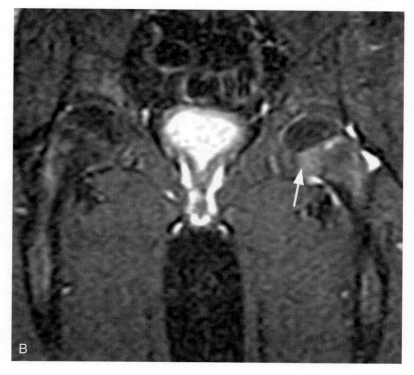

abduction and external rotation of the arm. The pathophysiology of this syndrome is entrapment of soft tissue, usually the supraspinatus tendon or the long head of the biceps tendon, between the humeral head and the anterior part of the acromion, AC joint, or the coracoacromial ligament. This can cause bursitis, rotator cuff tendinitis, fibrosis, and tearing of the rotator cuff. Neer postulated that 95% of rotator cuff tears are the result of chronic impingement on the supraspinatus tendon.

Impingement can occur as a result of degenerative disease and other abnormalities of the coracoacromial arch. The latter is composed of the clavicle, acromioclavicular arch, anterior acromion, coracoid, and coracoacromial ligament. Abnormalities in any of the components of the arch (osseous, ligamentous [Fig. 13-42], or soft tissue) may cause impingement. Degenerative changes include subacromial bone proliferation, spurring, or capsular hypertrophy at the inferior AC joint

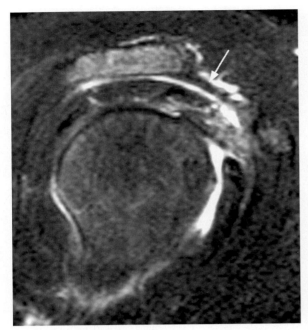

FIGURE 13–42. Impingement. A fat-suppressed T$_2$-weighted sagittal image reveals a hypertrophied coracoacromial ligament (*arrow*).

overuse of the shoulder and who develop hemorrhage and edema in the supraspinatus tendon. This stage is reversible, and it is treated conservatively. Stage II typically occurs in patients 25 to 40 years old who had repeated episodes of minor trauma leading to fibrosis and thickening of the rotator cuff and subacromial bursa. Stage III occurs most often in patients older than 40 years and manifests as a complete rotator cuff tear. Patients with stage III injuries require surgical correction. The goal of MRI is to diagnose impingement at stages I and II before a complete rotator cuff tear has occurred and to detect and quantify cuff tears to aid surgical planning.

MRI accurately detects rotator cuff tears. The most common site for a rotator cuff tear is a hypovascular zone located approximately 1 cm proximal to the site of insertion of the supraspinatus tendon on the greater tuberosity. Before MRI, radiographic evaluation of impingement syndrome and rotator cuff tear had limited success. Plain films are unreliable early, with the classic findings of decreased space (<7 mm) between the acromion and the humeral head and a high position of the humeral head only occurring late in the disease process. Arthrography and CT arthrography cannot detect stage I or II lesions.

The ability to differentiate tendinitis/tendinosis, partial tears, and small full-thickness tears may not always be possible because these entities represent a continuum of disease, and their MRI appearances overlap. The necessity of distinguishing these entities depends on the treatment philosophy of the referring orthopedist. From the work of Carrino, grade 1 tendons have increased signal intensity on T$_1$- or proton density-weighted scans 1 cm from the insertion. These changes do not increase or are less obvious on T$_2$-weighted scans. Grade 2 tendons (tendinitis/tendinosis) have increased signal inten-

(Fig. 13-43), and spurring of the humeral head. Acromial configuration (type 1 straight, type 2 curved, type 3 hooked) and anterior or lateral angulation of the acromion can also cause impingement (Figs. 13-44 and 13-45). Rarely, the impingement syndrome is due to a tumor or other mass. Neer believed that rotator cuff injuries represent a continuum of disease that progresses through three stages. Stage I usually occurs in patients younger than 25 years who have a history of acute

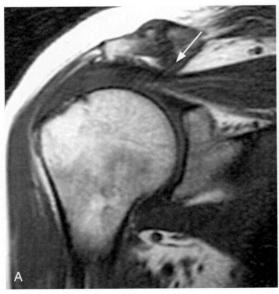

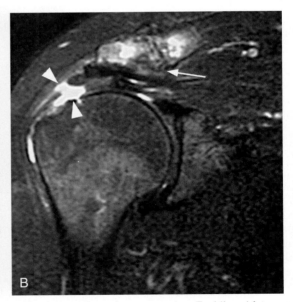

FIGURE 13–43. Impingement. Prominent acromioclavicular joint hypertrophic changes (*arrow*) are present on T$_1$- (*A*) and fat-suppressed T$_2$-weighted coronal (*B*) views of the shoulder. Mass effect on the musculotendinous junction of the supraspinatus is present, and a small full-thickness tear (*arrowheads*) is evident on the T$_2$-weighted image.

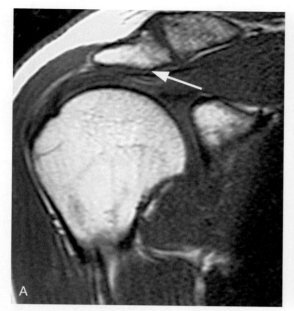 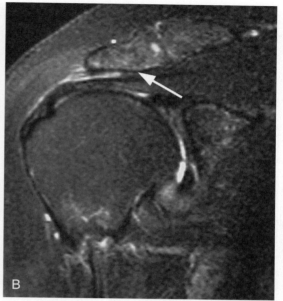

Figure 13–44. Impingement. An inferior offset of the acromion (*arrow*) relative to the distal clavicle is present on T_1- (*A*) and fat-suppressed T_2-weighted (*B*) images, resulting in decreased space for the underlying rotator cuff, thus predisposing this patient to impingement syndrome.

sity on T_2-weighted scans (Fig. 13-46), but this does not involve the inferior or superior surface of the tendon, thus not meeting the criteria for a partial tear. At this stage, high signal intensity on T_2-weighted images representing fluid should not be seen in the subacromial or subdeltoid bursa. The high-signal-intensity fat pad of

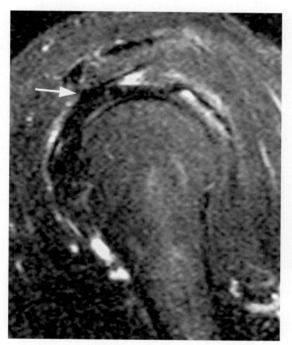

Figure 13–45. Impingement. A fat-suppressed T_2-weighted sagittal image reveals a case of positive acromial slope, in which the anterior edge (*arrow*) of the acromion lies significantly inferior to the posterior edge.

these bursae should be seen on T_1- and proton density-weighted images. The diagnosis of a partial tear is made when, in addition to the findings seen in tendinitis, there is abnormal high signal intensity on the T_2-weighted scan involving either the inferior or superior surface of the rotator cuff (Fig. 13-47). A potential pitfall is that a previous site of steroid or local anesthesia injection can also appear as a bright area on T_2-weighted images. The diagnosis of a small full-thickness tears is made when there is abnormal increased signal intensity on the T_2-weighted scan in the full thickness of the tendon (Fig. 13-48). Long term, the tear may fill in with scar or granulation tissue. There may be accompanying fluid in the subacromial and subdeltoid bursae, presumably representing extension of intra-articular fluid through the cuff tear into the bursa. Full-thickness tears may spare a few fibers of the tendon, involve the full thickness of the tendon without retraction, or be associated with retraction (Fig. 13-49).

Other findings seen on MRI in the impingement syndrome are spurs off the inferior acromion or AC joint, capsular hypertrophy of the AC joint, inferior displacement of the anterior acromion with respect to the distal clavicle, and pressure effect on the supraspinatus muscle or tendon. After massive rotator cuff tears, inactivity and instability of the shoulder, along with leaking of synovial fluid, can produce atrophy of the glenohumeral articular cartilage and resorption of subchondral bone, ultimately causing humeral head collapse. Another late finding is atrophy of the rotator cuff, which presents as decreased muscle bulk and increased signal intensity within the muscles on T_1-weighted images as a result of fatty infiltration. Timely acromioplasty can retard the progression of rotator cuff deterioration, and early diagnosis with MRI should facilitate appropriate therapy before the disease progresses to an irreversible stage.

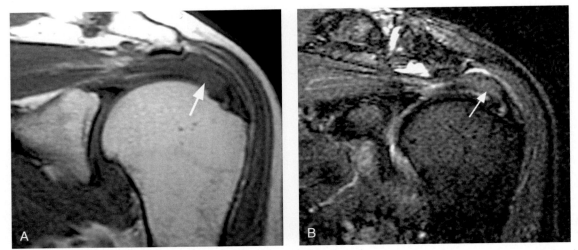

FIGURE 13–46. Rotator cuff tendinosis. The supraspinatus tendon (*arrow*) appears thickened and demonstrates increased signal intensity within its substance on T₁- (*A*) and fat-suppressed T₂-weighted coronal (*B*) images.

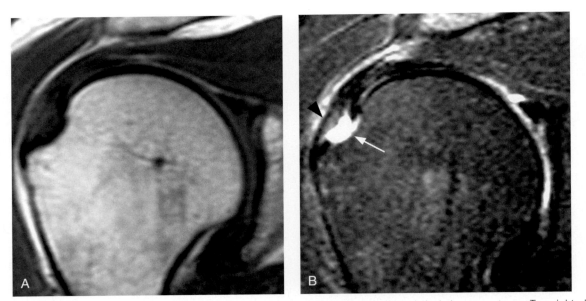

FIGURE 13–47. Partial rotator cuff tear. *A,* A partial articular surface tear of the rotator cuff is relatively inapparent on a T₁-weighted coronal image. *B,* On the fat-suppressed T₂-weighted coronal view, the partial tear (*arrow*) is readily apparent as a region of marked hyperintensity. Preserved bursal surface fibers (*arrowhead*) are evident.

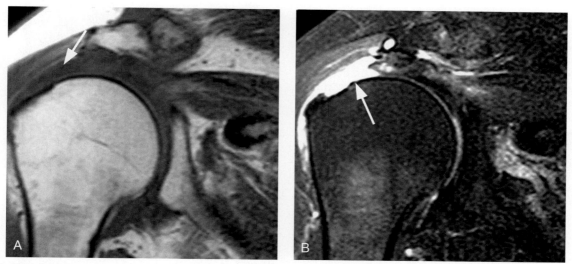

FIGURE 13–48. Full-thickness tear. *A*, On the T$_1$-weighted coronal image, a full-thickness tear (*arrow*) of the supraspinatus tendon demonstrates diffusely decreased signal intensity. *B*, The fluid-filled gap of the tear (*arrow*) is much more apparent on the corresponding fat-suppressed T$_2$-weighted coronal view.

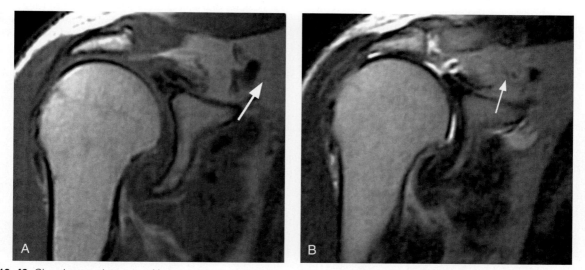

FIGURE 13–49. Chronic complete tear with retraction. T$_1$- (*A*) and T$_2$-weighted (*B*) coronal images demonstrate a massive, chronic full-thickness rotator cuff tear. The humeral head is high riding, contacting the undersurface of the acromion. Severe atrophy of the supraspinatus muscle is present; very few residual muscle fibers are seen in the expected location of the supraspinatus (*arrow*).

Occasionally, the long head of the biceps tendon is injured in the impingement syndrome as it travels with the supraspinatus tendon under the anterior acromion. The tendon is best evaluated in the axial plane. MRI can help by showing disruption of the tendon and the location of the tendon break.

Instability

The glenohumeral joint is the most mobile joint in the body; therefore, it is also the most unstable joint. The surrounding soft tissues, consisting of the glenoid labrum, synovium, joint capsule, and the rotator cuff muscles and tendons, are vital to joint stability. Instability of the joint most often causes anterior dislocation, pain, weakness, and decreased range of motion. Anterior dislocation can cause tearing of the anterior glenoid labrum and anterior joint capsule.

The capsular structures of the joint are best evaluated by MRI arthrography (Fig. 13-50), which is performed immediately followed by direct injection of a small amount of very dilute contrast media (gadolinium chelate). MRI arthrography is a topic beyond this textbook. There are many excellent articles and specialty texts that cover this technique and film interpretation in detail. On a routine shoulder evaluation obtained without injection of the joint, the thin-section axial gradient echo images provide a survey of the capsular structures. If a joint effusion is present, these scans can be even more informative. Anatomic variations in the labrum are common and can create confusion. The most frequent configuration is a triangular anterior and posterior labrum. Although less frequent, either labral structure may be rounded in appearance. Most authors believe that this is more common posteriorly. A small cleft is normally seen between the labrum and the adjacent articular cartilage. The labrum normally has low signal intensity on all pulse sequences. The MRI appearance of glenoid labrum tears (Figs. 13-51 and 13-52) can manifest as attenuation, irregularity, and indistinct borders of the labrum. Abnormal diffuse or linear areas of increased signal in-

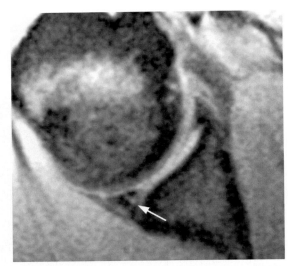

FIGURE 13–51. Labral tear. A T_2*-weighted axial image (obtained without administration of contrast) reveals a vertical tear (*arrow*) of the posterior glenoid labrum.

tensity may also be seen within the substance of the glenoid labrum on T_1- and T_2-weighted images. The term SLAP refers to superior labral tear with anterior and posterior extension (Fig. 13-53). SLAP lesions have been categorized into many different types, although there is no evidence that this categorization provides improved prognostic information. SLAP lesions are associated with rotator cuff tears and anterior instability in up to 25% of all patients and generally respond to arthroscopic repair.

Recurrent dislocation can produce bony lesions, the Hill-Sachs deformity and the Bankart lesion. Hill-Sachs deformity produces an abnormal contour of the lateral aspect of the humeral head at the level of the coracoid

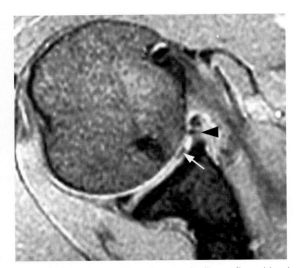

FIGURE 13–52. Labral tear. An arthroscopically confirmed bucket-handle tear of the anterior glenoid labrum is seen on a T_2*-weighted axial image (obtained without administration of contrast). A small, displaced labral fragment (*arrow*) is evident within the joint, and the residual anterior labrum (*arrowhead*) is abnormally small.

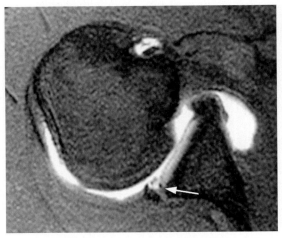

FIGURE 13–50. Labral tear. The posterior glenoid labrum has an ill-defined and fragmented appearance (*arrow*) on a fat-suppressed T_1-weighted axial magnetic resonance arthrographic image of a posterior labral tear.

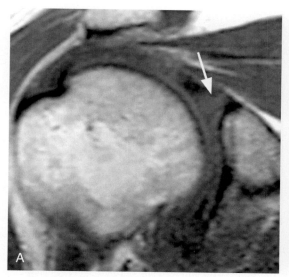 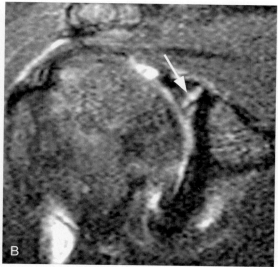

FIGURE 13–53. *A,* A SLAP (superior labral with anterior and posterior extension) lesion demonstrates diffusely increased signal intensity within the superior labrum (*arrow*) on the T_1-weighted coronal image. *B,* On the T_2-weighted coronal image, abnormal linear hyperintensity (*arrow*) undercuts the base of the superior labrum.

process. The Bankart lesion manifests as high-signal-intensity fluid along the base of the glenoid labrum or along the border of the scapula, indicative of capsular stripping. Fractures of the glenoid rim compatible with Bankart lesions can be identified.

MRI OF THE TEMPOROMANDIBULAR JOINT

The TMJ is a synovial joint that is the articulation between the mandibular condyle, the glenoid fossa, and the articular eminence of the temporal bone. Abnormalities of the TMJ occur in about one third of the adult population. These present as facial pain, joint click, or decreased range of motion of the jaw.

There are several methods for imaging the TMJ, including plain films, arthrography, and CT arthrography. Arthrography and CT arthrography are adequate techniques, but they are invasive, require specialized technical skill, and deliver a substantial radiation dose. MRI has become the preferred imaging modality for evaluating most abnormalities of the TMJ, especially the position of the meniscus (disk). MRI provides direct visualization of the meniscus, is noninvasive, has excellent soft tissue contrast, is easy to interpret, and does not use ionizing radiation. Reimbursement issues today generally dictate whether MRI of the TMJ is commonly performed in a specific radiologic practice.

Technique

To obtain the desired soft tissue resolution and SNR, images must be acquired using a surface coil. Bilateral TMJ coils, permitting simultaneous imaging of both joints, are available for most instrumentation. Spin echo pulse sequences are used for static imaging of the joint; "dynamic" studies use gradient echo technique. A standard exam includes first acquisition of sagittal spin echo

images with the mouth closed to determine the position of the meniscus. Open-mouth images are then obtained to determine whether a dislocated meniscus is reducible and to evaluate the degree of condylar translation. Images should be acquired using a T_1-weighted technique with a slice thickness of 3 mm or less, a matrix of 256×256 or greater, and a small FOV (12–16 cm). If inflammatory disease, joint fluid, or meniscal degeneration is suspected, T_2-weighted images should also be acquired. T_2-weighted scans are used to detect abnormal signal intensity in the disk or joint space and also help to assess the stage of AVN, if present, of the mandibular condyle. Strict attention should be paid to MRI technique so that images with appropriate SNR and resolution are obtained.

Functional, "dynamic" information concerning the joint can be obtained by acquiring gradient echo images at incremental stages of mouth opening (1–3 mm steps). The images are then displayed for interpretation in cine mode. When interpreting these images, however, it should be kept in mind that they simply represent a single cycle of opening and closing and that they are nonphysiologic, indeed not truly "dynamic." In some institutions, coronal spin echo T_1-weighted images are added to the standard exam to increase the accuracy in determining the disk position, specifically mediolateral displacement. Three dimensional volume gradient echo techniques are also used in some practices because the slices obtained can be thinner (1 mm) and are truly contiguous. Both joints should always be imaged because as many as 50% of patients have bilateral joint disease. The high incidence of bilateral disease suggests that the mechanical dysfunction of one side may affect the other.

Anatomy

The mandibular condyle is located anterior to the external auditory meatus. The head of the mandible articulates with the glenoid fossa and articular eminence of

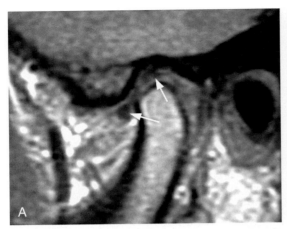
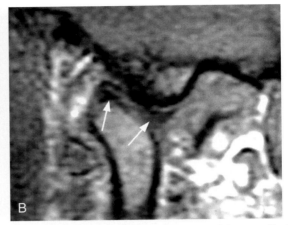

FIGURE 13–54. *A,* The normal temporomandibular joint meniscus (*arrows*) lies along the superior-anterior aspect of the mandibular condyle on a T_1-weighted sagittal closed-mouth view. *B,* With mouth opening, the mandibular condyle moves anteriorly, and the meniscus moves to the one- or two-o'clock position.

the temporal bone. The meniscus divides the joint space into upper and lower compartments. The meniscus has a biconcave configuration, with a thick anterior band, a slightly thicker posterior band, and a thin intermediate zone. The normal meniscus has lower signal intensity than the surrounding soft tissues on both T_1- and T_2-weighted images. The posterior aspect of the meniscus is attached to the retrodiscal bilaminar zone, which connects the meniscus to the temporal bone behind the condyle. The bilaminar zone contains elastic tissue and fat and has slightly higher signal intensity than the meniscus.

The lateral pterygoid muscle, located anterior to the meniscus, divides into two heads. The superior belly of the lateral pterygoid muscle inserts into the anteromedial aspect of the meniscus and applies traction on the normal meniscus during forward movement of the condyle. The inferior belly of the lateral pterygoid muscle inserts at the anatomic neck of the mandibular condyle and pulls the condyle forward during contraction.

Normal TMJ Motion

With the mouth closed, the mandibular condyle lies centered in the glenoid fossa, with the disk located between the condyle and the glenoid fossa. Normally, the posterior band of the disk lies at "12 o'clock" relative to the mandibular condyle. On opening the mouth, the mandibular condyle translates anteriorly to a position under the articular eminence of the temporal bone (Fig. 13-54). Occasionally, the mandibular condyle will translate anterior to the articular eminence in a normal TMJ. The meniscus also moves anteriorly on opening the mouth and should remain between the articular eminence and the mandibular condyle.

TMJ Dysfunction

The most common symptoms of an abnormal TMJ are facial pain, click, and decreased range of motion of the jaw. Anterior dislocation of the disk is the most common cause. In an anterior reducible dislocation (Fig. 13-55),

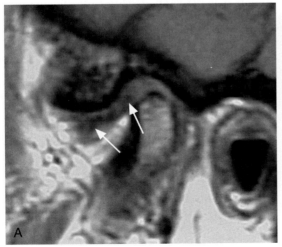
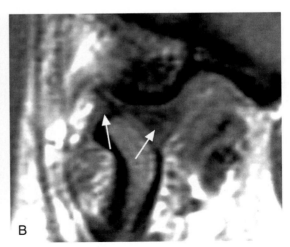

FIGURE 13–55. Anterior meniscal dislocation with reduction. *A,* The closed-mouth T_1-weighted sagittal image reveals an anteriorly displaced temporomandibular joint meniscus (*arrows*). *B,* With mouth opening, the meniscus (*arrows*) is recaptured, returning to a normal position atop the mandibular condyle.

the meniscus is located anterior to the mandibular condyle, with the condyle resting on the retrodiscal tissue in the closed position. On opening, the condyle translates anteriorly under the posterior band of the meniscus with a resultant click. The condyle then assumes a normal position, with the mandibular condyle located under the intermediate zone of the meniscus in the open-mouth position.

With a fixed (nonreducible) anterior dislocation (Fig. 13-56), the meniscus is located anterior to the mandibular condyle when the mouth is closed and often has a deformed, bunched-up appearance. In the open-mouth position, the disk remains dislocated anterior to the condyle. Often there is also mechanical obstruction to condylar translation, producing a locked condyle. Sideways displacement of the meniscus, most often medially, commonly accompanies anterior displacement of the meniscus and advanced internal derangements of the TMJ. Coronal images can help in demonstrating medial or lateral displacement, but sagittal images are often sufficient.

It is postulated that when the disk is anteriorly displaced, the condyle articulates with the posterior attachment of the disk rather than with the disk itself. This

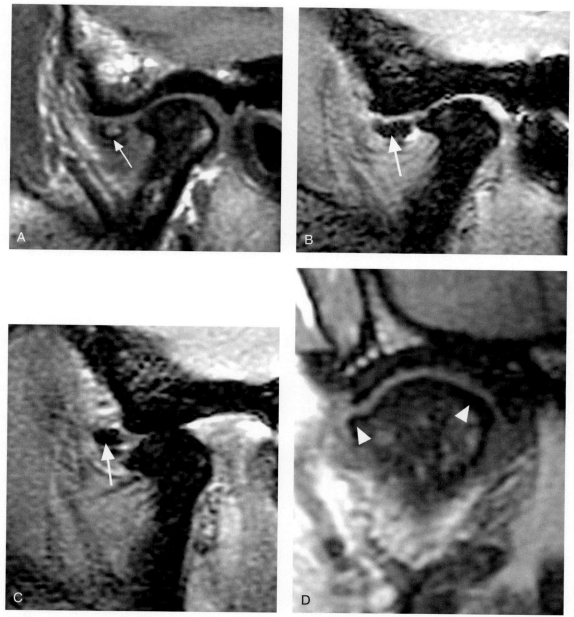

FIGURE 13–56. Anterior meniscal dislocation without reduction. T_1- (A) and T_2^*-weighted (B) sagittal images in the closed-mouth position demonstrate an anteriorly dislocated meniscus (*arrow*). The meniscus is severely degenerated and, in fact, ossified in this case and has lost normal morphology. Prominent osteoarthritic changes are evident at the joint; anterior osteophyte formation at the mandibular condyle and pronounced periarticular sclerosis are noted. C, The open-mouth T_2^*-weighted sagittal image reveals persistent anterior dislocation of the meniscus (*arrow*) and limited anterior translation of the mandibular condyle. D, The degenerative sclerosis at the joint (*arrowheads*) is readily apparent on a T_1-weighted coronal image obtained in the closed-mouth position.

leads to inflammation and often to perforation of the posterior meniscal attachment. Once perforation has occurred, the direct contact between the articular surfaces of the mandibular condyle and the temporal bone erodes the articular cartilage and causes degenerative arthritis.

Perforations of the meniscus are easily diagnosed by arthrography by demonstrating contrast entering the substance of the meniscus or contrast filling the superior joint compartment after injection of the inferior compartment. MRI has only marginal success in demonstrating perforations. Currently, only large perforations with separation of the disk fragments can be reliably demonstrated. Many smaller tears that could be seen with arthrography go undetected with MRI. One study demonstrated several false-positive perforations diagnosed by MRI. This was caused by an attenuated appearance of the stretched bilaminar zone in chronic anterior disk displacement. Because disk perforation is often a relatively late occurrence in the abnormal TMJ, the diagnosis of internal derangement of the TMJ should be based on earlier findings, such as anterior disk displacement. MRI is very accurate in determining the disk position and, therefore, has become the procedure of choice for evaluating TMJ meniscal abnormalities.

Chronic anterior disk displacement can lead to changes in the meniscus, muscles, and adjacent bony structures. Myxoid degeneration of the meniscus fibrocartilage may cause increased signal intensity in the substance of the abnormal meniscus on T_2-weighted images. Fibrosis, atrophy, and contracture of the superior belly of the lateral pterygoid muscle can occur after chronic anterior disk dislocation and present as fatty replacement (increased signal intensity on T_1-weighted images) and attenuation of the muscle. Thickening of the fascia in the inferior belly of the lateral pterygoid muscle may indicate chronic anterior disk displacement. Later, osteoarthritic changes can be seen in the mandibular condyle and along the glenoid fossa, which manifest as osteophytes and bony deformities.

Internal derangement of the TMJ may induce osteochondritis or AVN of the mandibular condyle. MRI findings of AVN include loss of the normal fatty marrow signal intensity, with resultant low signal intensity in the marrow of the mandibular condyle on T_1-weighted scans. Early and reparative AVN have increased signal intensity in the marrow on T_2-weighted scans, whereas late AVN has decreased signal intensity in the marrow. There is often associated contour deformity of the mandibular condyle. Osteochondritis presents as a focal subarticular bone defect, which often has a low signal intensity centrally, surrounded by high signal intensity on both T_1- and T_2-weighted scans.

Surgical procedures for patients with meniscal degeneration include meniscectomy, disk repositioning, lysis of adhesions, condylectomy, reduction osteotomy of the articular eminence, and replacement by autologous grafts or allografts. The postoperative TMJ is a challenge to MRI. Typically, after meniscectomy, the amputated posterior and anterior meniscal attachments are seen at the margins of the articular space. There is often some remodeling of the TMJ, with thickening of the articular cartilage surfaces of the glenoid fossa and man-

dibular condyle and often slight flattening of these structures. The articular space is maintained by the surface fibrocartilage, although often relatively narrowed, but without functional disturbance. If a prosthesis is placed, it can be identified as an area of signal void between the mandibular condyle and the temporal bone. Prostheses may fragment or fracture. Any discontinuity of the prosthesis should be interpreted as a fracture. Other complications of failed Proplast-Teflon implants include erosions, foreign body reactions, and AVN. Erosions can affect both the mandibular condyle and the temporal bone. Foreign body granulomatous reactions and AVN of the condyle are not uncommon. Either of these processes can present as decreased signal intensity in the marrow of the condyle. Granulomatous reactions often have accompanying soft tissue masses and cortical erosions. AVN is distinguished by bony deformity and collapse. Other complications after surgery include joint fluid, bony ankylosis, and adhesions, often seen as thick, fibrous connective tissue bands that are isointense with soft tissue.

MRI OF THE WRIST AND HAND

As in most other joints, high-resolution scans of the wrist or hand with adequate SNR require surface coil imaging, preferably performed at high field strength (1.0-1.5 T). Current indications for MRI of the wrist include evaluation after trauma (for both osseous abnormalities such as AVN and soft tissue injuries), soft tissue masses, infection, and carpal tunnel syndrome.

Technique

The patient should be placed in the MRI gantry with the wrist positioned in a comfortable manner to minimize motion. Surface coil imaging, typically with a flexible wrap around coil, is mandatory for adequate SNR and spatial resolution. T_1-weighted spin echo scans should be obtained in both the coronal and axial planes. Fast T_2-weighted scans should be obtained in the scan plane that best delineate the abnormality. Generally, coronal planes are best for osseous abnormalities, such as AVN, and axial planes are best for the carpal tunnel and to evaluate the extent of soft tissue masses. The exam may be supplemented with other scan techniques, such as fast STIR and 3D gradient echo scans. A small FOV is essential for attaining good spatial resolution. The slice thickness should be 3 mm or less.

Anatomy

The tendons and ligaments of the wrist usually have low signal intensity on all pulse sequences. Bone marrow has high signal intensity on T_1-weighted images because of fat, which is surrounded by low-signal-intensity cortical bone. Muscles and nerves have intermediate signal intensity on all pulse sequences.

Coronal images best show the relationship of the carpal bones to the metacarpal bones, the ulna, and the radius. The course of nerves, vessels, and tendons is also clearly visualized. The triangular fibrocartilage is seen on coronal images as a triangular region of low signal intensity on T_1- and T_2-weighted images.

The axial plane is superior for imaging the carpal tunnel. The tendons of the flexor muscles of the hand and the median nerve lie within the carpal tunnel. Carpal bones form the dorsal surface of the carpal tunnel. A ligamentous band called the flexor retinaculum forms the palmar surface. The flexor retinaculum extends medially from the hook of the hamate and pisiform bone laterally to the scaphoid and trapezium. The flexor retinaculum appears as a thin band of low signal intensity on all pulse sequences. Just deep to the flexor retinaculum are the tendons of the flexor digitorum superficialis muscles, which divide into four tendons as they pass through the carpal tunnel. Lateral and deep to these tendons is the tendon of the flexor pollicis longus muscle. Lateral to the flexor pollicis longus tendon is the flexor carpi radialis tendon, which actually lies outside and adjacent to the carpal tunnel. The deepest tendons in the carpal tunnel are the four tendons of the flexor digitorum profundus muscles, which lie deep to the flexor digitorum superficialis tendons. The tendons in the carpal tunnel have low signal intensity on all pulse sequences and are outlined by higher-signal-intensity sheaths. The median nerve usually is located against the flexor retinaculum near the second flexor digitorum superficialis tendon. The median nerve has intermediate signal intensity on all pulse sequences, paralleling that of muscle, in contrast to the low-signal-intensity tendons.

The sagittal plane is usually the least informative. It can help in evaluating the digits, especially the insertion of tendons on the phalanges. Sagittal images also offer an additional view of the relationship of the radius and ulna with respect to the carpal bones.

Pathology

Ganglion cysts are the most common "tumors" of the hand, often presenting with wrist or hand pain. Ten to 20% occur in close proximity to a major vessel, which must be avoided during aspiration. MRI can demonstrate the relationship of the ganglion to adjacent vessels and nerves (Fig. 13-57). Most ganglion cysts have typical MRI signal characteristics with intermediate signal intensity on T_1-weighted images and high signal intensity on T_2-weighted images. Often ganglion cysts splay the adjacent tendons.

AVN commonly occurs in the wrist after trauma and presents with local wrist pain. Fractures of the proximal or middle portion of the scaphoid bone often lead to AVN of the proximal pole of the scaphoid (Fig. 13-58). Minor repetitive trauma can cause AVN of the lunate bone (Kienböck's disease; Fig. 13-59) or rarely may involve other carpal bones. MRI is very sensitive for AVN and often shows abnormalities before radiographic changes. MRI is more specific for AVN than radionuclide bone scans. Marrow edema seen with AVN has abnormal low signal intensity on T_1-weighted scans compared with normal marrow and, conversely, abnormal high signal intensity on T_2-weighted scans. Fracture lines and adjacent reactive marrow have low signal intensity on T_1-weighted scans.

Radiographically occult fractures (Fig. 13-60), clearly demonstrated by MRI, have been reported in many anatomic areas, including fractures of the hook of the hamate. MRI reveals pannus formation around the carpal and interphalangeal joints in patients with rheumatoid arthritis. Acutely inflamed pannus has decreased signal intensity on T_1-weighted images and increased

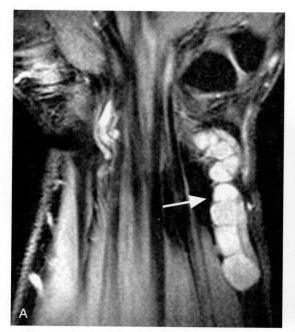
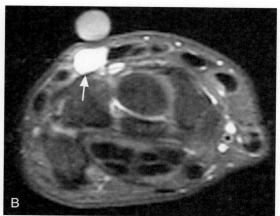

FIGURE 13–57. Ganglion cyst (wrist). Two cases of ganglion cyst formation at the wrist are illustrated. *A,* A T_2*-weighted coronal image reveals a multilobulated ganglion cyst (*arrow*) along the volar/ulnar aspect of the wrist. *B,* A fat-suppressed proton density-weighted image, from a different patient, reveals a dorsal ganglion cyst (*curved arrow*) at the level of the proximal carpal row.

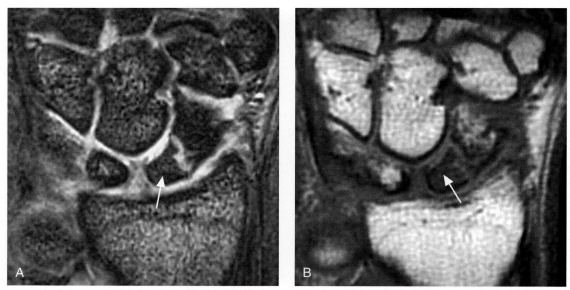

FIGURE 13–58. A fracture of the scaphoid waist resulting in avascular necrosis of the proximal pole (*arrow*) is noted on T_2^*- (*A*) and T_1-weighted (*B*) coronal images. The necrotic proximal pole demonstrates diffusely decreased signal intensity on the T_1-weighted image.

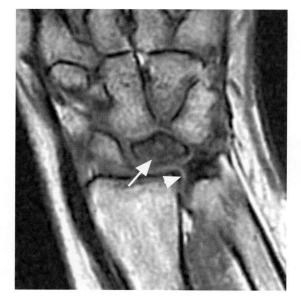

FIGURE 13–59. Wrist avascular necrosis of the lunate (Kienböck's disease). Diffusely decreased signal intensity within the marrow of the lunate (*arrow*) is apparent on a T_1-weighted coronal image. Negative ulnar variance (*arrowhead*) is also present.

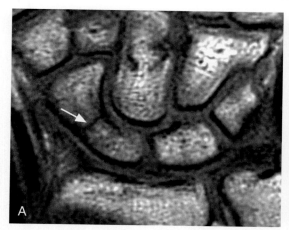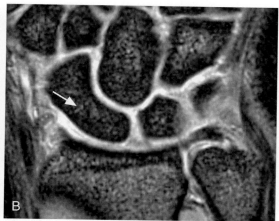

FIGURE 13–60. Occult scaphoid fracture. Plain films on this collegiate basketball player appeared normal after injury. T_1- (*A*) and T_2*-weighted (*B*) coronal magnetic resonance images subsequently obtained reveal a subtle linear signal abnormality (*arrow*) within the midscaphoid compatible with an occult scaphoid waist fracture.

signal intensity on T_2-weighted images, and chronic pannus has decreased signal intensity on both T_1- and T_2-weighted scans.

The carpal tunnel syndrome is caused by numerous pathologic conditions, including thickening and fibrosis of the flexor tendon sheaths, scar tissue, tumor compressing or involving the median nerve (Fig. 13-61), and inflammation producing swelling of the median nerve (Fig. 13-62). The normal size of the median nerve is 4.5 × 2.0 mm at the level of the pisiform bone and 4.9 × 2.1 mm at the level of the hook of the hamate. Abnormalities of the median nerve, causing the carpal tunnel syndrome, should be suspected when the median nerve measures more than two standard deviations above the mean. Increased signal intensity may be seen within the median nerve on T_2-weighted images, indicating

swelling or edema. Scar tissue, fibrosis of tendon sheaths, and tumors displacing and distorting the median nerve are easily identified with MRI. Comparison with the contralateral normal wrist can make the diagnosis easier.

Thin-section high-resolution imaging is particularly critical for demonstrating injuries of the interosseous ligaments and triangular fibrocartilage (TFC). Variations in signal intensity and configuration of these structures can be confused with partial or complete tears. Although MRI is accurate for the diagnosis of TFC tears, conventional arthrography continues to be used in many centers, given the complex anatomy and small size of the involved structures. T_2- or T_2*-weighted images are used to demonstrate tears of the TFC complex and clearly delineate these when they involve the ulnar portion (Fig.

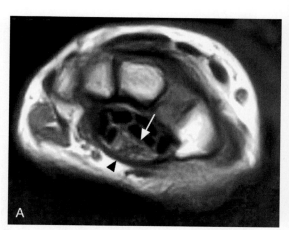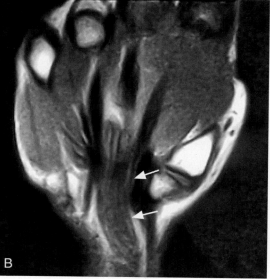

FIGURE 13–61. Carpal tunnel syndrome. Fibrolipomatous hamartoma of the median nerve, a rare but characteristic cause of carpal tunnel syndrome, is illustrated. T_1-weighted axial (*A*) and coronal (*B*) images reveal fusiform enlargement of the median nerve (*arrows*), which demonstrates heterogeneous intermediate signal intensity. The flexor retinaculum (*arrowhead*) has an outwardly bowed appearance.

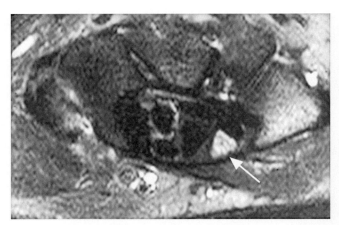

FIGURE 13–62. Idiopathic carpal tunnel syndrome. The median nerve (*arrow*) has an enlarged and edematous appearance on a fat-suppressed T₂-weighted axial image.

13-63). Defects near the radial attachment (Fig. 13-64) may be more difficult to define because of the smaller size (thickness) of the TFC complex at this level.

MRI of scapholunate (Figs. 13-65 and 13-66) and lunotriquetral ligament tears is a challenging area; accuracy rates are lower than that reported for tears of the TFC complex. If the scapholunate ligament is not seen in its entirety on high-resolution images, a tear can be implied. This rule does not apply, however, to the lunotriquetral ligament.

Tendon injuries include tears (partial or complete) and tendinitis. The latter is far more common in the wrist. The most common cause of carpal tunnel syndrome in the United States is flexor tendinitis. Tendinitis may be due to infection or overuse or the result of bone injury. The tendons are normally low signal intensity. In tendinitis, MRI may demonstrate abnormal signal intensity of the tendon or fluid surrounding it (Fig. 13-67).

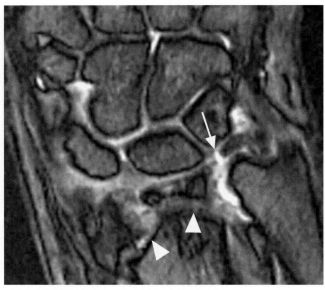

FIGURE 13–64. Triangular fibrocartilage complex lesion. A posttraumatic vertical tear (*arrow*) is evident near the radial insertion of the triangular fibrocartilage on a T₂*-weighted coronal image. A complex fracture of the distal radius (*arrowheads*) is also apparent in this case.

MRI OF THE ELBOW AND FOREARM

As with MRI of the wrist and hand, imaging of the elbow and forearm requires special attention to technique and choice of coil. Normal bone, soft tissue anatomy, and disease are clearly defined. Clinical information and, in particular, the type of disease suspected are critical in planning the MRI exam.

MRI is particularly well suited to delineate tendon injuries, which are more common in the upper than lower extremity. The most commonly injured tendon in

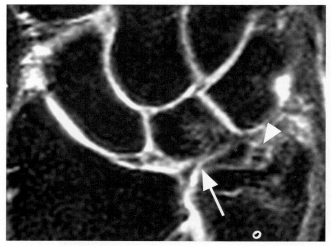

FIGURE 13–63. Triangular fibrocartilage complex lesion. A complex tear of the triangular fibrocartilage is seen on this T₂*-weighted coronal image of the wrist. Fluid extending through a central perforation (*arrow*) is noted near the radial insertion, and the ulnar insertion (*arrowhead*) has an irregular and fragmented appearance.

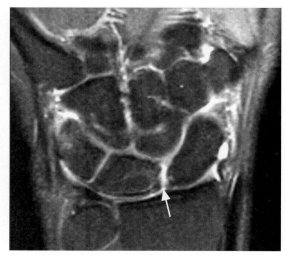

FIGURE 13–65. Scapholunate ligamentous tear. Fluid extends into the ligamentous defect (*arrow*) in this fat-suppressed proton density-weighted image depicting a radial-sided tear.

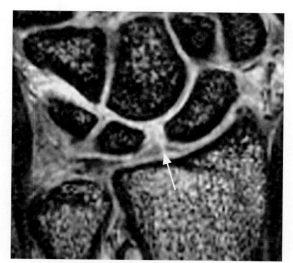

FIGURE 13–66. Scapholunate ligamentous tear. The scapholunate interval is abnormally widened on a T$_2$*-weighted coronal image of the wrist. A vertical full-thickness tear (*arrow*) near the scaphoid insertion of the scapholunate interosseous ligament is present.

from repetitive trauma or overuse (Fig. 13-69). The spectrum of MRI findings includes thickening and abnormal intermediate signal intensity in the common extensor origin, thinning (partial disruption), and complete rupture.

The ulnar collateral ligament (UCL) complex is critical for elbow stability. Athletes such as pitchers frequently injure the UCL because of excessive valgus stress. The anterior bundle of the UCL is the primary stabilizer and is best imaged in the coronal plane (Figs. 13-70 and 13-71).

Osteochondritis dissecans is the result of direct trauma to the elbow, with lateral impaction forces. Chronic lateral impaction results in a lesion of both bone and cartilage, involving the central or anterolateral surface of the capitellum (Fig. 13-72). Lesions typically occur in boys aged 12 to 15 years and occur more commonly on the dominant side. The lesion may progress to fragmentation and destruction of both articular cartilage and bone. It is important to define these changes because treatment is dictated by imaging appearance.

the elbow is the distal biceps tendon. Injuries occur at its insertion on the radial tuberosity (Fig. 13-68) from catching a heavy object with the arm flexed and supinated. In comparison, ruptures of the triceps tendon are rare. Lateral epicondylitis ("tennis elbow") involves injury to the common extensor tendon origin resulting

MRI OF THE ANKLE AND FOOT

The ankle is a commonly injured joint primarily imaged with plain radiographs or radionuclide bone scans and less commonly examined by arthrography and CT. MRI plays a limited role in evaluating ankle abnormalities, although it is very capable of delineating the complex

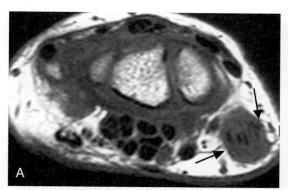

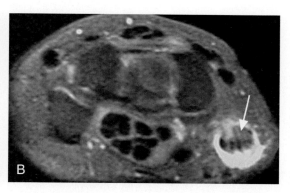

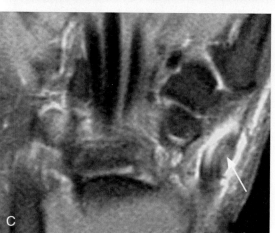

FIGURE 13–67. Tenosynovitis. The abductor pollicis longus tendon (*arrows*) is markedly enlarged and edematous in appearance on T$_1$-weighted axial (*A*), fat-suppressed proton density-weighted axial (*B*), and fat-suppressed proton density-weighted coronal (*C*) images of a case of de Quervain's tenosynovitis, one of the most common sites of tenosynovitis in the wrist. Fluid surrounding the inflamed tendon is apparent.

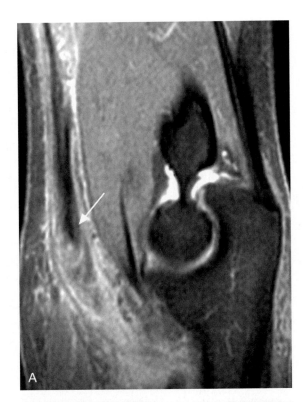

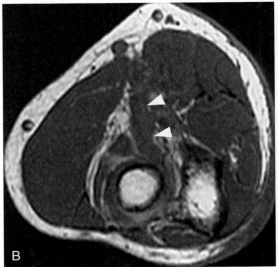

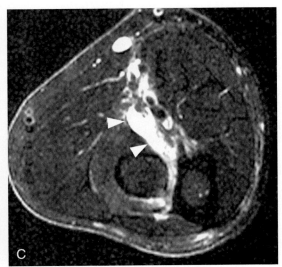

FIGURE 13–68. Biceps tendon tear. *A,* The distal biceps tendon insertion (*arrow*) is completely torn and retracted on the fat-suppressed proton density-weighted sagittal image. T_1- (*B*) and fat-suppressed T_2-weighted (*C*) axial images reveal only fluid and edema (*arrowheads*) along the expected course of the distal biceps tendon near its insertion on the radial tuberosity.

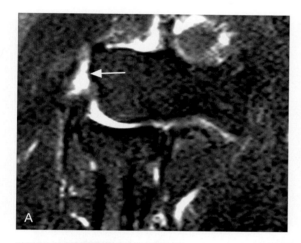

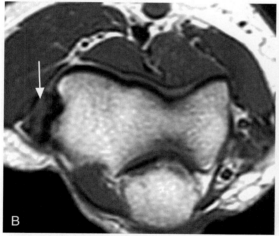

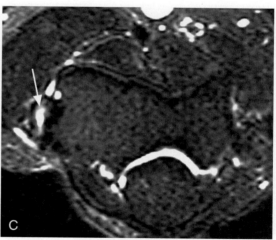

FIGURE 13–69. Lateral epicondylitis (elbow). The origin of the common extensor tendon (*arrow*) from the lateral epicondyle is thickened and edematous on fat-suppressed T_2-weighted coronal (*A*), T_1-weighted axial (*B*), and fat-suppressed T_2-weighted axial (*C*) images.

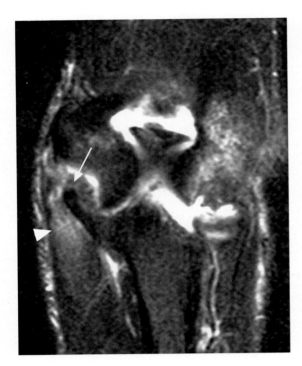

FIGURE 13–70. Ulnar collateral ligament tear. The ulnar collateral ligament is completely torn at its proximal attachment (*arrow*) on a fat-suppressed T_2-weighted coronal image. Edema is also apparent within the flexor digitorum superficialis muscle (*arrowhead*), a common ancillary finding in such cases.

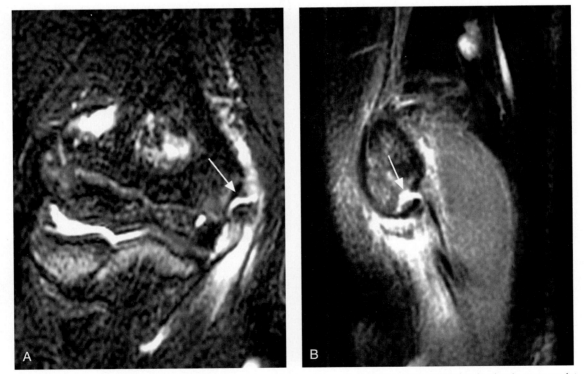

FIGURE 13–71. Ulnar collateral ligament tear. Another case of complete ulnar collateral ligament disruption is clearly seen on fat-suppressed T_2-weighted coronal (*A*) and fat-suppressed proton density-weighted sagittal (*B*) images of the elbow of an acutely injured teenage baseball player. An avulsion fracture from the medial epicondyle (*arrow*) is also apparent in this case.

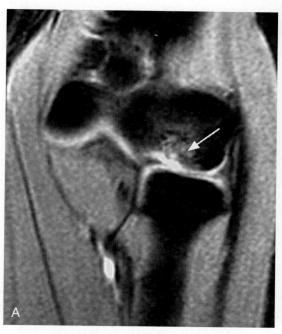

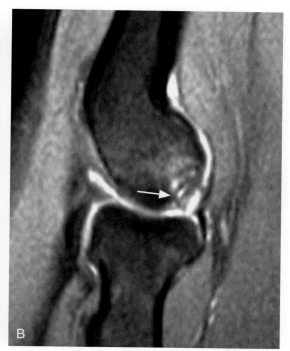

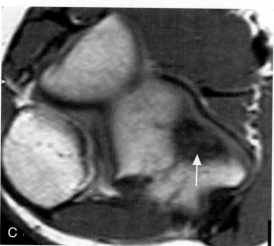

FIGURE 13–72. Osteochondritis dissecans of the capitellum. A typical case of osteochondritis dissecans of the capitellum is clearly seen on T_2^*-weighted coronal (*A*), fat-suppressed proton density-weighted sagittal (*B*), and T_1-weighted axial (*C*) images. Marrow edema and mild irregularity of the articular surface are apparent at the site of the osteochondral lesion (*arrow*).

anatomy of the ankle joint. As in other locations, MRI is useful for evaluating soft tissue masses, bone marrow abnormalities, ligaments, tendons, and articular cartilage.

Technique

The attainment of adequate SNR and spatial resolution requires the use of local coils. The ankle or foot may be placed within a small volume coil, such as the knee or head coil, with the patient lying supine in the gantry. Alternatively, a flexible wrap-around surface coil can be used. The ankle should be immobilized to minimize motion during the scan. The choice of imaging technique and plane is largely determined by the clinical question. Slice thickness should be 3 mm or less, and a small field of view should be used.

Anatomy

The excellent soft tissue contrast of MRI clearly delineates the complex anatomy of the ankle joint. The tendons and ligaments have very low signal intensity on all pulse sequences and are quite distinct because of the high signal intensity of adjacent fat. Bone marrow has increased signal intensity on T_1-weighted images and is surrounded by the decreased signal of cortical bone. Muscles have intermediate signal intensity on all pulse sequences. Hyaline cartilage also has intermediate signal intensity on most pulse sequences and is well visualized against the neighboring black (low intensity) cortical bone.

Coronal images show the relationship of the tibia and fibula to the adjoining tarsal bones, particularly the talus. The collateral ligaments are also clearly visualized on coronal images.

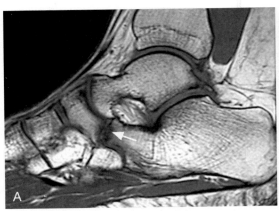
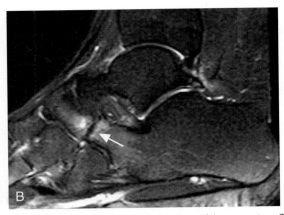

FIGURE 13–73. Tarsal coalition (calcaneonavicular). Fibrous coalition at the calcaneonavicular articulation (*arrow*) is present on T_1-weighted (*A*) and fat-suppressed T_2-weighted (*B*) sagittal images of the ankle.

Sagittal images optimally show the course of the tendons. The tibialis anterior, peroneus tertius, extensor hallucis longus, and extensor digitorum longus tendons reside anteriorly, and the peroneus longus and brevis tendons are seen laterally. Seen medially are the tibialis posterior, flexor hallucis longus, and flexor digitorum longus tendons. The Achilles tendon lies posteriorly. The tendons normally have low signal intensity on all pulse sequences. Sagittal images also demonstrate the articular surfaces of the tibia, fibula, and talus.

Axial images are useful for characterizing soft tissue masses and determining their extent. The Achilles tendon and the other ankle tendons are seen in cross-section on axial images.

Pathology

Soft tissue masses and bone tumors are well depicted by MRI along with the extent of involvement. Complex fractures and osteochondral fractures are well demonstrated by MRI. Other imaging modalities often fail to recognize the degree of abnormality, such as nonviability of a fracture fragment. AVN of the talus or other tarsal bones is not uncommon. Cartilaginous defects, thinning of the cartilage, and synovial abnormalities, as well as ligamentous injuries, may be seen on MRI. Although not frequently used in the evaluation of foot deformities, MRI is very capable of demonstrating unossified bones and developing ossification. MRI is also useful in the evaluation of patients with suspected tarsal coalition, whether fibrous (Fig. 13-73) or osseous (Fig. 13-74) in nature.

One entity unique to the ankle for which MRI has been shown to be extremely useful is injury to the Achilles tendon. The normal Achilles tendon has low (black) signal intensity on all pulse sequences with no intratendinous signal. The Achilles tendon is best visual-

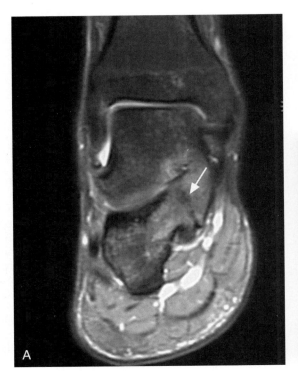

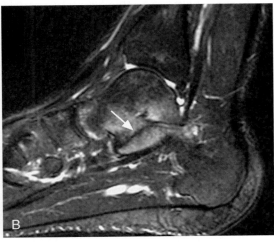

FIGURE 13–74. Tarsal coalition (talocalcaneal). Marrow edema and sclerosis (*arrow*) are present at the site of a talocalcaneal osseous coalition on fat-suppressed proton density-weighted coronal (*A*) and fat-suppressed T_2-weighted sagittal (*B*) images.

ized on sagittal and axial images. In cross-section, on axial images, the normal Achilles tendon is flat with a slight concavity anteriorly and slight convexity posteriorly. The lateral and medial margins have a rounded configuration. The incidence of Achilles tendon injuries is increasing. Injuries can be seen in joggers and gymnasts and other athletes, or after blunt trauma. The most common site of injury is 2 to 3 cm proximal to its insertion on the calcaneus.

The hallmark of an Achilles tendon injury is thickening and swelling of the tendon with or without increased intratendinous signal intensity. Acute complete tendon tears show disruption of the tendon fibers (Fig.

13-75). There are foci of increased signal intensity on T_2-weighted images adjacent to the tear, representing edema or hemorrhage. Partial tears of the tendon produce thickening of the tendon, partial discontinuity of the tendon fibers, and abnormal increased signal intensity within the tendon on T_2-weighted images and intermediate signal intensity on T_1-weighted images. Tendinitis manifests as diffuse tendon thickening (Fig. 13-76), with a rounded configuration, with or without abnormal intratendinous signal.

The other tendons of the foot and ankle, including the peroneal tendons, the medial tendons, and the anterior tendons, are also well evaluated by MRI. Of all imaging

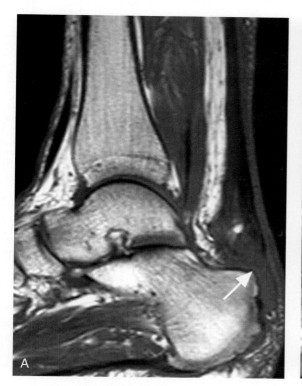
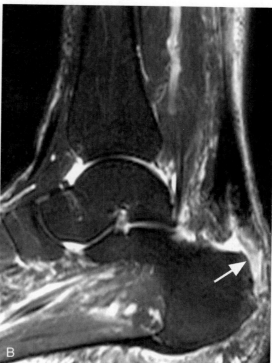
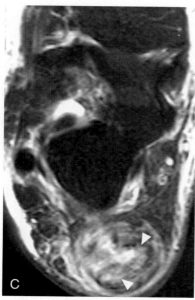

FIGURE 13–75. Achilles tendon rupture. A fluid-filled gap (*arrow*) is seen at the distal insertion of the Achilles tendon on T_1-weighted (*A*) and fat-suppressed T_2-weighted (*B*) sagittal images of a complete Achilles tendon rupture. *C,* The distal tendon is markedly thickened and edematous (*arrowheads*) on the corresponding fat-suppressed T_2-weighted axial view.

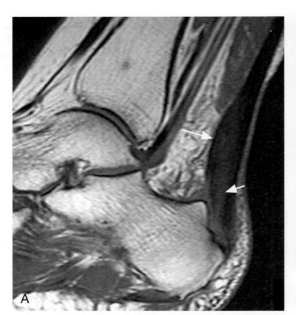 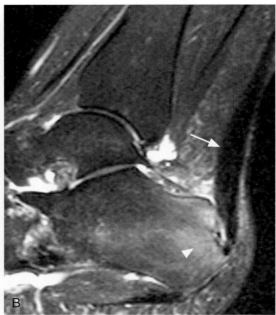

FIGURE 13–76. Chronic Achilles tendinitis. The distal Achilles tendon (*arrow*) is markedly thickened on T$_1$-weighted (*A*) and fat-suppressed T$_2$-weighted (*B*) sagittal images. Diffusely increased signal intensity is seen within the distal tendon on the T$_1$-weighted image (*short arrow*), and reactive marrow edema (*arrowhead*) is noted within the calcaneus on the fat-suppressed T$_2$-weighted image.

modalities, MRI is the most useful for the peroneal tendons because it can identify the multiple different disorders involving these structures most effectively. T$_2$- (and T$_2$*-) weighted images are typically used to delineate subtle subluxations or dislocations. Peroneal tendon tears (Fig. 13-77) are classified as degenerative, partial, and complete; the latter is uncommon. Most tears of the peroneal tendon are partial and longitudinal in configuration. As with other tendons, peroneal tendinitis causes thickening with increased signal intensity in the tendon and sheath typically, peripherally. The medial tendon group is composed of the posterior tibial, flexor digitorum longus, and flexor hallucis longus tendons. Of the three medial tendons, the posterior tibial tendon is most commonly injured (Fig. 13-78). Type 1 tears are incomplete with thickening and vertical slits. (The latter appear as scattered areas of high signal intensity on T$_2$-weighted images.) Type 2 tears are partial tears with areas of attenuation (thinning) of the tendon. Fluid surrounding the tendon can be due to tendinitis, peritendinitis, or tenosynovitis. The anterior tendons include the anterior tibial, hallucis longus, and extensor digitorum longus tendons. Injury of the anterior tibial tendon is not uncommon in runners.

Ligament injuries, like tendon injuries, can be well depicted by MRI. As with the examination of smaller tendons, thin-section imaging is critical. Care is needed to exclude false-positive findings caused by partial volume imaging. MRI can accurately detect injuries in the lateral and medial ligaments. Ligament injuries in the ankle and foot resemble ligament injuries in other areas. Grade 1 injuries have subtle increased signal intensity and slight thickening. Grade 2 injuries involve about a half thickness with more obvious signal changes and thickening. Grade 3 injuries are complete tears with

high signal intensity on T$_2$-weighted images between the two fragments (Figs. 13-79 and 13-80).

The most common cause of plantar heel pain is plantar fasciitis. Repetitive microtrauma during heel strike and prolonged pronation stresses lead to degeneration and inflammation. MRI is superior to all other modalities for diagnosing this entity and excluding other causes of posterior heel pain. T$_2$-weighted images are used for diagnosis, with demonstration of abnormal high signal intensity in or adjacent to the plantar fascia. The most common finding is perifascial edema, both superficial and deep to the plantar fascia. The second most common finding is marrow edema in the calcaneus at the insertion site (Fig. 13-81).

The sinus tarsi or tarsal canal is the hollow formed by the groove of the talus and calcaneus. The canal contains fat, neurovascular structures, and several ligaments. The sinus tarsi syndrome is most commonly caused by inversion injury. Patients present with lateral foot pain and tenderness over the tarsal canal. Identification of ligament injury is important if surgery is contemplated. On MRI, inflammatory soft tissue is seen within the canal replacing fat, with low signal intensity on T$_1$- weighted images and high signal intensity on T$_2$-weighted images (Fig. 13-82). There may also be erosions of the adjacent bones.

MUSCULOSKELETAL TUMORS, MARROW DISEASE, AND INFECTION

MRI is commonly used to detect and evaluate bone and soft tissue tumors, especially for preoperative planning.

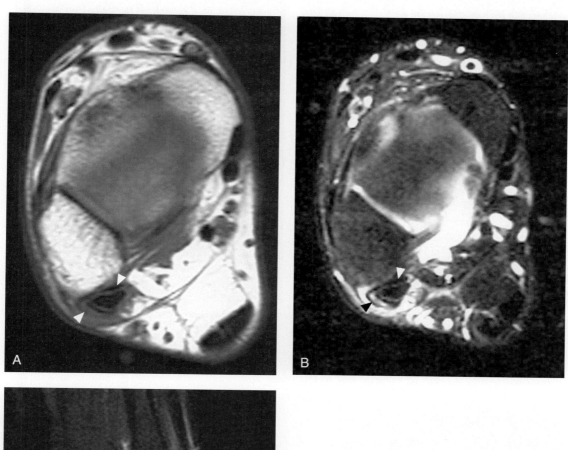

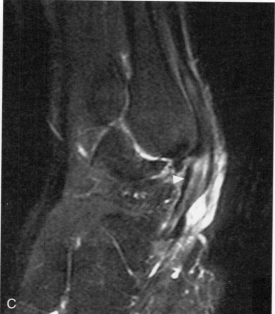

FIGURE 13–77. Peroneal tendon tear. Two separate components (*arrowheads*) of a split peroneus brevis tendon are apparent on T$_1$- (*A*) and fat-suppressed T$_2$-weighted axial (*B*) images at the level of the lateral malleolus. *C,* The edematous, split peroneous brevis (*arrowhead*) is also well visualized on a fat-suppressed T$_2$-weighted sagittal view.

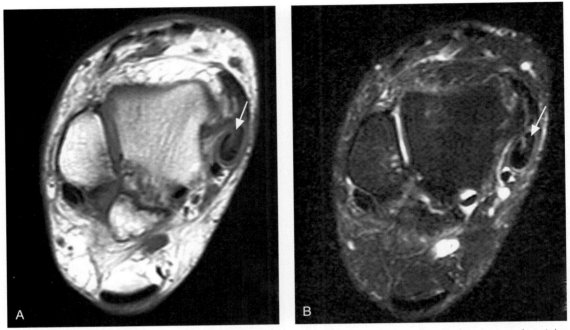

FIGURE 13–78. Posterior tibial tendon tear (type 1). The posterior tibial tendon (*arrow*) is enlarged and edematous and contains a longitudinal split on T$_1$- (*A*) and fat-suppressed T$_2$-weighted (*B*) axial images.

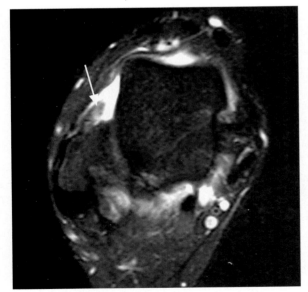

FIGURE 13–79. Anterior talofibular ligament tear. A fat-suppressed T$_2$-weighted image reveals a complete tear of the anterior talofibular ligament from its talar insertion. The thickened and retracted tendon (*arrow*) is clearly seen on this axial image.

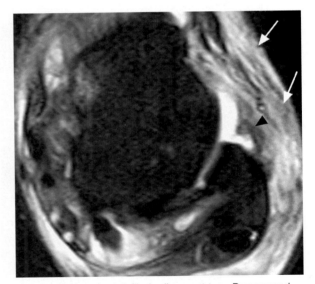

FIGURE 13–80. Anterior talofibular ligament tear. Pronounced lateral edema and soft tissue swelling (*arrows*) are apparent on a fat-suppressed T$_2$-weighted axial image demonstrating a complete tear of the anterior talofibular ligament (*arrowhead*).

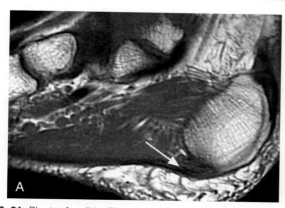 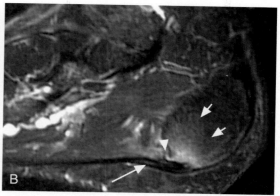

FIGURE 13–81. Plantar fasciitis. The plantar fascia is thickened and edematous at its calcaneal insertion (*arrow*) on sagittal T$_1$- (*A*) and fat-suppressed T$_2$-weighted (*B*) images demonstrating plantar fasciitis. Reactive marrow edema (*short arrows*) and a plantar calcaneal spur (*arrowhead*) are also apparent on the T$_2$-weighted image.

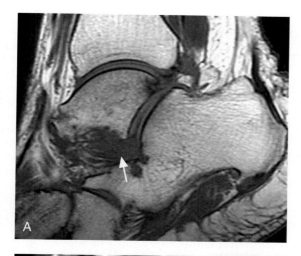

FIGURE 13–82. Sinus tarsi syndrome. Edema and soft tissue thickening (*arrow*) are evident throughout the tarsal sinus on T$_1$-weighted sagittal (*A*), T$_1$-weighted axial (*B*), and fat-suppressed T$_2$-weighted (*C*) axial images from a patient with severe tarsal sinus syndrome. The axial images also demonstrate a markedly enlarged and degenerated-appearing posterior tibial tendon (*arrowhead*), compatible with a type 1 tear. This is a common associated finding in patients with tarsal sinus syndrome.

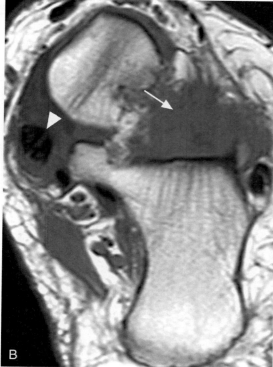 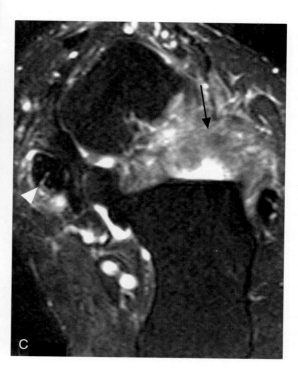

The multiplanar capability, excellent signal contrast between neoplastic and normal tissue, lack of artifacts from dense bone, and absence of ionizing radiation are desirable features. MRI is very sensitive for detecting and defining the extent of soft tissue and bone marrow disease.

Anatomy and Technique

Normal bone marrow contains a large amount of fat and, therefore, has intermediate or high signal intensity on T_1-weighted images depending on the marrow composition. The surrounding bone cortex has very low black signal intensity on all pulse sequences. Most pathologic lesions lead to replacement of marrow fat, causing decreased signal intensity on T_1-weighted images. Normal soft tissue, such as muscle, has intermediate to low signal intensity on T_2-weighted scans. Most pathologic soft tissue lesions have greater fluid content, producing increased signal intensity on T_2-weighted images.

Spin echo pulse sequences are ideal for differentiating normal bone marrow and soft tissue from pathologic conditions. Short TR/time to echo (TE) (T_1-weighted) sequences emphasize the difference between normal and abnormal marrow fat composition. Long TR/TE (T_2-weighted) sequences distinguish normal from abnormal soft tissues. T_1- and T_2-weighted axial images through a tumor best show the characteristics of the mass, specifically the signal intensity of the lesion, soft tissue extension, and cortical involvement. Sagittal or coronal T_1-weighted images are ideal for showing the extent of bone marrow involvement and skip lesions. Sagittal and coronal T_2-weighted images can help in delineating the cephalocaudad extent of soft tissue abnormalities.

MRI is the most sensitive imaging modality for detecting soft tissue and bone marrow lesions. Most osteolytic lesions have low signal intensity on T_1-weighted images and high signal intensity on T_2-weighted images. Tumors that produce bone or elicit a sclerotic response, such as sclerotic osteosarcoma and blastic metastases, often have low signal intensity on both T_1- and T_2-weighted images. Low-signal-intensity tumors on T_2-weighted images tend to be fibrotic and hypocellular. Most soft tissue lesions have decreased signal intensity on T_1-weighted images and increased signal intensity on T_2-weighted images. The ability to distinguish between malignant and benign soft tissue masses is limited, but malignant lesions often have a more heterogeneous signal intensity. Despite these advantages, a major criticism of MRI is its lack of lesion specificity.

Soft Tissue Masses

Several characteristic findings improve the diagnostic specificity of MRI with soft tissue lesions. Lipomas have increased signal intensity on T_1-weighted images and intermediate signal intensity on T_2-weighted images, paralleling normal fat. Well-differentiated liposarcomas account for more than half of all liposarcomas. On MRI, a well-differentiated liposarcoma will be seen as a predominantly fatty mass with irregular, thickened linear or nodular septa. Although lipomas that are completely homogeneous and fatlike in signal intensity can be distinguished from a well-differentiated liposarcoma on MRI, overlap in imaging appearances does occur. (Some lipoma variants may not be completely characteristic in their appearance on MRI.) Myxoid liposarcomas, the next most common type, often do not contain substantial amounts of fat and thus are easily distinguished on MRI from a lipoma. When fat is present, it may be linear, clumplike, or amorphous in appearance.

Hematomas have various signal intensities, depending on the stage of hemoglobin degradation, and sequential scans can show progression of clot resorption. Unlike hematomas within the brain parenchyma, chronic soft tissue hematomas have the signal characteristics of fluid and usually do not contain hemosiderin. Hemangiomas (Fig. 13-83) and lymphangiomas are usually well circumscribed and have decreased signal intensity on T_1-

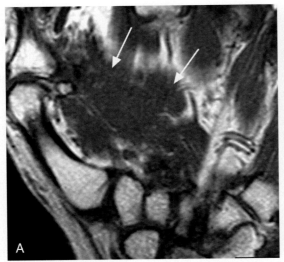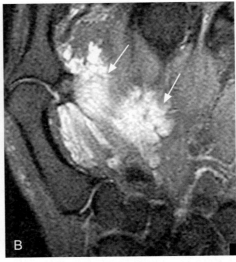

FIGURE 13–83. Soft tissue hemangioma. *A,* On the T_1-weighted coronal image, a soft tissue hemangioma (*arrows*) is difficult to visualize because it remains relatively isointense to muscle. *B,* The hemangioma is much more readily apparent as a lobulated, hyperintense lesion (*arrows*) on the fat-suppressed proton density-weighted coronal view.

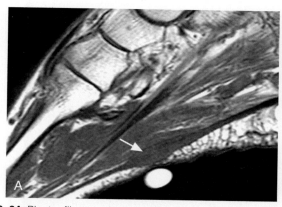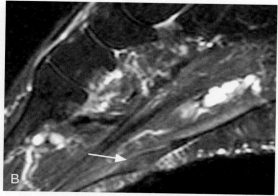

FIGURE 13–84. Plantar fibroma. A plantar fibroma presents as an area of nodular soft tissue thickening (*arrow*) on T$_1$- (*A*) and fat-suppressed T$_2$-weighted (*B*) sagittal images of the foot. Only mild hyperintensity is apparent on the T$_2$-weighted exam, a typical appearance in cases of plantar fibroma.

weighted images and very high signal intensity on T$_2$-weighted images.

Neurofibromas may have mildly increased signal intensity on T$_1$-weighted images and markedly increased signal intensity on T$_2$-weighted images, often with a central area of decreased signal intensity resulting from dense fibrous tissue condensations. Aggressive fibromatosis is a rare soft tissue lesion that usually has low signal intensity on T$_1$- and T$_2$-weighted images because of dense fibrous tissue. Depending on the degree of cellularity, aggressive fibromatosis may have high signal on T$_2$-weighted images. Benign soft tissue cysts are typically well defined, with homogeneous signal intensity equal to or less than muscle on T$_1$-weighted images and hyperintense on T$_2$-weighted images. Proteinaceous cysts have increased signal intensity on both T$_1$- and T$_2$-weighted scans.

Fibrous lesions span the spectrum from benign (such as a fibroma [Fig. 13-84], or fasciitis) to malignant (fibrosarcoma). Fibromatosis is an entity that is intermediate in biological behavior; such lesions are characterized by proliferation of benign fibrous tissue. The fibromatoses are classified by anatomic location as superficial or deep. Plantar fibromatosis is within the superficial group. Superficial fibromatoses are in general small, slow-growing lesions. The MRI appearance of plantar fibromatosis is relatively characteristic, being isointense to muscle on T$_1$-weighted images and slightly hyperintense to muscle on T$_2$-weighted spin echo images.

Malignant fibrous histiocytoma is the most common malignant soft tissue tumor of adults. Presentation is usually in the sixth to eight decades, with location in the extremities or retroperitoneum. The typical clinical presentation is that of a painless, rapidly growing mass. Treatment is by radical resection; however, recurrence and metastasis to the lungs are frequent. The tumor is locally infiltrative and carries a poor prognosis. The MRI characteristics are nonspecific other than the infiltrative nature (Fig. 13-85). Intravenous contrast administration can be used to improve delineation of tumor margins.

The most common soft tissue tumor of children younger than 15 years is rhabdomyosarcoma (Fig. 13-86). This tumor can also be seen in older adolescents and young adults. It is a malignant lesion and can metastasize to lymph nodes. Treatment is by radical resection and chemotherapy. On MRI, rhabdomyosarcomas have heterogeneous low signal intensity on T$_1$-weighted images and high signal intensity on T$_2$-weighted images. Infiltrating margins and peritumoral edema are also seen, similar to other malignant soft tissue tumors, including malignant fibrous histiocytoma. The role of MRI, as with other soft tissue lesions, is to determine the extent of involvement and response to therapy or recurrence.

Bone Tumors

The hallmark of a benign bone tumor on MRI is a well-defined peripheral margin of decreased signal intensity on all pulse sequences, separating the lesion from the adjacent normal marrow. Some specific findings for bone tumors have been published. Hyaline cartilage matrix lesions, including enchondromas (Fig. 13-87), osteochondromas, and most chondrosarcomas (Figs. 13-88 and 13-89) may have a unique appearance on T$_2$-weighted scans. Various sizes of lobules of homogeneous increased signal intensity separated by thin, low-intensity septa are characteristic of these lesions. The septated appearance and homogeneity of the signal intensity allow differentiation of hyaline cartilage lesions from most other masses with increased signal intensity on T$_2$-weighted images.

Fibroxanthomas typically have predominantly decreased signal intensity on T$_1$- and T$_2$-weighted images because of hemosiderin pigment or increased amounts of collagen. Osteoid osteoma classically has low signal intensity in the nidus of the lesion on T$_1$- and T$_2$-weighted scans, with a surrounding area of increased signal intensity (edema) on T$_2$-weighted scans (Figs. 13-90 and 13-91). Osteochondromas show continuity of the cortex of the lesion with the parent bone and of the parent medullary cavity with the lesion. A bright signal intensity cartilage cap can be demonstrated on T$_2$-weighted images. As a general rule, the thicker the cartilage cap, the more likely it is that the lesion has undergone malignant change. Most cartilage caps less

Text continued on page 445

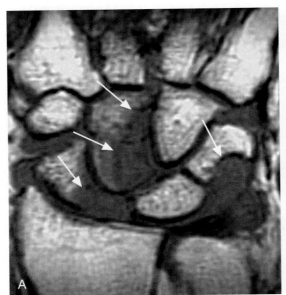

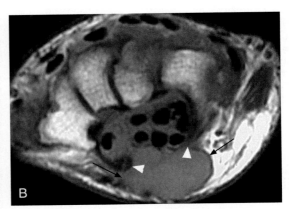

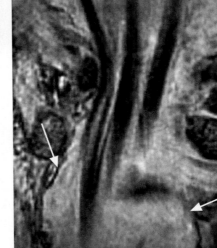

FIGURE 13–85. Malignant fibrous histiocytoma. This patient presented with volar wrist swelling and pain years after a carpal tunnel release. *A,* Numerous carpal erosions (*arrows*) are noted on the T_1-weighted coronal image. T_1-weighted axial (*B*) and T_2*-weighted coronal (*C*) images reveal a lobulated signal abnormality (*arrows*) surrounding the flexor tendons. The abnormality extends through the defect (*B, arrowheads*) from the patient's prior retinacular release. At surgery, a diagnosis of malignant fibrous histiocytoma was confirmed.

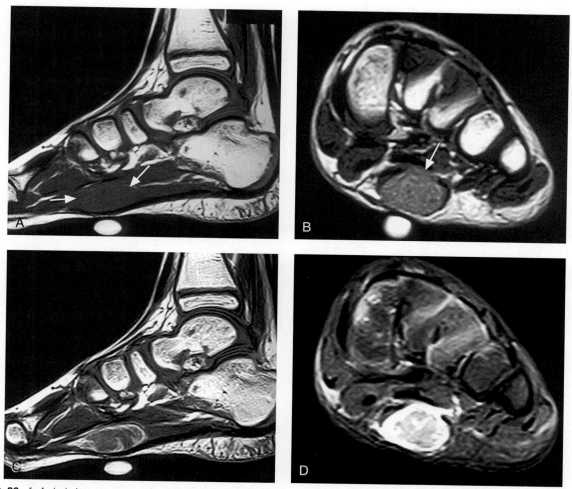

FIGURE 13–86. *A,* A rhabdomyosarcoma (*arrows*) arising within plantar musculature deep to the anterior aspect of the plantar fascia appears isointense to muscle on the T$_1$-weighted sagittal image. *B,* The lesion demonstrates intermediate signal intensity on the T$_2$-weighted coronal view. *C,* Peripheral enhancement is seen within the lesion on the postcontrast T$_1$-weighted sagittal image. *D,* A postcontrast T$_1$-weighted coronal view obtained with fat suppression reveals a more intense and prominent pattern of enhancement within the tumor.

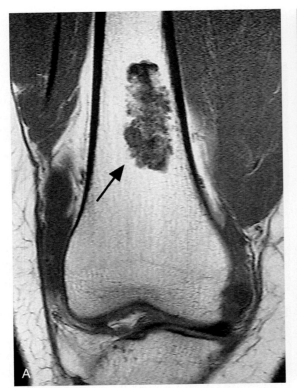

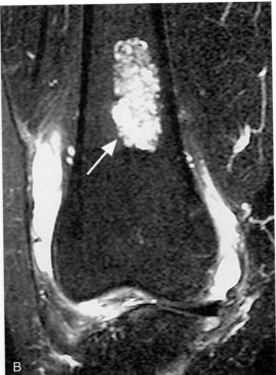

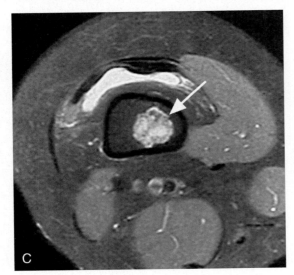

FIGURE 13–87. Enchondroma. An enchondroma of the distal femur (*arrow*) is clearly seen on T_1-weighted coronal (*A*), fat-suppressed T_2-weighted coronal (*B*), and fat-suppressed proton density-weighted axial (*C*) images. These lesions are typically intramedullary, lobulated, and markedly hyperintense on T_2-weighted images.

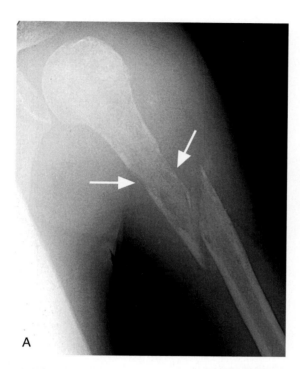

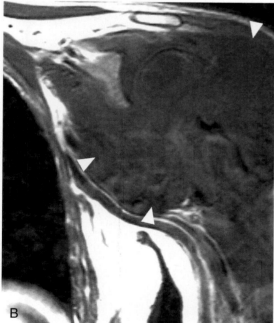

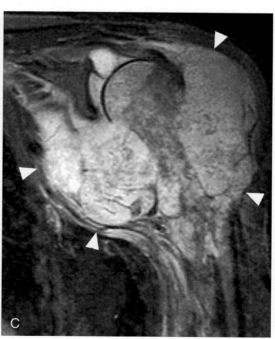

FIGURE 13–88. Chondrosarcoma (humerus). *A,* A lytic lesion (*arrows*) and pathologic fracture are present on the anteroposterior plain film of the left humerus. T_1- (*B*) and fat-suppressed proton density-weighted (*C*) coronal images reveal a large soft tissue mass (*arrowheads*) causing bony destruction in this region. The pathologic diagnosis in this case was chondrosarcoma.

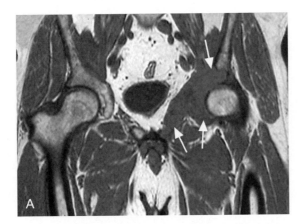

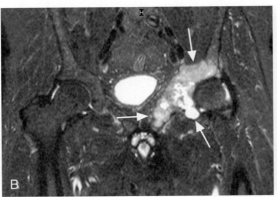

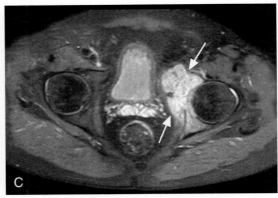

FIGURE 13–89. Chondrosarcoma (acetabulum). An expansile, destructive chondrosarcoma of the left acetabulum (*arrows*) is readily apparent on T_1-weighted coronal (*A*), fat-suppressed T_2-weighted coronal (*B*), and fat-suppressed proton density-weighted axial (*C*) images of the pelvis.

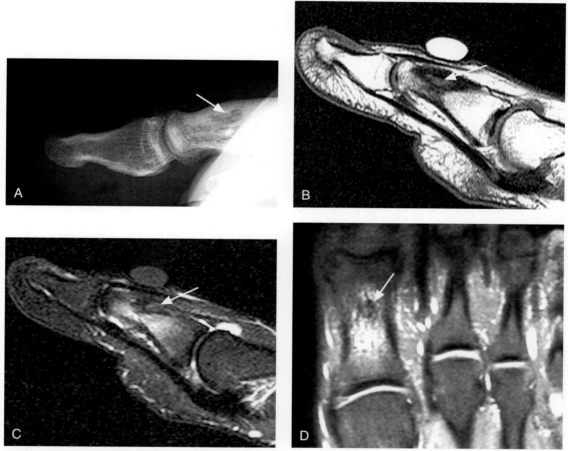

FIGURE 13–90. *A,* An osteoid osteoma involving the proximal phalanx of the great toe presents as a lytic lesion with a sclerotic nidus (*arrow*) on a lateral plain film. *B,* The lesion (*arrow*) is clearly visualized on a T_1-weighted sagittal image. The low-signal-intensity central nidus (*arrow*) with surrounding marrow edema is clearly seen on fat-suppressed T_2-weighted sagittal (*C*) and proton density weighted (*D*) coronal views.

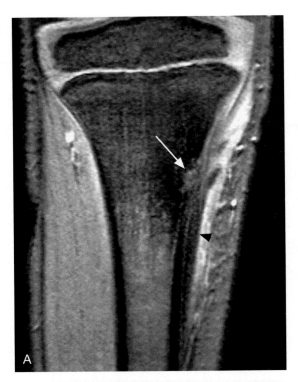

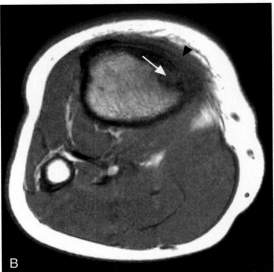

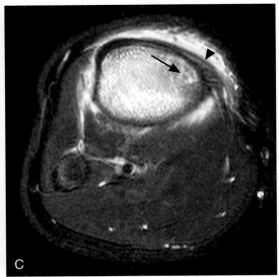

FIGURE 13–91. The central nidus (*arrow*) of an osteoid osteoma of the tibia is apparent on fat-suppressed proton density-weighted coronal (*A*) and T$_1$-weighted axial (*B*) images of the proximal tibia. *C*, Periosteal elevation (*arrowhead*) and surrounding bone marrow and soft tissue edema are better seen on the fat-suppressed T$_2$-weighted axial view.

than 3 mm thick are benign. A dark-rimmed perichondrium can be seen around the cartilage cap. It is important to delineate this preoperatively because incomplete removal of the perichondrium can allow tumor regrowth postoperatively.

Aneurysmal bone cysts (Fig. 13-92) and giant cell tumors (Fig. 13-93) frequently have increased signal intensity on T_1-weighted images as a result of central areas of hemorrhage. On T_2-weighted images, these lesions have increased signal intensity and may contain fluid-fluid levels. Vertebral hemangiomas have a unique MRI appearance, with mottled, rounded areas of increased signal intensity on T_1-weighted and T_2-weighted

scans interspersed with areas of decreased signal intensity. The increased signal intensity on T_1-weighted images represents fatty components of the lesion. Despite these specific findings, plain films continue to play an important role in the differential diagnosis of most bone tumors.

Chondroblastoma, an uncommon primary cartilage tumor, occurs in adolescents and young adults. This lesion arises in the ends of long bones; half occur around the knee. On radiographs, the lesion is round to oval with well-defined margins and often a sclerotic rim. Chondroblastomas have a lobulated appearance, with signal intensity similar to that of fat on T_2-weighted

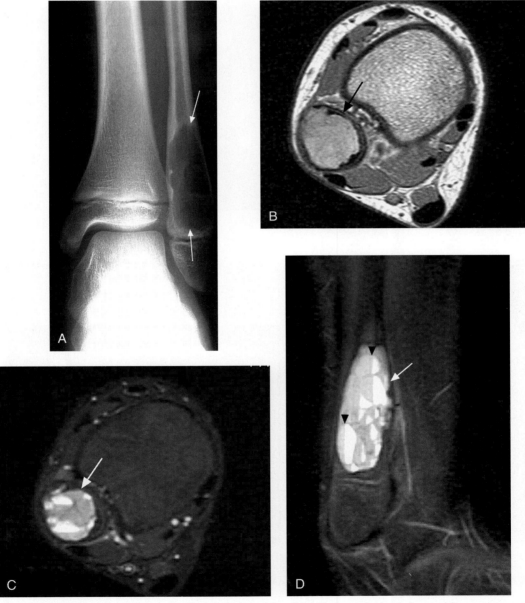

FIGURE 13–92. Aneurysmal bone cyst. *A,* An expansile, lytic lesion of the distal fibular metaphysis (*arrows*) is present on an anteroposterior plain film of the ankle. The lesion (*arrow*) displays fluid signal intensity characteristics on proton density-weighted (*B*) and fat-suppressed T_2-weighted (*C*) axial images. *D,* Pockets of hemorrhagic fluid, with fluid-fluid levels (*arrowheads*), within this multiloculated lesion are more readily apparent on the fat-suppressed T_2-weighted sagittal image.

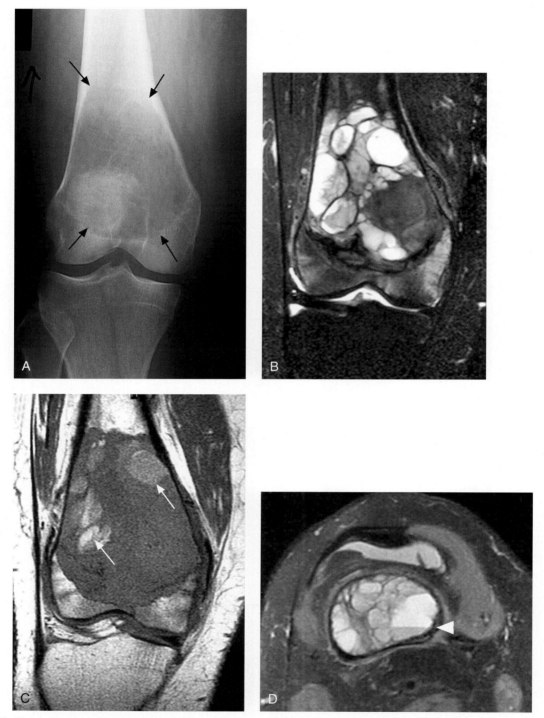

FIGURE 13–93. Giant cell tumor. *A,* A lytic, expansile lesion (*arrows*) extending from the metaphysis into the epiphysis is seen on the anteroposterior plain film from this patient beyond the age of epiphyseal closure. The abnormality is hemorrhagic (*arrows*) and multicystic in appearance on fat-suppressed T$_2$-weighted coronal (*B*), T$_1$-weighted coronal (*C*), fat-suppressed proton density-weighted axial (*D*) images. A fluid-fluid level (*arrowhead*) is also apparent on the axial image. Tissue pathology (after surgery) revealed this lesion to be a giant cell tumor.

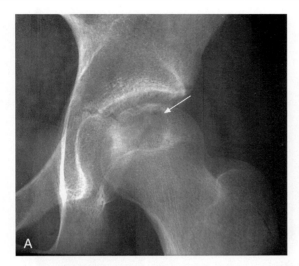

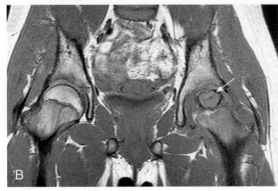

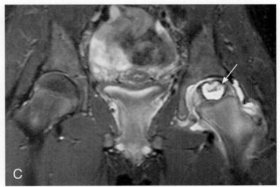

FIGURE 13–94. Chondroblastoma. *A,* A lytic lesion (*arrow*) confined to the epiphysis is present on a plain radiograph of the left hip. *B,* The lesion (*arrow*) demonstrates intermediate signal intensity on a T_1-weighted coronal image. *C,* On the fat-suppressed T_2-weighted coronal image, the abnormality (*arrow*) is markedly hyperintense and remains well defined. Surrounding marrow edema and a reactive joint effusion are also evident on the T_2-weighted scan. The epiphyseal location and the signal characteristics similar to cartilage are typical for a chondroblastoma, the pathologic diagnosis in this case.

images and isointense to muscle on T_1-weighted images (Fig. 13-94). The appearance on T_2-weighted images is often heterogeneous, with scattered areas of increased signal intensity resulting from small foci of hemorrhage or hyaline cartilage.

Osteosarcoma (or osteogenic sarcoma) is the second most common primary tumor of bone with plasma cell myeloma the most frequent. Histologically, the tumor contains cells that produce osteoid and immature bone. The MRI appearance depends on the predominant cellular component (Fig. 13-95).

As with MRI in other areas of the body, imaging findings may be characteristic for the pathologic diagnosis (Fig. 13-96) or very nonspecific (Fig. 13-97). Benign lesions can generally be differentiated from malignant.

The primary use of MRI in bone tumors is for staging. MRI is superior to other imaging modalities in determining intramedullary tumor extent. MRI also detects the skip lesions that occur with bone sarcomas. T_1-weighted coronal or sagittal images are often best for showing the intramedullary tumor extent. Assessment of invasion or breakthrough of the bony cortex is important

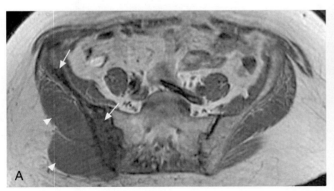

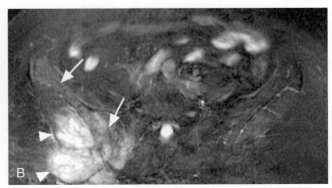

FIGURE 13–95. Osteogenic sarcoma. Abnormal marrow replacement (*arrows*) and a bulky extraosseous soft tissue mass (*arrowheads*) are present on T_1-weighted (*A*) and fat-suppressed T_2-weighted (*B*) axial images from a case of osteogenic sarcoma involving the medial right iliac wing. In this case, the osteogenic sarcoma arose from a site of preexisting Paget's disease, which is suggested by the cortical thickening and low signal intensity within the right iliac wing on the T_1-weighted image.

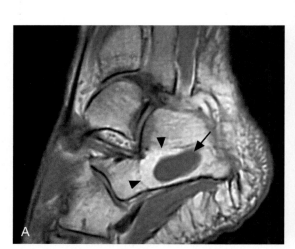

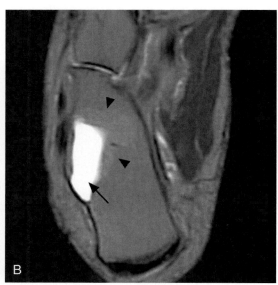

FIGURE 13–96. Calcaneal lipoma. A cyst-appearing central zone (*arrow*) with a surrounding fat signal intensity region (*arrowheads*) is noted on T₁-weighted sagittal (*A*) and T₂-weighted axial (*B*) images demonstrating a calcaneal lipoma. Intraosseous lipomas such as this often have cystic components, unlike their soft tissue counterparts, which are typically homogeneously fatty.

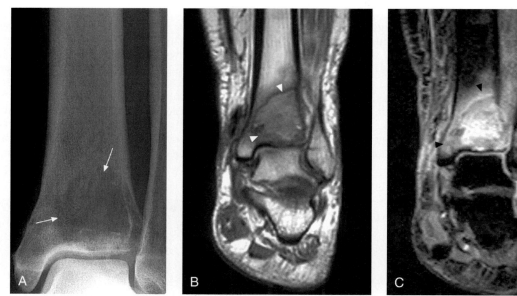

FIGURE 13–97. Primary lymphoma. *A*, A permeative lytic lesion (*arrow*) is noted within the distal tibia on the anteroposterior radiograph. Proton density-weighted (*B*) and short TI inversion recovery (*C*) coronal images confirm the presence of a large lesion with marrow replacement (*arrowheads*) and surrounding marrow edema.

preoperatively. Bone cortex invasion manifests as slightly increased signal intensity compared with the normal signal void of cortical bone on proton density- and T_2-weighted images. Gross cortical destruction produces interruption of the normal cortical signal void.

MRI is superior to other imaging modalities in detecting and demonstrating the extent of soft tissue involvement. The local soft tissue extension of tumor is best seen on T_2-weighted axial images. Gadolinium chelates using intravenous contrast administration enhance viable tumor, further improving tumor conspicuity and visualization of the extent of soft tissue involvement on T_1-weighted images. MRI may also permit differentiation of soft tissue tumor extension from reactive edema in the muscles. Both of these conditions present as increased signal intensity in the muscle adjacent to a tumor on T_2-weighted scans. If the tumor is well demarcated from the adjacent increased signal intensity in the muscle, the muscle signal is most likely caused by edema. If the distinction between the muscle and the mass is poor, it more likely represents tumor invasion. Contrast enhancement can also improve differentiation of tumor from edema, although edematous muscle does enhance.

MRI is superior to other imaging modalities in detecting joint involvement and neurovascular encasement, obstruction, and displacement. MRI can obviate the need for angiography by offering sufficient information about vascular involvement. One downfall of MRI is the poor detection of calcifications and ossification of tumor matrix, which limits the specificity of the technique. Thin, bony rims and subtle cortical breaks may not be seen with MRI.

Postoperative Tumor Detection

MRI can be valuable for assessing the success of bone tumor surgery and for evaluating postoperative masses; MRI is also useful for evaluating the response of tumors to chemotherapy. A satisfactory chemotherapeutic response is seen as decreased tumor volume; decreased signal intensity on T_2-weighted images as a result of dehydration of the tumor, calcification, or fibrosis; or marked increased signal intensity on T_2-weighted images as a result of necrosis or hemorrhage. An unsatisfactory response manifests as stable signal intensity and tumor volume or as increased tumor volume.

Bone Marrow Disease

Normal bone marrow is composed of red marrow, which is hematologically active, and yellow (fatty) marrow, which is hematologically inactive. Fatty marrow has increased signal intensity on T_1-weighted spin echo images and intermediate signal intensity on T_2-weighted images. Red marrow MRI signal characteristics are formed by a combination of lipid and water. The T_1-weighted signal intensity of red marrow is less than that of yellow marrow.

During growth, there is continual conversion of red to yellow marrow. At birth, almost the entire marrow space contains red marrow. Conversion to yellow marrow begins in the appendicular skeleton. An adult pattern is reached by 25 or 30 years of age. The normal adult pattern has red marrow in the axial skeleton (skull, vertebrae, ribs, sternum, and pelvis) and in the proximal appendicular skeleton (proximal femur and humerus). Epiphyses and apophyses contain fatty marrow, even in infants. Slow, progressive conversion of red to yellow marrow continues throughout adulthood. This is most noticeable in the vertebral bodies in which focal fatty conversion is a common finding with increasing age.

Several specific MRI techniques exist for evaluating the marrow. STIR is a form of inversion recovery that obliterates the signal from yellow fatty marrow. Pathologic lesions can be readily detected in fatty marrow as bright areas. Limitations of STIR are poor anatomic definition and SNR. Fast STIR has replaced conventional STIR sequences, much as fast spin echo has replaced spin echo imaging for T_2-weighted scans. Although fast STIR is markedly superior to its predecessor, images still generally suffer from poor SNR. Chemical shift imaging is another technique that can enhance the differences among fatty marrow, hematopoietic marrow, and abnormal marrow by forming "fat minus water" images or exclusively fat or water images.

When using spin echo pulse sequences, the differentiation of fatty marrow, hematopoietic marrow, and pathologic marrow depends on detecting the fat content in the marrow. Highly T_1-weighted images, which ideally show fat, are essential. The shorter the TR, the better the T_1-weighted contrast will be. Images should therefore be acquired with TR less than 500 msec.

Pathologic processes involving the bone marrow replace normal marrow fat cells and produce decreased signal intensity on T_1-weighted spin echo images. MRI is very sensitive to bone marrow infiltration, but it is nonspecific. Lymphoma, leukemia, myelofibrosis, metastatic disease, multiple myeloma, Gaucher's disease, and severe anemias can present similarly as focal or diffuse areas of decreased signal intensity in the bone marrow on T_1-weighted images. MRI can distinguish between hypercellular and fibrotic marrow. Marked increased signal intensity in the bone marrow on T_1-weighted images, resulting from fatty replacement, can be seen with aplastic anemia and after radiation therapy.

Osteomyelitis

The diagnosis of osteomyelitis is a clinical dilemma. Radionuclide bone scans are the primary imaging modality for diagnosing osteomyelitis, but they have poor spatial resolution and require hours to be completed. MRI is a useful adjunctive imaging modality that is very sensitive to osteomyelitis (Figs. 13-98 and 13-99). Osteomyelitis appears as decreased signal intensity on T_1-weighted scans and increased signal intensity on T_2-weighted scans. Enhancement after intravenous gadolinium chelate administration is prominent. The specificity of MRI is poor in the absence of clinical information and does not allow differentiation from other conditions, such as neoplasm or trauma. Osteomyelitis tends to be less well defined than tumors. MRI is useful for determining the extent of bone and soft tissue involvement (Fig. 13-100).

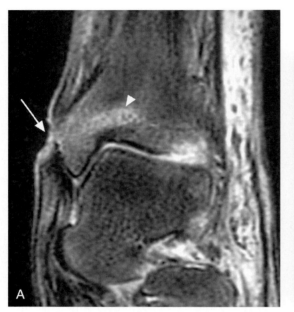

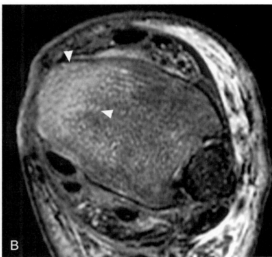

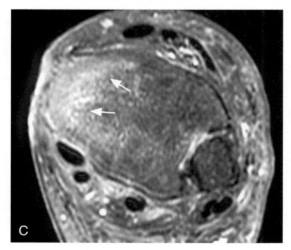

FIGURE 13–98. Osteomyelitis (ankle). *A*, A skin defect (*arrow*) is seen on a fat-suppressed T$_2$-weighted coronal image from a diabetic with a nonhealing ulceration at the medial malleolus. Underlying marrow edema (*arrowheads*) is apparent on this image and on the corresponding fat-suppressed T$_2$-weighted axial image (*B*). The marrow edema indicates osteomyelitis. *C*, The infected bone is seen to enhance (*short arrows*) on the fat-suppressed T$_1$-weighted axial image obtained after administration of a gadolinium chelate.

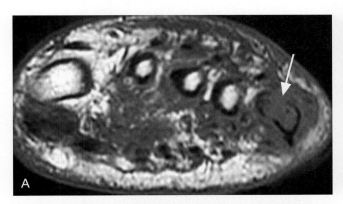

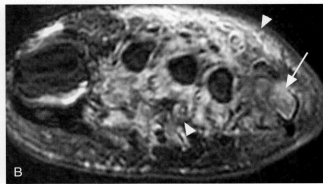

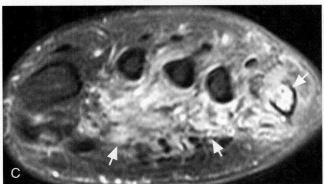

FIGURE 13–99. Osteomyelitis (foot). T_1- (*A*) and fat-suppressed T_2-weighted (*B*) axial images reveal marrow edema and bony destruction (*arrow*) at the fifth metatarsal. Soft tissue edema (*arrowheads*), most apparent on the fat-suppressed T_2-weighted axial image, is compatible with associated cellulitis. *C*, Intense enhancement (*short arrows*) is noted on the postcontrast fat-suppressed T_1-weighted axial view.

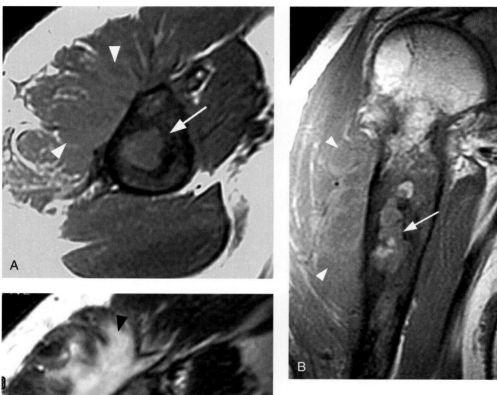

FIGURE 13–100. Chronic osteomyelitis was diagnosed in this patient years after a fracture of the proximal humerus. Intraosseous (*arrow*) and soft tissue (*arrowheads*) abscess formation are apparent on the T_1-weighted axial (*A*), T_1-weighted coronal (*B*), and T_2-weighted axial (*C*) images.

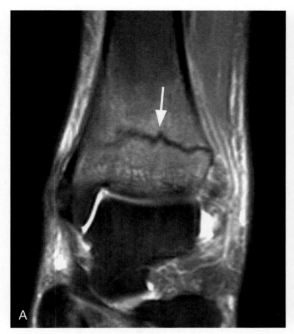
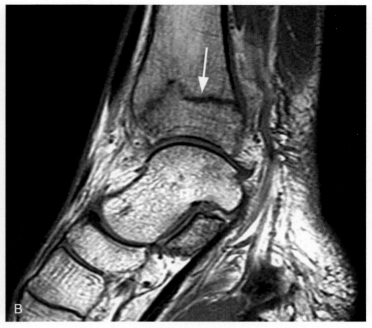

Figure 13–101. Distal tibial stress fracture. A linear signal abnormality (*arrow*) oriented perpendicular to the cortex is seen on fat-suppressed proton density-weighted coronal (*A*) and T₁-weighted sagittal (*B*) images. Surrounding marrow edema is evident on the fat-suppressed examination.

Stress Fracture

Stress fractures are most often caused by repeated minor trauma and present with focal pain. They are usually located in the metaphysis or diaphysis of long bones. Radiographs are notoriously poor for diagnosing stress fractures. Radionuclide bone scans are very sensitive for detecting stress fractures but are nonspecific. MRI is at least as sensitive as radionuclide bone scans but much more specific for diagnosing stress fractures.

MRI findings of stress fracture are a thin band of very low signal intensity in the bone marrow, which extends to the cortical surface and is seen on both T_1- and T_2-weighted images (Fig. 13-101). This represents microfracture or bone sclerosis. A larger surrounding area of relatively decreased signal intensity is also seen in the bone marrow on T_1-weighted images. On T_2-weighted images, there is an area of increased signal intensity in the marrow around the thin band of low signal. This represents hemorrhage or edema.

14

Contrast Media

The mechanisms responsible for image contrast in magnetic resonance imaging (MRI) are many, as are the methods used to produce a clinically useful MRI image. MRI contrast media design requirements, contrast mechanisms, relaxivity theory, and imaging techniques are reviewed first. This is followed by an in-depth discussion of the agents that are currently available and those that will soon come to market, focusing on diagnostic utility and clinical safety. Contrast media add an additional dimension to the manipulation of inherent contrast in MRI. Their application leads to improved sensitivity and specificity in clinical MRI.

BASIC PRINCIPLES

By 1990, just 10 years after its clinical introduction, MRI had become the imaging modality of choice for the study of central nervous system (CNS) disease. Additional broad applications in the abdomen, pelvis, and musculoskeletal system were subsequently established. Concurrent development of contrast media, now in widespread use, aided the rapid expansion of this field. Contrast-enhanced scans offer important additional diagnostic information in many instances. MRI provides high spatial resolution and soft tissue contrast, with sensitivity to contrast media greater than that of x-ray computed tomography (CT). First-pass brain studies now also make possible the assessment of regional cerebral blood volume. New hardware developments, together with advances in contrast media design, continue to drive the expansion of contrast media applications. These build on the large base of current clinical use.

MRI provides excellent soft tissue contrast on unenhanced images. Thus, it was initially speculated that there would be no need for a contrast agent. In the early 1980s, it became apparent that contrast enhancement could substantially improve the sensitivity and specificity of scans. For example, many brain metastases can only be visualized after contrast enhancement. As the benefits of MRI contrast agents became more obvious, their use increased exponentially. Currently, contrast agents are commonly used in clinical practice for a broad range of indications.

Design Requirements

Certain criteria need to be met in the design of an MRI contrast agent. First and foremost is its ability to alter

the parameters responsible for image contrast. MRI is unique in that there are multiple parameters responsible for signal intensity. The contrast agent must be efficient in its ability to influence these parameters at low concentrations to minimize dose and potential toxicity.

Second, the contrast agent should possess some tissue specificity in vivo so that it is delivered to a tissue or organ in a higher concentration than to other areas in the body. Once delivered to the desired tissue or organ, it must remain localized for a reasonable period of time so that imaging can be performed.

Third, the contrast agent must be substantially cleared from the targeted tissue or organ in a reasonable period of time, usually several hours after imaging, to minimize potential effects from chronic toxicity. The contrast agent must also be excreted from the body, usually by renal or hepatobiliary routes.

Fourth, the contrast agent must have low toxicity and be stable in vivo while being administered in doses that can affect the MRI relaxation parameters sufficiently to result in visible contrast enhancement. The dose levels of the contrast agent required to meet these criteria must be evaluated for acute and subacute systemic tolerance, potential mutagenicity, teratogenicity, and carcinogenicity. Many other tolerance tests are also required, depending on intended use.

Finally, the contrast agent must possess a suitable shelf life for storage. It must remain stable in vitro for a reasonable period of time while being stored. A shelf life of years is desirable.

Contrast Mechanisms

In conventional radiography and CT, image contrast is generated by differential attenuation of the x-ray beam. The degree of attenuation is directly related to the mass absorption coefficient of the tissue being imaged. The use of a contrast agent with a high mass absorption coefficient (e.g., any of the iodinated agents) results in attenuation of the x-ray beam to a greater degree. This produces contrast enhancement. The mechanisms responsible for contrast enhancement in MRI are multiple, not singular. The large inherent differences in signal intensity between normal tissues also make MRI unique compared with other imaging modalities. To further complicate matters, the appropriate selection of operator-dependent imaging parameters is critical so that these signal intensity differences are exploited to optimize MRI contrast.

The parameters that determine MRI signal intensity

Portions of this chapter are reprinted with permission from Runge VM: Findings advise against lower MRI contrast doses. Diagnostic Imaging 1998, April, pp 23–24.

and contrast are many. The first of these, and the easiest to understand, is spin density. Spin density refers to the fraction of protons that exists in the voxel of tissue being imaged and determines the maximum potential MRI signal intensity that can be realized from that volume of tissue. Most protons in tissue are water protons. These far outnumber the protons that are associated with organic compounds in tissue. Because a contrast agent cannot easily alter the in vivo water content of tissue, compounds that affect spin density have received little attention.

Another common parameter exploited in the generation of MRI contrast is relaxivity. There are two relaxivity parameters that are unique to each tissue: T_1 and T_2. Longitudinal or spin-lattice relaxation time, known as T_1, refers to the amount of time it takes for the tissue magnetization to return to its equilibrium state in the longitudinal direction of the main magnetic field after excitation with a radiofrequency (RF) pulse. The excess energy that is absorbed by the magnetic spins from the RF pulse is transferred back to the environment during the relaxation process. The second relaxivity property of tissue is transverse or spin-spin relaxation, referred to as T_2 relaxation. In this relaxation process, the excess energy deposited in the tissue by the RF pulse is subsequently transferred between magnetic spins. This transferred energy results in loss of spin phase coherency in the transverse plane and spin dephasing.

Contrast agent enhancement that is based on alteration of these two relaxivity parameters can be categorized according to the relative change it imparts on either T_1 or T_2. A contrast agent that predominantly affects T_1 relaxation is referred to as a positive relaxation agent. This is because reducing T_1 results in increased signal intensity on a T_1-weighted image. By comparison, a contrast agent that predominantly affects T_2 relaxation is considered a negative relaxation agent. This is because reducing T_2 results in decreased signal intensity on a T_2-weighted image.

Another determinant of signal intensity in MRI is magnetic susceptibility. Susceptibility describes the ability of a substance to become magnetized in an external magnetic field. There are four categories of magnetic susceptibility. Most organic compounds are diamagnetic substances and have a small, negative magnetic susceptibility when placed in an external magnetic field. Paramagnetic substances have a net positive magnetic susceptibility, whereas superparamagnetic and ferromagnetic materials have very large net positive susceptibilities. Diamagnetic susceptibility has a negligible effect in clinical MRI; therefore, diamagnetic substances are of little interest as contrast agents.

Paramagnetic substances afford the greatest flexibility in contrast agent design and have, therefore, received the greatest attention in contrast media development. The presence of a paramagnetic ion, such as gadolinium, can strongly influence the relaxation properties of nearby protons, leading to changes in tissue contrast. Paramagnetic contrast agents are predominantly used as positive T_1 relaxation contrast agents, with little effect seen on T_2 relaxation, and then only at high concentrations. The positive net magnetic susceptibility of a paramagnetic ion actually has little influence as an actual enhancement mechanism in conventional MRI studies. This effect is important in one application: the assessment of cerebral perfusion. Here the contrast is injected as a bolus and observed during its first pass through the tissue. The concentration of the agent is then sufficiently high to permit observation of the susceptibility effect.

By comparison, the large net magnetic susceptibility of superparamagnetic and ferromagnetic compounds more directly influences tissue contrast, with little effect on relaxation per se. Superparamagnetic substances are individual particles that are large enough to be a domain. When these particles are exposed to an external magnetic field, they align with the field, resulting in a large net positive magnetization. When removed from the magnetic field, they return to random orientations and lose their magnetization. By comparison, ferromagnetic compounds are large collections of interacting domains in a crystalline matrix. They exhibit an extremely large net positive magnetization in an external magnetic field and maintain this when removed from the field. Both superparamagnetic and ferromagnetic compounds have received substantial attention in regard to their application as MRI contrast agents. These agents function as negative contrast agents, because the large positive magnetic moment induces spin dephasing in tissue, with resulting signal loss.

The final two parameters that provide image contrast in MRI are diffusion and perfusion. The intensity of the MRI signal is based on the magnitude of the bulk magnetization lying in the transverse plane. It is maximal when all the transverse spins are in phase coherence. Movement or diffusion of water on a microscopic level leads to spin dephasing and loss of phase coherence in the transverse plane. This subsequently results in the loss of MRI signal intensity. Similarly, perfusion of blood in the microcirculation of the tissue being imaged also contributes to spin dephasing and a decrease in the intensity of the MRI signal. In this manner, different degrees of diffusion and perfusion within tissue contribute to contrast in the MRI. The use of a relaxivity or susceptibility contrast agent to manipulate diffusion coefficients, and thus serve as a contrast agent, has received little attention. The presence of a susceptibility agent in the blood pool can cause large changes in signal intensity. This approach, as previously noted, is used in one instance as a means of contrast enhancement, specifically for the assessment of cerebral perfusion.

Relaxivity Theory

Most of the attention in the development of MRI contrast agents has focused on the use of paramagnetic compounds. The most commonly used paramagnetic ion is the gadolinium ion, which is complexed with various ligands (such as diethylenetriamine pentaacetic acid [DTPA] in gadopentetate dimeglumine [Magnevist, Berlex Laboratories] and HP-DO3A in gadoteridol [ProHance, Bracco Diagnostics]) that act as chelating agents. Although an extensive review of relaxivity theory is beyond the scope of this chapter, a basic conceptual understanding is important to appreciate the physics involved in paramagnetic contrast agent enhancement.

The presence of unpaired electrons in the paramagnetic ion is a mandatory component to cause a change in the T_1 and T_2 relaxation rates of water protons. The magnetic dipole moment created by the unpaired electrons can thereby enhance the relaxation rates of water protons either by direct interaction with the water protons or by its local magnetic field influence. Only paramagnetic ions with exceptionally slowly relaxing unpaired electrons are effective. The relaxivity contributions of a paramagnetic ion are highly dependent on its spin state. If S denotes the spin quantum number of the total electron spin of the paramagnetic ion, then the relaxation rate is proportional to $S*(S + 1)$. A paramagnetic ion with the highest spin quantum number is desirable, provided it has slowly relaxing electrons. The gadolinium ion (Gd^{3+}) of the lanthanide metal group has a high spin quantum number of 7/2, making it a desirable relaxivity contrast agent. Other ions that have received attention as potential MRI contrast agents include Fe^{3+}, Dy^{3+}, and Mn^{3+} (all with $S = 5/2$). Although a high spin quantum number is theoretically desirable, it is not the only factor that determines the efficacy of an MRI contrast agent.

The interactions that occur between a paramagnetic contrast agent and protons of water molecules can be classified into two categories. Inner-sphere relaxation refers to the formation or dissociation of a coordinate covalent bond between a water molecule and the paramagnetic ion. A chemical exchange occurs, leading to catalyzed relaxation of the water protons. It follows that the more water molecules that can bind with the paramagnetic ion, the greater is its influence on relaxation enhancement. A short residence time allows the paramagnetic ion to interact with more water molecules. In contrast agent design, a rapid exchange ($= 10^6$ seconds^{-1}) between water molecules and the paramagnetic ion is a desirable feature because it allows for greater relaxation enhancement. This factor is important only up to the point at which the exchange contributes as a correlation time.

Outer-sphere relaxation is a more complex concept. It does not involve a direct bonding or chemical exchange mechanism. It is the result of the relative rotational and translational diffusion of water molecules and the paramagnetic ion. Basically, the more water molecules that can approach the paramagnetic ion and interact with its dipole, the greater will be the relaxivity influence of the paramagnetic ion. The more the paramagnetic ion can move through space, the greater will be its ability to interact with other water protons. The closer the water protons can approach the paramagnetic ion, the more efficient the relaxation enhancement will be. This interaction of the dipole moments of the paramagnetic ion and the water molecules in the environment has been termed a dipole-dipole relaxation process. Inner-sphere relaxation for Gd^{3+} is also a dipolar process ("through space") because Gd^{3+} has no scalar relaxation ("through bond").

These factors are critical in contrast agent design. For example, if the paramagnetic ion is complexed with a ligand such as DTPA, the molecular complex will rotate slower and translate slower in space. This will not allow as many water proton–paramagnetic ion interactions to occur, thereby limiting the relaxation effect. By complexing the paramagnetic ion, there will be increased distance between the water proton dipole and the paramagnetic ion dipole, decreasing the paramagnetic ion's relaxation enhancement effect.

The Solomon-Bloembergen-Morgan equation is a mathematical expression that describes the relaxation of water protons in the presence of a paramagnetic ion species. This equation is used as a predictor of the relaxation efficiency of a paramagnetic ion species in contrast agent design. The Solomon-Bloembergen-Morgan equation consists of two parts. The first part, the dipole-dipole term, expresses a distance factor between interacting species. In one dimension, this is a statement of the inverse square law in that the magnitude of the paramagnetic effect is related to the reciprocal of the square of the distance (d^{-2}). In three dimensions, this becomes d^{-6} expressed as r^{-6} ($r = $ radius). The dipole-dipole component is critically affected by the distance factor. Simply, the more closely a water molecule approaches the paramagnetic ion species, the more efficient will be the relaxation enhancement effect. Because the dipole-dipole component is critically affected by distance, it is important in contrast agent design to use carrier ligands that minimize this effect. Some of the carrier ligands, however, may be quite large. These ligands cause an undesirable effect from the standpoint of relaxation enhancement. The use of chelates is required because of the high toxicity of paramagnetic ions, such as gadolinium, when free in the body. Large carrier ligands and their surrounding water molecules of hydration tend to displace free or bulk water molecules from the surrounding inner sphere of influence of the paramagnetic ion, decreasing proton relaxation enhancement effects. Of all factors, this has the greatest negative impact.

The second part of the Solomon-Bloembergen-Morgan equation contains the scalar component. This term describes the probability of contact (correlation time) between the paramagnetic ion and the water proton. The total correlation time (t_c) between the two interacting species can be expressed mathematically for both dipole-dipole and scalar interactions as follows:

$$1/t_c = 1/t_r + 1/t_s + 1/t_m,$$

where t_r is the correlation time of rotation, t_s is the correlation time of electron relaxation, and t_m is the correlation time of chemical exchange. Relaxivity is directly proportional to t_c. The critical feature of this mathematical expression is that the component of the smallest magnitude will be the most important in determining the total correlation time of interaction.

Correlation times are important in paramagnetic agent design. For example, the larger the carrier ligand to which the paramagnetic ion is bound, the slower it will rotate and translate in space, thereby increasing the magnitude of t_r. The total correlation time of interaction is thus increased in most instances of a large carrier ligand molecule, somewhat offsetting the distance factor for these large carrier ligands. Correlation times will always reflect the interaction possessing the shortest time characteristic or the fastest dynamic behavior of the paramagnetic contrast agent, provided that chemical exchange is fast enough ($= 10^6$ seconds^{-1}).

Imaging Technique

As is now evident, the mechanisms responsible for MRI contrast are multiple, including spin density, T_1 and T_2, susceptibility, diffusion, and perfusion. Similar to the intrinsic MRI properties of the tissues themselves, the methods of measurement of these parameters in clinical MRI are multiple. The type of MRI pulse sequence used to generate a clinical MRI image and its associated parameters profoundly affects the contrast that is visualized from the tissues.

The ultimate goal when optimizing MRI scan technique for contrast agent visualization is to suppress the contrast from unchanged tissue parameters and accentuate the contrast based on the parameter that is altered by the contrast agent. This requires knowledge of the mechanism of contrast agent enhancement, the MRI pulse technique being used to measure that parameter, and how the operator-dependent parameters can be altered to optimize the enhancement of the contrast agent being used. What follows is a discussion of the MRI pulse sequences that are commonly used in conjunction with clinical MRI contrast agents and the issues that are related to their optimization.

Conventional spin echo imaging continues to be the principal technique for visualization of contrast agents. This approach can provide images with T_1, T_2, and spin density information. In spin echo imaging, a 90-degree RF pulse is followed by a 180-degree pulse. The latter generates an MRI signal or echo at an operator-specified echo time (TE). This measurement is repeated at a repetition time (TR) also specified by the operator. In spin echo imaging, short TR and short TE times produce an image with T_1-weighted contrast. For example, a scan with TR = 500 msec and TE = 10 msec is T_1-weighted. The enhancement effect of the gadolinium chelates is typically visualized on such T_1-weighted scans (Fig. 14-1). Long TR and TE times produce images with T_2-weighted contrast. A scan with TR = 3000 msec and TE = 100 msec is thus T_2-weighted. During the same long TR interval used to produce a T_2-weighted image, an additional image can be obtained with a short or intermediate echo time. This image will have spin density or intermediate T_2-weighting. One of the major disadvantages of conventional spin echo imaging when used to produce T_2-weighted scans is the long imaging time. Imaging time is directly proportional to TR, which is long for a typical T_2-weighted pulse sequence.

In the mid-1990s, imaging techniques using magnetization transfer (MT) were introduced. The application of MT in spin echo imaging can improve the enhancement effect produced by a gadolinium chelate in the brain (Fig. 14-2). Water protons in tissue exist in three distinct pools. The protons in the free water pool exist in a narrow range of resonant frequencies and possess a long T_2. It is these protons that account for most of the MRI signal recorded in clinical MRI. In the brain, protons in the second pool, fat, are few. The third pool of protons is the restricted pool. These protons represent structural or bound water protons associated with large molecules. Protons in the restricted pool have a large range of resonant frequencies and an extremely short T_2. Because the signal from this pool decays so quickly during MRI imaging (as a result of the short T_2), it contributes little to the image. With the application of MT, magnetization is transferred from the restricted pool to the freely mobile pool. The result is a shortening of T_1, with lower overall available magnetization and signal intensity. In theory, enhancement with gadolinium chelates is not mediated by macromolecular interactions and thus not suppressed by the application of MT. Accordingly, MT pulses preferentially suppress the signal from background tissue, usually improving the conspicuity of gadolinium-enhanced regions. This can lead to improved visualization of contrast enhancement at standard doses.

In areas of the body with abundant fat, scan techniques that combine T_1-weighting with fat suppression provide improved depiction of contrast enhancement (Fig. 14-3). Short TI inversion recovery (STIR) is one such approach. STIR suffers from poor signal-to-noise ratios and long scan times. Techniques that use a fat saturation pulse are currently more common. Frequency selective or spectral saturation exploits the slight difference in resonance frequency between fat and water. The signal from fat is saturated (removed) by the application of a frequency selective pulse. This approach can be adapted to any imaging technique and is similar in principle to spatial saturation.

Fast or turbo spin echo imaging became widely available in the mid-1990s. This approach permits T_2-weighted scans to be acquired in a much shorter time. With fast spin echo techniques, multiple echoes are acquired with different phase encoding values during each TR interval. Images with both proton density– and T_2-weighted information can be obtained in times from one fourth to one sixteenth that required for conventional spin echo techniques. The images generated from this approach arise from multiple TE data measurements, which are then averaged together for an effective TE image. Thus, image contrast is somewhat different from a conventional spin echo sequence. For example, the MRI signal from fat is more intense on a T_2-weighted image obtained with fast spin echo technique, reflecting in part the brighter signal that fat produces on short TE images. Despite these and other minimal shortcomings of fast spin echo sequences, they have gained widespread popularity in clinical MRI.

Another pulse technique popular in both spine and body applications is gradient echo imaging. This offers an alternative imaging approach with substantially reduced imaging time and RF power deposition. A gradient echo sequence differs from a spin echo sequence in that a 180-degree RF pulse is not used. The initial RF pulse also typically uses a flip angle of less than 90 degrees. Signal is generated after this initial pulse by manipulation of the gradient magnetic fields. By changing the operator-dependent parameters of the flip angle, TR and TE, image contrast with T_1, T_2^*, and

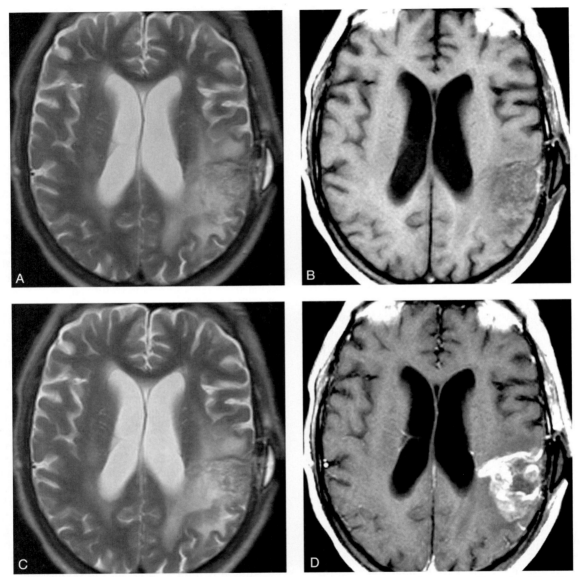

FIGURE 14–1. Glioblastoma illustrating the utility of T_1-weighted scans for detection of lesion enhancement. Precontrast T_2- (*A*) and T_1-weighted (*B*) scans are compared with postcontrast T_2- (*C*) and T_1-weighted (*D*) scans. Gadolinium chelates (ProHance in this instance) are detected in most instances using T_1-weighted scans. *D*, On the postcontrast T_1-weighted scan, positive lesion enhancement is noted in the region of blood-brain barrier disruption (marking the bulk of tumor mass). The contrast agent causes little or no change in signal intensity on the postcontrast T_2-weighted scan (*C*).

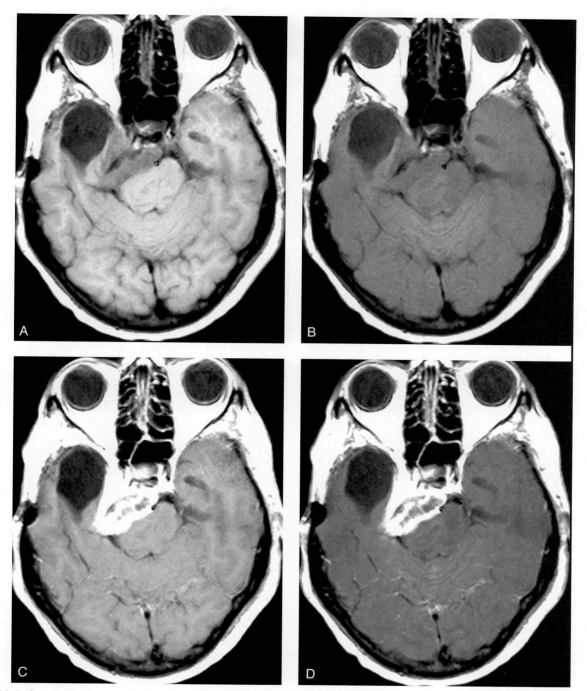

Figure 14–2. Cavernous sinus meningioma illustrating the use of magnetization transfer (MT) suppression. Precontrast T_1-weighted scans without (*A*) and with (*B*) MT are compared with postcontrast T_1-weighted scans without (*C*) and with (*D*) MT. The addition of an MT pulse shortens the T_1 of the freely mobile hydrogen pool, decreasing the signal intensity of normal brain. The effect is less on areas that demonstrate contrast enhancement, thus improving the depiction of lesion enhancement in most cases when MT is used.

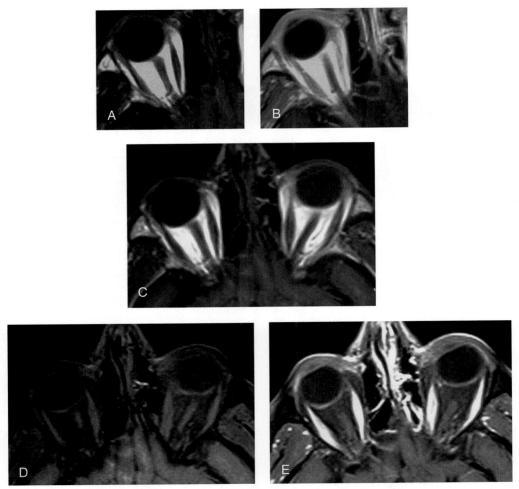

FIGURE 14–3. Normal orbital magnetic resonance exam illustrating the use of fat saturation to improve visualization of contrast enhancement. The scans shown are all T_1-weighted (and specifically spin echo in type). When comparing conventional pre- (*A*) and postcontrast (*B*) scans without fat saturation, it is difficult to appreciate the normal enhancement of the rectus muscles because of the high signal intensity of adjacent fat. The subsequent three scans are precontrast without fat saturation (*C*), precontrast with fat saturation (*D*), and postcontrast with fat saturation (*E*). The marked enhancement of the rectus muscles, and to a lesser extent other normal structures, is well depicted on the postcontrast scan with fat saturation (*E*). In areas of abundant fat, such as the orbit and soft tissues of the neck, acquisition of postcontrast scans with fat saturation is highly recommended to improve visualization of contrast enhancement and thus the conspicuity of enhancing lesions.

spin density information can be generated. One of the major disadvantages of gradient echo imaging is that susceptibility effects become prominent. This enhanced susceptibility effect can be exploited to advantage, however, in certain clinical situations. For example, the high magnetic susceptibility of blood degradation products, such as deoxyhemoglobin, results in increased conspicuity of hemorrhage on gradient echo scans.

Echo planar imaging (EPI) became widely available for clinicians in the late 1990s. EPI-based techniques are used to decrease motion artifact with uncooperative patients by shortening scan time and to acquire brain perfusion studies. High-quality images can be acquired in seconds as opposed to minutes. Fast spin echo scans, for example, require several minutes for acquisition. EPI scans can be proton density–, T_1-, or T_2-weighted. In combination with bolus contrast injection, EPI is used to view the first pass of a gadolinium chelate through the brain. Tissue perfusion can thus be assessed.

For perfusion imaging, the contrast medium (typically one of the approved extracellular gadolinium chelates) is injected as a bolus using an MRI-compatible power injector. Images are acquired very rapidly, about one per second, during and immediately after injection. This makes possible observation of the first pass of the contrast agent through the brain. In all other applications, T_1-weighted scans are used to detect a gadolinium chelate. In brain perfusion studies, T_2^*-weighted scans are used. These scans provide the high temporal resolution needed and also are quite sensitive to the very concentrated contrast medium within the vascular bed. On T_2^*-weighted scans, the gadolinium chelates cause a reduction in signal intensity as opposed to the increase in signal intensity seen on T_1-weighted scans. After acquisition, processing software can be used to produce relative cerebral blood volume (rCBV) and relative mean transit time (rMTT) images. Perfusion imaging can detect brain ischemia far sooner than standard T_2-weighted

FIGURE 14–4. Whole body residual gadolinium after intravenous administration of radiolabeled gadolinium (Gd) chelates. Gd edetic acid (EDTA) dissociates rapidly in vivo and is poorly tolerated. The residual Gd at each time point reflects the stability of each chelate and the degree to which in vivo dissociation occurs. More stable chelates, with less release of gadolinium in vivo, leave less free metal ion. Of the agents approved for clinical use in the United States, Omniscan shows the greatest residual Gd. Free Gd accumulates in liver, brain, and bone marrow. The toxicity of this heavy metal, when free (not chelated), is well known from industrial accidents. (Adapted from Tweedle MF: Physicochemical properties of gadoteridol and other magnetic resonance contrast agents. Invest Radiol 1992;27:S2–6).

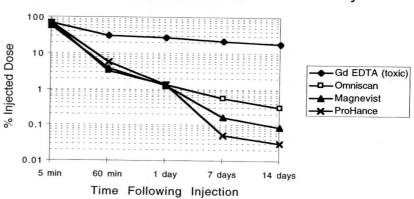

scans, with important clinical applications in infarct detection and evaluation.

Development History

Before 1982, the relaxation effects of the paramagnetic metals, which include gadolinium, were well known. However, the toxicity of these metals in their ionic forms appeared to prevent their use in humans. To design a safe agent, it was proposed that the metal ion be tightly bound by a chelate. Thus, the paramagnetic effect could be expressed, yet toxicity limited, by achieving rapid and total renal excretion. The gadolinium ion emerged as the most favorable choice because of its large paramagnetic effect or, more specifically, enhancement of T_1 relaxation.

The clinical safety of these agents is largely dependent on the stability of the chelate in vivo (Fig. 14-4). Key factors determining safety include thermodynamics, solubility, selectivity, and kinetics. There must be a high affinity of the chelate for the metal ion, which is reflected by the thermodynamic binding constant of the complex (K_{eq}). If the agent is not sufficiently soluble, precipitation of the gadolinium ion can occur, with potential toxicity. The chelate must also have high selectivity for the gadolinium ion itself. This requirement is such that metal exchange with endogenous ions, such as zinc and copper, does not occur. Last, but not least, the compound must exhibit slow kinetics in regard to release of the gadolinium ion. This makes possible near-complete excretion of the complex in the setting of normal renal function. One way to assess kinetics is by the rate of dissociation of the complex in acid solution. Table 14-1 presents a comparison of the three agents available

in the United States on the basis of these and other chemical characteristics. High thermodynamic stability, slow kinetics of dissociation (small $k(obs')s^{-1}$), low osmolality, and low viscosity are favorable features.

The gadolinium chelates, the major class of contrast agents currently used in MRI clinical practice, enhance T_1 relaxivity. Positive lesion enhancement is seen on T_1-weighted scans. Changes on T_2-weighted scans are generally not appreciable. Although these agents primarily affect T_1 relaxation rates, producing positive enhancement, they also affect T_2. In most clinical situations, T_2 effects have little contribution. However, at very high concentrations, negative enhancement can be seen. For example, on postcontrast scans of the bladder, some urine may be of low signal intensity. This occurs as a result of layering of contrast and hyperconcentration posteriorly when the patient is supine. The low signal intensity reflects the T_2 contribution.

Administration of a gadolinium chelate can substantially improve lesion identification and characterization. Within the CNS, lesion enhancement occurs as a result of disruption of the blood-brain barrier (BBB). For extra-axial abnormalities and lesions outside the CNS, contrast enhancement is governed by differences in tissue vascularity. At a standard dose (0.1 mmol/kg), lesion enhancement on MRI using a gadolinium chelate is equivalent or slightly superior to that on x-ray CT using an iodinated agent. However, unlike CT, adjacent bone or calcification does not obscure abnormal contrast enhancement.

Over the past decade, research has focused in part on the development of new gadolinium chelates with improved tolerance. Increased emphasis has been placed on physicochemical properties, including osmolality, viscosity, and stability of the metal chelate in vivo. Agents with lower osmolality and viscosity can be administered faster and generally at higher doses, important features for first-pass perfusion studies. Other avenues of research include development of compounds with higher relaxivity. Both approaches seek to lower the toxicity of the agent for a given effective dose. One step in development has paralleled the history of the iodinated agents. Nonionic (neutral) compounds, such as Pro-Hance, have been perfected since the initial develop-

☐ TABLE 14–1. Physicochemical properties of the gadolinium chelates in clinical use in the United States

Trade name	log K_{eq}	$k(obs')s^{-1}$	Osmolality (mOsm/kg)	Viscosity (cP)
ProHance	23.8	6.3×10^{-5}	630	1.3
Magnevist	22.1	$>1 \times 10^{-3}$	1960	2.9
Omniscan	16.9	$>2 \times 10^{-2}$	783	1.4

ment of Magnevist, an ionic (charged) compound. Another evolution in design has been from linear chelates (initially) to macrocyclic chelates. Macrocycles, such as ProHance, exhibit higher thermodynamic and kinetic stability, leading to lower long-term heavy metal (Gd^{3+}) deposition. Although only one macrocycle is currently approved in the United States, another (Dotarem) is in use outside the United States, and a third (Gadovist, gadobutrol, Schering AG), from the manufacturer of Magnevist, is awaiting approval in Europe. Gadolinium chelates targeted in part to the liver (MultiHance, gadobenate dimeglumine, Bracco Diagnostics) are also in clinical use; agents that bind to human serum albumin to increase blood pool residence time are being evaluated in clinical studies. The latter class of agents may have utility in MRI angiography.

Contrast agents that principally affect T_2 have received less attention. One factor that discouraged development early on was the long imaging time for T_2-weighted scans. With the advent of fast spin echo scans, this factor has become less important. Gradient echo scans can also be done, but their sensitivity to bulk susceptibility artifacts limits their usefulness. One of the more promising groups of intravenous T_2 contrast media is the iron particle group. The size of the particles determines their distribution. Larger particles are phagocytosed by macrophages of the reticuloendothelial system, with uptake in normal liver and spleen. Smaller particles are taken up by lymph nodes and bone marrow and have a long residence time in the bloodstream.

In the presence of a sufficient concentration of iron particles, there is selective T_2 shortening with profound signal loss. Because MRI signal intensity is decreased in normal liver and spleen (with large iron particles), focal areas of replacement, such as metastatic disease, are seen as areas of higher signal intensity. Iron particles exhibit a monophasic effect on signal intensity because progressively larger doses can only further reduce signal intensity until the level of background noise is reached.

GADOLINIUM CHELATES

This discussion is limited to gadolinium chelates that have been developed for use as contrast media in MRI and the intravenous application of these agents. In the past, clinical trials were conducted in Europe examining the oral use of gadolinium chelates. However, no agent is currently approved for such an indication in the United States. The gadolinium chelates are paramagnetic agents, developing a magnetic moment when placed in a magnetic field (the scanner). The large magnetic moment enhances the relaxation rates of water protons in the vicinity of the agent. On T_1-weighted images, there is a resultant increase in signal intensity when sufficient contrast material is present. T_1-weighted scans are used largely for the detection of these agents. In routine clinical practice, both pre- and postcontrast T_1-weighted scans are acquired. This enables certain identification of the presence of contrast material postinjection. T_2^*- (susceptibility) weighted scans are used for

visualization of these agents in one application only, that being first-pass brain imaging. In this instance, because T_2 relaxation is enhanced (with T_2 shorter), the result is a decrease in signal intensity.

Agents in Current Clinical Use

Because of their molecular size, the agents in current clinical use do not cross an intact BBB. Disruption of the BBB or abnormal vascularity allows accumulation of a gadolinium chelate in lesions, thus providing contrast enhancement. As a group, these agents have a good overall safety profile. The majority of adverse reactions are mild and transient. Although they are rare, severe anaphylactoid reactions have been documented. Diagnostic use should be carried out under the direction of a physician, with adequate preparation for treatment of a major untoward event. The possibility of a reaction is considered to be higher in patients with previously documented sensitivity to iodinated agents, gadolinium chelates, or multiple drugs or with history of asthma. The gadolinium chelates are given according to weight. The standard dose is 0.1 mmol/kg, which is equivalent to 0.2 ml/kg. Magnevist, ProHance, and Omniscan (gadodiamide, Nycomed) are all formulated at a 0.5 mol/L concentration. Except for dose, the clinical approval for these three agents is similar. Broad indications exist for their use in the CNS and body. None are formulated with antimicrobial preservatives. Most vials sold are for single-patient use only.

Magnevist is known to be excreted in breast milk. This is believed to be true, although not studied, for the other gadolinium chelates. If given to lactating mothers, the recommendation has been historically that breast-feeding should be discontinued for several days. One study demonstrated that the actual dose delivered to the infant is very low; thus, this recommendation (to discontinue breast-feeding) is now in question. The gadolinium chelates do cross the placenta and should not be used during pregnancy except under extenuating circumstances. There are no adequate, well-controlled studies examining safety in pregnant women.

Gadolinium is a metal of the lanthanide series, which are rare-earth elements. The safety of this class of agents is based on the use of chelates, firmly holding the gadolinium ion and ensuring rapid and complete excretion. If dechelated, the gadolinium ion can be deposited in liver, brain, and bone marrow. Gadolinium toxicity is known from industrial accidents. From a theoretical perspective, based on stability in vivo, ProHance is the safest agent and Omniscan the least. An increase in urinary zinc excretion has been documented after Omniscan injection (far greater than that observed with any other agent), reflecting in vivo transmetallation and release of free gadolinium ion.

Magnevist

In 1988, Magnevist was approved by the U.S. Food and Drug Administration (FDA) for intravenous injection. This agent was the first gadolinium chelate evaluated in humans and served as the model for development of the agents that followed. It is a linear chelate with a net charge of -2, counterbalanced by the two N-methylglucamine salts. The osmolality is 1960 mOsm/kg water at 37°C and the viscosity 2.9 cP. Thus, Magnevist has an osmolality 6.9 times that of blood plasma and is markedly hypertonic. The agent, like ProHance and Omniscan, is distributed in the extracellular space and excreted exclusively by glomerular filtration (in the urine). Approval is for adults and children (2 years of age and older). This approval is for the intracranial space (adults and children), spine (adults and children), and body (chest, abdomen, and pelvis, but excluding the heart, and in adults only). Nausea is reported as an adverse reaction with an incidence of 2.5% (according to the package insert). An intravenous injection rate of not more than 10 ml per 15 seconds is recommended.

ProHance

ProHance was approved for clinical use in the United States in 1992. This agent was the first ring chelate developed, accounting for its high stability in vivo and favorable safety margin. The ligand carries a charge of -3 and the gadolinium ion a charge of $+3$, with the combination (or chelate) carrying no charge. Thus, ProHance is a neutral or nonionic agent. The osmolality is 630 mOsm/kg water at 37°C and its viscosity 1.3 cP. Thus, ProHance has an osmolality only 2.2 times that of blood plasma. The agent is much less viscous than Magnevist, a difference quite noticeable to the individual performing the injection. Approval is for adults and children (2 years of age and older) in the brain (intracranial), spine, and associated tissues. ProHance is also approved for use in adults to visualize lesions in the head and neck. Nausea and taste perversion are reported as adverse reactions with an incidence of 1.4% (according to the package insert). In adults, there is approval for an additional dose of 0.2 mmol/kg, supplementing the initial dose of 0.1 mmol/kg (for a total of 0.3 mmol/kg). In clinical practice, scans are typically performed either after a standard dose or a single high-dose injection. The latter is most commonly used in the evaluation of intracranial metastatic disease (Fig. 14-5). In the multicenter U.S. trial (published in 1994) comparing 0.1 and 0.3 mmol/kg ProHance for the detection of brain metastases, an improvement of 32% in number of lesions detected was demonstrated at high dose. These trials established not only the greater efficacy for lesion detection but also the overall cost-effectiveness of this approach. Additional diagnostic value for high-dose administration has been demonstrated for a broad range of poorly enhancing disease. ProHance is approved for bolus injection. Single-dose (prefilled) syringes have also become available, with the field moving in this direction for packaging of all MRI contrast media.

Omniscan

Omniscan was approved for clinical use in the United States in 1993. This agent features a variant of the linear chelate used in Magnevist. The ligand carries a charge of -3, with the gadolinium chelate itself thus carrying no charge. Neutrality is achieved, however, at the cost of a substantial decrease in the stability of the chelate in vivo. The osmolality is 783 mOsm/kg water at 37°C and the viscosity 1.4 cP. Thus, Omniscan has an osmolality 2.8 times that of blood plasma. CNS (brain and spine) approval is for adults and children (2 years of age and older). Approval for use in the body is restricted to adults and includes the intrathoracic (noncardiac), intra-abdominal, pelvic, and retroperitoneal regions. An adverse effect on embryofetal development has been shown with Omniscan in rabbits. Nausea, headache, and dizziness occurred in clinical trials in 3% or less of patients (as reported in the package insert). In adults, there is approval for an additional dose of 0.2 mmol/kg. Omniscan, like ProHance, is approved for bolus injection.

OptiMARK

OptiMARK successfully completed phase III clinical trials in the late 1990s and received FDA approval for a dose of 0.1 mmol/kg (with limited indications) in the year 2000. OptiMARK is similar in design, distribution in the body, and use to the three extracellular gadolinium chelates previously approved by the FDA. Results from U.S. clinical trials were reported in 1999. Adverse events were seen in 73% of patients who received OptiMARK. In this trial, 163 patients received OptiMARK and 42 patients received a placebo. Adverse events were reported in 50% of the placebo group. The rate of adverse events increased with dose (doses of 0.1, 0.3, and 0.5 mmol/kg were evaluated). In a second trial, also published in 1999, OptiMark was compared with Magnevist. In this trial, 37 of 99 patients (37%) receiving OptiMARK experienced an adverse event; events in 9 patients (9%) were considered likely related to the contrast agent. Reaction rates were similar with Magnevist. Forty-five of 94 patients (48%) receiving Magnevist experienced an adverse event; events in 13 patients (14%) were considered likely related to the contrast agent. The most common reported adverse event attributed to either OptiMARK or Magnevist was taste perversion (6%). Urticaria occurred with an incidence of less than 2%.

Adverse Reactions

Although the gadolinium chelates are commonly thought not to be associated with any adverse reactions, this is not true. Other than pain at the injection site, which may or may not, in reality, be related to contrast injection, the two most common mild reactions encountered (attributed to contrast injection) are nausea and hives. On the basis of U.S. clinical trials published in the journal *Radiology*, there is no statistically significant difference between the agents in terms of incidence of these two adverse reactions. Nausea is reported in 1.5% of patients receiving Magnevist, 1.2% of patients receiving ProHance, and 1.6% of patients receiving Omniscan. With regard to hives, these were reported in 0.3% of patients receiving Magnevist, 0.2% of patients receiving ProHance, and 0.7% of patients receiving Omni-

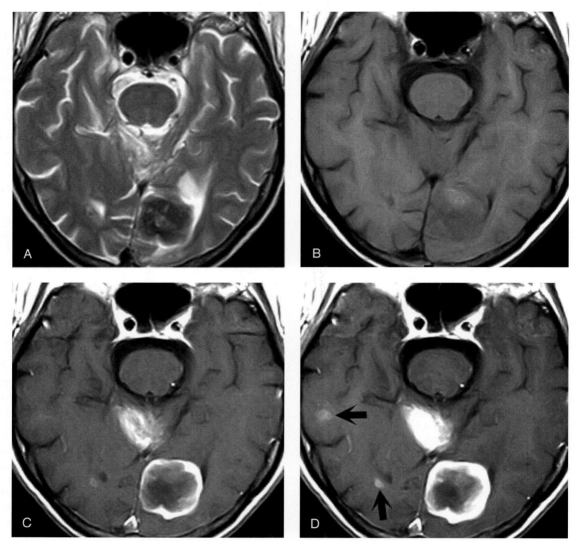

FIGURE 14–5. Brain metastatic disease illustrates the use of high contrast dose. Precontrast T_2- (*A*) and T_1- (*B*) weighted scans are compared with postcontrast T_1-weighted scans using doses of 0.1 (*C*) and 0.2 (*D*) mmol/kg. High dose improves the detectability of two small metastases (*D, arrows*): one near the right occipital horn and the other in the right temporal lobe. All lesions show greater contrast enhancement at high dose. Although ProHance or Omniscan could have been used in this manner, the results were obtained with MultiHance, a new agent already approved in Europe (with Food and Drug Administration approval pending). (From Runge VM, Nelson KL: Contrast agents. In DD Stark, WG Bradley Jr. [Eds]: Magnetic Resonance Imaging. St. Louis, Mosby Year Book, 1999, 3rd ed.)

scan. Severe anaphylactoid reactions occur, but are very rare, with all agents. Patients with asthma, multiple allergies, or known drug sensitivities (including to iodinated contrast media) are at increased risk. Health care personnel should be aware of the potential for severe anaphylactoid reactions in association with the use of gadolinium chelates and be prepared should complications arise. All agents for intravenous use in MRI should only be administered to a patient when a physician is readily available, in the near vicinity, in case such an untoward event is encountered.

Agents in Clinical Trials

Contrast media currently in clinical trials include new extracellular gadolinium chelates (similar to Magnevist,

ProHance, and Omniscan), hepatobiliary gadolinium chelates, and intravascular agents. Of this group, MultiHance is somewhat unique, with intended applications including both the CNS and body. MultiHance is excreted principally by the kidneys and to a small extent by the liver. The latter feature markedly improves the performance of this agent in the liver. MultiHance also binds slightly to proteins, improving its relaxivity (enhancement effect) regardless of location in the body. Thus, at an equivalent dose, it exhibits a superior contrast effect compared with other chelates regardless of body region.

Of the agents with some hepatobiliary excretion, MultiHance is the farthest along in regard to approval status. This agent is currently awaiting approval in the United States. However, MultiHance is already approved and in clinical use in most of Europe. When used in the liver, both dynamic and delayed scans provide valuable information. Before its clinical approval, dynamic imaging with the extracellular gadolinium chelates will continue to play a major role in liver MRI.

MultiHance

MultiHance is the first agent in a new class of gadolinium chelates with initial extracellular distribution, weak protein binding, and subsequent renal and hepatobiliary excretion. A substantial increase in enhancement is seen with MultiHance, when compared at the same concentration with the three gadolinium chelates in current clinical use, because of the weak protein binding. In one experiment, peak signal intensity enhancement in brain tumors was 87% after 0.1 mmol/kg MultiHance versus 64% after 0.1 mmol/kg Magnevist, which has no protein binding. A similar increase in enhancement has been observed in an infarct model. In the CNS, MultiHance at a dose of 0.2 mmol/kg should provide roughly the same lesion enhancement as seen with 0.3 mmol/kg of a conventional agent (see Fig. 14-5).

Phase I, II, and III clinical trials have been performed in Europe and Japan, with 975 individuals receiving MultiHance. These trials included imaging of the CNS, chest (heart), and abdomen. In Phase IIb-III studies, nausea was reported in 1.1% of subjects. In addition to being an excellent extracellular contrast agent for application in the CNS, MultiHance is a superior agent for liver imaging because of its hepatobiliary excretion (Fig. 14-6). With its clinical introduction, MultiHance will replace conventional extracellular gadolinium chelates for liver applications. In addition to dynamic scans, as acquired with conventional agents, delayed scans can also be obtained after MultiHance injection (for liver imaging). On delayed scans, there is clearance of the agent from the extracellular space with uptake in hepatocytes and biliary excretion. Delayed scans are particularly useful for the detection of small liver metastases. Liver-lesion contrast is highest 60 to 120 minutes after injection, and detection of lesions less than 1 cm in size is markedly improved. MultiHance is the lead agent in this class in terms of both clinical experience and stage of evaluation. MultiHance is currently approved for clinical use in most of Europe.

Phase II U.S. clinical trials with MultiHance have also been completed. The agent was evaluated in both the liver and CNS. In the former trial, which was a study of focal liver lesions, 222 patients were enrolled at 14 sites. Based on the judgment of the on-site investigator, postcontrast scans improved diagnostic confidence to a degree sufficient to change patient management in 22% and 41% of patients, depending on the dose administered. Dynamic and delayed postcontrast scans proved complementary; both were of substantial diagnostic value (Fig. 14-7).

Gadovist

Clinical trials with Gadovist have been performed in Europe and Japan since 1992. Gadovist, like ProHance,

demonstrates high in vivo stability as a result of the ring shape of the chelate. As with ProHance, this enables safe injection of up to 0.3 mmol/kg and formulation at twice the normal concentration (1.0 molar vs. 0.5 mol/L). Gadovist was approved in Switzerland in 1998 for CNS use in adults (at doses of 0.1 and 0.3 mmol/kg). Both the 0.5 and 1.0 mol/L formulations were approved. The latter has advantages for perfusion studies, specifically for the diagnosis of stroke, detection of focal cerebral ischemia, and evaluation of tumor perfusion.

Eovist

Eovist is a new gadolinium chelate that, like MultiHance, has renal and hepatobiliary excretion. Eovist has been evaluated in European clinical trials; the focus has been for liver use. As with MultiHance, both dynamic (extracellular phase) and delayed (hepatobiliary phase) scans can be acquired when imaging the liver. Eovist provides improved detection of hepatic lesions over conventional extracellular gadolinium chelates, such as Magnevist.

AngioMARK

The ligand in AngioMARK is a derivative of that used in Magnevist, with an additional protein-binding diphenylcyclohexyl group attached to the chelate by a phosphodiester linkage. The agent binds strongly to plasma albumin after injection, achieving greater signal enhancement for longer periods of time when compared with a conventional extracellular gadolinium chelate. The slower molecular tumbling of the albumin-bound chelate affords a five- to 10-fold enhancement in relaxivity over existing gadolinium chelates. AngioMARK is designed for vascular indications, including peripheral, carotid, and coronary artery disease. In phase I, doses from 0.05 to 0.15 mmol/kg were evaluated. No clinically significant adverse events were reported in 63 normal individuals. A phase II safety and efficacy trial (for peripheral and carotid disease) has been completed in the United States using a dose of 0.05 mmol/kg. In a more recent phase II feasibility trial for imaging coronary arteries, the agent was administered at a dose of 0.1 mmol/kg.

Low Dose

The choice of contrast dose for screening MRI exams of the head and spine is now discussed, focusing on the issue of low (half) dose: 0.05 mmol/kg. The discussion is pertinent to the use of the gadolinium chelates (approved worldwide) with extracellular distribution and renal excretion (only). Data from clinical trials strongly support a dose not lower than 0.1 mmol/kg for screening MRI exams of the head and spine. The use of a lower dose, with proven lower efficacy, places the patient at risk of adverse reactions because of contrast administration, yet does not ensure the one result for which contrast was administered: improving lesion detection and differential diagnosis. The choice of dose in certain specialty applications, specifically for the study of pitu-

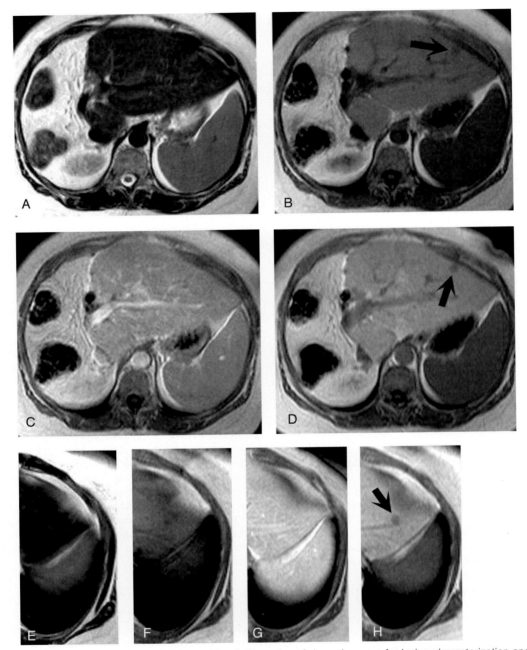

FIGURE 14–6. Metastases (adenocarcinoma, unknown primary). The value of dynamic scans for lesion characterization and delayed scans for lesion detection (using MultiHance, a gadolinium chelate with both renal and hepatobiliary excretion) is evident. A lesion adjacent to the anterior margin of the left lobe is questioned on the precontrast T_2-weighted scan (*A*) and confirmed on the precontrast T_1-weighted scan (*arrow*) (*B*). The lesion enhances to isointensity with normal liver on dynamic imaging (consistent with a metastasis) (*C*) and is best identified on the delayed scan at 80 minutes after MultiHance injection (*D, arrow*). Closer to the dome of the diaphragm, precontrast T_2- (*E*) and T_1-weighted (*F*) scans appear normal prospectively, as does the dynamic postcontrast scan (*G*). However, an additional metastasis (*arrow*) is clearly visualized on the delayed scan at this level (*H*). In retrospect, the lesion is seen (albeit poorly) on the precontrast T_2-weighted scan (*E*). No additional metastatic lesions were noted.

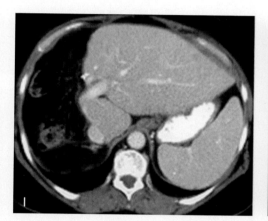 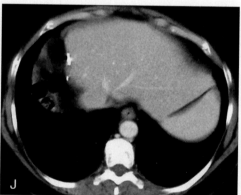

FIGURE 14–6 *Continued. I* and *J*, Both metastases were poorly detected by enhanced spiral computed tomography.

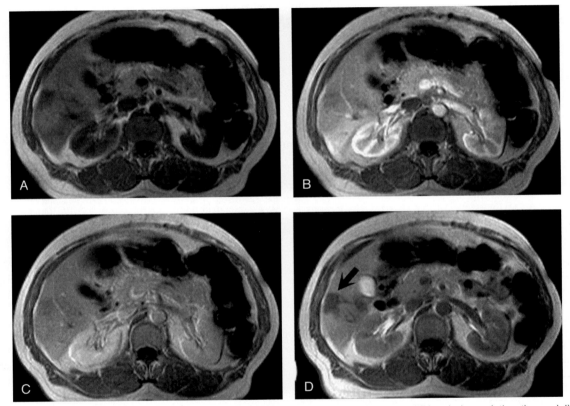

FIGURE 14–7. Metastases from colon carcinoma. The value of delayed postcontrast scans in additional planes (other than axial) using MultiHance is evident. No abnormality was noted on the precontrast T_2-weighted scan (not shown). *A,* Two areas of abnormal low signal intensity are seen in the liver on the precontrast T_1-weighted scan. *B,* The more posterior of the two enhances on the dynamic scan obtained immediately after contrast injection, consistent with normal liver (focal sparing from fatty infiltration). The lesion more laterally demonstrates mild inhomogeneous enhancement that progresses slightly from immediately (*B*) to 5 minutes (*C*) postcontrast. Lesion margins are also indistinct on the dynamic scans. These features are consistent with a metastasis. *D,* This metastasis (*arrow*) is clearly seen on the delayed scan obtained 80 minutes after MultiHance injection.

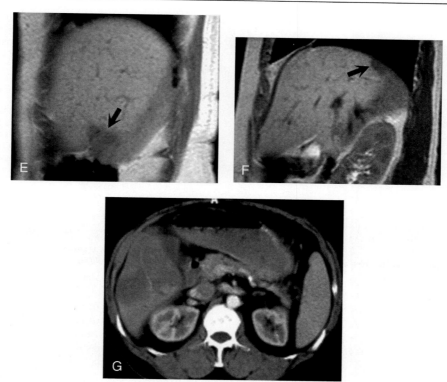

FIGURE 14–7 *Continued. E* and *F,* Acquisition (in the delayed time frame) of additional breathhold images in the sagittal plane led to a change in patient management. These scans show clearly the metastasis (*E, arrow*) noted on axial imaging but also identify an additional metastasis (*F, arrow*) adjacent to the diaphragm. *G,* The enhanced computed tomography scan was difficult to interpret prospectively (without reference to the magnetic resonance image) because of extensive focal fatty infiltration.

itary microadenomas and acoustic schwannomas, is also discussed. Excluded from commentary is the choice of dose for contrast-enhanced magnetic resonance angiography (CE-MRA), an area of current controversy. However, in CE-MRA, doses higher than 0.1 mmol/kg are commonly used. The reason for addressing the issue of dose in some depth is the practice at some MRI sites of splitting a 20-ml vial of contrast (intended for single-patient use) into two doses of 10 ml, each for different patients. This practice cannot be justified on a scientific basis and raises important ethical and legal issues.

Clinical Trial Experience

In the referenced literature, only a small number of studies exist that compare results in the CNS over a range of contrast dose, from very low (0.025 mmol/kg) to high (0.3 mmol/kg). In 1987, the first experience with a gadolinium chelate (Magnevist or gadolinium DTPA) in intracranial tumors was published. This study, which evaluated doses of 0.05 to 0.2 mmol/kg in 11 patients, concluded that a dose of 0.1 mmol was both safe and suitable. Also noted was that a dose of 0.2 mmol/kg increased diagnostic yield in selected cases. In a follow-up 1990 report, which evaluated doses of 0.025 to 0.2 mmol/kg, a dose of 0.1 mmol/kg was recommended for routine study of intracranial tumors. This study also noted that the use of 0.2 mmol/kg further increased tumor-brain contrast. In the largest series published with gadolinium DTPA, doses of 0.025, 0.05, and 0.1 mmol/kg were evaluated in 88 patients. This study, which

appeared in 1992, confirmed the conclusion of earlier investigations that a dose of 0.1 mmol/kg was more effective for enhancing intracranial tumors than lower doses (on both mid- and high-field units).

The advent of clinical trials with ProHance in the late 1980s provided a second opportunity to examine dose and efficacy. In a study of 14 patients, doses of 0.05 to 0.3 mmol/kg were evaluated. The authors concluded that lesion enhancement was sufficient for clinical diagnosis in all cases at a dose of 0.1 mmol/kg. However, doses higher than 0.1 mmol/kg further improved lesion enhancement. A 1991 study examined 40 patients given doses of 0.05 to 0.3 mmol/kg. The authors concluded that lesion contrast improved with dose and that the lowest dose evaluated, 0.05 mmol/kg, was inadequate for the evaluation of most CNS tumors.

Thus, phase II and III clinical trials, which are the only dose-ranging studies to date, conclude that a dose of 0.1 mmol/kg (using a gadolinium chelate with extracellular distribution and renal excretion) is sufficient for screening the CNS. No data are provided to support a lower dose, and indeed the evidence points to this being markedly inferior. Figures 14-8, 14-9, and 14-10 show the difference between lesion enhancement with half-dose (0.05 mmol/kg) and full dose (0.1 mmol/kg). Metastases can be readily missed at doses lower than 0.1 mmol/kg (see Fig. 14-8). Other intra-axial lesions may not enhance sufficiently at doses lower than 0.1 mmol/kg to permit the identification of BBB disruption, the very reason for contrast injection (see Fig. 14-9). Simi-

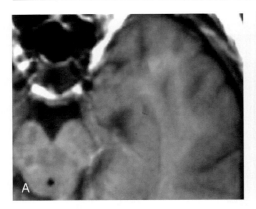
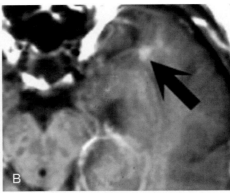

FIGURE 14–8. Metastatic disease, comparison of half- (*A*) and standard dose (*B*) postcontrast scans. A single brain metastasis (*B, arrow*) is well seen when the standard dose (0.1 mmol/kg) of contrast is administered. Enhancement after half-dose is poor; the metastasis is difficult to identify. This lesion was also not clearly seen on the precontrast T$_2$-weighted scan (not shown), as is often the case with small brain metastases.

larly, extra-axial abnormalities may not be recognized at half-dose (see Fig. 14-10).

Phase II and III clinical trials also provided the impetus for the examination of high doses in selected patient populations. It is important to note that extensive clinical experience exists with high contrast dose (0.3 mmol/kg with ProHance or Omniscan) in the study of brain metastases. Clinical trials examining this issue have established not only the greater efficacy for lesion detection (with a dose of 0.3 mmol/kg) but also the overall cost effectiveness of this approach.

Specialty Applications

Limited clinical trials have been published in only two specialty areas regarding possible use of doses lower than 0.1 mmol/kg. In a 1995 study limited to acoustic schwannomas, with a sample of 39 patients, it was suggested that a dose of 0.1 mmol/kg may not be necessary for detection of acoustic schwannomas, and that half-dose might be sufficient. This result is to some extent expected, given the intense enhancement (often 1000%) of acoustic schwannomas on MRI after gadolinium chelate injection (using standard dose). Of all brain lesions, acoustic schwannomas display by far the greatest magnitude of contrast enhancement.

In a 1991 study of pituitary adenomas, 11 microadenomas and 12 macroadenomas were evaluated with half-dose only. There was no comparison with full-dose exams. On the basis of this limited number, it was stated that the half-dose study appeared comparable to full-dose techniques for the detection of micro- and macroadenomas. Again, theoretical considerations support the choice of a lower dose in this area, given the intense enhancement of the normal anterior pituitary and infundibulum, two structures that lie outside the BBB.

It should be noted that even in these two specialty areas the support for half-dose is limited. Both studies commented on the need for confirmation of their results, which has never been done, in larger populations.

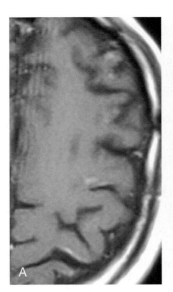
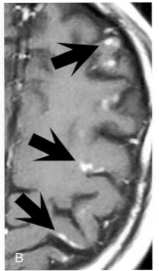

FIGURE 14–9. Subacute infarction, comparison of half- (*A*) and standard (*B*) dose. The patient presented 12 days previously with a left hemispheric stroke. Precontrast scans were normal, including both fast T$_2$-weighted and fluid-attenuated inversion recovery sequences. In subacute brain infarction, there may be sufficient resolution of vasogenic edema to make the lesion difficult to identify on precontrast scans. In this setting, the lesion can be identified on postcontrast scans as a result of blood-brain barrier disruption. The scan obtained after standard dose contrast administration (*B*, 0.1 mmol/kg) demonstrates multiple areas of abnormal cortical enhancement (*arrows*), confirming the clinical diagnosis. At half-dose, enhancement is subtle and less widespread; identification of the abnormality is not assured.

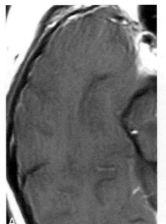
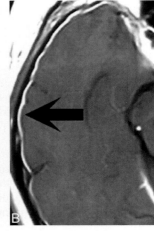

FIGURE 14–10. Dural inflammation, comparison of half (*A*) and standard (*B*) dose. *A*, Enhancement of extra-axial abnormalities can also be poor with half-dose. Dural enhancement, in this instance resulting from previous hemorrhage, is clearly seen (*arrow*) at standard contrast dose (0.1 mmol/kg).

Neither study addresses contrast dose at low fields. One study was performed at 0.5 and 1.5 T and the other at 1.0 and 1.5 T. Low-field systems are poor candidates for thin-slice high-resolution imaging, as required in the pituitary and internal auditory canal. High-quality imaging at low field requires careful selection of imaging technique; higher dose is typically advocated, not lower dose. Both of the publications referenced also examined half-dose in patient populations with a specific known diagnosis. In real-world imaging of the sella and internal auditory canal, other diseases need to be considered and would likely not be as well depicted at a lower contrast dose.

OTHER APPROVED AGENTS

Feridex (ferumoxides, Berlex Laboratories) is a reddish-brown colloid of superparamagnetic iron oxide particles that also contain dextran formulated for intravenous use. The agent is taken up by cells of the reticuloendothelial system (RES). Its principal use is as a liver agent. The iron enters the normal body iron metabolism cycle after injection. Feridex shortens T_2, producing signal loss on T_2-weighted scans. Tissues with decreased RES function (e.g., tumors, cysts, and other benign lesions) retain their signal intensity, so contrast between normal liver and lesions is increased. Feridex is approved in the United States for intravenous use in adults only and only for liver imaging. The dose is diluted in 100 ml and given over 30 minutes. Feridex is contraindicated in patients with known allergic or hypersensitivity reactions to parenteral iron or dextran. Anaphylactic-like reactions and hypotension have been seen after injection. Acute severe back, leg, or groin pain can occur within 1 to 15 minutes after injection alone or with other symptoms, such as hypotension and dyspnea. In clinical trials, this pain was severe enough to cause interruption or discontinuation of the infusion in 2.5% of patients (12.5% of patients with cirrhosis).

Teslascan (Mn DPDP, Nycomed) is a manganese chelate approved for liver imaging at a dose of 5 μmol/kg (0.1 ml/kg). The dose is given by intravenous administration over 1 minute. Postcontrast images are typically acquired with a slight delay, 15 minutes or longer, after injection. The ion responsible for enhancement, manganese, is different when compared with the gadolinium chelates. The agent was designed to be incorporated into hepatocytes. Postcontrast, moderate enhancement of normal liver parenchyma is seen, improving, in some instances, lesion conspicuity and differential diagnosis. In phase I, facial flushing and warmth were observed in 35 of 40 individuals. Dose-dependent increases in heart rate and blood pressure were also seen.

Subsequent clinical trials were conducted with lower doses and slower intravenous injection, resulting in fewer side effects. Mild to moderate adverse events were reported in 17% of patients in a phase III study published in 1997. Mn DPDP dechelates in vivo, accounting for the high incidence of flushing and enhancement of the intestinal mucosa and pancreas. The DPDP ligand does not facilitate transport of manganese into any organ, except the kidney, but does reduce distribution to the heart. The instability of the complex in vivo has raised concerns regarding potential toxicity from free manganese (known to accumulate in the brain and leading to a parkinsonism-like syndrome). In preclinical evaluation, Teslascan injection caused skeletal abnormalities in fetal rats; Mn^{2+} was the causative agent. There was also an increased rate of fetal demise in rabbits at 10 times the recommended clinical dose.

The market acceptance in the United States of Feridex and Teslascan has been poor. Reasons for low utilization of these agents include the inability to obtain dynamic postcontrast scans, limited diagnostic value, and the high number of adverse reactions (relative to the gadolinium chelates).

ORAL CONTRAST MEDIA

Four different oral contrast media have been approved for clinical use in the United States. In Europe, but not in the United States, an oral formulation of Magnevist is also available. Imagent (PFOB, Alliance) was approved in the early 1990s but is no longer marketed. Gastro-MARK (AMI 121, Mallinckrodt) was the second agent to market. LumenHance (Bracco Diagnostics) and Ferri-Seltz (Nyomed) were approved by the FDA in 1999. Imagent was highly effective in producing low signal intensity in the bowel. It is tasteless, water insoluble, and nontoxic. However, complete bowel opacification was difficult and side effects were high because of the rapid transit of the agent through the bowel. The majority of the agent is eliminated rectally within the first few hours after administration.

GastroMARK is a dark-brown aqueous suspension of superparamagnetic iron oxide. The recommended dose is 600 ml (900 ml maximum) administered orally at a rate of 300 ml over 15 minutes. Depending on the section of the bowel that is to be opacified, imaging is performed from between 30 minutes to several hours postadministration. A substantial time delay after administration (4-7 hours) is recommended for delineation of the lower gastrointestinal tract. GastroMARK is approved for oral use in adults only to enhance delineation of the upper gastrointestinal tract. The approval (according to the package insert) states that usefulness in the lower gastrointestinal tract is limited by transit time and dilution. With pancreatic and gastric masses, clinical trials demonstrated increased confidence in delineating the mass in 44% to 49% of cases. In clinical reports, efficacy in bowel marking was significant for the small bowel and cecum but not significant with all scan sequences for the sigmoid colon.

The formulation for LumenHance contains manganese (Mn^{2+}) chloride as the active ingredient. The agent is supplied as an off-white powder with strawberry flavoring. Each packet is dissolved to yield 300 ml; the instructions for use specify that the first packet be given 45 to 90 minutes, the second packet 30 to 45 minutes, and the third packet less than 30 minutes before imaging. LumenHance is approved for oral use in patients older than 16 years for enhanced delineation of the upper gastrointestinal tract. Clinical trials demonstrated that there was additional information on the postdose scans in 50% to 54% of patients. The agent provides both improved lesion visualization and the ability to distinguish the bowel from other normal and abnormal structures. On imaging, LumenHance has a dual T_1 and T_2 effect. The agent is hyperintense on T_1-weighted scans; clinical trials report good to excellent bowel marking on such scans. The agent is hypointense on T_2-weighted scans; clinical trials also demonstrate improved bowel marking on such scans. The latter feature (low signal intensity on T_2-weighted scans) makes LumenHance useful in MRI cholangiography. The agent lowers the signal intensity of the duodenum and small bowel, which might otherwise interfere with visualization of the biliary system on cholangiographic-type sequences.

The active ingredient in FerriSeltz is ferric ammonium citrate. The package insert states that two packets (6 g) are to be dissolved in 600 ml of water and administered orally over 15 to 30 minutes. Imaging is to be initiated within 5 to 20 minutes after administration. FerriSeltz is approved for use only in adults for enhanced bowel delineation of the upper gastrointestinal tract. T_1-weighted scans are used to visualize the agent. In clinical trials, investigators found increased intraluminal signal intensity, improved contrast enhancement of the gastrointestinal tract, and improved signal homogeneity in 89% to 98% of patients after ingestion. New or additional radiologic information was provided in clinical trials in 64% of patients and information that changed diagnosis, management, or surgical approach in 15%.

OFF-LABEL CONTRAST USE

The definition of off-label use, as it pertains to diagnostic radiology, is the use of an approved contrast agent for a clinical purpose not stipulated in the package insert. Off-label use is common in clinical practice in the United States. Addressing legal issues, off-label use is not a violation of U.S. law, provided that the use is in the course of routine medical practice and not part of an investigation into safety or effectiveness and not commercialized through advertising. Off-label use is possible because the FDA does not have the authority to regulate the use of approved contrast media in any manner that radiologists believe, in their professional judgment, would best serve the patient. Furthermore, the use of an approved contrast agent for a clinical purpose not explicitly contained in the labeling does not expose the radiologist to malpractice liability. Reimbursement, however, limits off-label use. Off-label use may or may not be reimbursed, depending on the specific application and local insurance carrier. In Europe, the situation is similar in regard to off-label use and the ramifications thereof.

Off-label use is important to ensure that the patient, in many situations, receives the best diagnostic exam. For example, no MRI contrast agent is approved in the United States for use in patients younger than 2 years. This is at odds with standard clinical practice. Published clinical trials have established safety and guidelines for the use of gadolinium chelates in young children and infants. Particularly in hospital settings, gadolinium chelates are commonly administered to patients younger than 2 years because contrast use can be important for lesion detection and appropriate differential diagnosis. An even more significant example of off-label use is the injection of gadolinium chelates for MRA exams (CE-MRA). No agent has specific approval for this indication. Off-label use of the gadolinium chelates for CE-MRA is common and accepted practice throughout the United States.

The subject of off-label use is very important in clinical practice; thus, the issue bears re-explaining, perhaps in a manner more understandable to the average user. Contrast media are approved with certain indications. This does not, however, limit how a physician can use an agent. Almost 85% of all MRI contrast use is in the head and spine, and all agents have approval here for patients older than 2 years. Comparatively, very few doses are used in other areas. Some agents have "whole body approval"; however, this refers specifically to the chest, abdomen, and pelvis. None of the agents are approved for the heart, breast, or musculoskeletal system or for MRA. Diagnostic radiologists commonly use contrast media in these and other off-label applications. Such use often constitutes the best of medical care.

CONCLUSION

The gadolinium chelates play a major role in the evaluation of patients by MRI. These agents improve both the sensitivity and specificity of the exam. In many cases, particularly in the CNS, lesions cannot be identified before contrast administration. Lesion delineation, assessment of lesion activity, and differential diagnosis are improved with the addition of postcontrast scans. The scope of applications continues to expand, as the modality and clinical experience mature. New agents on the horizon include gadolinium chelates with enhanced relaxivity (greater contrast effect at the same dose), hepatobiliary distribution, and intravascular distribution.

15

Contrast-Enhanced Magnetic Resonance Angiography

ontrast-enhanced magnetic resonance angiography (CE-MRA) is a stunning new application of magnetic resonance that has gained widespread clinical acceptance and application in a very short time. Clinical applications exist in all areas of the body; this subsequent discussion focuses on applications in the brain, carotid arteries, branch vessels of the aortic arch, pulmonary arteries, aorta (thoracic and abdominal), portal vein, renal arteries, and extremities. There are four major applications within this group, in terms of total number of exams, because of the large patient populations with vascular disease involving these critical areas. The major applications involve the carotid arteries, aorta, renal arteries, and arteries of the lower extremity.

Vascular imaging is performed in CE-MRA by visualization of the first pass of a contrast agent, typically a gadolinium chelate, immediately after bolus intravenous (IV) contrast injection (Fig. 15-1). A 10- to 25-fold reduction in blood T_1 occurs during the first pass of the contrast bolus in arteries and veins. This produces a large signal intensity difference between vessels and background tissues. The consequence of this reduction in T_1, with appropriate imaging techniques, is that vessels have (transiently) very high signal intensity. Scans are acquired using rapid three-dimensional (3D) gradient echo technique; both multiplanar reconstructions and maximum intensity projection images are viewed for diagnostic purposes. Trying to make the scan as fast as possible places a premium on gradient performance; the latest 1.5-T scanners produce markedly superior scans. The trend in evolution of scan technique has been toward ever shorter time to repetition (TR) and time to echo (TE). Proper timing of image acquisition relative to contrast injection can be achieved by using a test dose (1 or 2 ml), with automatic bolus detection techniques, or by continuous acquisition of sequential (very rapid)

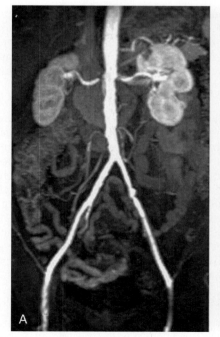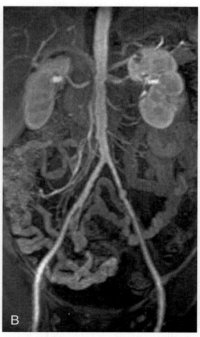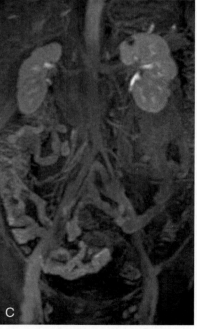

FIGURE 15–1. Timing of image acquisition. In contrast-enhanced magnetic resonance angiography (CE-MRA), timing is critical to achieve arterial phase images. In this patient with bilateral renal artery stenosis, three sequential scans were acquired. Arterial enhancement is maximum in the first scan (*A*), decreased in the second (*B*), and virtually absent in the third (*C*). A simple renal cyst is incidentally noted in the left kidney. Early venous return of contrast is evident in the third scan. (Images courtesy of K. Bis.)

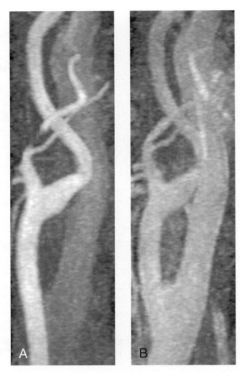

FIGURE 15–2. Image degradation resulting from incorrect timing. In the carotid arteries, timing of imaging acquisition is particularly critical. The first scan (A) was obtained immediately after contrast injection and the second (B) 25 seconds later. The carotid bulb is well visualized (A). The quality of the second study (B) is compromised by the temporal decrease in arterial signal intensity and marked enhancement of the jugular vein. (From Saloner D: Determinants of image appearance in contrast-enhanced magnetic resonance angiography. A review. Invest Radiol 1998;33:488–495.)

scans. Both body weight and area of investigation influence contrast dose. Unlike all other applications, in CE-MRA the gadolinium chelates are typically given according to volume, not weight. Currently, injection of 40 ml is most common; 20 ml is used in some applications and by some institutions. The injection rate is typically 2 to 4 ml/second. Vessel contrast in CE-MRA is critically dependent on the timing of the contrast bolus (Fig. 15-2), the bolus geometry, and the choice of sequence parameters (Fig. 15-3). The bolus geometry is defined by flow rate, dose of contrast, and volume of saline flush. Consistent results require the use of a power injector for contrast administration.

The attributes of CE-MRA are many. First and foremost is the short scan time. Images can be acquired on high-performance systems using current software in 5 seconds or less. This enables imaging during breath-holding, which is critical for high-quality exams of the chest and abdomen. Other attributes include high (relative) spatial resolution, improved depiction of true vessel lumen, more accurate estimation of stenoses, and less sensitivity to turbulent flow. Unlike time-of-flight (TOF) MRA, the depiction of flow is independent of the orientation of the acquisition plane. Selection of scan orientation is dictated by the body part being examined, not by the orientation of the major vessels. In

terms of visualization of the vessels, CE-MRA shares much more in common with x-ray–based digital angiography than with noncontrast MRA techniques. In CE-MRA, it is the blood (containing a contrast agent) that is imaged. In TOF and phase-contrast MRA, it is the flow (or movement) of blood that is imaged.

BRAIN

Although CE-MRA has replaced TOF MRA in almost all areas of the body, it has not done so to date in the brain. TOF MRA performs well in the brain because of the presence of the blood-brain barrier and the rapid transit of blood from the arteries to the veins. TOF MRA continues to be used in most clinical practices for aneurysm screening. The improvement in vessel visualization offered by CE-MRA is incremental and tempered by the inability to separate (in time) the arterial and venous anatomy (Fig. 15-4). Applications of CE-MRA have focused on acquiring very high-resolution images, with long scan times (5 minutes), in which both arteries and veins are visualized (Figs. 15-5 and 15-6). This is unlike the application of CE-MRA techniques in the rest of the body, in which images are acquired only during the first pass of the contrast agent and the arterial and venous anatomy are routinely separated.

CAROTID ARTERIES

Conventional MRA, although widely used, suffers in the carotid arteries from motion artifacts (because of long scan times) and overestimation of stenotic lesions (as a result of turbulent flow). Both factors are much less of a problem with CE-MRA. The latter approach has thus gained widespread acceptance for imaging of the carotid arteries (Figs. 15-7 and 15-8). Of all anatomic areas, here imaging timing is likely the most critical. Rapid filling of the jugular veins occurs after bolus contrast injection, with the potential to obscure arterial anatomy.

Technique

The mean transit time of blood through the carotid arteries is less than 10 seconds. Thus, imaging time must be kept to a minimum. Scan times of 5 to 7 seconds are possible with the use of very short TRs. Other pulse sequence modifications include temporal interpolation, view sharing, and zero filling. The result is an approach called "time-resolved MRA." Scans are acquired sequentially from just before contrast injection for up to 50 seconds. Scan timing errors with this approach are practically impossible. One disadvantage to this technique is the lower spatial resolution compared with conventional MRA and x-ray angiography.

Atherosclerotic Disease

With time-resolved CE-MRA, it is possible to visualize the carotid arteries consistently without venous overlay. The use of longer scan times (up to 20 seconds) provides higher spatial resolution; the trade-off is possible image degradation as a result of jugular opacification. In the

FIGURE 15–3. Reduction of background signal intensity (SI) by subtraction of the precontrast image. Maximum intensity projection images are compared from images after contrast injection (*A*) and before injection (*B*) and from subtracting the pre- from the postcontrast data (*C*). The use of image subtraction reduces background SI and can eliminate some artifacts, such as the central radiofrequency spike in this example. (From Saloner D: Determinants of image appearance in contrast-enhanced magnetic resonance angiography. A review. Invest Radiol 1998;33:488–495.)

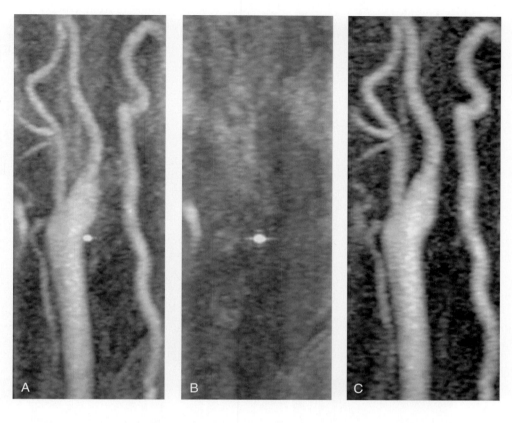

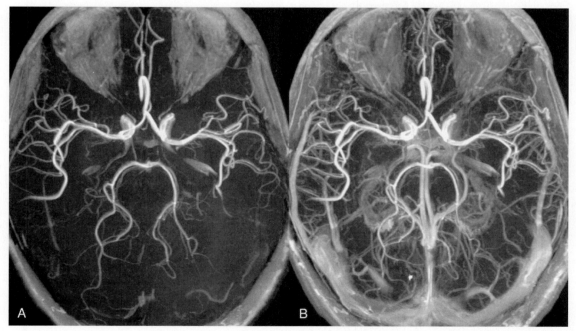

FIGURE 15–4. Intracranial magnetic resonance angiography (MRA) performed before (*A*) and after (*B*) intravenous contrast administration (normal patient exam). In the brain, after the first pass of a contrast agent, the T_1 of blood remains relatively constant. The contrast agent remains intravascular because of the presence of the blood-brain barrier. Thus, there is greater time for acquisition of high-resolution three-dimensional MRA images. Postcontrast images will, however, demonstrate substantial enhancement of venous structures. (From Parker DL, Tsuruda JS, Goodrich KC, et al: Contrast-enhanced magnetic resonance angiography of cerebral arteries. A review. Invest Radiol 1998;33:560–572.)

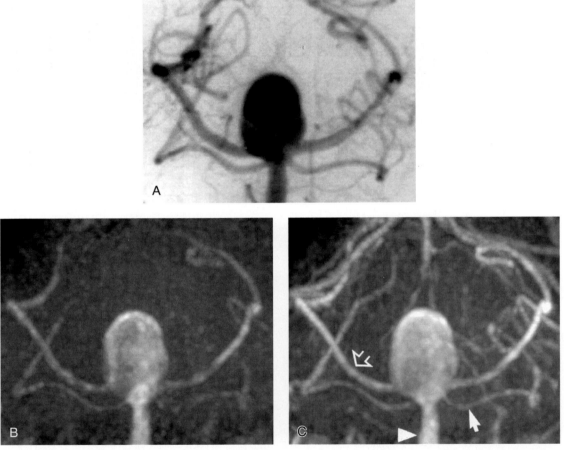

FIGURE 15–5. Basilar tip aneurysm. Note the improved arterial detail on high-resolution postcontrast three-dimensional magnetic resonance angiography (MRA). Conventional x-ray angiography (*A*) is compared with MRA exams obtained before (*B*) and after (*C*) contrast administration. The postcontrast exam was obtained in a nondynamic fashion. Postcontrast, there is improved visualization of the superior cerebellar (*C, arrow*) and posterior cerebral (*open arrow*) arteries, the terminal branches of the basilar artery (*arrowhead*). The postcontrast MRA exam is comparable to the conventional x-ray angiogram for visualization of arterial vessels. (From Parker DL, Tsuruda JS, Goodrich KC, et al: Contrast-enhanced magnetic resonance angiography of cerebral arteries. A review. Invest Radiol 1998;33:560–572.)

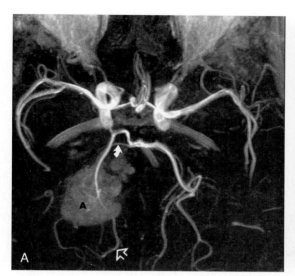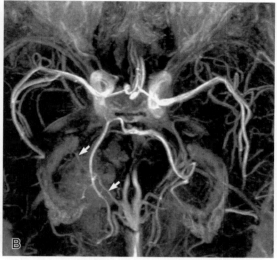

FIGURE 15–6. Cavernous angioma. Postcontrast magnetic resonance angiography (MRA) confirms a normal deep venous system (*B, arrows*). Specifically, there is no associated venous anomaly. Maximum intensity projections from pre- (*A*) and postcontrast (*B*) exams are presented. The precontrast exam clearly depicts the adjacent superior cerebellar (*curved arrow*) and posterior cerebral (*open arrow*) arteries. Hyperintense methemoglobin is present within the angioma (*A*). In this patient, acquisition of the postcontrast three-dimensional MRA exam ruled out the presence of a possible associated venous angioma. (From Parker DL, Tsuruda JS, Goodrich KC, et al: Contrast-enhanced magnetic resonance angiography of cerebral arteries. A review. Invest Radiol 1998;33:560–572.)

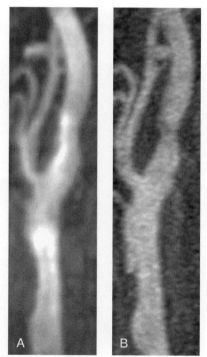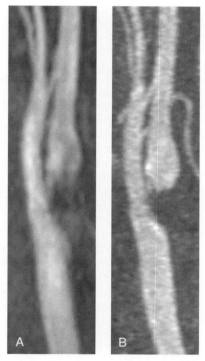

FIGURE 15–7. Improved depiction of atherosclerotic plaque with contrast-enhanced magnetic resonance imaging (CE-MRA). Maximum intensity projection images of the carotid bifurcation are presented from conventional three-dimensional time-of-flight (TOF) MRA (*A*) and CE-MRA (*B*) exams. Acquisition times were 10 minutes 45 seconds (*A*) and 21 seconds (*B*). Blurring is markedly reduced as a result of the short scan time of the CE-MRA exam, with resultant improved depiction of plaque in the common carotid artery. (From Saloner D: Determinants of image appearance in contrast-enhanced magnetic resonance angiography. A review. Invest Radiol 1998;33:488–495.)

FIGURE 15–8. Improved depiction of high-grade stenosis of the internal carotid artery with contrast-enhanced magnetic resonance angiography (CE-MRA). Maximum intensity projection images are presented from conventional three-dimensional time-of-flight MRA (*A*) and CE-MRA (*B*) exams. Turbulent flow causes signal dropout on the conventional MRA exam, with poor delineation of the proximal internal carotid artery. (From Saloner D: Determinants of image appearance in contrast-enhanced magnetic resonance angiography. A review. Invest Radiol 1998;33:488–495.)

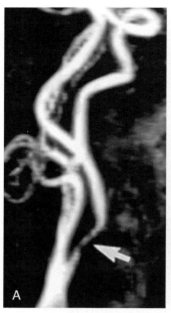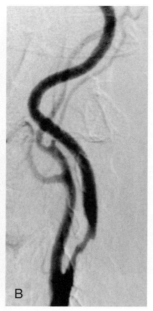

FIGURE 15–9. Comparable depiction of high-grade stenosis (*arrow*) of the internal carotid artery by contrast-enhanced magnetic resonance angiography (CE-MRA) (*A*) and intra-arterial digital subtraction angiography (*B*). Slight overestimation of a stenosis can occur with CE-MRA, as in this case. However, using North American Symptomatic Carotid Endarterectomy Trial (NASCET) criteria, CE-MRA does accurately depict carotid artery morphology and degree of stenosis. (From Steffens J-C, Link J, Heller M: Contrast-enhanced magnetic resonance angiography of the cervical arteries. A review. Invest Radiol 1998;33:573–577.)

evaluation of atherosclerotic disease of the carotid arteries, there is excellent agreement between CE-MRA and intra-arterial digital subtraction angiography (Fig. 15-9). The sensitivity and specificity of CE-MRA are high for the identification of surgical and nonsurgical disease (<50% stenosis). Plaque morphology is clearly demonstrated. Despite marked improvement compared with conventional 3D TOF MRA, CE-MRA may still overestimate high-degree stenosis. Across the United States, CE-MRA has largely replaced 3D TOF (noncontrast) MRA for the evaluation of the carotid and vertebral arteries.

The possibility of using a large field of view (FOV) represents another major advantage of CE-MRA (Fig. 15-10). Although this choice limits spatial resolution, use of a large FOV can be clinically advantageous, permitting depiction of vessel origins from the aortic arch. Disease of the subclavian vessels can thus also be visualized on a single exam (Fig. 15-11).

PULMONARY VASCULATURE

Respiratory and cardiac motion, saturation problems, long imaging times, and low spatial resolution have hampered the use of MRA in the pulmonary vasculature. These problems have been largely overcome with the advent of CE-MRA, making routine clinical studies possible. The major application of CE-MRA in the lungs is for the demonstration of pulmonary emboli. High sensitivity and specificity can be obtained. Complementary information is available from MRA evaluation of

the pelvic and femoral veins. In the not too distant future, clinical evaluation of lung ventilation and perfusion by MRA may also be possible.

Technique

Several special problems exist in imaging of the pulmonary vasculature. Flow may be slow, especially if right ventricular failure is present. Short imaging times are paramount, given the typical clinical presentation of pulmonary emboli with dyspnea. Although these present significant problems for conventional MRA, CE-MRA is much more robust. Very short TR (<5 msec) and TE (<2 msec) times are advised. The short TR makes breath-hold scans possible. The short TE is critical to minimize susceptibility artifacts caused by air-tissue interfaces in the lung. The flip angle is not critical; values between 20 and 60 degrees are used. High spatial resolution is, however, critical; 512 matrices are used together with a rather large FOV (320 mm). Phased-array coils are advised because of the importance of the signal-to-noise ratio. To avoid wrap-around artifacts, the arms are placed above the head. Scans are typically acquired in a coronal or coronal oblique plane. Excluding the most anterior and posterior portions of the lungs can minimize section thickness. An alternative approach (offering higher resolution) is the use of the sagittal plane, with separate scans of the right and left lungs. Electrocardiographic (ECG) triggering is generally not used.

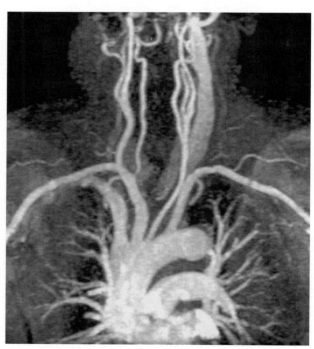

FIGURE 15–10. Illustration of the large field of view possible with contrast-enhanced magnetic resonance angiography (CE-MRA). Maximum intensity projection image displays the arterial vasculature from the aortic root to the skull base. Major advantages of CE-MRA compared with conventional MRA include short scan time, large anatomic coverage, and reduced flow artifacts (in part because of the use of short echo times). (From Saloner D: Determinants of image appearance in contrast-enhanced magnetic resonance angiography. A review. Invest Radiol 1998;33:488–495.)

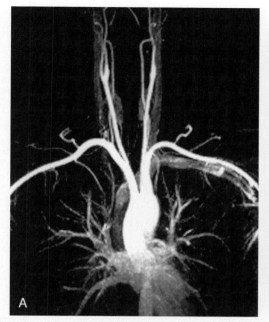
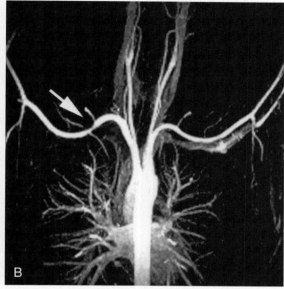

FIGURE 15–11. Thoracic outlet syndrome diagnosed with contrast-enhanced magnetic resonance angiography. Two exams were performed: the first in neutral position (A) and the second with elevation of the arms (B). In the latter, compression (arrow) of the right subclavian artery is evident. (From Boos M, Lentschig M, Scheffler K, et al: Contrast-enhanced magnetic resonance angiography of peripheral vessels. Different contrast agent applications and sequence strategies. A review. Invest Radiol 1998;33:538–546.)

The scan should be timed to maximize opacification of the pulmonary arteries. Because of rapid blood circulation, some venous opacification is often present. In high-quality exams, both central and peripheral (segmental and subsegmental) pulmonary arteries should be visualized without superimposition by pulmonary veins or the aorta and its branches. CE-MRA has led, in particular, to improved visualization of smaller pulmonary arteries compared with noncontrast MRA techniques.

Acute Pulmonary Embolism

Because the gold standard for diagnosis of pulmonary embolism is an invasive procedure (x-ray pulmonary angiography), there is a need for a highly sensitive and specific, widely available, readily performed, cost-effective noninvasive test. Currently used tests include computed tomography angiography (CTA) and ventilation-perfusion nuclear medicine lung scans. Currently, CE-MRA stands as an alternative to these procedures, possibly displacing CTA in the future.

Pulmonary emboli are diagnosed on CE-MRA by the detection of intraluminal filling defects or abrupt vascular cutoffs (Fig. 15-12). Maximum intensity projection (MIP) images permit assessment of the total thrombotic burden. For clot detection, however, multiplanar reconstructions are superior to MIP images. Observer experience is particularly important for accurate interpretation of CE-MRA in cases of possible pulmonary embolism.

Chronic Thromboembolic Disease

CE-MRA has also been successful in the diagnosis of chronic pulmonary thromboembolism (Fig. 15-13). Features of chronic pulmonary thromboembolism (with accompanying pulmonary hypertension) include dilation of the central arteries, direct visualization of wall adherent thrombotic material, wall vessel thickening, absence of peripheral vessels, abnormal proximal to distal tapering, and inhomogeneity of enhancement of the lung parenchyma.

Other Clinical Applications

CE-MRA can be used to evaluate the involvement of central pulmonary arteries by bronchogenic carcinoma (Fig. 15-14). ECG-triggered studies have been used to evaluate pulmonary arteriovenous malformations (AVMs). Clear separation of arterial and venous phases has not been possible. Utility has also been shown in pulmonary sequestrations.

CE-MRA versus CTA

CE-MRA offers many advantages over CTA. Smaller volumes of contrast are needed. The contrast agent is not considered to be nephrotoxic, and the osmotic load is less. With spatial resolution key to lesion detection, MRA offers the capability of direct image acquisition, with high in-plane resolution, in the coronal and sagittal planes. In addition, CE-MRA of the pulmonary vasculature can be complemented by MRA venography of the pelvic and femoral veins; the latter has been shown to be highly accurate.

THORACIC AORTA

CE-MRA is a powerful tool to evaluate both congenital and acquired disease of the thoracic aorta. In many institutions, this technique has replaced aortography for the study of nontraumatic aortic disease and is used for screening of suspected arch vessel disease.

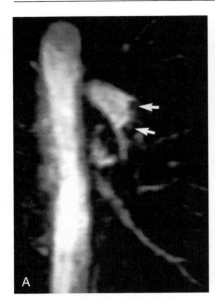

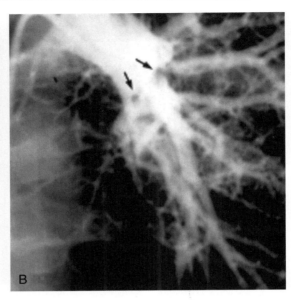

FIGURE 15–12. Acute pulmonary emboli, diagnosis by contrast-enhanced magnetic resonance angiography (CE-MRA) (*A*) with confirmation by x-ray angiography (*B*). Coronal CE-MRA image demonstrates multiple intravascular filling defects and vessel cut-offs (*arrows*). Pulmonary emboli (*arrows*) are confirmed by selective arteriography. (Courtesy of J. Debatin.)

FIGURE 15–13. Chronic pulmonary thromboemboli. *A,* Axial contrast-enhanced magnetic resonance imaging demonstrates thrombotic material adherent to the wall of the left main pulmonary artery (*arrows*). CE-MRA maximum intensity projection image reveals narrowing of the left main pulmonary artery (*curved arrow*) and peripheral segmental arterial cut-offs. CE-MRA, however, underestimates the amount of wall adherent thrombotic material. (From Kauczor H-U: Contrast-enhanced magnetic resonance angiography of the pulmonary vasculature. A review. Invest Radiol 1998;33:606–617.)

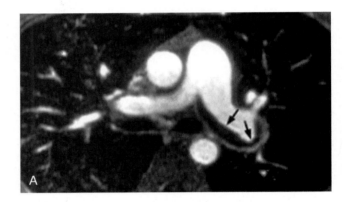

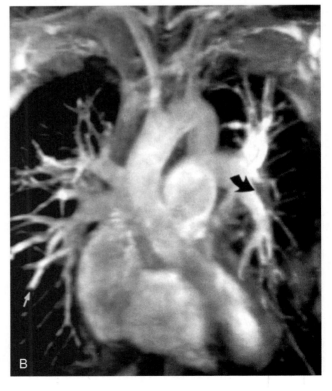

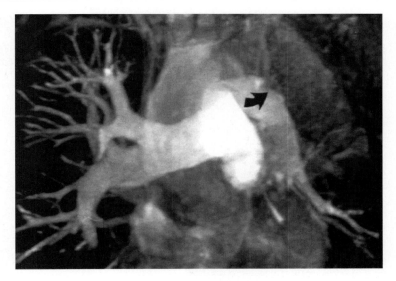

FIGURE 15–14. Occlusion of left upper lobe arteries in a patient with bronchogenic carcinoma illustrated by contrast-enhanced magnetic resonance angiography. Maximum intensity projection image demonstrates normal vascularity in the right lung with invasion of the left main pulmonary artery (*arrow*) and rarefaction of left upper lobe vessels. (From Kauczor H-U: Contrast-enhanced magnetic resonance angiography of the pulmonary vasculature. A review. Invest Radiol 1998;33:606–617.)

Technique

A timing exam with a test bolus or an alternative method to ensure optimal arterial enhancement (without overlying venous enhancement) is required. The use of a phased-array coil is recommended over the body coil. The latter is suboptimal for evaluation of small vessels, in particular the vertebral arteries. The patient's arms are placed at the side, avoiding possible compression of the subclavian artery and vein against the first rib. Contrast should be administered via the right antecubital vein because enhancement of the brachiocephalic vein from an injection on the left may degrade visualization of the arch vessels. A more general recommendation is that contrast be administered on the side opposite the anticipated disease. If disease is suspected bilaterally, the injection can be performed using a vein in the lower extremity. Dedicated arch vessel studies should use a smaller field of view than thoracic aortic studies. Acquisition of a mask image for subsequent subtraction is helpful, eliminating bright subcutaneous fat. Scans are acquired during breath-holding. For most patients, 20 ml of contrast is adequate; 40 ml is recommended in heavy patients. The use of an adequate saline flush (30 ml) after contrast injection is important to minimize artifacts from concentrated contrast in the vein injected. A power injector should be used. A second image acquisition 10 to 15 seconds after the first is recommended in dissections to better opacify the false lumen. Black blood images (using a technique such as HASTE) are acquired before the CE-MRA exam because these better delineate the aortic diameter and mural disease. Both multiplanar reformations and MIP images should be viewed to improve diagnostic accuracy and minimize interpretive errors. MIP images alone can be poor in the evaluation of thrombus or dissection and may overestimate stenoses.

Congenital Disease

Congenital arch vessel variants are readily demonstrated by CE-MRA. Most, however, are of little clinical significance, unless surgery is indicated because of occlu-sive, aneurysmal, or embolic disease. Frequently seen variants include a common origin of the innominate and left carotid artery, direct origin of the left vertebral artery from the aortic arch, and an aberrant right subclavian artery.

In aortic coarctation, there is focal narrowing of the thoracic aorta, usually in the region of the ductus arteriosus. CE-MRA provides excellent anatomic images of the extent of a coarctation and collateral circulation if present. The ability to view the images in 3D is quite helpful for surgical planning. Imaging follow-up on a regular basis is recommended after corrective surgery to look for recurrent coarctation and aneurysm formation (Figs. 15-15 and 15-16).

Occlusive (Acquired) Disease

In the United States, atherosclerotic disease is the most common cause of stenosis or occlusion involving the proximal great vessels. A substantial number of cases are also caused by arteritis; Takayasu's arteritis is the most common type.

The most common arch vessel lesion is occlusion of the proximal vertebral artery. Clinical symptoms result from lack of appropriate blood flow without adequate compensation from the carotid circulation.

The second most common proximal arch vessel lesion is stenosis or occlusion of the subclavian artery (Fig. 15-17). This is three times more frequent on the left side than the right. These lesions are often clinically silent because of excellent collateral circulation. The subclavian steal syndrome occurs when use of the upper extremity increases the demand for blood and diverts this from the cerebral circulation through the vertebral or innominate artery. Posterior fossa symptoms and arm claudication are seen clinically. Not all patients are symptomatic. Concomitant arch vessel occlusive disease is seen in 80%. Rapid serial CE-MRA scans readily demonstrate stenosis of the subclavian artery and subclavian steal.

Patients with innominate artery disease can present with right upper extremity ischemia or neurologic symp-

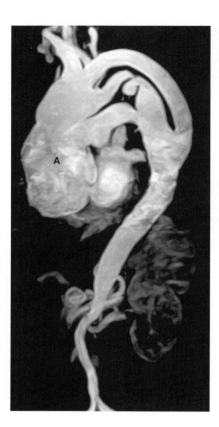

FIGURE 15–15. Patent aortic bypass graft in a patient with aortic coarctation illustrated by contrast-enhanced magnetic resonance angiography. Maximum intensity projection image depicts extra-anatomic bypass graft from the ascending to the descending aorta. Also noted is a juxtaductal pseudoaneurysm and ascending aortic aneurysm (A). (From Krinsky G: Gadolinium-enhanced three-dimensional magnetic resonance angiography of the thoracic aorta and arch vessels. A review. Invest Radiol 1998;33:587–605.)

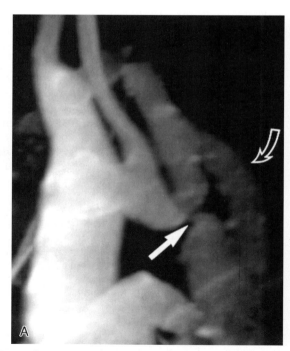

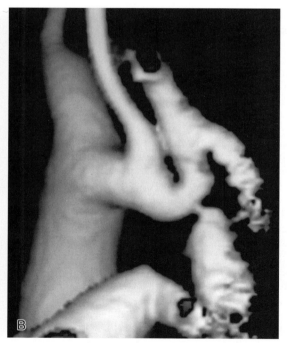

FIGURE 15–16. Severe focal aortic coarctation (*arrow*) depicted by contrast-enhanced magnetic resonance angiography. Both maximum intensity projection (*A*) and surface rendered (*B*) images clearly depict the focal stenosis distal to the left subclavian artery. The bucket-handle graft (*open arrow*) is not well visualized because of signal drop-off from the use of a surface coil. (From Yamada CY, Grygotis LA, Kaufman J: Gadolinium-enhanced magnetic resonance angiography of the aorta. A review. Invest Radiol 1998;33:618–627.)

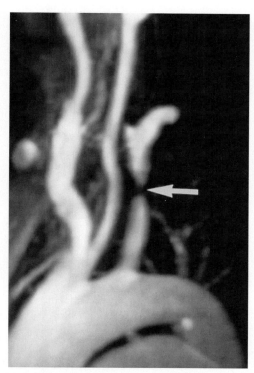

FIGURE 15–17. Severe focal stenosis of the left subclavian artery (*arrow*), proximal to the origin of the vertebral artery, depicted by contrast-enhanced magnetic resonance angiography (maximum intensity projection image). (From Yamada CY, Grygotis LA, Kaufman J: Gadolinium-enhanced magnetic resonance angiography of the aorta. A review. Invest Radiol 1998;33:618–627.)

toms. The latter may involve either the anterior or posterior circulation or both.

Thoracic Aneurysm

Thoracic aneurysms occur from the aortic root to the diaphragm and may be fusiform or saccular in shape (Fig. 15-18). Concomitant infrarenal abdominal aortic aneurysms are common, mandating evaluation of the entire aorta in patients with nontraumatic thoracic aneurysms. The most serious complication is death from rupture. Median diameter at rupture or dissection is 6 cm for ascending and 7 cm for descending aortic aneurysms. Similar to abdominal aortic aneurysms, size at presentation can be used to assess risk of rupture. In operative candidates, ascending aortic aneurysms of 5.0- to 5.5-cm diameter and arch or descending aortic aneurysms of 5.5 to 6.5 cm are electively repaired. The surgical approach depends on the extent of involvement, which is readily demonstrated by MRA. Limitations of MRA include the inability to evaluate the blood supply to the spinal cord and the coronary arteries. Both CE-MRA and black blood scans are required; the former provide anatomic information concerning the aneurysm and the latter are used to detect thrombus and mural disease (and assess size and extent). With thoracoabdominal aneurysms, the evaluation must include the renal and visceral vessels because involvement by the aneurysm or occlusive disease of these may alter the surgical approach.

Aortic Dissection

Aortic dissections are classified by extent of involvement. Seventy-five percent of all dissections involve the ascending aorta (Fig. 15-19) or transverse arch (Stanford A, DeBakey I and II). Immediate repair of acute proximal dissections is indicated. Such patients are often unstable with diagnosis and surgery based on transesophageal echocardiography. Acute dissections distal to the left subclavian artery (Stanford B, DeBakey III) are initially treated medically. A small percentage of these will eventually require surgery. MRA evaluation for dissection requires imaging from the aortic root to the iliac arteries. The location of the flap, aortic diameter, patency of branches, and presence or absence of associated hematomas should be determined. The false lumen usually is larger, has slower flow, is crescentic in shape, and lies along the outer curvature of the aorta. It often contains thrombus. Black blood techniques should be used in addition to CE-MRA; the latter is insensitive to intramural hematoma and extraluminal disease. Image quality is sufficient with breath-hold CE-MRA to also determine from which lumen the native coronary arteries, or bypass grafts, originate.

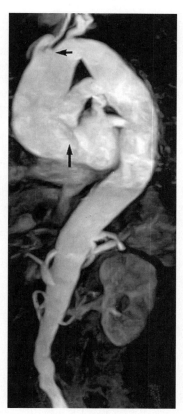

FIGURE 15–18. Ascending aortic aneurysm, sparing the sinotubular segment (*long arrow*) and extending into the proximal arch (*short arrow*), depicted by contrast-enhanced magnetic resonance angiography (maximum intensity projection image). This type of aneurysm is typical for atherosclerotic disease and long-standing aortic valvular disease. (From Krinsky G: Gadolinium-enhanced three-dimensional magnetic resonance angiography of the thoracic aorta and arch vessels. A review. Invest Radiol 1998;33:587–605.)

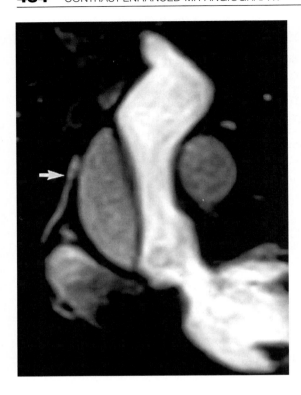

FIGURE 15–19. Type A aortic dissection diagnosed on a coronal reformatted, contrast-enhanced magnetic resonance angiography image. There is differential enhancement of the true and false lumen, with greater enhancement of the true lumen (because of the first pass nature of the exam). A coronary artery bypass graft (*arrow*) is noted to arise from the false lumen. (From Krinsky G: Gadolinium-enhanced three-dimensional magnetic resonance angiography of the thoracic aorta and arch vessels. A review. Invest Radiol 1998;33:587–605.)

Other Clinical Applications

Penetrating ulcers are seen in the elderly with severe atherosclerotic disease (Fig. 15-20). The ulcer penetrates into the media (middle layer) of the aorta. There is always an associated intramural hematoma. Rarely, these lesions rupture. A complete MRA exam includes both black blood imaging (to demonstrate the hematoma and to look for possible pleural or pericardial blood) and CE-MRA (to best depict the ulcer crater). Penetrating ulcers progress in size with time and may eventually result in a saccular or fusiform aneurysm or a pseudoaneurysm.

Intramural hematoma, without associated dissection, is an entity with clinical findings and risk factors similar to classic aortic dissection. Hemorrhage is confined to the aortic media. The appearance on MRA is that of circumferential wall thickening without mass effect on the lumen. The lesion can progress to a dissection at any time, necessitating imaging follow-up at regular intervals.

ABDOMINAL AORTA

CE-MRA provides sufficient information for presurgical planning in abdominal aortic aneurysms. The size and extent of the aneurysm should be evaluated (Fig. 15-21). The presence or absence of associated disease, including branch vessel occlusion/stenosis and mural thrombus, should also be determined.

RENAL ARTERIES

X-ray angiography has long been the standard of reference for the diagnosis of renovascular disease. This is despite substantial limitations as a result of the invasive nature of the study, its cost, and the use of nephrotoxic agents. Advances in MR technique have altered this situation; CE-MRA is now a viable alternative to catheter angiography.

Technique

With careful attention to technique, CE-MRA of the renal arteries is a robust, highly reliable exam. Timing of image acquisition is critical to obtain a high-quality angiogram without venous contamination (Fig. 15-22). As with applications in other areas, various timing strategies have been successfully used. Higher spatial resolution scans, in combination with high contrast dose (0.2 mmol/kg), can markedly improve depiction of the renal arteries (Fig. 15-23). Analysis of both MIP images, which provide an overview, and multiplanar reconstructions are recommended. Final diagnosis should be made on the basis of the latter.

Atherosclerotic Disease

Atherosclerotic disease generally affects the proximal renal arteries, lending it to study by CE-MRA (Fig. 15-24). This is unlike fibromuscular dysplasia, which often affects only the distal vessel and in which imaging findings are subtler. A study of 103 patients with atherosclerotic disease used intra-arterial contrast angiography as the gold standard. The sensitivity and specificity of CE-MRA for the assessment of significant renal arterial stenosis were 93% and 90%, respectively. Thirty-one of 33 accessory renal arteries were also correctly identified by CE-MRA. Two very small accessory vessels were missed.

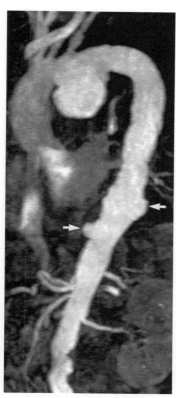

FIGURE 15–20. Saccular aortic arch aneurysm and smaller atherosclerotic ulcers (*arrows*) depicted by contrast-enhanced magnetic resonance angiography (maximum intensity projection image). (From Krinsky G: Gadolinium-enhanced three-dimensional magnetic resonance angiography of the thoracic aorta and arch vessels. A review. Invest Radiol 1998;33:587–605.)

Renal Revascularization

Beyond the arterial stenosis in renovascular disease, flow is turbulent and the vessel dilated. Renal perfusion pressure is also diminished. Conventional magnetic resonance imaging (MRI) scans as well as CE-MRA demonstrate delayed enhancement of the affected kidney and a decrease in the intensity of parenchymal enhancement. CE-MRA can be used to evaluate the technical success of renal arterial revascularization. Caliber change of the vessel after percutaneous transluminal angioplasty or renal artery endarterectomy can be documented, and surgical extra-anatomic reconstructions demonstrated. Preliminary studies point to the change in parenchymal thickness as a possible early predictor of clinical success. A major limitation of MRA currently is the inability to adequately evaluate arterial flow after intravascular stent placement.

PORTAL VENOUS SYSTEM

Precise delineation of portal venous anatomy is essential before liver transplantation and portosystemic shunting. Visualization of the portal venous system is also useful in evaluating patients with cirrhosis and portal hypertension. Doppler ultrasonography plays a major role in evaluation of the portal system. CE-MRA offers a viable alternative and is considered the modality of choice in

many clinical situations. On occasion, CE-MRA can be superior to indirect portography, the latter requiring, of course, arterial catheterization.

Technique

In normal individuals, on conventional MRA scans, the portal vein is often seen as a flow void because of its large size. When flow is slow, as in portal hypertension, high signal intensity may be seen mimicking thrombus. MRA techniques circumvent this problem, permitting distinction between slow flow and thrombus. Quantification of portal venous flow can be achieved using bolus-tracking methods. In this approach, a saturation band is placed across the portal vein; blood velocity is determined from the distance this moves. CE-MRA overcomes many previous problems with MRA in this region, in particular by permitting acquisition of breath-hold scans. Unlike other MRA techniques, it also permits simultaneous evaluation of the liver parenchyma.

CE-MRA of the portal venous system is best performed in the coronal plane. The arms should be positioned over the head to prevent aliasing. Care should be exercised when selecting the imaging volume, particularly with regard to anterior extent, to encompass the entire relevant venous anatomy (including the mesenteric veins). Choice of TE with fat and water out of

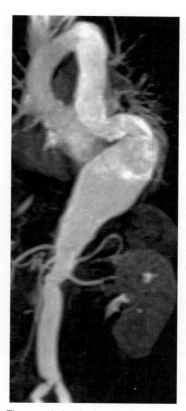

FIGURE 15–21. Thoracoabdominal aortic aneurysm depicted by contrast-enhanced magnetic resonance angiography (maximum intensity projection image). Critical to operative management is the position of the mesenteric and renal arteries, which are clearly depicted in this exam, relative to the aneurysm. (From Krinsky G: Gadolinium-enhanced three-dimensional magnetic resonance angiography of the thoracic aorta and arch vessels. A review. Invest Radiol 1998;33:587–605.)

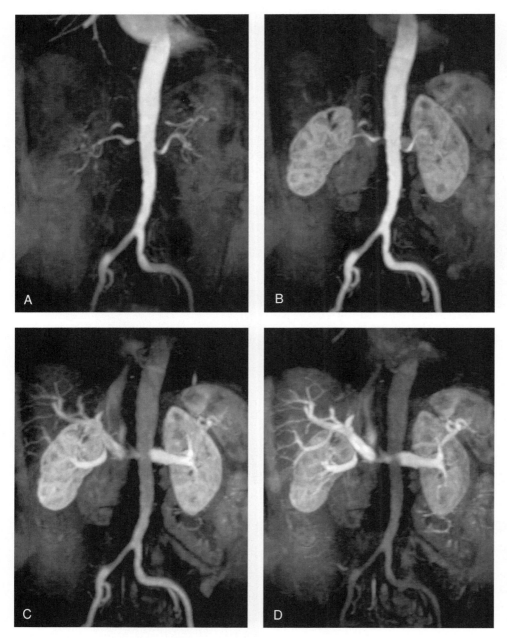

FIGURE 15–22. Multiple time sequential contrast-enhanced magnetic resonance angiography acquisitions (maximum intensity projection images) in a patient with bilateral renal artery stenosis. *A,* In the early arterial phase, there is complete visualization of the renovascular tree. *B,* Slightly later, arterial enhancement is at a maximum, accompanied by prominent renal parenchymal enhancement. *C,* In the early venous phase, the proximal renal vein is visualized in its entirety. *D,* Slightly later, venous enhancement is maximum; the renal arteries are no longer visualized. (From Schoenberg SO, Knopp MV, Prince MR. Arterial-phase three-dimensional gadolinium magnetic resonance angiography of the renal arteries. Strategies for timing and contrast media injection. Original investigation. Invest Radiol 1998;33:506–514.)

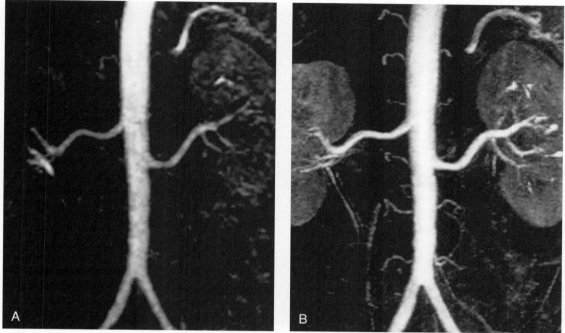

FIGURE 15–23. Contrast-enhanced magnetic resonance angiography exams (maximum intensity projection images) of the renal arteries performed with low resolution and standard contrast dose (0.1 mmol/kg) (*A*) compared with high resolution and double dose (*B*). The visualization of distal renal artery branches is markedly improved in the latter because of higher spatial resolution and the 0.2-mmol/kg contrast dose. Note also the visualization of lumbar arteries in *B*. A standard body coil was used in *A* and a phased array coil in *B*. (From Boos M, Lentschig M, Scheffler K, et al: Contrast-enhanced magnetic resonance angiography of peripheral vessels. Different contrast agent applications and sequence strategies. A review. Invest Radiol 1998;33:538–546.)

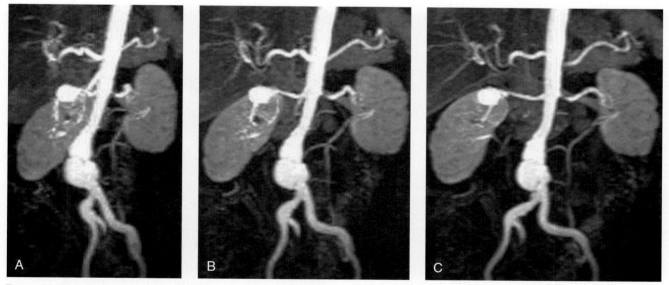

FIGURE 15–24. Left renal artery stenosis and a right renal artery aneurysm on contrast-enhanced magnetic resonance angiography (maximum intensity projection images). *A–C,* Three projections from a single 3D exam are presented. Note the importance of appropriate projection angle for visualization of the renal artery origins. Also visualized is a lower abdominal aortic aneurysm. (Images courtesy of K. Bis.)

phase can help to decrease the signal from fat. Slice thickness should be 3 mm or less. Because contrast is diluted by the time it reaches the portal system, the use of triple dose (0.3 mmol/kg) is recommended. As with other CE-MRA exams, the use of a saline flush immediately after the contrast bolus is important. Both arterial phase and portal (or late venous) phase scans are acquired. Bolus timing is critical for the arterial phase scan. Review of multiplanar reconstructions, in addition to coronal MIP images, has been shown to increase the sensitivity in identifying abnormalities of the main portal vein.

Liver Transplantation

Preoperative evaluation of liver-transplant candidates is aimed at providing anatomic information for surgical planning and excluding patients for whom surgery is not feasible or will not be of benefit. For selection of candidates, direction and velocity of flow are generally not important. Surgical techniques now also exist for patients with portal vein thrombosis. Prior knowledge of the hepatic arterial anatomy is, however, useful, with variants common. It is also important to identify celiac axis stenosis, if present, because these patients are predisposed (if uncorrected) to posttransplant ischemia.

Vascular complications after liver transplantation most commonly involve the hepatic artery. Doppler ultrasonography is used as the initial screen, with CE-MRA used in equivocal or nondiagnostic cases. Vascular complications well delineated by CE-MRA include hepatic arterial thrombosis, portal vein stenosis or thrombosis, and vena cava stenosis. Nonvascular complications, including infarction, abscess, and biloma, are well depicted by conventional MRI scans.

Shunt Evaluation

Transjugular intrahepatic portosystemic shunting (TIPS) is often used for decompression of portal hypertension in patients with bleeding from esophageal varices unresponsive to sclerotherapy or with intractable ascites. Using a percutaneous approach, a communication is opened between the right hepatic vein and the right portal vein. The tract is dilated and a metallic stent placed. Before performing such a procedure, patency of the hepatic and portal veins should be demonstrated. CE-MRA has been used successfully for this assessment and is a useful technique when ultrasound is equivocal. The role of MRA after TIPS is, however, limited, because of the metallic artifact from the stents currently available.

Surgical shunts are less common today but, when present, are well assessed by CE-MRA (Fig. 15-25). An important advantage of CE-MRA is its 3D nature. Conventional angiography is on occasion inadequate because of the projection used or vessel overlap (which can obscure a stenosis). CE-MRA is also useful for visualization of splenorenal shunts, which cannot be easily examined by ultrasonography because of bowel gas. Metallic artifact from surgical clips can, however, compromise the MRA exam.

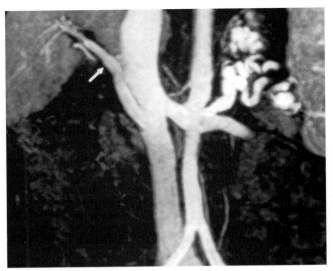

FIGURE 15–25. Patency of a portocaval shunt (*arrow*) in a patient with cirrhosis established by contrast-enhanced magnetic resonance angiography (maximum intensity projection image). Note the extensive varices. (From Stafford-Johnson DB, Chenevert TL, Cho KJ, Prince MR: Portal venous magnetic resonance angiography. A review. Invest Radiol 1998;33:628–636.)

Other Clinical Applications

Vascular encasement (of veins or arteries) can occur with pancreatic carcinoma and cholangiocarcinoma (Fig. 15-26). Hepatomas tend to grow into the portal vein or, less frequently, the hepatic vein. CE-MRA can be used preoperatively to demonstrate vascular encasement or invasion. Its final role in this area awaits greater clinical experience.

In the Budd-Chiari syndrome, CE-MRA plays an important role in both diagnosis and therapeutic planning. Hepatic vein occlusion is easily demonstrated. In this syndrome, the liver displays heterogeneous enhancement and the hepatic veins' "feathery" enhancement.

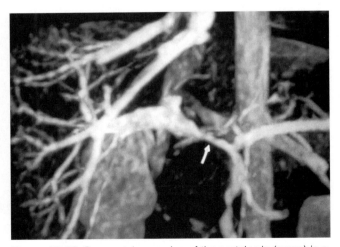

FIGURE 15–26. Segmental narrowing of the portal vein (*arrow*) in a patient with pancreatic cancer illustrated by contrast-enhanced magnetic resonance angiography (maximum intensity projection image). This finding suggests venous encasement by tumor. (From Stafford-Johnson DB, Chenevert TL, Cho KJ, Prince MR: Portal venous magnetic resonance angiography. A review. Invest Radiol 1998;33:628–636.)

MESENTERIC VASCULATURE

Disease of the mesenteric circulation can lead to acute and chronic bowel ischemia. The incidence of acute bowel ischemia is rising in the United States, and mortality rates remain high. Chronic ischemia is less common but increasingly recognized. Most acute mesenteric ischemia is caused by arterial occlusive disease; embolic occlusion of the superior mesenteric artery (SMA) accounts for 50% of cases. The SMA occlusion is usually within the first 10 cm of the vessel. Thrombotic arterial occlusion accounts for 25% of cases. Venous thrombosis is less common and accounts for 10% of all cases of mesenteric ischemia. CE-MRA can be used to visualize both the arterial and venous mesenteric vasculature. Occlusive disease of the major vessels is well visualized. Segmental ischemia is diagnosed on the basis of delayed mesenteric or bowel wall enhancement.

Acute mesenteric ischemia may present quickly, with severe abdominal pain, or more slowly over several days. Early diagnosis is essential before irreversible ischemia occurs. X-ray angiography is the definitive diagnostic exam for occlusive and nonocclusive ischemia but is invasive and expensive (particularly as a screening tool in a disease process in which symptoms are often nonspecific). Clinical symptoms of chronic mesenteric ischemia include weight loss and postprandial pain. This disease is caused by atherosclerotic stenosis or occlusion of mesenteric arteries; both the SMA and celiac axis are involved in 85% of cases. Anatomic information alone is not sufficient to diagnosis chronic mesenteric ischemia because asymptomatic vessel stenosis or occlusion is common.

Technique

As with other CE-MRA exams, the correct timing of image acquisition after bolus contrast injection is critical. A power injector is helpful in this regard. Both automated bolus-tracking and test bolus methods have been used. Contrast dose at most centers remains high, approximately 0.2 to 0.3 mmol/kg. Arterial, capillary, and venous phase images should be obtained. Caloric stimulation has been suggested and demonstrated in normal volunteers. This provides improved visualization of smaller vessels, including the inferior mesenteric artery (IMA). Both multiplanar reconstructions and MIP images should be viewed. The use of CE-MRA should be confined to patients who can hold their breath for the duration of the exam.

Acute Mesenteric Ischemia

With CE-MRA, the celiac axis and SMA are well visualized. However, in some patients, the IMA may not be well seen. Sensitivity and specificity for significant stenoses are very high. In animal models, it has been demonstrated that CE-MRA can detect quite small areas of acute bowel ischemia. Diagnostic signs include vessel cut-off, delayed enhancement, and lack of a capillary blush.

Chronic Mesenteric Ischemia

As previously discussed, anatomic information alone (such as that supplied by CE-MRA) is not sufficient for the diagnosis of chronic mesenteric ischemia. Two approaches have been proposed to examine postprandial changes in blood flow: cine phase contrast MRI and in vivo measurement of oxygen extraction. It is hypothesized that mesenteric blood flow increases after meal challenge in normal individuals; this response is inadequate in symptomatic patients for the increased metabolic demand, resulting in pain. Both of the MRA techniques just noted have been used successfully in initial clinical trials.

LOWER EXTREMITY

Using bolus chase MRA, the vessels of the lower extremity can be imaged in their entirety in less than 2 minutes (Fig. 15-27). Overlapping 3D gradient echo images are acquired during arterial transit of a single intravenous contrast injection (using a gadolinium chelate). Atherosclerosis of the lower extremities is common, affecting more than 20% of those individuals older than 75 years. The disease is diffuse in nature and characterized by multiple arterial stenoses and occlusions. Angiographic examination must include the infrarenal aorta, iliac arteries, femoropopliteal arteries, and tibioperoneal arteries. CE-MRA is particularly well suited for study of the aortoiliac arteries, which are often tortuous and thus poorly depicted by TOF MRA techniques. CE-MRA also readily demonstrates retrograde filling of patent arteries distal to an occlusion, allowing better assessment of the length of occlusion (Fig. 15-28).

Bolus chasing was originally developed for conventional x-ray angiography. Before the advent of digital subtraction angiography (DSA), a test bolus was used for timing. DSA permits real-time control of imaging and table motion by the operator. This technique (bolus chasing) has been successfully adapted to CE-MRA and is the method of choice for imaging of the arteries of the lower extremity. With current generation MRA scanners, automated table motion and automated bolus detection are both used. Typically, the distance between the infrarenal aorta and tibioperoneal arteries is divided into three stations; each station is imaged twice during the total imaging time of 2 minutes. Each station can be acquired in as little as 10 to 15 seconds. The second set of images at each station is acquired in a delayed fashion (during the equilibrium phase). The delayed scan can be useful in patients with asymmetric lower extremity arterial flow. Image subtraction is used for background suppression. A superior alternative is frequency-selective fat presaturation; such scan sequences are under development for CE-MRA. Phased-array coils specifically designed for lower extremity MRA produce markedly superior exams compared with the standard body coil. Bolus chase techniques have improved lower extremity MRA to the point at which this technique is a viable clinical tool for the work-up of peripheral atherosclerosis, with the potential to replace diagnostic x-ray angiography (Fig. 15-29).

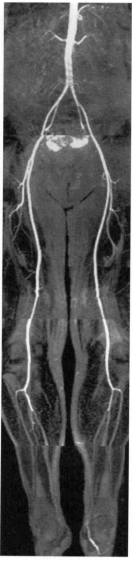

FIGURE 15–27. Lower extremity contrast-enhanced magnetic resonance (MR) angiography (maximum intensity projection image) using MR SmartPrep and automated table motion for multistation bolus chasing. A 40-mL contrast bolus was chased successfully from the abdominal aorta to the distal extremities. The image presented is a mosaic created from four time sequential (and anatomically adjacent) scan acquisitions. (From Ho VB, Foo TK: Optimization of gadolinium-enhanced magnetic resonance angiography using an automated bolus-detection algorithm (MR SmartPrep). Invest Radiol 1998;33:515–523.)

Technique

With current hardware and software, the lower extremity (iliac, femoral, popliteal, tibial, and fibular arteries) is imaged after a single contrast injection. Multistation bolus chasing, as this approach is termed, requires very fast scan acquisition (<12 seconds per station), automated bolus detection, and rapid, automated table motion. If the hardware or software to accomplish this is lacking, then the lower extremity can be examined in its entirety by performing three injections (dividing the region to be studied into three sections in the craniocaudal dimension). The latter approach restricts the con-

trast dose to 0.1 mmol/kg for each injection; the approval for total dose in any one setting is a maximum of 0.3 mmol/kg. Overlap of vessels resulting from venous return can be a problem, regardless of imaging technique, in imaging of the lower leg and foot. Dedicated peripheral angiographic coils, if available, provide superior exam quality.

Atherosclerosis

In atherosclerotic disease of the lower extremities, CE-MRA is used to determine the location, degree, and length of arterial stenoses and to reliably distinguish these from occlusions. CE-MRA competes directly with conventional contrast angiography in this application. When occlusive disease is present, flow within the tibial and fibular arteries is slow and the peripheral run-off delayed. Acquisition parameters must be adjusted to take into account these conditions.

UPPER EXTREMITY

The most common clinical indication for arteriography of the upper extremity (and hand) is ischemia, which may be either acute or chronic. Causes include atherosclerotic disease, thromboembolism, vasculitis, and vasospasm. Arteriography is also used in cases of trauma and

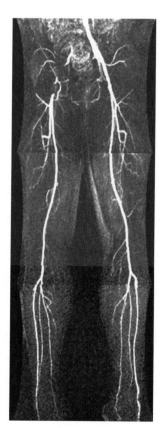

FIGURE 15–28. Lower extremity contrast-enhanced magnetic resonance angiography (maximum intensity projection image) demonstrating occlusion of the right external iliac artery with reconstitution of the femoral artery by collateral vessels. (Image courtesy of V. B. Ho.)

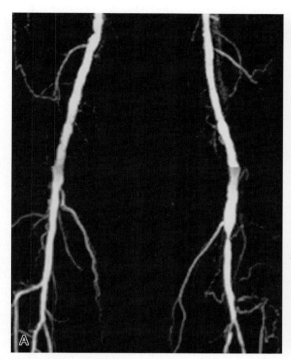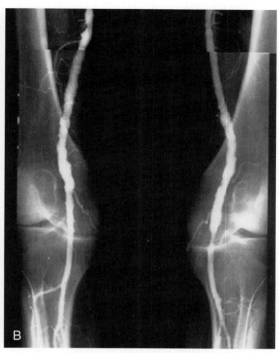

FIGURE 15–29. Improved depiction of atherosclerotic disease by contrast-enhanced magnetic resonance angiography (CE-MRA) (maximum intensity projection image) (*A*) as compared with intra-arterial x-ray angiography (*B*). Both exams demonstrate a high-grade stenosis of the left popliteal artery. Higher vessel contrast with the CE-MRA exam provides clearer depiction of the occlusion of the left anterior tibial artery. (From Boos M, Lentschig M, Scheffler K, et al: Contrast-enhanced magnetic resonance angiography of peripheral vessels. Different contrast agent applications and sequence strategies. A review. Invest Radiol 1998;33:538–546.)

FIGURE 15–30. Normal contrast-enhanced magnetic resonance angiography (maximum intensity projection image) of the hand. The *curved arrow* points to enhancement of an incidental granuloma, and the *straight arrow* to the junction between the deep palmar arch and the ulnar artery. E indicates a vitamin E capsule, and v indicates early venous enhancement. Clinical applications in the hand include vasospastic disorders, trauma, and vascular malformations. (From Lee VS, Lee HM, Rofsky NM: Magnetic resonance angiography of the hand. A review. Invest Radiol 1998;33:687–698.)

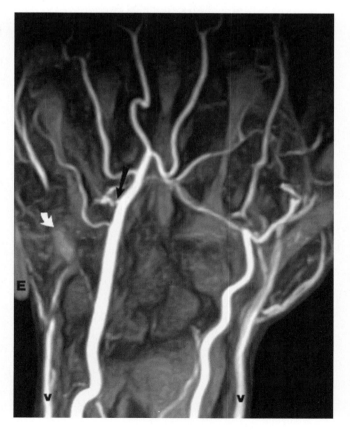

with vascular malformations. Conventional arteriography is technically challenging. The vessels are very sensitive to stimuli (such as pain and catheter manipulation) and react by constriction and vasospasm. The clinical efficacy of CE-MRA in the upper extremity has yet to be established. In the hand in particular, visualization of the extremely small diameter arteries represents a substantial challenge (Fig. 15-30).

Technique

To minimize the number of phase encoding steps, CE-MRA is performed in the coronal plane. A precontrast acquisition is important to confirm adequate anatomic coverage and may also be used as a subtraction mask for the subsequent contrast enhanced scans. The intravenous catheter for contrast injection should be placed in the contralateral arm.

Atherosclerosis

Symptomatic atherosclerotic disease is much less frequent in the upper extremity than in the lower extremity. Subclavian steal, a complication of atherosclerotic disease of the upper extremity (with subclavian obstruction proximal to the origin of the vertebral artery), is well demonstrated by CE-MRA. Embolic disease is best examined with conventional angiography, which can be used not only for diagnosis but also to initiate thrombolytic therapy.

Trauma

In acute trauma, conventional angiography is the procedure of choice. In addition to providing a diagnostic exam, temporizing measures are possible before surgery. Damage from penetrating wounds can, however, be initially occult. Such complications include aneurysm, arteriovenous fistula, thrombosis, and embolism. It is in these patients that CE-MRA may play a role.

Vascular Malformations

MRA provides a more accurate definition of the extent of AVMs and is rapidly gaining acceptance. Soft tissue extent is typically underestimated by conventional angiography. MRA also depicts the relationship of the malformation to adjacent muscle, nerves, and fascial planes.

CONCLUSIONS

The high temporal and spatial resolution possible with contrast-enhanced MRA improves markedly the diagnostic accuracy of MRA in vascular imaging. CE-MRA has largely replaced noncontrast MRA techniques for imaging of both the arterial and venous systems. Flow-induced signal loss is much less of a problem than with noncontrast MRA vascular techniques. Also of much less importance is vascular saturation because of the use of a contrast agent, thus allowing large fields of view. Current advances in MRA hardware and software make contrast-enhanced MRA an attractive alternative to catheter angiography. CE-MRA provides high-contrast images of the vasculature. The technique is easy to execute and minimally invasive. As opposed to x-ray angiography, neither arterial catheterization nor a nephrotoxic contrast agent is required.

Index